)02

3

)

RESEARCH METHODS FOR NURSES AND THE CARING PROFESSIONS
Second edition

SOCIAL SCIENCES FOR NURSES AND THE CARING PROFESSIONS

Series Editor: Professor Pamela Abbott
University of Teesside, Middlesbrough, Cleveland, UK

Current and forthcoming titles

Psychology for Nurses and the Caring Professions
Sheila Payne and Jan Walker

Sociology for Nurses and the Caring Professions
Joan Chandler

Social Policy for Nurses and the Caring Professions
Louise Ackers and Pamela Abbott

Research Methods for Nurses and the Caring Professions (Second edition)
Pamela Abbott and Roger Sapsford

Research into Practice: A Reader for Nurses and the Caring Professions (Second edition)
Edited by Pamela Abbott and Roger Sapsford

Community Care for Nurses and the Caring Professions
Nigel Malin

Race and Ethnicity for Nurses and the Caring Professions
Ahmed Andrews and Lovemore Nayatangi

Nursing People in Psychiatric Systems
Chris Stevenson, Phil Barker and Shaun Parsons

RESEARCH METHODS FOR NURSES AND THE CARING PROFESSIONS
Second edition

Pamela Abbott and
Roger Sapsford

OPEN UNIVERSITY PRESS
Buckingham • Philadelphia

Open University Press
Celtic Court
22 Ballmoor
Buckingham
MK18 1XW

email: enquiries@openup.co.uk
world wide web: http://www.openup.co.uk

and
325 Chestnut Street
Philadelphia, PA 19106, USA

First Published 1998

Copyright © Pamela Abbott and Roger Sapsford 1998

A catalogue record of this book is available from the British Library

ISBN   0 335 19697 7 (pb)   0 335 19698 5 (hb)

Library of Congress Cataloging-in-Publication Data
Abbott, Pamela
     Research methods for nurses and the caring professions / Pamela Abbott and Roger Sapsford. — 2nd ed.
       p.   cm
     Rev. ed. of: Research methods for nurses and the caring professions / Roger Sapsford. 1st ed. 1992.
     Includes bibliographical references and index.
     ISBN 0-335-19698-5 (hb)   — ISBN 0-335-19697-7 (pb)
     1. Nursing—Research—Methodology.   2. Social Service—Research—Methodology.   3. Nursing—Research—Evaluation.   4. Social service—Research—Evaluation.   I. Sapsford, Roger.   II. Sapsford, Roger. Research methods for nurses and the caring professions.   III. Title.
     RT81.5.S26 1998
     610.73'07'2—dc21   97-42886
                                                              CIP

Copy-edited and typeset by The Running Head Limited, London and Cambridge
Printed in Great Britain by Redwood Books, Trowbridge

CONTENTS

SERIES EDITOR'S PREFACE

It is now widely recognized that an understanding of research and research methodology is essential for caring professionals. However, while it is argued that nursing, for example, must become research-based, it is less certain that this is being achieved. Until caring professionals have an understanding of research methodology that enables them to evaluate research findings and utilize them in their own research, the aspiration for practice to be based on research will not be realized. Research-based practice relies on practitioners reading the research literature and implementing the findings in their own practice. It is now also necessary for them to be able to evaluate their own practice and the practice of others. Not all practitioners will become researchers – carrying out large-scale research is a specialized task that requires a high level of training. All, however, should be able to appreciate the research of others and understand how to incorporate research findings into their own professional practice.

This is a book on the appreciation and evaluation of other people's research and on the conduct of your own. It stands by itself but may also be read in conjunction with Pamela Abbott and Roger Sapsford (1997) *Research into Practice: A Reader for Nurses and the Caring Professions* (2nd edition), also published by Open University Press, which contains many of the examples which are discussed here. Both have been revised for this new edition; some of the examples have been changed, and the material on research into one's own professional practice has been strengthened.

One of the book's main aims is to 'de-mystify' research – to distinguish the often complex techniques from the basically fairly simple logic which underlies research projects. The focus is explicitly on social research: there is no attempt to cover research methods in biology, nor research into the efficacy of drugs. The principles are the same, however (except that social research tends to face more complex questions, because of the great variability of its subjects and the fact that the researcher is a part of the social world which he or she is investigating). Most of the examples are small-scale studies, in the sense that they could be (and in many cases were) carried out by one or two people rather than large and well resourced teams. Particular emphasis is given to evaluative research of various kinds and the attempt to assess the efficacy of one's own professional practice. (The term 'evaluative research' is preferred to 'action research' as defining the methodology for researching professional practice.)

Part of the target audience for this book is the nursing profession – people taking nursing degrees and diplomas, people taking post-qualificatory diplomas and certificates, and practising nurses who want to undertake research or the evaluation of their practice. For this reason a good proportion of the examples are based around the concepts of health and treatment. The book is also appropriate, however, for other community and institutional practitioners and trainees – for example, social workers, family workers, community workers. The intended level is introductory, and you should not imagine that reading it will fully equip you to carry out research of all kinds. (In particular, no attempt has been made to deal with getting funding for research.) There should be enough here to get you started, however, and the rest comes with practice, further reading and competent supervision by others who are already experienced.

Pamela Abbott

ACKNOWLEDGEMENTS

We should like to acknowledge our colleagues at the Open University, the University of Plymouth and the University of Derby, and elsewhere, with whom we have been teaching this material and discussing these issues over a long period of years. We are not aware of having 'borrowed' any of their ideas, but all academic work is an unacknowledged collaboration, and we have benefited greatly from having talked and worked with them. We can at least be sure, however, that the mistakes and unorthodoxies are mostly our own.

INTRODUCTION

FINDING OUT AND MAKING SENSE

'Research' is often presented as something mysterious and technical, something beyond the capability of those who have not undergone long training. It is what is done by scientists, it requires the use of computers and abstruse mathematics, and ordinary untrained people sometimes cannot even understand the questions, let alone the answers. However, 'doing research' is just an extension of what we all do in our daily lives. We are continually coming to conclusions on the basis of what we experience plus what we know already – to recognize something as a tree, or a post box or a person is to take knowledge which we have already and apply it to what appears to be in front of us. We all have occasion, every day, to try to find out more about something in order to act more appropriately – to look up an address, to take a closer look at the tree, to explore whether this person is really to be trusted. When something puzzles us and we cannot quite make it out, we generally set about looking for evidence about it which will help us to make sense of it. The researcher does no more. Research starts as an extension of common sense – finding out about things, looking for information about them, trying to make sense of them in the light of evidence and working out what evidence is needed.

Common sense has its limitations, however, which the researcher tries to overcome. In our everyday thinking and decision-making we often act on poor evidence. Indeed, we have to do so; events will not wait until the evidence is in, even if we were prepared to collect it. We come to quite hasty judgements about people, for instance, on the basis of one incident; we classify them as sympathetic or unsympathetic on the basis of how they behave when we first meet them, and behave accordingly. We judge whole classes of people on the basis of single examples. Common sense is full of 'facts' for which it has little or no evidence. What has been heard on the radio or television, or in the pub or the bus queue, or what is believed and announced by opinion leaders such as politicians, churchmen or scientists, becomes 'the truth' without further examination. Finally, common sense is influenced by a wide range of stereotypes and ideological presuppositions of which we are hardly ever aware. Our attitudes to the stranger, to the deviant minority, to those who might be seen as attacking our interests, are so well rooted as to be often impervious to the penetration of logic and evidence. The way we view the world is itself often open to question: our particular culture's construction of social class, gender and age as supposedly innate or inevitable stratifying principles – together with all the implicit assumptions about people and their wants and needs – are taken for granted as common sense.

Good research tries not to take for granted what is assumed by common sense. It tries to argue rigorously, according to the 'rules of evidence' which we shall be exploring in the rest of this book. At the same time, it requires a degree of imagination, and the power to put the taken-for-granted to one side and 'make the familiar strange'. It is not the *techniques* of research which make it hard work, as you will see in the rest of this book, but the strain of trying to see topic areas simultaneously from all possible angles.

The book falls into four sections. The first chapter is a 'mini-course', looking at most of the major ways of collecting data and structuring research and evaluation; it raises many of the issues to which you will come back again and again as you progress through the book. Chapters 2–7 are about reading and evaluating other people's research – Chapter 2 is about the structure of research reports in general; the others each take a type of research design and examine it through two or three major projects which have used it. Then Chapters 8–13 are on various aspects of the practice of research. The examples range more widely here, but some of them are drawn from the kinds of project that have been undertaken by students and could be carried out by you. Finally there is a chapter on the writing of research reports and a final summary chapter which also raises and pulls together more fundamental questions about ideology, discourse and the way in which the taken-for-granted aspects of everyday life are also taken for granted in research and evaluation studies.

We have provided practical exercises to back up the text wherever we can. If you are able to fit them into your lives, we strongly recommend trying to carry out the exercises, at the point at which they occur in the text; no amount of descriptive rhetoric is as illuminating as even a small-scale attempt at actually doing the research. The exercises are often quite short. Many of them either take no real time at all – they can be fitted into time spent travelling from one place to another, for example, or they can be accomplished in 10–20 minutes. Very few of them require any special arrangements or disturbance to your life, except when it is required that you ask someone direct questions, in which case you have to line up someone who is prepared to answer them – often a spouse or friend or working colleague. (The 'taken-for-granted' in the exercises is that you are able to leave the home in order to go to work or to the shops. If you are entirely housebound then you may need to modify some of them – e.g. observing family interaction rather than the interactions in shops or hospitals – but the exercises so modified will still make the points for which they were designed.) The exercises provided in Chapters 1 and 8–13 are practical activities. In Chapters 3–7 the exercises involve reading and commenting on particular research reports. These may mostly be obtained in academic libraries, or all of them may be found in Abbott and Sapsford (1997), the Reader mentioned in the Preface.

Various of the chapters also end with 'Further reading'. This is not necessary for the understanding of the text, but it is intended to expand your horizons beyond what we have written. In Chapters 3–7 the 'Further reading' suggests other articles or books you might like to examine if the subject area of one of the examples is particularly relevant to your interests or to your area of professional expertise – in other words, to research which you might be interested in carrying out. In Chapters 8–13 we mostly suggest further textbooks or articles which offer a more detailed treatment of the relevant research techniques than space permits here – plus a few studies worth reading because they use non-standard and imaginative ways of applying the method. These are not 'required' reading for the chapters, but additional material you will find useful if you go on to do research for yourself in the relevant area and/or style.

This chapter begins the book with a brief and cursory review of a wide variety of research activities, organized around the ideas of 'looking to see what is going on', 'asking questions' and 'trying something out'. We shall mostly be concerned here with questions of structure in research – structure in the way that questions are asked, or observations or measurements carried out, and structure in the sense of planned **comparison** between one group and another to illuminate their differences. (Throughout, words in bold are defined in the Glossary.) These are two dimensions along which research studies may differ. (A third major factor – how **typicality** or **representativeness** is guaranteed so that you can assert that what is true in the research context is true of the wider population – is left for consideration elsewhere in the book.)

Research is carried out for a wide variety of audiences. Much of what people think of as research – the kind of work carried out by 'researchers' – is to do with the evaluation of new or existing practices. Research is carried out to evaluate the outcome of a policy initiative or the functioning of an existing policy. For example, there will be a fair amount of research published in the next few years on how cash-limited budgets affect the practice of medicine, and on the functioning of hospitals before and after opting to become hospital trusts. In today's political climate of demand for 'value for money', research is undoubtedly also being carried out into the effectiveness of the health visitor policy of doing home visits to all homes with young children and on whether the expense is justified by what they do there. The effectiveness of treatments is evaluated by controlled research projects: the use of these is most obvious in the clinical trial of new drugs, but similar projects have also been run on the effectiveness of forms of psychological counselling, the introduction of new nursing practices and on innovations in social work practice. 'Before-and-after' projects are also carried out on social innovations (changes in forms of welfare benefits, for example) and gross demographic changes (such as the increased life-span of the population) on the 'clients' who are affected by them and the work of the professionals who try to help them.

A second major audience for research is the academic world. Much research is carried out not with the immediate aim of informing policy or practice, but to build an understanding of the field of study and to test

theories about it which are derived from more general sociological, psychological or economic models of how the social world is structured and how
people function within it. Much of the classic work on health inequalities
by region, class and gender, for example, may have been commissioned by
government or more local authorities, but it has as its aim the discovery of
factors associated with poor health, specifically whether the state of health
of a group is more affected by their personal actions or by their position
within society as defined by structural variables, such as class, gender and
material deprivation. (This kind of research blurs into the more 'practical'
work discussed in the last paragraph, of course; much social theory is
directly concerned with the implementation of social policy.)

A third kind of work involves the evaluation of professional practice. (A
fourth kind, less often thought of as 'research', but requiring all the same
techniques, is the work of *self*-evaluation.) Research techniques can be used
to evaluate the effectiveness of our own practice or that of others, and to test
the effects of altering some aspect of it. They can be used to explore the
wants and needs of client groups, so that practice can be better informed.
They can be used in a vaguer but still rigorous way just 'to find out a bit more
about' client groups and working environments, to see if any ideas are generated which may be of use in our practice. This is something we all do
without thinking of ourselves as 'carrying out research', but we can do it
better if we apply a little rigour and logic. In many ways what distinguishes
research from the common-sense use of argument and evidence is a certain
'cast of mind' – an openness to evidence and a distrust of presuppositions,
even when taking this critical stance can be personally uncomfortable.
When evaluating the work of others – whether their usual way of doing
things or some innovative technique – we must clearly be seen to pass
judgement fairly, without preconceived ideas, and on the basis of evidence.

In the rest of this chapter we shall be looking at some of the main ways in
which evidence is gathered – **observation**, asking questions, and **controlled trials**. Practical exercises are provided for you to carry out, and you
should try to find time for them if you possibly can; words on paper are no
kind of substitute for actually doing some practical work and experiencing
both the pleasures and difficulties of research. If possible, the practical
activities should be carried out at the point in the chapter at which they
occur, as the experience of doing them often acts to introduce or reinforce
some teaching point which we want to make.

Observation

The most obvious way of getting to know a situation is to go and observe it,
and observation is a major way by which research data are collected. Just
how to do observation, however, is not quite as obvious as it might at first
appear. Events are not just 'there' for us to note as if we were cameras taking
pictures. On the contrary, in a sense we construct our world as we observe
it, seeing what we do as a result of the knowledge which we already have.
The same 'event' could be a parent disciplining a child in one frame of
observation, a case of child abuse in another, and a piece of play-acting in a

third. It could also be analysed in terms of local norms of parental discipline, patterns of communication or even patterns of physical movement. (One can – just about! – imagine a sports physiotherapist who was more interested in whether the muscles of the arm were working smoothly than in whether the hand was causing pain.) Similarly, there are many different ways of observing in research, ways which are good for different purposes and with different drawbacks.

Exercises 1–6: Observation

These exercises will take about 30 minutes, not including time spent taking notes. They do not have to be done all at once; they are split up into five-minute 'sessions', and each session could be done on a different day if that were more convenient for you.

Find yourself somewhere where the general public gather for some purpose and interact with someone who is in some kind of service or regulatory role. If you work in a hospital or general medical practice or in a social services department you may be able to observe a 'reception area' where people wait around for their appointments. If you are a health visitor you may be able to do your observation in a clinic. Parents may be able to observe other parents at 'mums and toddlers' groups. Otherwise, a good location is a large self-service shop where people take their own goods from shelves and queue at a cash desk to pay for them. Whatever the location, you want to find somewhere where you can stand around for five minutes at a time without drawing attention to yourself; those under observation must not know that you are observing, and if you are observing in a shop you will not want to be suspected as a potential shoplifter.

All the sessions require you to take notes. For the first two you will want to go away somewhere to do this – sit outside, or go and have a cup of coffee. The others require you to record numbers of various kinds, so you will need to take notes while actually doing the observation. Work out how to do this unobtrusively beforehand – in a small notebook, perhaps, or on what might be taken for a shopping list, or on a magazine or the margins of a book.

Exercise 1
Spend five minutes just looking round and seeing what is going on in general. At the end of the five minutes, go and sit down somewhere, and write some notes on what you have seen – not more than a page, but at least eight or ten lines, describing what was going on.

Exercise 2
Spend another five minutes focusing on the cashier or receptionist (without attracting his or her attention), looking at how he or she deals with people, how the people behave and whether they appear satisfied, disconcerted or annoyed by the interchange. Again, go somewhere and write some notes on what you have seen.

Exercise 3
Now spend another five minutes (or as long as it takes to get at least ten interchanges between the cashier/receptionist and a member of the public) looking at what is done in each interchange. Count how many of the interchanges involve one or both parties speaking, whether the cashier/receptionist appears to treat them in a friendly, distant or haughty manner, and whether the members of the public appear polite, rude, brusque or neutral to him/her.

Exercise 4
For another five minutes (or ten interchanges), count the total amount of time spent speaking in the interchanges by (a) the cashier/receptionist, (b) male members of the public and (c) female members of the public. Count slowly to yourself at a constant speed while any speech is occurring and jot down the numbers in three columns, to be totalled later.

Exercise 5
Spend five minutes concentrating on the cashier/receptionist, and count the number of seconds he or she spends looking at the face of the member of the public with whom he or she is interacting.

Exercise 6
Finally, go to another kind of location and repeat the count you have just done on a different cashier/receptionist. If you used a waiting room of some kind for your main location, go to a shop for this last part of the exercise. If you used a shop, try observing in a library or a garage or at the ticket office of a large railway station.

The notes from the first exercise, where you were recording simply 'what was going on', would probably tell us more about you than about the events which you were observing. What we asked you to do, effectively, was to make sense of the situation, and you will have done so largely in terms of your own well tried and pre-existing categories. It is possible that what actually happened may have surprised you, but nonetheless you will have described the situation in terms which came readily to you and made sense to you. You can see, however, that this kind of 'holistic' observation – trying to make sense of situations as a whole – is not as easy as it looks, and that more careful work needs to be done before the conclusions are readily acceptable as evidence. When we come to look at this kind of observation later in the book, you will see that it generally involves quite long periods of immersion in a situation, as a person with a role within it rather than just as a 'neutral' observer.

The second exercise may have taxed you more, because we asked you to concentrate on one participant for five minutes, a longer span of attention by far than you would normally grant to one person with whom you were not in interaction. This being so, we suspect you probably came to regard what was going on as to some extent strange – to start describing it to yourself in different terms from the ones that you would use in everyday life – and to that extent you may have come up with something which surprised you and would surprise us. Making the familiar strange is one stance regularly adopted by researchers who wish to penetrate below the taken-for-granted aspects of the situation. However, note that the closer focus on the cashier/receptionist in itself imposes structure on what you may have 'seen'; you were asked to focus on an individual, so you undoubtedly came up with notes bearing on the actions of that individual and the actions taken towards him or her, and with very little on the more general and structural features of the situation.

Exercises 3–6 introduced a new dimension by asking you to count something. What you counted became increasingly more specialized. What the numbers allow you to do is to provide a more convincing and 'available' description of the situation. We no longer have to rely on your judgement as to what was going on, however good and reliable that might be; you present us with figures on some aspect of the situation, and we can look at them for ourselves. In Exercise 4, for example, we can see whether men spoke more than women, not just accept your judgement that one or the other gender was more active, and we can compare the activity of clients with the activity of the 'gatekeeper'. Comparing Exercises 5 and 6, we can look at the different behaviour of 'professionals' in two contrasting situations, as judged from an aspect of behaviour which has been shown to be very important in the regulation of face-to-face relationships.

Looking back over what you have collected, you will probably find that the data from the later exercises were much more 'definite' than what was collected in the earlier ones. ('Data' means 'what has been collected for analysis' – in the early exercises your notes on what happened, and in the later exercises the counts that you made.) Figures seem somehow to carry more weight in an argument than one's vaguer general impressions, to look more like 'proof', to seem somehow more 'neutral' than more general descriptions. You will realize already, however, that there is nothing magic about numbers as such. Numbers can, indeed, be more precise, and it is certainly easy to argue from them that something is more common than something else, or that two somethings are related. The value of the numbers, however, is created at the stage of data collection, and it depends entirely on your accuracy (how good were you at counting seconds?) and on what we decided to count in the first place. If what we decided to count was not important, then the data will be of no importance, irrespective of how neatly laid out in numbers they are. We constructed the situation as one in which speech and eye contact were 'the important thing that was going on'. All manner of interesting actions may have taken place during the interactions, but in the later exercises you will not know what they were. (At least, you may know what went on, but they do not appear in your data and are, therefore, not available for subsequent analysis.) Different frames of analysis – in terms of economic exchange, multi-person systems, personal histories, structural inequalities, etc. – are effectively ruled out by the way in which we elected to collect the data in the earlier exercises.

Thus there are many forms of observation, ranging from the very general and unstructured to the very structured and numerical. None of them is necessarily the 'right' way to proceed; each has advantages and disadvantages for particular situations, depending on your aims as a researcher and what you know already. We shall explore observation techniques in more detail in later chapters.

Asking questions

Another obvious and everyday way of proceeding, if you want to know what is going on and what people are thinking, is to ask them. A great deal of social science research is concerned with the asking of questions, and a substantial technology, folklore and body of expertise has grown up around the art and science of asking them. We ask a lot of questions as part of our everyday conversations. Ordinary everyday conversation can be a prime source of information, and you might well be taking advantage of it as part of a relatively unstructured piece of observation research. If you were studying a hospital ward without the people there knowing you were doing research – pretending to have an official role there, for example, or actually being a nurse and observing your own workplace – then part of the data you would collect would be what people said to you. If you were participating but being open about the fact that you were a researcher you could ask more questions, and more obvious ones; indeed, you would be expected to do so by the other participants. The strength of this kind of ordinary, everyday questioning is that you get what the participants want to say, in their own words and using their own concepts.

The problem with ordinary conversation is that you contribute as much to it as does the person to whom you are talking. Indeed, as it is you who are asking the questions, you will probably contribute more of the ideas that matter; it will be you that 'starts the ball rolling' with each topic, and the terms in which you do so are likely to structure the subsequent exchanges. So, far from getting the participant's own ideas in his or her words, you will get your own words and ideas fed back to you. An example which springs to mind is a student whom one of us was supervising on a methods course who was asking questions about social class and how the informant saw the social world as being structured. The informant used a categorization of working-class people into 'rough' and 'respectable', which the student found quite exciting, because it duplicated a set of categories which have been in use for over a hundred years and underlies the practice of charitable and state welfare – the distinction between the deserving and the undeserving poor. Checking back over the transcript of the interview, however, he found that he had been the first person to introduce this distinction, without thinking or noticing. The informant had found it a useful one and had used it consistently thereafter. So the student had no notion of how the informant would have described the world if this set of categories had not been made available.

When we 'interview' people rather than just chatting to them, we tend to play down our own part in the interview, to say as little as possible, to put across as few ideas new to the informant as possible and to concentrate on eliciting the pre-existent ideas of the informant in the informant's own words. This kind of interviewing is a very common means of research into social topics. It is often used to contrast groups of people who differ in some key respect or to compare the same people over time, and before and after major policy changes or 'social landmarks'. You will find it referred to in the literature as 'ethnographic', 'qualitative', 'semi-structured' or 'unstructured' interviewing. We did not like any of these terms, so we have coined the term 'open interviewing' to describe it.

So much for 'open' interviewing. There is also a more systematic and structured way of asking questions – you will probably be most familiar with it from being stopped by market-research interviewers in the street – which uses predesigned questionnaires or schedules. (A **questionnaire** is a list of questions for self-completion by the respondent; an **interview schedule** is a list of questions to be asked by an interviewer, face to face or on the telephone.) These are used in national **survey**s such as the Census for obtaining factual information from respondents – number of people in household, number of rooms in the house, etc. Their purpose is to collect exactly comparable information from every respondent, on a large scale. It is obviously important in the Census, for example, that the interviewers and respondents have a precise definition of what constitutes a household, and the same definition for every respondent. Otherwise, if the same group of people sharing a flat might be classified as one household in one part of the country and a number of co-resident single households in another, then we would be collecting information not about patterns of domestic living, but about whether people think of themselves as a household or not. Even an apparently simple question such as the number of rooms in house needs very precise definition. Does the bathroom count as a room? What about a separate and very small w.c., or a shower cubicle *en suite* to a bedroom? Is a breakfast room with a kitchen alcove to count as one room or two?

Structured questionnaires and interview schedules are also used for the collection of information about attitudes, beliefs and intentions, for example market-research interviews – 'What do you think of this product?' – and political opinion polls – 'Which political party would you vote for if there were a general election today?' Similar kinds of questionnaires are also used extensively by social psychologists and sociologists to test theories about the relationship of attitudes to each other, and they are one standard way of assessing likely popular reaction to policy changes. Their merit is that a great deal of data can be collected relatively quickly, and that the same questions are asked of everyone, allowing comparisons to be drawn. It is also possible, under certain conditions, to generalize with some degree of precision from a sample to the population as a whole; this is discussed in Chapters 6 and 9. There are corresponding disadvantages, however, as the following exercises may help to make clear.

Exercises 7 and 8: Interviewing

Exercise 7
Find someone who is prepared to sit down with you in a quiet place for a quarter of an hour or so – a friend or spouse will do – and ask him or her the following list of questions (for questions a–c, do not offer definitions

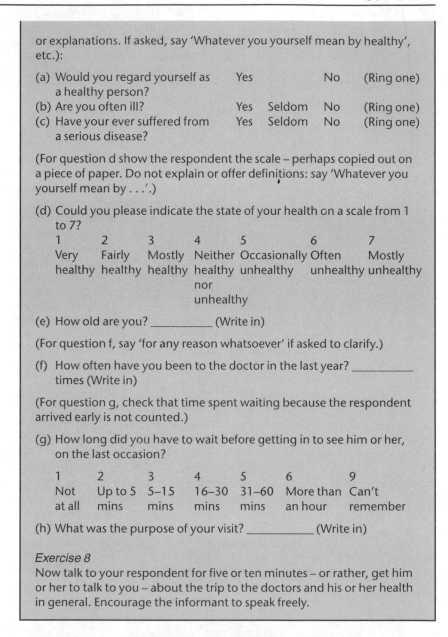

or explanations. If asked, say 'Whatever you yourself mean by healthy', etc.):

(a) Would you regard yourself as   Yes   No   (Ring one)
    a healthy person?
(b) Are you often ill?   Yes   Seldom   No   (Ring one)
(c) Have your ever suffered from   Yes   Seldom   No   (Ring one)
    a serious disease?

(For question d show the respondent the scale – perhaps copied out on a piece of paper. Do not explain or offer definitions: say 'Whatever you yourself mean by . . .'.)

(d) Could you please indicate the state of your health on a scale from 1 to 7?

1	2	3	4	5	6	7
Very healthy	Fairly healthy	Mostly healthy	Neither healthy nor unhealthy	Occasionally unhealthy	Often unhealthy	Mostly unhealthy

(e) How old are you? _____ (Write in)

(For question f, say 'for any reason whatsoever' if asked to clarify.)

(f) How often have you been to the doctor in the last year? _____ times (Write in)

(For question g, check that time spent waiting because the respondent arrived early is not counted.)

(g) How long did you have to wait before getting in to see him or her, on the last occasion?

1	2	3	4	5	6	9
Not at all	Up to 5 mins	5–15 mins	16–30 mins	31–60 mins	More than an hour	Can't remember

(h) What was the purpose of your visit? _____ (Write in)

Exercise 8
Now talk to your respondent for five or ten minutes – or rather, get him or her to talk to you – about the trip to the doctors and his or her health in general. Encourage the informant to speak freely.

The interview schedule you used in Exercise 7 is obviously a very short one, made up for the occasion, but it does display the major forms of question used. Questions a–c are essentially yes/no questions, though b and c offer a midpoint. (Did you have difficulty trying to get the respondent to say 'yes' or 'no' to question a?) Question d is an attitude scale. Questions e and f ask for a straightforward number. Question g again asks for a number, but the answer is recorded as a *code*, a number standing in for a range of possible answers. In question h you just write down (in summary form) whatever reason the respondent gives; this would be coded afterwards into categories.

The importance of clear instruction to ensure comparable responses is also evident. In most of the questions you were instructed not to offer definitions or explanations, but to force the respondent to make up his or her own mind what the questions meant. This would mean that the answers would have to be interpreted in terms of whether respondents think themselves healthy, not against some absolute standard of health. (We could have obtained further information which would have helped the interpretation of the data, however, by asking whether they had suffered from any of a list of diseases and ailments during the last year. Most people would describe themselves as healthy even if they have had a cold, for example, but only some would describe themselves as healthy, but suffering from arthritis.) We were careful to exclude 'unnecessary waiting time' in question g – time spent waiting because the respondent was early for an appointment. There are still ambiguities left in, however; for example, what about home visits from doctors, or times when the respondent visited the surgery, but saw the practice nurse, or visited only to deliver a specimen. At least one of the apparently simple counts is, in fact, fraught with potential error, because it asks for 'number of times in the last year'; people's memories are very unreliable for time periods such as this. (It might have been better to anchor the time period to a memorable event – 'how often since Christmas?', for example.) In that same question, you may have had difficulty coding the answer. What did you do, for example, with respondents who initially said 'not very long', or 'absolutely ages', or '15 to 20 minutes'? We didn't give you instructions on whether to probe or not – to ask follow-up questions. Did these responses go down as 'can't remember', or did you probe further to get a figure out of them? What confidence do you have in the figure, if they were vague initially? And note that if several interviewers were all using this schedule on different respondents, and they used different probes, then the answers to this question would not strictly be comparable. Designing structured questionnaires and schedules is not as easy as it may look at first sight.

When you talked with the informant afterwards, in Exercise 8, did you get the feeling that the definition of 'health' and 'healthy' was not the simple, cut-and-dried matter that the interview schedule seems to suggest? Did you, in fact, spend a certain amount of time *negotiating* with the informant what together you were prepared to count as 'being healthy', 'being unhealthy', 'being ill'? Did you find yourself swapping experiences with your informant and describing your own views on health? As you can see, the structured interview data are not nearly as rich and full as what can be collected by open interviewing, nor do they give one complete confidence that the respondent's complex views and life-circumstances are fully recorded. On the other hand, it would not be possible to use open interviewing on a very large sample: it takes too long. Also, you will have seen for yourself just how very difficult it is not to suggest to the informant what you are prepared to count as an acceptable answer – which would mean you were to some extent collecting your own views, not theirs.

Controlled trials

We have repeatedly talked about measurement before and after a change, and this is the key to the more systematic research design known as the **'controlled trial'** or **'experiment'**. If we want to try out a drug which is expected to reduce pulse rate, for example, it would not be much evidence of its effectiveness just to give people the drug and then measure their pulse rate; we could accidentally have picked people whose normal pulse rate was abnormally low or high. The minimum which would count as reasonable evidence of effectiveness, therefore, is measurements before administering the drug and afterwards, so that we could document a decrease. This is the essence of the experimental approach: a pre-test, a treatment or manipulation, and a post-test. Everything else that is built into experimental design represents the experimenter's attempts to show that the change is actually produced by what he or she says it is produced by – that there is no other plausible explanation for it.

In the simple drug experiment which we have just described, the evidence for a change is good, but the evidence that it is the drug which produced it is not very good. Almost anything might be responsible for it; for example, the group could have been taking exercise just before the administration of the drug, in which case we would have expected their pulse to decline from an initial high reading whether or not they took the drug. This kind of obvious physical feature can be controlled for – we simply make sure that it does not occur – but it is impossible to guard against every **confounded variable**, including those which have not even occurred to us. Normal practice, therefore, is to select a second group who go through exactly the same procedures as the first, but do not receive the drug. If pulse declines in the experimental group (the one that received the drug) and not in the **control group** (the one that did not), then we are on fairly firm ground in arguing that it is the drug that produced the effect.

However, this argument holds only to the extent that the two groups are exactly similar and undergo exactly the same procedures except for the experimental treatment. The experimenter goes to great length to ensure this similarity. Similarity of people is ensured by: **'matching'** cases (selecting pairs of people who are the same in key respects) and allocating one from each pair **randomly** to an experimental or control group; or by jumbling up the names of all the selected subjects, and drawing out an experimental and a control group at random; or sometimes by using the same subjects as control and experimental group. The merits of the three different approaches are discussed in Chapter 10. Similarity of treatment is guaranteed by careful duplication of procedures and by using a little imagination as to what might go wrong.

We have used a drug trial as an example of an experiment because such trials are easy to describe and understand. Precisely the same principles are applied in social experiments, however. Experimental social psychologists run just the same kind of procedure, with experimental and control groups measured beforehand on the variable which the experimenter intends to change, a 'treatment' applied to the experimental group but not the control group, and a post-test to assess the extent of the change produced in one group and not the other. You might use a similar procedure to assess the effects of an innovative nursing or social-work practice or the efficiency of a new teaching method. In the 'scientific' style of experiment, a key question is the accurate measurement of 'variables' – producing numbers which mean something, for subsequent analysis. The same design logic, however, would underlie an evaluation study carried out by one of the more **holistic** and less measurement-obsessed methods, such as unstructured observation or open interviewing. You would still want to assess how things were before the onset of whatever it was whose effects you were evaluating, and then again afterwards, and you might well include among the people you observed or interviewed a group who were not exposed to the change, to make changes among those who did experience it more interpretable by comparison.

Indeed, the same logic underlies many research reports which are not experimental. A frequent form of research involves looking at something which has occurred in one region – a new way of doing health visiting, say – and comparing some supposed outcome of it with how things were in the same region before the change and with how things were at the same points of time in a region where the change has not occurred. This cannot class as an experiment because there is no guarantee that the two groups which are being compared are like each other; regions may differ in the sort of people who live in them. You do have pre-tests and post-tests in both regions, however, and a 'treatment' administered in one region and not the other. The same form of argument would be used in interpreting the results, therefore, except that more care and investigation would have to go into demonstrating that it was fair to compare the two regions. (We sometimes call this kind of research **quasi-experimental**: it is *like* the experiment and shares its logic, but lacks some of its more important strengths.)

Exercise 9: Field experiment

At some time when you are likely to pass a fair number of people – on your way to work in the morning, for example – try controlling your own behaviour systematically and see if it has any effect on the behaviour of those whom you pass. With the first five people whom you pass, smile at them and look them in the eye. Note whether they smile back or greet you, and jot down the number unobtrusively – perhaps on the margin of a newspaper. (If you pass a group of people, focus on only one of them and do not count the others.) Now, with the next five, do not smile, and look at their chins instead of their eyes. Again, count how many smile at or greet you. Carry on doing this, smiling at five and not smiling at the next five, until you have at least 20 of each. Compare the number who smiled or greeted you in the 'smiling' condition with the number who did so in the 'not smiling' condition.

'Not smiling' is the control condition and 'smiling' the experimental treatment, in this exercise. As it was the same person who did both, we have no problems about comparing them in that respect. However, your journey to work is not uniform in terms of whether you are likely to meet people who already know you. Typically, people start off walking down a street where most people are known to them at least by sight, then get into territory less well frequented by acquaintances, then begin to recognize people again as they get near to where they work. This is why we asked you to do five 'smiles' and five 'no smiles', alternating: that way there is less likelihood that all of the people you pass in the 'smiling' condition would be known to you and all of the others unknown, or vice versa. Although only a small exercise, with a trivial 'manipulation', this design in fact shows many key features of the traditional field experiment of social psychology (i.e. one carried out 'in the real world', not in a laboratory or other artificial setting). It might have been set up to test a theory about the control of one person's behaviour by rewarding features of the others. On the other hand, it might have tested what happens when you initiate or do not initiate socially constructed 'greeting sequences' by catching someone's eye and smiling. Note that even where an experiment is technically well constructed, the interpretation of its results may not be unambiguous; in this case, the 'treatment' could be interpreted as two different things – administering a reward or initiating a 'social script' – depending on the theory from which you approach it.

You may also want to think whether the experiment was quite ethical. No particular harm was done to anyone, but it must have been disconcerting to some people to be, in a sense, greeted warmly by a complete stranger who then passed on down the street without following through into conversation. A charge often rightly levelled against those who carry out experimental research is that they are callous or unimaginative about the harm which their procedures might do to their subjects.

On the other hand, the overall logic of experimental design underlies all serious attempts to evaluate policy or practice. As we argued above, the *logic* of experimentation is not particularly tied to one method of data collection; it can be applied as readily to unstructured observation or open interviewing as to the more structured methods traditionally associated with it. Indeed, it also underlies a fair amount of conventional practice in the caring professions. The Nursing Process, or the Health Visiting Process, are modelled on evaluation studies and draw on their logic. They consist of a pre-test (assessment of a 'case' and his or her needs), a decision as to what is to be done, its implementation, and reassessment to determine the outcome. All that is lacking is a control group or condition. Social-work practice and teaching follow similar lines though in less explicit form; their practice consists of assessment of a situation, action in accordance with the assessment, and reassessment to evaluate the effects of action.

This process of evaluation, when used in research, has been referred to as '**action research**' by some commentators. However, we find this confusing and prefer the term 'evaluation research' – evaluating practice. Any of the research methods discussed in this book can be used to evaluate and inform practice. We prefer to restrict the term 'action research' to research structured so that its findings are continually fed back into the continuing practice situation and themselves become part of what is being evaluated. Again, any of the methods described in this book may be used. 'Action research', in this sense, is a sub-type of evaluation research.

Research ethics and Research Ethics Committees

In the previous section we asked you to consider whether the experiment we asked you to carry out was ethical. We are now going to consider the question of research ethics and the procedures for obtaining ethical approval in more detail, for virtually all research has potential ethical considerations – even when the research itself does not involve human subjects. This is especially the case for research findings, something over which the researcher has little or no control. Oppenheimer, after the United States dropped nuclear bombs on Hiroshima and Nagasaki, is reputed to have said that he would not have done research on splitting the atom if he had anticipated how the findings would be used. Similarly, social and health research can be used in ways which would be offensive to the researchers; for example, the results of research designed to find the most efficient and effective way of providing community care could be used by 'management' to justify reducing the nucleus of qualified district nursing staff and increasing the numbers of home care assistants. Researchers cannot always anticipate how the findings of their research will be taken up and used by others. The motives of a given research team may have been to improve patient care, but the findings might be used by management to impose new working practices and reduce staffing levels or modify the skills mix – something the researchers might believe would actually *harm* patients. It is important to consider how research findings might be used, but we would probably not do **applied research** at all if we refused to do research which could be used to justify actions other than those we intended.

What we are mainly concerned with here are the ethical considerations that need to be taken into account at the planning stage and the process of gaining ethical approval for research involving patients. All research that involves patients has to have Research Ethics Committee (REC) approval. Each district health authority has an REC, and approval has to be obtained for research from the committee(s) in whose district the research is being carried out. This may mean having to obtain 'ethical approval' from more than one committee. At an early stage in the planning of research it is a good idea to consult the secretary or chair of the committee and find out about the procedures for obtaining approval, which vary from committee to committee. Some universities also have ethical committees concerned with research on human subjects, and in some cases this committee or a sub-committee established for the purpose may have delegated authority from the health district's REC to approve the research proposals of staff and students.

The primary role of the REC is to review all proposals for research which involve any contact with patients or the medical records of present or past patients. The committee will be concerned about a number of ethical issues related to the proposed research. The University of Derby Research Ethics Committee, for example, has delegated authority at the time of writing from Southern Derbyshire Health Authority and uses the criteria in Table 1.1.

The Committee will also need to be assured that you have negotiated the

Table 1.1   Criteria used for ethical screening

How, if at all, will the health of subjects be affected?

Does the study have merit, is it feasible and practicable, thus ensuring that it does not waste subjects' time and effort?

Are there any possible hazards? If so, are facilities adequate to deal with them?

Is the investigation adequately supervised?

Are there acceptable procedures for obtaining consent from the subjects or, where necessary, their parents or guardians?

Will the subjects be given appropriate information on which to base their agreement to take part?

Are there adequate procedures for obtaining approval from the responsible consultant or general medical practitioner where appropriate?

Source: School of Health and Communities Studies, the University of Derby, School Ethics Screening Committee 1996.

necessary access with line managers before they give approval. In some health authorities there is also a Scientific Review Committee who screen proposals for the design and method of research and its likely contribution to knowledge.

Ethics are concerned with norms and values – standards of behaviour. They involve balance and judgement based on personal and professional knowledge and expertise. In research, ethics also relates to 'good practice'. There are no absolute ethical standards, but there are guidelines that can help us in deciding how to carry out research ethically and in evaluating the ethics of other people's research. Nurses have to adhere to the code of professional conduct of the UKCC (United Kingdom Council for Nursing, Midwifery and Health Visiting 1984). This states that

> Each registered nurse, midwife and health visitor shall act at all times in such a manner as to justify public trust and confidence, to uphold and enhance the good standing and reputation of the profession, to serve the interests of society and, above all, to safeguard the individual patient and client.
>
> (UKCC, quoted in Hammick 1996)

In addition the Royal College of Nursing issued a Code of Conduct for Nursing Research in 1977, the International Council of Nurses issued Guidelines for nursing research and development in 1985, and the Royal College added supplementary guidelines on confidentiality in 1987. A number of professional associations have guidelines for members: for example, the BSA (British Sociological Association), the BPS (British Psychological Society) and BERA (the British Educational Research Association). All of these documents can be useful in helping you to think about ethics and ethical principles when planning, carrying out and reporting on your research.

Hammick (1996) has devised a 'Research Ethics Wheel' divided into four quarters – practicalities of the research, the principles of the research, the duty of the researcher and the outcomes of the research. Issues to be considered under 'practicalities' include resourcing, the ability of the researcher to carry out the project, professional codes and the law. Those to be considered under 'principles' include the extent to which original knowledge will be obtained, respect for participants in the research and respect for authority. The issues relating to the duty of the researcher include veracity (truth), consent of participants, confidentiality and the weighing-up of risk versus benefit. In terms of outcomes, issues to be considered include the aims of the research, what happens to those who refuse to participate (or to those who form 'control groups'), the hazards and consequences, and the dissemination of findings. Hammick suggests that in reaching their decisions RECs pay most attention to issues surrounding informed consent and anonymity. These are key concerns because patients are vulnerable – they are unwell, often confused, and possibly compliant because the researcher or the promoter of the research is in a position of authority. It is essential, she argues, not only that informed consent is obtained but that those who are approached are informed in writing that non-participation in the research will in no way impair the care/treatment they receive, and that they can withdraw from participation at any stage. Patient Information Sheets written in lay language and readily understandable should be given to those who are asked to consider taking part. All those who agree to participate should complete a consent form. The REC would scrutinize the Patient Information Sheet and Consent Form before 'ethical approval' was given to the research. Another crucial issue is confidentiality/anonymity. Anything that a patient says when participating in research is confidential – it should not be passed on to others without the express consent of the patient. Similarly, research should always be written up in such a way that the anonymity of participants is preserved.

It is, however, necessary to recognize at the end of the day, as we said above, that ethics is about balance and judgement, and about justification. A key dilemma is whether the end can ever justify the means – for example, whether it is ever ethically justified to risk harming some people for the good of the majority. This has long been identified as a key issue in animal experimentation – whether it is justifiable to 'try out' cosmetics on rabbits to ensure that they are safe for humans. It also arises in medical research on humans, however – for example, in experiments where either a potentially beneficial treatment is withheld from one group or a potentially harmful treatment is administered to one group. In recent years the balance has tended towards ensuring that no human is harmed by research, but there can be no absolute guarantee of this, and if it were used as an ethical absolute it would prohibit all applied research. There are many other ethical dilemmas, and there are seldom 'right' or 'wrong' answers to them. However, whatever choices are taken, it is necessary that there be sound arguments in justification of them.

Exercise 10: Ethical questions

Consider the following questions and make notes on your responses. If possible, discuss your answers with colleagues.

1 Is it ever justifiable to withhold from participants the aims of the research?
2 Is it ever justifiable to carry out research when the subjects of the research cannot give informed consent?
3 Is it justifiable to use people as the objects of research?
4 Is it justifiable to carry out research that will solely or mainly benefit the researcher by, for example, leading to a PhD?
5 Is it justifiable to carry out research when the funders of the project retain the right to censor the findings?
6 Is it justifiable to accept funding for health research from the tobacco industry?
7 Is it justifiable to carry out research when the findings might be used to reduce staffing levels or to withdraw treatment from certain categories of patients?

Note: you need to give more than a 'yes' or 'no' answer to these questions. If you are inclined to say that a course of action *can* usually or often be justified, try to think of cases where it might *not* be justifiable. If you are inclined to think that it is *never* justifiable, try to think of valuable kinds of research which its prohibition would render impossible.

The research imagination

We have tended to talk on occasions, as everyone does, as if 'research' were a set of skills to be brought out and applied to the particular problem. This is true, of course, but a training in research entails more than this. As we suggested earlier, the 'research stance' is more a frame of mind, an openness and neutrality at the point of immediate argument, a kind of imagination. Few research projects are definitive in the answers they offer, and the unit of research is generally not the particular project – the **controlled trial**, the interview study, the period of observation – but the whole programme of related studies which explore and expand the question. Our notional drug trial, for example, would not be possible until the drug had been developed as a result of a large series of experimental studies in the pharmaceutical laboratory. Nor would one study be enough to show that it worked and had no harmful side-effects. The good research team would **replicate** – run the study again, to check that the results did not come up positive by chance alone. They would try the drug out on a wide range of people, to make sure it was safe for all and not just some of them. They would think about possible side-effects and run specific studies to try to detect them in a harmless form before they occurred in clinical practice with potentially fatal consequences. They would follow up all the people who had received the drug, over time, and look for longer-term effects. One question suggests another.

One aspect of the research imagination – particularly important in the more structured and 'quantified' styles of research – is having the imagination to know what data to collect. Open studies (participant observation, open interviewing) can often 'change their own agenda' by highlighting ideas as important which had not occurred to the researcher. More structured studies (questionnaire surveys, structured observation, controlled trials) solely collect the data they propose to collect, and are not open to surprises. To take an obvious example: if the classic **epidemiological** research on cancer had not collected information on whether people smoked, it *could not* have shown an association between smoking and lung cancer.

Studies may also lead to the research question being modified and expanded. In the case of the small field experiment you ran on the effect of smiling on the way to work, for example, we came up with two possible explanations – the 'reward characteristics' of smiling, and its function as the beginning of a well learned social script. If we were developing theory in this area we would want to run at least one further study to determine which of these, if either, was the more useful explanatory concept. In the process we might throw up further possible competing explanations which would need to be explored. We would also be developing our theory of the functions of smiling at the same time, and the developed theory might well suggest further questions which necessitated research. Where the questioning stops is an arbitrary decision; if the theory has merit, it is probably capable of indefinite expansion and refinement.

The researcher who does commissioned research also learns to widen the frame of reference when considering questions of research design. If you had been commissioned by management to study how cashiers in a large shop could improve the impression they gave to customers, or health receptionists the impression they gave to clients, you might well have carried out some or all of the observation studies which we tried out as Exercises 1–6. Management would have framed the questions in terms of what cashiers/receptionists do and how they behave, and social psychology's past research on the functions of eye contact and speech-sharing as satisfying aspects of interaction might well have led you to the kind of studies we proposed in the exercises. The underlying question, however, is not the narrow 'What can cashiers/receptionists do?', but the broader 'How can things be improved for customers/clients?', and you might well direct your research to this wider question rather than the narrower way in which management had framed it. The cashier/receptionist and her behaviour is only one element in the situation. You would have looked at her physical circumstances and whether they were conducive to friendly behaviour. You would have looked at the number of interchanges she had to manage – her workload – to see whether it was excessive. You would have looked at her rates of pay, and the rates of pay of comparable jobs, and the possibilities for promotion. You might even have regarded long queues as inevitable and looked at what was offered to clients/customers while they were waiting, to 'serve them up' as friendly people at the point of interaction. You would almost certainly have talked to everyone relevant to the interaction – the cashier/receptionist, the customers/clients, other 'professionals' involved in the scene – to get their views and explore their satisfactions and dissatisfactions.

The broader the frame of reference, within the practical constraints of what can be managed within the available time, the broader the understanding, and broader understanding leads mostly to better solutions. It takes a measure of imagination to conceptualize a problem widely enough to make it really worth doing research on it. It is now some time since the medical profession realized – occasionally – that more needs to be taken into account in drug research than just the biochemical action of the drug. (A famous series of experiments demonstrated that some doctors get better results than others with the same drug, and that some doctors get better results with placebos – inactive pills – than others get with the active drug.) It is now commonplace in the teaching of nurses and health visitors to stress that medical 'facts' about patients exist as just one part of complex social lives and networks of understanding, and that what may seem a good pattern of care from the medical point of view may not be the best form of approach if the 'total patient' is taken into account.

Nonetheless, we lapse into simple thinking – not least in the sphere of medicine and nursing – if we run simple studies based on preconceived ideas of what 'must' be the right course of action.

The rest of this book is devoted to studying a range of good research which has already been carried out, and to looking for ways in which 'good practice' in research can be applied to the kinds of situations that you might find yourself wanting to explore. We hope that you will bring your widest imagination to the reading and not let anything be 'taken for granted'.

Summary

1 'Doing research' is an extension of what we do in our daily lives – observing, asking questions, trying things out, in order to make sense of what is about us. Research starts as an extension of common sense.

2 Common sense has its limitations, however – particularly, it is full of 'facts' for which there is no evidence, and it takes for granted, embodies and reproduces our cultural habits of assigning people and events to categories and taking prescribed action on the basis of them.

3 The researcher tries to overcome these problems by arguing rigorously, according to rules of evidence.

4 A more important difference between research and common sense is that the 'research imagination' requires an openness to negative evidence and a neutrality at the point of immediate argument, however committed the researcher may be to particular outcomes.

5 All social research has effects on human beings – by the way the research is administered, by the selection of problems for research and/or by the use made of the findings – and so all researchers face ethical problems.

Broad ethical principles are that the researcher should not misuse any power he or she might have, that subjects/participants should not be harmed or inconvenienced, that their interests should be taken into account, that their *informed* consent should be obtained, that their anonymity should be preserved and that every attempt should be made to see that the research findings are not used to their disadvantage. Nursing bodies and other professional associations have issued guidelines and codes of conduct which elaborate on these principles and offer more precise advice. All research involving NHS patients or their records is subject to scrutiny by Research Ethics Committees, and the same is true in many universities for research on human subjects. At the end of the day, however, there are no right or wrong answers, and the problems remain for the researcher to tackle.

Further reading

Hammick, Marilyn (1996) *Managing the Ethical Process in Research*. Salisbury: Quay Books.

ASSESSING RESEARCH

READING RESEARCH REPORTS

The structure of research reports
Assessing research reports
Ethical and political questions
Summary

In this section of the book we shall be considering a range of different kinds of research through reading and analysing a number of published research reports. The current chapter stands as an introduction to this work and looks at the structure of research reports and how best to go about reading them. Some of what we say may seem abstract and difficult on first reading, However, the research skills which we are trying to get across will become clear as you carry on with the rest of the section, read our evaluations of the papers and start to evaluate research reports for yourself.

When we look at particular research reports in Chapters 3–7, a starting point will be a checklist of the topics which we shall discuss briefly in this chapter and consider in more detail in the remainder of the book:

1 Does the design of the research lend itself to the arguments which are based on it – can the conclusions follow logically from what has been done?

2 Could there be other explanations of the results, alternative theorizations which might characterize what has been found in quite different ways?

3 Could the results be due to variables which are '**confounded**' in the design, accidentally confused with what we really want to measure? Or could they be an artefact of the research situation?

4 What is measured? Are the measuring instruments **valid** and **reliable**? Does the choice of 'quantities' to measure close off certain kinds of explanations and predispose us from the start to other kinds? (This is a series of questions, but they are all closely interrelated.)

5 To what population may the results be generalized?

6 Was anyone harmed, embarrassed or even inconvenienced by the research?

7 To what extent are people treated as objects by the research?

8 In whose interests is the research carried out?

9 Does the way in which the research is framed embody **ideological** presuppositions such that the outcome is 'written in' or 'predetermined' by the original conceptual analysis and design?

10 Are the results of any conceivable interest? Can I use them in my practice?

This is a checklist of the questions that can be asked of research reports. Not all of them are relevant to all reports. What we have tended to do in this section when discussing each paper is to concentrate on the questions that are most relevant for evaluating that type of research, not every question that could conceivably be raised. (It is also important to bear in mind that the questions we ask of a research report are, in part, determined by the purpose for which we are reading it.)

The structure of research reports

A formal research paper is expected to have a simple and readily comprehensible structure. Every paper outlines, in order: what the question or field of investigation is (and, probably, why it is interesting and/or what is already known about it); how the researcher or research team have gone about looking at it; what the results are; and what the results mean. Thus you can reasonably expect that a published paper aimed at an academic/research/professional audience will consist of:

1 an *Introduction* which sets up the question or problem, explains why it is of interest to theory, policy and/or practice, and probably reviews the 'literature' (previously published reports, etc.) relevant to it;
2 a *Methods* section – how the problem or area is to be explored;
3 a *Results* section – what was found out;
4 a *Discussion* section – what the results mean, what they imply, and any major reasons for treating them with caution.

Books vary more in their precise organization, but you would expect a similar ordering of content (except that some of the Methods material is often relegated to an Appendix at the end of the work, to save 'ruining the narrative flow').

The form of this kind of report will be familiar to you from school science: it is the format of the school laboratory report ('Method: a pipette was taken . . .'). Not all 'social science' research would think of itself as 'scientific' in this sense, but the form of the scientific report is, nonetheless, a good one for presenting research results and showing what may be concluded from them, and it is widely used. This kind of report fits in most naturally with 'quantitative' research – **experiments**, **controlled trials**, **surveys**, systematic observation – but a similar *logic* is followed by reports of research in more 'qualitative' or 'appreciative' styles – open interviews, unstructured participant **observation**. What these latter tend to add is a greater narrative element, telling the story of the research process in more realistic detail.

Those who adopt a more 'qualitative' research design tend to be more aware of their data as the outcome of a process in which they themselves participated, and in which their own attempts to make sense of the situation and those of other participants will necessarily have had a great effect on what is produced. Thus qualitative reports tend to display greater **reflexivity**: they reflect more on the process of the research, on how the participants made sense of it, on their own preconceptions and on how detailed events may have shaped the nature of the data. In fact, you will now find an increasingly reflexive stance taken even in the more scientific style of report, as the proliferation of formal methods courses makes a generation of researchers more aware of the extent to which people make sense of their situation and how that can shape the nature of the data collected. Reflexivity is a quite essential component of the more qualitative research report, however; it is the major means by which we can assure ourselves of the quality of the evidence, given that we were not there when it was collected.

The majority of reports and accounts of research, of course, are not 'research reports'. Most are written for administrators who need to use the results, or for commercial companies, or presented to a relevant audience in one of the 'popular' professional publications (e.g. *Nursing Times*, *Social Work Today*, *The Health Visitor*, *The Magistrate*) or reported in the popular press or on radio or television for everyone's consumption. Many of the reports you come across in these ways will not cover all the sections that we outlined above. In particular, 'popular' reports tend to give little or no detail of how the evidence was collected; this is seen as tedious for the lay audience and therefore to be avoided. To the extent that such detail is not given, however, we should be very chary of giving more than a tentative and provisional acceptance to what is claimed to be the conclusions of the research. Popular reports tend to expect you to accept conclusions on the authority of the researcher; you are not given the resources to form your own judgement of their validity.

Assessing research reports

In reading a research report and assessing the worth of its conclusions,

1 your first steps will be to look at the Introduction, to see what the researchers were looking for and why it is supposed to be interesting;
2 secondly, you will look at the Discussion/Conclusions (and perhaps the end of the Results section) to see what the authors claim to have found and what they think it means;
3 with this established we can go on to look a little under the surface of the results and assess the quality of the evidence as well as the quality of the arguments based on it.

Looking at the arguments and the evidence, the first step is clearly to assess their overall validity: do the conclusions follow validly from the initial arguments, given the evidence that is presented? At the same time you need to look at the research part of the paper – the Methods and Results sections – and see if *they* constitute a valid argument. The paper will be arguing that certain kinds of results will be obtained or not be obtained, if an initial line of theory is to remain plausible. Or it will be claiming that an account of what a given social setting is like, based on survey methods or on open interviewing or on participant observation, is to be accepted as a valid characterization of what it is actually like. In either case there is an implicit argument in the project: 'given what I have measured or recorded, the best interpretation of it is the one which I am advancing'. You will be examining this claim very carefully to see whether alternative explanations could be put forward – alternative theories, or explanations based on inadequacies in the design of the research. Questions of reflexivity arise here; is the researcher well enough aware of the likely effect of the procedures on the data, and has he or she given us enough information to judge this? A part of the examination will also cover the question of measurement: are the measuring instruments or methods of recording and classifying observations valid – do they measure what the authors claim they measure? and are they reliable? are they likely to produce consistent results rather than values which are much at the mercy of chance? These are some of the questions we shall be exploring with you in the next five chapters, where we look in detail at a relatively small number of concrete research studies.

Another question which will arise in reading some papers – particularly the more 'scientific' ones – revolves around the question of **operationalization**. Many of the phenomena which the social scientist wants to measure are not readily and obviously available for measurement. What we actually have to measure is something which acts as a 'symptom' of the underlying characteristic – ability to answer questions on paper as an indicator of 'intelligence', job and/or attitudes (verbal expressions) as an indicator of 'social class', what patients say and what they do as indicators of 'depression'. From these we deduce a measurement for the underlying characteristic. The problem of validity which we mentioned in the last paragraph obviously applies: in translating the theoretical characteristic into something operational that can be measured, do we succeed in producing something which really does measure it? A further problem arises, however. Psychologists take the concept of intelligence for granted, for example, as we all tend to do nowadays, but the idea that people can be placed on a continuum of general ability in this way is a fairly recent invention (see Rose 1985) and one which embodies as 'fact' a range of politically very contentious ideas and practices (see Kamin 1974). Sociologists take their ability to place people in social classes for granted, and measures of social class are a commonplace in very down-to-earth projects such as the analysis by **market researchers** of what newspapers different kinds of people read. The way the concept is used, however, often presents as facts some very contentious statements about social inequalities (see Abbott and Sapsford 1987a, for example, for a discussion of the problems and consequences of assigning social class in different ways to married women). So, part of the assessment of a piece of research may involve **critical analysis** of its basic concepts – the apparently unproblematic 'things' which it sets out to measure – to see whether ideological presuppositions are being put forward unwittingly as unproblematic 'facts', biasing the outcome of the research from the outset. This kind of critical analysis is an aspect of the 'research imagination' about which we talked at the end of Chapter 1.

The other 'methods' question you would ask of any piece of research is to what population its conclusions are meant to generalize – of what is it supposed to be an example? Very little published research, even on single cases, is meant to tell us about just that single person or setting. (In this respect it differs from the case reports of the clinician or the social enquiry reports of the probation officer; these may be informed by the principles of research and, indeed, constitute a form of research, but they are seldom of sufficiently general interest to be worth wider publication.) Where a single case is researched, it is often chosen as being **typical** of some class of cases or at least as casting light on some class of cases; for example, an ethnographic study of one school will aim to tell us something about schools in general, or at least schools of that type. (Alternatively, the single case may be deliberately extreme and chosen to test a theory – 'if it is happening *anywhere*, then it is happening here'. The 'Affluent worker' study in Luton in the 1960s (Goldthorpe *et al.* 1969) was research of this type, selecting Luton as somewhere *un*typical of traditional working-class communities.

Most research extends beyond the single case to the sample – large or small according to the type of design – which is to be taken as **representative** of a designated population of cases. However, to take an obvious example, if all your research subjects are men then you would be unwise to generalize about 'the human race'; women might be different. Quite a lot of research has based conclusions about a culture or even about people in general on research into White males – either students or volunteers – and neglected questions of gender, race, age, class/wealth, geographical location, degree of physical or mental impairment, and all the other characteristics which might have made a difference to the results if only they had been considered. In assessing a piece of research we often have to be aware of quite subtle ways in which a sample might appear typical of a given population; it can in fact be unrepresentative because of the way in which it has been selected. So, another aspect of the 'research imagination' is that, if we are satisfied that the conclusions hold up for the case or sample under consideration, we still have to think about the extent to which they also hold up for the wider population of which the case or sample is said to be representative or typical.

Having assessed whether the methods and arguments of the paper are valid, you will want to return, with more confidence, to the paper's contents. Research is ultimately about substance – about the problems and questions which it explores – and not about its methods. Taking into account any reservations you may have as a result of your analysis of methods, what you will want to know is whether the paper tells you anything new and interesting. Does it add to or elucidate theory? Does it inform or criticize the operation of policy? Does it suggest anything which you can use to improve or modify your own professional practice?

Ethical and political questions

Finally, a further set of questions will also need to be considered as we build up an assessment of a piece of published research – Questions 6–9 on the checklist at the beginning of the chapter. Whether anyone was harmed or inconvenienced by the research is the basic 'minimum question' of research ethics: did the researchers act responsibly, leaving the world no worse a place by pursuing their investigation? We may reasonably go on to ask whether there is any benefit to the 'subjects' or 'informants' of the research, and whether the research is justified if there is none. This means, for example, asking in whose interests the research was carried out. Is it obviously commissioned by management, for example, to look into how workers can best be exploited – or dominated by that perspective, even if not formally commissioned? Is it to do with the social control of working-class people, or youths, or women? Is it set up to explore how the convenience of doctors or nurses or hospitals can best be served? More fundamentally, we may ask whether the research paid proper attention to the fact that it was *people* who were involved in it. Some feminists (see, for example, Reinharz 1979) have likened conventional social research to the act of rape: researchers go into a situation, take out of it what they need for their own ends (publication, academic esteem, promotion) and leave the subjects/respondents/informants at best not much harmed; they certainly obtain no benefit from the process but are there merely to satisfy the needs of the researcher.

These three questions do not affect the results – though they may affect our opinion of the researcher – but they lead quite naturally into a yet more fundamental one: does the way in which the research is framed embody ideological presuppositions such that the outcome is written in or predetermined by the original conceptual analysis and design? In other words, is there a very bad failure of the 'research imagination' in this research?

Summary

1 A very common way of structuring research reports is into the sections of the traditional 'scientific practical' report – Introduction, Methods, Results, Discussion. Research in qualitative traditions may depart from this ordering, but the same kinds of information will have to be delivered.

2 A logical way of approaching research reports is to look at: the Introduction to see what question is being posed and what the aims of the research are; the Discussion/Conclusions to see what answer is being given and the extent to which the aims have been achieved; and then at the Methods and Results to examine the evidence which sustains these conclusions.

3 Important 'methods' questions which will be asked of any research reports are whether the conclusions follow logically, whether the measurement procedures are valid, to what population the results can validly be generalized.

4 We would also want to ask ourselves whether anyone was harmed or embarrassed by the research, and in whose interests it was carried out.

READING OPEN INTERVIEW RESEARCH

The research paper: Abbott and Sapsford (1987b) 'Leaving it to Mum' (on mothering children with learning difficulties)
Discussion
Summary: points for evaluation
Further reading

> ### Exercise 11
>
> This chapter is based around Section 2 of Abbot and Sapsford (1987b) *Community Care for Mentally Handicapped Children* – ' "Leaving it to Mum": motherhood and mental handicap'. If you can get hold of this, you might like to read through it quickly before proceeding. A slightly shortened version is reproduced in the Reader which is designed to accompany this volume – Abbott and Sapsford (1997) *Research into Practice: A Reader for Nurses and the Caring Professions*.
>
> While reading, bear in mind the list of questions suggested at the beginning of Chapter 2; it will also form the basis of our comments below. (However, we shall not try to answer every one of the ten questions for every one of the research papers on which we comment.) Also, make a list of the questions that you would have liked to ask us, if you had the opportunity, about how we did the research.

The research paper: Abbott and Sapsford (1987b)

This paper describes an interview study which we carried out in a new town in the middle 1980s, plus some data drawn from Abbott's earlier doctoral work (Abbott 1982). It is part of a longer monograph which also sets mental handicap in its historical context and traces the development of government policy towards people with learning difficulties. (These were most commonly called 'mentally handicapped people' at the time when it was written; terminology changes as sensitivity develops and as situations are re-theorized.) As you would expect, the paper starts with a brief exposition of the 'problem' and why it is interesting:

The policy of 'community care' for mentally handicapped children has non-financial costs for families: work which in institutions would be wage-labour becomes unpaid work for 'Mum' when the burden of care is transferred to the family. This paper looks at the nature and extent of such work and at the extent to which it alters the nature of the mother's life. We look also at the price which is paid by the whole family for the fact of having a mentally handicapped child . . . (The 'price' differs markedly from family to family, depending at least in part on the degree of handicap, the extent of associated physical handicaps and the social and economic situation of the family: what follows is a composite, not necessarily true to the experience of any one mother.)

(Abbott and Sapsford 1987b: 45–6)

We are reminded, right from the start, that even though this is detailed 'open' interviewing of a very small number of 'cases', nonetheless what is to be presented is an average or typification, with some idea of the range of variability around that average, and not straightforward life histories of particular mothers.

The method of the joint interview study is described thus:

Sixteen families were contacted from a list extracted for us from the school rolls of two Special Schools in the new city (one designated for the mildly handicapped and one for the severely). We carried out two interviews with each mother separated by about a year, not using a formal questionnaire but rather trying for the atmosphere of a friendly chat about life and work between neighbours. Although the interviews were tape-recorded, it seems to us that this atmosphere was readily attained in most cases . . . These data are contrasted with a parallel series of interviews with mothers of children who have not been labelled mentally handicapped.

(p. 46)

So we know that the method was 'open interviewing' cast in a 'life-history' mould – asking women to describe their current and past lives, but steering them towards topics of particular interest to the researchers. We note that the 'sample' is not statistically **representative** – one would not wish to say that because half or a quarter of the sample said or felt something, then half or a quarter of the corresponding population were likely to do so. However, it is a reasonably **typical** sample in the sense that it shows a reasonable range of cases, in terms both of the ages of the children and of the degree and type of their condition, so any major problems (or any conspicuous lack of them) would probably be represented somewhere in it.

The account was written for a particular publication format, and its length had to be kept down, so many of the details which might have appeared have been omitted. The paper does not mention some of the strengths of the procedure. For example, we failed to record in the paper that we went in with an 'agenda' of basic questions which we wanted to cover somewhere in the interview. Though the questions were seldom or never asked explicitly, they served to make sure that key topics were covered by everyone, and that we did not form conclusions on the fact that someone had failed to talk about something important to us, when the fact of the matter was simply that it had failed to come up in the conversation. Chief among the strengths was the sheer **naturalism** of the situation. The interviewers were very evidently a couple, having 'got together' not all that long ago, and some of the atmosphere of a 'family visit' was sometimes achieved; it is remarkably natural for one couple to be talking to another mother about children and the experience of bringing them up. Pamela's pregnancy helped here. By the time Pamela had been settled comfortably in a chair and cushions arranged to support her, and Roger had been taken to one side and asked how she liked her coffee (a curious variant on the 'Does she take sugar?' phenomenon), some degree of acquaintance seemed already to have grown up. Later in the interview series some of the same effect was unwittingly achieved by the small child we brought with us in a carrycot, owing to the lack of babysitting facilities.

Among what is not recorded is some of the detail of the informants, the interviewing and how it progressed – this might have helped the reader judge its **validity**. The paper does not record, for instance, that the tape recorder did not work for the first interview, so that we were reduced to sitting down afterwards and writing out, independently, everything we could remember that was said. It does not record the number of tapes which were difficult to decipher afterwards because of the noise of children playing in the room or building work going on outside. It does not talk about the interviews which were difficult to 'get going', nor give much detail about the roles in which informants tended to cast us and how these changed. We do not talk much about the individual mothers, in fact, and this detracts from the richness of the presentation.

One of the findings we report, as you might expect, is that the mothers to whom we talked are very aware of their children's status as 'handicapped' and very aware of other people's reactions to it. Apart from the obvious reactions of strangers, even more difficult to deal with are the 'ignorant' reactions of friends and neighbours:

> When I talk to people and I say 'Mark is mentally handicapped', and as soon as they know he is coming up to sixteen, you see, you know what I mean? . . . You see it before they even say it . . . It is an unspoken look . . . there is that fear of danger to 'my daughter'.
>
> (Abbott and Sapsford 1997: 62)

Such reactions can be looked for even from within the family:

> Let's put it this way, there were relations we have not seen since we found out about Trevor . . . [and] we have only been invited to tea with Trevor once to my brother-in-law. He thinks we should put Trevor away.
>
> (Abbott and Sapsford 1997: 61)

The mother's life comes very much to centre round the 'handicapped' child, in a majority of cases. The amount of sheer physical labour – washing and cleaning – is immense, with children who will normally not become 'house trained' till substantially after other children – in their teens or never, in the most severe cases. Another part of the burden is constant supervision; as one mother pointed out, you expect to have to be home to supervise a 5-year-old, but not a 15-year-old. In many different ways these mothers' children caused extra work and took up extra time, and the fact that the labour was freely and lovingly given did not diminish its extent. In all this it was clear that the concept of 'community care' basically meant 'care by mother'. Some had help from neighbours, some from immediate household, some from wider family, but in many cases the help was intermittent or trivial, and in many cases it did not occur. Eight of the 16 families had no help from neighbours, and six of these also received little or no help from kin.

We also attempted a tentative typology of 'coping strategies' – trying to find a characterization of women's (or families') lives as a whole which would differentiate some families from others (in terms of the general style of their self-placement with regard to the outside world) and some women from others (in terms of the constructs they used to characterize and justify their lives). We noted a difference between those families which seemed determined that life should go on 'as normal' and those which conceded that there was something with which to 'cope'. Within the latter class we noted the 'bare copers' – those who managed from day to day and year to year – and those who seemed to have formed some stable kind of 'adaptation' to their situation. Within the latter class again we noted that some women seemed to have adopted the 'wife and/or mother' designation – seen as a positive role, not a form of constraint – as a preferred characterization of their current lives and as a description of their life goals. That is, they found themselves satisfied with what they were doing and appeared not to desire for any form of change.

We went on in this study – unusually for research into 'social problem' categories – to attempt a comparison with the 'normal':

> Shortly after the second interviews . . . one of us conducted a series of interviews with a 'sample' of mothers whose children had not been labelled as mentally handicapped, roughly **matched** for size of family and area of residence (which **correlates** well, in the new city, both with social class and with availability of 'social resource'). The sample is of course too small and haphazard to be representative of mothers in general . . . but the two samples match closely enough for some tentative conclusions to be drawn. One can after all say little about what is distinctive in the experience of mothering mentally handicapped children except by comparison with the general experience of mothering.
>
> (Abbott and Sapsford 1987b: 65)

Overall we found similar kinds of work being done by the two samples, with a similar lack of help from both community and kin, but the work was greater in extent and more demanding for the mothers of children with learning difficulties, and they received even less help from kin and community.

The biggest difference between the two samples of families came in the kind of future that they could foresee. In the normal course of events children grow up and leave home, and women receive back their power to dispose of their daily time. Children with learning difficulties do not necessarily leave home unless the parents actively determine that they shall do so, and the feelings of guilt and apprehension which are associated with the child's teenage years colour the whole view of the future. For some families the decision will effectively be taken for them by events: one or two of the children were so severely physically handicapped that they were not expected to live into their twenties. For others it was clear that a decision would have to be taken, in the child's interests. Some families were adamant that their child would stay with them, for ever if need be: 'When you think what her mental age is, say four or five, by the time she's nineteen she won't be more than that. You wouldn't stick a five year old in a hostel, would you?' (p. 74).

For many, however, the decision is a mixture of the child's interests, the convenience of the family and a feeling that in some way the problems of an adult 'child' are beyond what the neighbourhood can cope with.

Finally, the paper summarizes the study's conclusions about

> the real cost of bearing and bringing up a mentally handicapped child in the community. Some of it – the day to day grind of 'child work' – falls largely on the child's mother . . . The rearing of a mentally handicapped baby does not differ in kind from the rearing of any other baby – itself a substantial social burden – but it differs in its density and its duration . . . The burden goes on, moreover, potentially for ever, unless the decision is made to send the child away . . . Specific to mental handicap . . . are the other range of major problems which families encounter: the reactions . . . among strangers and also within the family and kin group.
>
> (Abbott and Sapsford 1987b: 74–5)

Discussion

In what purports to be an evaluation of research methods we have spent a fair amount of time looking at the substantive findings of the study – what it has to say about mothering children with learning difficulties. We have also given you additional information which was not in the report but which might be thought vital if the research is to be properly evaluated. This will not, of course, be possible when we are discussing the research of others. We cannot generally, when reading a report, ask researchers questions which might provide additional information about their methods and methodologies. It is therefore important, when writing up research, to consider what material about the methods has to be included to answer possible questions. Limitations of space often cause problems, however, and researchers often respond to them by leaving out the information which is vital for an informed evaluation of the research.

We read research studies mostly to look at what they have found out, not to study their methods. The study of methods comes in, however, when we need to determine whether we believe what is stated, whether it accords with the evidence as given, and whether the conclusions are possible ones given the ways in which the data have been collected. We need to look then to the strengths of each method, in general and in the particular case under examination, and to the corresponding weaknesses of logic of that type of research in general or this particular example of it.

One very definite strength of 'open' approaches to research – just talking to people, or observing and participating in their lives (discussed in the next chapter), without imposing much structure on what is collected – is the immediacy, the vivacity, the feeling of actually 'being there'. The Abbott and Sapsford (1987b) piece carries the actual words of the informants and lets them tell their own stories, often better than we could tell them for them. No amount of second-hand description can convey what it may be like to have a mentally handicapped child nearly as powerfully as the words of Mrs Miller:

> For about a month after I found out I didn't have any feeling for her any way – she wasn't my baby, she was just a baby that had got to be looked after and fed and kept clean . . . [And then] I walked past the pram one day and she looked up at me and she smiled at me . . . she just smiled . . . After that I was all right.
>
> (p. 47)

The price that is paid for this power and immediacy, which comes from the detailed study of a few cases or a single setting, is a necessary doubt about the representative nature of the 'sample'. To what extent does an interview study of less than 20 mothers of mentally handicapped children in one geographical location tell us anything about the problems nationwide of this kind of community care? In our study we did our best to 'cover the range' – to include as wide a range of 'cases' and social settings as was possible. We sampled, for instance, mothers from both a 'severe' school and a 'mild' school, so we could reasonably expect to contact cases ranging from near-total physical and mental inability to children who could have passed for 'just a bit stupid' at ordinary schools (and we did, in fact, contact cases covering this entire range). Our sample was well scattered through a new city in which geographical locality is fairly well correlated with social class and material circumstances, and we had everything from a mother permanently on social security to one in a substantial rural house set in its own grounds. Some of the sample were 'immigrants' of recent date to the new town, some had moved there in the 1940s and 1950s from London, and some were locally born and still to a large part involved in the original local 'village' community. However, we do not know how representative the new city is of places where parents whose children have learning difficulties might be living. Thus even if we are fairly confident that the results generalize to all families with a child with learning difficulties in that city, we would probably be less confident that they would generalize to families living in other parts of the country. Also, we do not know the extent to which looking after a child with learning difficulties is typical of caring for other groups of dependants.

We would certainly not want to assert that a particular percentage of all such mothers held this or that belief, or experienced this or that problem, on the basis of our handful of cases, but the problems experienced by our informants are probably not far different from those experienced by all such mothers. Nonetheless, all were 'customers' of the same schools and health and social service provision, so a study carried out elsewhere might well come up with different experiences depending on how much service differs across the country. Our study was also tied to a particular historical time, since when there have been major changes: we do not know how the newer policy of integrating mentally handicapped children into the 'normal' schools has affected the lives of mothers.

The other question which must be asked of this kind of research, where so much depends on the building of relationships and so much is apparently 'left in the hands of the informants', is the extent to which the findings are specific to those particular relationships, or even 'created' by something that the researchers did or said. The only guard against this, and the only warrant of validity, is constant **reflexivity** in the research and in the report of it – constant attention paid to what is going on, and detailed discussion of all aspects of the social situation and the procedures in the report. Our report is weak in this respect; it is characteristic of short reports of 'open' research that what is omitted in order to keep length down is the reflexive account, important as it is, and while reflexive material has been supplied, there is not as much of it here as we would have liked.

One aspect of reflexivity which you should look for in research reports is an awareness of the crucial importance of role and audience in the construction of interview data. 'What is expected' differs according to setting: the accounts we give when we are 'doing a public performance' are different from those we might produce in the privacy of the home. Similarly, a male interviewer may be faced with a different kind of account from what would be produced for a female, and the same goes for young *v.* old, Black *v.* White, able-bodied *v.* disabled . . . The account which we produce is very much conditioned by who we see the interviewer as being and, therefore, what is to be seen as 'relevant' or 'useful'.

Informants *have* to make sense of the situation before they can function within it, and how they do so is much conditioned by our presentation of the situation. They have to use the clues we provide to work out what we are after and what we see as relevant. One common way of introducing this kind of research task, for instance, is to present it as one which a student has to do as a requirement of the degree. The risk here is that to present the interviews as just a student task may devalue the work and lead the informants to produce accounts which are easy, memorable and picturesque, but not necessarily 'true' in any usual sense. The major alternative tack is to present the work as 'research', as in the Abbott and Sapsford (1987b) study, but the problem here is that the term 'research' is ambiguous in common language and has no single clear meaning. Our informants were quite clear as to why they were being interviewed: they knew they had been approached because their children had learning difficulties. Most started off by identifying us with some branch of the support services – as doctors, psychologists, social workers – and assumed that we were in some way checking up on the efficiency of provision. When they realized that these identifications did not hold up, we tended to become (in their view) the other kind of researcher – people writing a book and looking for useful material. (The mothers knew they had a story worth telling.) When this role transition took place, the nature of the accounts tended to change. The informants became more relaxed. The conversation became more general and it was easier to probe for detail not immediately relevant to the question of mental handicap. On the other hand, the informants were often less precise and less analytic in stating what they had experienced and what they felt they needed.

A problem with accounts, which you need to look out for in evaluating published research of this kind, is that we all have many different ways of accounting for ourselves, many different stories to tell. There are, for instance, public '**rhetorics**' which people tend to produce in a rounded, rehearsed form when asked direct questions. Some of them are minimal, polite, 'safe', problem-avoiding accounts, what Cornwell (1984) calls 'public accounts': something uncontroversial which is always safe to produce when questioned on this topic. Others are learned rhetorics: the first response on the subject of social class from anyone who has studied sociology, for instance, tends to recapitulate some part of the course studied. Others again are 'class-markers' – to state certain kinds of beliefs communicates membership of a class or group, or sympathy with it. Others again are just well rehearsed stories, polished and perhaps partly falsified or simplified by frequent telling. All or any of these rhetorics may truly be held as beliefs by the informant, and any or all may be acted out in practice, but the chances are that they are sincerely held but purely verbal beliefs, unconnected in any way to action. One always strives to get underneath these rhetorics, to get the informant analysing his or her own life in a fresh way and producing 'true' accounts. However, one should note that these 'private' accounts are equally a product of a particular social situation – the informant striving to make sense of his or her life in the light of his or her perception of what is relevant and useful for the interviewer – so we cannot treat these as necessarily 'more true' than the rhetorics and polished stories.

The points which are important here as guidelines for the evaluation of research are:

1 that informants do not 'give interviewers the facts', but work out the purpose of the interview and give accounts that will make sense and be relevant in the context of that purpose;
2 that they are constrained by what they think is acceptable (as well as relevant) to say to different kinds of people, in different kinds of tasks;
3 that we all have accounts of common topics which 'roll easily off the tongue', but we may have other and possibly contradictory things to say about them if one can get behind the rhetoric; and
4 that any given account may be a rhetoric in this sense, but nonetheless not 'rhetorical' – well practised verbal accounts may or may not be accurate descriptions of behaviour and attitudes.

You would expect to find enough reflexive material in a good account of open interviewing to enable you to form some view on these questions: whether the situation partly dictated the response, whether the interviewer has taken a rhetoric for a reality, whether a well practised account, nonetheless, describes a reality of the informant's life. To the extent that such material is not present, you may have to suspend judgement on the credibility of the results – not necessarily to disbelieve them, but to give them less credit than if their validity was well established.

A second question when evaluating the scope of a piece of research – the opposite of the question of how far it can be generalized – is how specific the findings are. In the Abbott and Sapsford (1987b) paper one important question was the extent to which the experiences of those who care for children with learning difficulties are different from those of other mothers (all mothering being, in a sense, a form of community care). For this reason we also interviewed a group of mothers whose children had not been labelled as having learning difficulties and so were able to distinguish the problems of having children with learning difficulties from the problems of having children in general. (Naturally we took pains to pick a **comparison group** as like the mothers of children with learning difficulties as possible, so that where differences were found they were not equally likely to be due to age or class/material circumstances or area of residence.)

It is worth noting that the interviews with the mothers whose children were not labelled as having learning difficulties were far more difficult than those with mothers whose children were so labelled. The mothers of children with learning difficulties 'knew' what they were being interviewed about – they knew that what we had picked out was mothers in their situation. The other mothers had far more difficulty making sense of the situation. There was no obvious 'social problem' which we might be investigating, and they could not see what it was about their situation which made it interesting for us to get them to 'tell their story'. They therefore had great difficulty working out what story to tell. As we said above, the sense which the informant makes of the situation is a key determinant of the accounts which are elicited in interview.

Summary: points for evaluation

1 When reading 'open interview' research, you need to know quite a lot about the interviewer, the situation and the course of the interviews, to judge the validity of the results. **Reactivity** – the production of material in response to loaded questions, or the reshaping of it to suit the expected prejudices of the interviewer – is a particularly strong possibility in this kind of research.

2 One might be suspicious of research reports based on one quick interview with each informant; the likelihood of the interviewer getting beyond the 'rhetoric' or 'public account' is not high (see Cornwell 1984, particularly p. 16).

3 At a more subtle level, you need to work out what sense the informants probably made of the situation, in order to see what they will have perceived as relevant and what they may have omitted or ignored in their accounts.

4 To the extent that there is insufficient reflexive material for you to make these judgements, you do not need to reject the research report entirely, but its conclusions should be handled with some caution.

5 Looking at the 'sample' you should ask yourself how far the results are likely to generalize beyond the immediate informants – of what are these informants typical?

6 You should also ask yourself how specific the results are to the type of person or setting which is being described – to what extent they might be equally true of quite different groups or settings.

> ### Exercise 12
>
> Now re-read the Abbott and Sapsford (1987b) paper in the light of this chapter, bearing in mind the points listed at the end. Note particularly how much extra material we have had to supply in this chapter in order to give you any real insight into the process of the interviews and the ways in which we were typecast by informants. Look back at the questions you thought you would have liked to ask us. How many of them have been answered by the 'extra' material we have provided in this chapter?

Further reading

On children with learning difficulties

Abbott, Pamela and Sapsford, Roger (1986) Diverse reports: caring for mentally handicapped children in the community, *Nursing Times*, 5 March, 47–9.

Bayley, M. (1973) *Mental Handicap and Community Care*. London: Routledge and Kegan Paul.

Glendinning, C. (1983) *Unshared Care: Parents and their Disabled Children*. London: Routledge and Kegan Paul.

Shearer, A. (1972) *A Report on Public and Professional Attitudes towards the Sexual and Emotional Attitudes of Handicapped People*. London: Spastics Society/National Association for Mental Handicap.

Voysey, M. (1975) *A Constant Burden: The Reconstitution of Family Life*. London: Routledge and Kegan Paul.

On 'normal' mothering

Abbott, Pamela and Wallace, Claire (1996) *An Introduction to Sociology: Feminist Perspectives* (2nd edition). London: Routledge.

Backett, K. (1982) *Mothers and Fathers*. London: Macmillan.

Boulton, M. (1983) *On Being a Mother*. London: Tavistock.

Kitzinger, S. (1978) *Women as Mothers*. London: Fontana.

Oakley, A. (1972) *Sex, Gender and Society*. London: Fontana.

Porter, M. (1983) *Home, Work and Class Consciousness*. Manchester: Manchester University Press.

On coping and coping strategies

Davis, F. (1963) *Passage through Crisis: Polio Victims and their Families*. Indianapolis, IN: Bobbs-Merril.

Goffman, E. (1961) *Asylums: Essays on the Social Situation of Mental Patients and Other Inmates*. Harmondsworth: Penguin.

Goffman, E. (1963) *Stigma: The Management of Spoilt Identities*. Harmondsworth: Penguin.

Roth, J. (1963) *Timetables*. Indianapolis, IN: Bobbs-Merril.

CHAPTER FOUR

READING OBSERVATION RESEARCH

Research paper 1: Kirkham (1983) 'Labouring in the dark' (observation of labour wards)
Research paper 2: Cayne (1995) 'Portfolios: a developmental influence?' (participant research on nurse professional development)
Research paper 3: James (1984) 'A postscript to nursing' (reflexive account of observation research in hospital)
Summary: points for evaluation
Further reading

This chapter deals with interpretative **observation** studies which involve varying degrees of participation; 'systematic' observation is dealt with under the heading of survey research. The chapter is built around three research papers: Mavis Kirkham (1983) 'Labouring in the dark'; Julia Cayne (1995) 'Portfolios: a developmental influence?'; and Nicky James (1984) 'A postscript to nursing'. All three are reprinted, two of them in slightly short-ened form, in Abbott and Sapsford (1997), the Reader associated with this text.

> **Exercise 13**
>
> Now would be a good time to read the first of these three, the paper by Mavis Kirkham, 'Labouring in the dark'.

Research paper 1: Kirkham (1983)

Mavis Kirkham's paper deals with the event of giving birth in hospital and the time leading up to it. Her focus of interest is the transmission – or non-transmission – of information from doctors, nurses and midwives to the pregnant woman, about the progress of her imminent delivery and the timescale that may be expected. She is interested in the hierarchical rela-tionship between nurses and midwives, and patients, and the way in which this may in fact impede delivery by failing to reassure patients and not allowing them to draw on their own strengths during the process.

What she did was to sit in on 90 labours in one consultant unit of a northern teaching hospital, take notes of what was said and done, and talk to the women after their babies had been born; she also talked to 85 patients in hospital before confinement. In addition, she observed five home confinements and 18 confinements in a neighbouring GP unit, and she interviewed a number of midwives. Her method was that of open, unstructured, participant observation:

> I wanted to see what issues were important to those involved as shown in their actions and words at the time. Observation was clearly an appropriate method . . . I came to this research as a midwife and a mother. But my observations were guided by those aspects of care in labour which the midwives and mothers I observed showed were important to them. Thus my observations and analysis were 'grounded' (Glaser and Strauss 1967) in the experiences of those observed as shown in their words and actions.
>
> (Kirkham 1983: 86)

The aim is to describe not necessarily a fully **representative** sample of confinements, but at least a sample of **typical** ones: 'These labours were chosen as normal labours, as far as anyone can tell this in advance. I therefore did not observe women with known medical or obstetric abnormalities' (p. 86).

Kirkham describes and illustrates the main tactics she sees the pregnant women using in order to get information. Straightforward questions are, of course, asked, but this is not always a good tactic for gaining information because questions are often deflected or blocked 'in the patient's interests' or 'because she wouldn't really understand'. Another tactic is to make what appears to be a statement, but which has the force of a question – for example:

> Patient: My backside's hurting. It'll be the cut. [*Silence*] . . . It's the episiotomy.
> Sister: It's not an episiotomy. It's a tear. But it hasn't gone anywhere it shouldn't.

Some patients try out statements in the form of jokes:

> Patient: Is there much water?
> Doctor: A normal amount.
> Patient: You imagine buckets!
> Doctor: You've not got that much when you get to term . . .
>
> (p. 90)

Some combine this with what Kirkham calls 'self-denigration':

> Student midwife [SM]: Let's see if the machine is playing silly beggars.
> [*Patient pulls up her gown to show the . . . connection to the monitor.*]
> SM: You're a right flasher, aren't you?
> Patient: And I've got such a wonderful body.
> [*Both laugh. SM listens to fetal heart. Patient asks if she can listen. SM lets her . . .*]
>
> (p. 91)

Passive watching and the active drawing of conclusions is a common tactic here as elsewhere – 'If it was going to be quick they wouldn't have given me Pethidine' – but it is limited by the extent to which what is seen is correctly understood. A certain amount can be gleaned from eavesdropping on teaching sessions, where sisters are instructing student midwives, for instance, but this essentially passive tactic does not lend itself to the patient gaining useful – usable and interpretable – information.

All of this is contrasted with deliveries in GP units and at home. On the GP units, not surrounded by senior medical staff, midwives were freer with information and found it necessary to solicit the patient's cooperation more. Patients giving birth at home tended to demand to know what was going on.

The author concludes that the women on the ward want and need information with which to orient themselves within the process of birth, and that what they receive is generally inadequate. The lack of information very much constrains their choices. A hierarchy of relations, and of control of information, runs from the patient at the bottom through midwives and sisters to doctors. Kirkham observes that the tactics which patients use to elicit information from midwives run remarkably parallel to those which midwives use to elicit information from doctors. She comments in conclusion that an awareness of problems shared by midwife and patient could do much to change midwives' behaviour, which in turn could fundamentally change the patient's experience of labour.

Exercise 14

Now read Julia Cayne (1995) 'Portfolios: a developmental influence?'

Research paper 2: Cayne (1995)

This paper describes **applied research** undertaken as part of the normal work of the researcher – as a nurse tutor in training in a particular unit, she set up a 'learning group' and monitored its progress.

> A situational analysis had demonstrated a need to help staff within an orthopaedic/trauma unit review past and plan future learning. An **action research** project was undertaken to explore two research questions: is the process of portfolio preparation in itself developmental? If so, what factors influence this developmental process?
>
> (Cayne 1995: 395)

The focus of the group was the actual preparation of portfolios – documentation of past learning – as a cooperative effort within the group (including Cayne, the facilitator).

The membership of the group was somewhat 'happenstance'. In principle, Cayne had permission to approach all qualified nurses on the unit, but in practice the vagaries of shift work determined who was on an early shift on Friday mornings and therefore able to participate, and staffing levels on some units proved a further constraint. In the event a group of six was achieved, one from each of four wards plus one from the accident and emergency department and one from the fracture clinic. The first session was structured to establish the 'contract' for the remaining sessions, but the remaining sessions dealt with problems raised by the group members themselves. Data collection was by the keeping of **field notes**, the taping of group sessions, and taped interviews following an exploratory question-naire (**open-ended questions** – see Chapter 6 below). Each individual was given the chance to comment on a written draft of the findings and to require information to be removed if she felt threatened by its inclusion.

The Results section of the paper begins with a description of the way in which the group facilitated reflection on an individual's career to date. This started as what might be termed 'a vague feeling of discomfort': as one participant put it,

> . . . it gives you – really I suppose a chance for reflection over every-thing, to sort of, I don't know, categorize what you have done and what you haven't done, what you need to do. But and, you feel that it ought to come out with, what I need to do now is this. And when you don't come out with anything specific . . . it feels like nothing's achieved.
>
> (p. 399)

Others described how completing their portfolios made them face up to difficulties in their practice and/or question and revise their self-image. One thing brought home to many of the participants was the value of their professional experience, as opposed to the courses they had taken. The researcher's conclusion was that there were indications that portfolio preparation is developmental in its own right but that the small numbers and short duration of the project make it difficult to provide evidence for this conclusion. Factors which affected the process were uncertainty about the validity of 'subjective' information, fear of failure and, on the other hand, the need to explore and comply with new regulations then coming into force.

The tone of the paper is very reflexive throughout, drawing heavily on the researcher's experience and not trying to any great extent to emulate the 'scientific' style adopted by some research reports:

> I have used the first-person pronoun in the writing of this report because I believe it is an ethical imperative to be open about one's own role in the shaping of events in a project such as this. Webb (1992) points out that the third-person pronoun is used in academic writing to convey 'an impression that the ideas being discussed have a neutral, value free, impartial basis [which] is rarely if ever the case'.
>
> (p. 395)

The belief that the researcher is a neutral scientist who can and should remain detached from what he or she is studying is something we shall dis-cuss elsewhere in this book; it is not a position we take ourselves.

Research paper 3: James (1984)

This concern with reflexivity – a sensitivity to the research as itself a social situation and a part of the researcher's biography – is very characteristic of 'open' research. Both authors are quite aware of their own position within the research, and Mavis Kirkham is explicit about how her position may have affected the behaviour of the women she observed:

> I sat during most of the labours level with the patient's head about six feet from her and took constant written notes. The question of the researcher's influence upon the research is raised by this method . . . The people I observed may well have been on their 'best behaviour' because I was observing them.
>
> (Kirkham 1983: 86)

(In the Cayne paper, despite its open stance, we might have expected to find more discussion of how the fact that she was running the groups might have affected what she found; her control of the topic of conversation, and presumably of its timing and routeing as well, would put her in a strong position to direct the outcome, and because of space constraints we have to take a lot of the conclusions on trust. We might also want to consider the extent to which knowing that they were part of a research project may have altered the participants' approach to the developmental task.) We know from Chapter 4, however, that there is more than the discussion of **reactivity** to a proper **reflexive** account. How the researcher is received and what sense the participants make of her are part of the story that needs to be told. We also need, however, to know more about the researcher herself, her theoretical perspectives, her professional expectations – anything which may affect the conduct of the research or the interpretation of the data.

The third paper to be considered in this chapter, Nicky James's (1984) 'A postscript to nursing', is not a report of research results, but an extended reflexive account, written for a book of articles on the research process. James describes what it was like, as a trained nurse, to return to the wards to do research on nursing for a higher degree. It raises many of the special problems (and the strengths) of the open participation method in an acute form.

Exercise 15

You might like to read the paper at this point: Nicky James (1984) 'A postscript to nursing'.

James went in 'labelled' as a researcher and had no role into which she could 'disappear from view'. Whether participant research should be open or **covert** (secret) is much debated. Covert research obviously disturbs what is going on less; if the researcher can pass as a natural member of the scene, then there is no 'researcher identity' to which participants might react. This obviously holds even more where the researcher is a natural participant in the context. (There are problems of detachment here, however;

it is very difficult to stand back from your own real-life involvement.) The disadvantage of covert research is that you tend to be 'stuck' in one part of the field and bound by the limitations of the adopted role: if you have 'become' a nurse, then you cannot also socialize with doctors on equal terms and experience what the patients experience. You are also limited in the number and type of questions you can ask about what is going on before you start looking unnaturally incompetent and ignorant for a true participant. Some might also consider covert research unethical, in that participants are deceived into revealing things about themselves which they might not have chosen to reveal to a researcher and an abuse of relationships is involved.

Open research has the converse disadvantage, that participants have to make sense of you and will generally try to consider what they do and say because they know it may be recorded. The presence of an explicit researcher may also be uncomfortable for the other participants because it forces them to question aspects of their behaviour which are normally taken for granted and may partially destroy the careful set of 'cognitive defences' which we all set up against the unpleasant or boring aspects of our jobs and our lives in general. To the extent that real involvement is achieved, moreover, the researcher will also acquire some of these defences, and breaking through them into analysis will become a real emotional problem. (This is also a problem for covert researchers, of course – sometimes more so.) James certainly found both problems during her research relationships with other nurses:

> A dysfunction built into the research . . . was the constant prodding at the defence mechanisms which are a means of continuing at the unit. If I pushed the others too far they would evade, avoid or tell me to shut up, but my own defences were also under scrutiny and the more I was perturbed by exposing them, the more my reluctance to write up at the end of the day grew. I was enjoying the nursing. For the research, philosophy, the structure of the National Health Service, and numbers became easier lines of thought. None of them had anything to do with people.
>
> (James 1984: 141–2)

One of the major problems of undertaking fieldwork, particularly in the role of 'the researcher', is to establish a role within the setting which is something other than sitting and taking notes. As a qualified nurse, Nicky James found it particularly difficult to be present on a ward for which she had no nursing responsibilities, as her field notes show:

> I didn't know what I was doing, and the lack of routine was very undermining, or rather the lack of knowledge of the routine . . . I felt that I had no independence on the ward because I nearly always had to ask people if I wanted to do, or thought I ought to do, something.
>
> (pp. 136–7)

> Confusion and doubt is part of any nurse's move to a new ward, but I had forgotten that and I found it difficult to make sense of things as a nurse, let alone a researcher.
>
> (p. 137)

Having acquired a role within the ward, she found it almost equally diffi-cult to dissociate herself from it again.

The problem for the participants is making sense of the researcher and assigning her a social role, and some of the solutions may not always be flattering or even useful, as James points out:

> Nicky, you're sort of like a PS in a letter. Not part of the main body of the nursing team, but still important.
>
> (Night nurse)

> This is our pet sociologist, who's working on the unit and studying us. She's found out all sorts of interesting things.
>
> (Continuing care unit sister) (p. 129)

What sense will be made is essentially unpredictable, so one has to be prepared to make changes 'on the run'. James had this problem right from the start, in her initial discussions with 'gatekeepers':

> In the proposal to the nursing administrators, submitted before I went to see them, I tried to 'sell' myself by predicting what they would like . . . my main doubt was whether they would tolerate an observer. Why should they? To try to overcome that, I made a commitment to working free, instead of being an onlooker . . . I had totally misjudged their reading of the proposal. Instead of being flexible, it looked as though I did not know what I was doing, and though they welcomed nursing research, there was some anxiety over someone who wanted to be integrated . . . I acquiesced to their suggestions . . . In the report on the meeting I noted that 'I went in optimistic and came out feeling like a grilled sardine – small, squashed and hot.'
>
> (pp. 133–4)

In conclusion, James's account of her research reinforces very strongly the importance of reflexivity. She describes how difficult it was to 'get in' with any freedom of movement, how difficult it was to find herself a role which was plausible to herself, and how difficult it was for others to find a place for her in their social world. She makes it clear that observing was not a neutral process, but one which trampled over her own preconceptions and led to considerable emotional turmoil, the more so because her investigations also tended to trample over the preconceptions and defences of others.

Summary: points for evaluation

1 Observation research, like open interviewing, needs to show a substan-tial reflexive element in the report if we are to be able to judge the effect of researcher and situation on the recorded data, and how the way in which both researcher and participants make sense of the situation affects what is produced.

2 In observation research even more than in open interviewing we need to know something of the researcher and his or her preconceptions, fears and capabilities, to put faith in the reported interpretations of the situation.

3 In covert research we need to know what kind of role the researcher took up, how convincing he or she was, and the extent to which the role may have tied him or her down to one segment or aspect of the situation and perhaps blinded him or her to interpretations which might seem **valid** from a different perspective. A common criticism of male studies of youth gangs, for instance, is that young women are 'seen' only through the eyes of young men and the male researcher.

4 In research where the researcher is a 'real' participant, carrying out his or her normal role as well as writing about the situation, we need to consider the extent to which it has been possible for him or her to step outside the professional assumptions of that situation for the purposes of the research analysis.

Exercise 16

Now re-read the papers by Kirkham and Cayne in the light of the James paper and our discussion.

Further reading

On maternity nursing

Cartwright, A. (1979) *The Dignity of Labour?* London: Tavistock.

Lorenson, Margarethe (1983) Effects of touch in patients during a crisis situation in hospital, in J. Wilson-Barnett (ed.) *Nursing Research: Ten Studies in Patient Care*. Chichester: Wiley.

Maternity Services Advisory Committee (1984) *Maternity Care in Action Pt II: Care during Childbirth*. London: HMSO.

Maternity Services Advisory Committee (1985) *Maternity Care in Action Pt III: Care of the Mother and Baby*. London: HMSO.

Metcalf, Clare (1983) A study of change in the method of organising the delivery of nursing care in a ward of a maternity hospital, in J. Wilson-Barnett (ed.) *Nursing Research: Ten Studies in Patient Care*. Chichester: Wiley.

Oakley, Ann (1980) *Women Confined: Towards a Sociology of Childbirth*. Oxford: Martin Robertson.

Oakley, Ann (1981) *From Here to Maternity*. Harmondsworth: Penguin.

Savage, Wendy (1986) *A Savage Enquiry: Who Controls Childbirth?* London: Virago.

Developmental learning for professionals

Barber, P. (1989) Developing the 'person' of the professional carer, in
  S. Hinchcliffe, S. Norman and J. Schober (eds) *Nursing Practice and Health
  Care*. Sevenoaks: Edward Arnold.
Brookfield, S. (1986) *Understanding and Facilitating Adult Learning*. Milton
  Keynes: Open University Press.
Rogers, A. (1992) *Adults Learning for Development*. London: Cassell.
Schön, D. (1987) *Educating the Reflective Practitioner*. San Francisco, CA:
  Jossey-Bass.

Research on general ward nursing

Brown, Roswyn (1989) *Individualised Care: The Role of the Ward Sister*.
  Harrow: Scutari.
Cope, David (1981) *Organisational Development and Action Research in
  Hospitals*. Aldershot: Gower.
Wilson-Barnett, Jenifer and Robinson, Sarah (eds) (1989) *Directions in
  Nursing Research*. Harrow: Scutari.

READING ABOUT CONTROLLED TRIALS

Research paper 1: Gordon (1986) 'Treatment of depressed women by nurses
  in Britain'
Research paper 2: Doll and Hill (1954) 'The mortality of doctors in relation
  to their smoking habits'
Summary: points for evaluation
Further reading

At the other extreme of the spectrum of research from open interviewing
and observation comes the controlled trial or experiment. The central
principle here is not finding out about the unknown, but testing known
principles. The medical controlled trial tests the efficacy of a drug or treatment by applying the drug to one group of people and withholding it from
another. To the extent that the first group are *exactly* like the second in
terms of personal characteristics and histories, and to the extent that they
receive *exactly* the same treatment in all ways except that the drug is
administered to the experimental group and withheld from the control
group, then logically any difference between the two which is present at
the end but was not present at the start must be due to the administration
of the drug. The four essentials are: a clearly defined 'treatment'; a clearly
defined 'outcome'; a comparison of outcomes between treatment and non-
treatment, or between different treatments; and control of anything else
which might otherwise have explained observed differences in outcome.

Generally, we associate experimental research with highly scientific subject areas – medicine, the more scientific kinds of psychology, etc. It is quite
possible, however, to apply precisely the same principles to much more
'woolly' topic areas, such as the treatment of mental conditions; the first
paper considered in this chapter is the evaluation of an experimental
nurse-administered treatment for women's depression – Verona Gordon's
'Treatment of depressed women by nurses in Britain'.

> **Exercise 17**
>
> You might now like to read the paper by Verona Gordon (1986). The full
> text, entitled 'Treatment of depressed women by nurses in Britain and
> the USA', can be found in Julia Brooking (ed.) *Psychiatric Nursing
> Research*, published by Wiley. A shortened version which omits the USA
> material will be found in Abbott and Sapsford (1997).

Research paper 1: Gordon (1986)

Verona Gordon's paper begins with a discussion of the extent to which depression can be considered one of the major health problems of women. Twice as many women as men are diagnosed depressed around the world and the incidence of the condition shows an alarming growth over time. (Whether an increased incidence of *diagnosis* of depression over time necessarily equates with an increased *incidence* of depression is questionable, however. We shall return to this point in a later chapter.)

Gordon suggests that current treatment practices are not satisfactory for women's depression:

> There are two concerns that remain with treatment and prevention issues. One is that traditional treatment approaches by male therapists perpetuate the passivity and negative self-image of women . . . The other is that while there are numerous programmes to treat depression, treatment usually begins after the depression has reached a serious level. This lack of early identification and intervention does not support nursing's commitment to prevention and health maintenance.
>
> (Gordon 1986: 95)

She suggests that a group approach is far superior to individual therapy for women, in that it allows for peer support and gives a safe and rewarding environment within which negative self-labelling can be unlearned. The (female) professional nurse, she suggests, is uniquely well placed to run such groups successfully: she is herself a woman (though possibly better educated than some of those she serves); she appreciates the problems of women's positions and the value to them of both family and work; she is not seen by the public as having a judgemental or diagnostic role; and she is popularly stereotyped as someone who cares and offers support.

This paper reports on an experimental treatment group for women's depression which Gordon set up in England. (Two earlier studies were carried out in the United States – see Gordon 1982; Gordon and Ledray 1984).

> Twenty women, 40 to 60 years of age, were selected for the study. These subjects had been recruited through a public service radio broadcast (BBC airwaves) seeking depressed women as participants . . . There was an overwhelming response to the broadcast from hundreds of women . . . The University of London's phone lines were flooded with calls, confirming the author's belief that depression in women is extensive.
>
> (p. 100)

'Information meetings' were set up, at which 119 women who showed interest and met the criteria filled out a descriptive questionnaire and took two standardized tests of depression and suicidal pathology. Eighty-one women showed up on these tests as mildly to moderately depressed, and 20 of these were randomly selected for the treatment group. A similar-sized group of women were selected from the 81 as a control group, and they filled in the same tests as these 20 at around the same time. However, women assigned to the control condition received no intervention between pre- and post-testing. At the first information meeting they had been asked to refrain from joining other therapy groups or seeking counselling while the study was going on unless necessary.

(p. 105)

(The women who were not to be used in the study were, nonetheless, informed of their test results by post. Gordon telephoned the six who showed up as very depressed; all of them agreed to consult their GP.)

Meetings were arranged for the 20 women in a comfortable central location in London, and the discussion group began to meet. In the first meetings all the women were encouraged to 'tell their story', but subsequently such working over past ground was discouraged. Instead, a topic was assigned for each meeting – signs and symptoms of depression, assertiveness, goal-setting, conflict management, etc. – and this was discussed, with Gordon introducing educational material into the discussion. Homework tasks were set and a workbook issued. At the start of the series of meetings, all subjects filled in five self-report tests, all of proven reliability and widely used in research, covering self-esteem, social adjustment, loneliness, depression/hopelessness and 'life events' occurring. The same tests were re-administered at the end of the 14 group sessions.

The results were fairly clear-cut. There were no significant pre-treatment differences between the experimental group and the controls. Three of the tests – depression, self-esteem and hopelessness – showed significant post-test differences between the experimental group and the control group. *Prima facie* the results suggest strongly that the treatment made a difference to the attitudes and internal states of those who received it.

The author's conclusions are:

1 that professional nurses . . . tend to be effective facilitators of depressed women's groups;
2 that coping strategies for women can be taught, tested and shared within a supportive group atmosphere;
3 that replication of the intervention model with increased numbers of women of a variety of ages and backgrounds could be useful future nursing research.

The significance of the intervention model is:

1 to help women cope effectively and take an active role in their own health;
2 to prevent possible severe depression in women;
3 to gain data about the complex phenomena of depression in women;
4 to strengthen the family unit by increasing self-esteem of women.

(pp. 112–13)

(The first conclusion is possibly stronger than the design of the study warrants: one may not conclude that 'nurses tend' on the basis of results from one or a few nurses. The best that can be said is that nurses *are able* to act as facilitators.)

As an example of a 'controlled trial', this experiment in therapy shows many of the classic features of the true experiment as used in medicine or psychology, but falls down in some respects and is questionable in others. (This is not a criticism of the particular study, but the general verdict on the use of this research approach to evaluate events which happen outside the 'pure science' laboratory.) Its strength is in the clean lines of its design – a treatment applied to one group and withheld from another, with demonstrably little pre-treatment difference between the groups and demonstrably significant differences after the treatment. (The concept of 'significance' will be dealt with in a later chapter. For now, accept as a suitable simplification that a result is described as 'significant' if the odds against it occurring by chance are very high.)

There are two questions which might sensibly be asked of this as an experiment, however, issues on which it perhaps fails to reach the rigour of the 'true' laboratory experiment or hospital controlled trial.

1 The 'manipulation' is somewhat vaguely defined. If someone were to try to duplicate the procedures and obtained the opposite effect we would not know whether this argued against Gordon's findings or merely demonstrated that the new researcher had not, in fact, managed to duplicate Gordon's procedures. This is a general point about the evaluation of therapies.

2 The second potential criticism concerns the measure of outcome – the questionnaires which the subjects filled in. At least in this study we have what purports to be an objective measure of outcome – as opposed to therapist's or patient's judgement, which are obviously suspect in this context. However, this fact that the 'measures' are predesigned questionnaires purporting to give a score for some predetermined mental trait, state or circumstance is always a reason for pausing to think about the research. We shall discuss such measures in the next chapter and elsewhere in the book. You might want to ask yourself, however, the extent to which you could realistically expect any kind of prestructured questionnaire to reflect people's real experience of the complex, social phenomenon which we call depression. (Note, however, that this criticism does not necessarily hold true for the test used to select the experimental and control groups. These did not purport to explain/describe depression, but merely to predict whether it was likely to occur, and even an ill-theorized test can turn out empirically to have considerable predictive value.)

Research paper 2: Doll and Hill (1954)

For the second paper in this chapter we go back 30 years, to a classic of health research. A number of studies (among them Doll and Hill 1950) had demonstrated that there were fewer non-smokers among patients with lung cancer and more heavy smokers than among patients suffering from other diseases. This kind of comparison has some of the structure of an experiment: if we think of cancer patients as the 'experimental' group and other patients as the 'controls', it would appear that there is an association between smoking and the likelihood of becoming a cancer patient. The temptation is to go beyond asserting just an *association*, to the supposition that it may be smoking that causes cancer (or at least *some* cancer): we have a prior factor – smoking – and a subsequent variation in incidence of cancer, so it seems not unreasonable that the cancer may be consequent on the smoking. The logic is weaker than that of the true experiment, however, because so many *other* differences could also have an effect. People who smoke may differ from people who do not smoke in any number of ways: personally they could be more anxious and tense, for example, or as a group they might tend to be in different kinds of occupations which put them into a higher risk category, or smokers might tend to be older on average than non-smokers, or there might be any number of other differences which might be responsible for the difference in cancer incidence.

Some of these had been eliminated by collecting data on them in the original survey. In their 1950 paper, for example, Doll and Hill were able to look at the gender, age and social class of cancer patients and non-cancer patients; the two groups did not differ in age or gender, so these are not likely to be causal factors (but there *were* some minor differences in social class, and quite large differences in place of residence). Another way of dealing with differences, if any had been found, would have been by statistical control: comparisons can be made in ways which are not affected by known differences on other variables. For example, it would have been possible to compare cancer rates among younger people, separately from older ones, and so do away with the effect of age on any perceived differences. Nonetheless, logical doubts must remain; we cannot control for everything – and certainly not for factors on which it has not occurred to us to collect information. Further, there is always the possibility that something about the situation leads to higher reporting (in this case of smoking) in one group than the other, or that something in the research procedures made a cancer patient's smoking more likely to be recorded.

> Another possibility to consider is that the lung-carcinoma patients tended to exaggerate their smoking habits . . . they would have known that they had respiratory symptoms, and such knowledge might have influenced their replies to questions about the amount they smoked . . . consideration must [also] . . . be given to the possibility of interviewer bias affecting the results (by the interviewers tending to scale up the smoking habits of the lung-carcinoma patients).
>
> (Doll and Hill 1950: 745)

The second of these was controlled, in the 1950 study, by looking at those cases thought to be cancerous at the time of interview whose diagnosis was subsequently changed, and they did not appear to have their smoking in any way exaggerated by the interviewers. The first can be argued against on the basis of other patients with respiratory diseases, who did not appear in the 1950 study to differ in their smoking habits from patients with other kinds of illness. Nonetheless some doubt must remain, and a different kind of study was needed.

> **Exercise 18**
>
> You may now like to read the paper – Richard Doll and A. Bradford Hill (1954) 'The mortality of doctors in relation to their smoking habits', in *British Medical Journal* (26 June, pp. 1451–5). It is also reprinted in Abbott and Sapsford (1997).

This study is a *prospective survey* in design: it identifies groups of people who differ in some respect and follows them up to see the outcome of their differences. In this case the researchers wrote to every member of the UK medical profession in October 1951 and asked them to fill in a short questionnaire giving name, address, age, and 'smoking behaviour' – whether they were current smokers, had smoked in the past but since given up, or had never smoked regularly (defined as 'as much as one cigarette per day or its equivalent in pipe tobacco for as long as a year'). Current smokers were asked the age at which they started smoking and the method of smoking, and ex-smokers were asked similar questions relating to the time immediately prior to giving up. Nearly 60,000 questionnaires were sent out, and about 41,000 were returned, of which 40,564 were sufficiently complete to be usable. (This gives a usable response rate of 68 per cent – in other words, the returned and usable forms covered two-thirds of the doctors in the UK.) Lung cancer is relatively rare in men younger than 35 and in women, however, so these forms were discarded, leaving 26,389 forms for analysis.

From the replies the doctors were classified into broad groups by age, amount of smoking, method of smoking and whether they were current smokers or had given up. Additional information was collected from the Registrar General for the United Kingdom – a form showing particulars of death for every doctor who had died since completing the questionnaire. Thirty-six deaths certified as from lung cancer were discovered in this way; checking on the evidence for the diagnosis by writing to the doctors who had signed the death certificates they found that 'there were firm grounds for the diagnosis in at least 33 of the cases, and in only three was the evidence limited to clinical examination'. Deaths from other cancers, respiratory diseases, coronary thrombosis, other cardiovascular diseases and 'other diseases' were also recorded. A total of 789 deaths occurred among the group in the 29 months after the questionnaire was sent out.

Death rates differed very markedly between smokers and non-smokers. No non-smokers died of lung cancer during the period, for example, but 0.48 men per thousand of the light smokers (i.e. about one man in 2000 in this category), 0.67 per thousand of medium smokers and 1.14 per thousand of heavy smokers died of lung cancer; in other words, the death rate for this disease was well over twice as high for heavy smokers as for light smokers, and immeasurably smaller for non-smokers. Differences for coronary thrombosis showed a similar but less marked pattern. Deaths from the other diseases did not show this pattern at all; for example, death rates from other cancers were *higher* for non-smokers than for smokers.

It was noted, however, that smoking habits varied considerably with age and that cancer incidence also varied with age, so age could be an

Table 5.1 Actual and expected lung-cancer deaths in the Doll and Hill research

	Non-smokers	Smokers		
		Light	Average	Heavy
Actual deaths	0	12	11	13
Expected deaths	3.77	14.20	10.73	7.33

Source: Doll and Hill (1954: 1453).

alternative explanation of the results: perhaps age was responsible for the cancer, and also responsible independently of the cancer for the amount people smoke. This was examined in the 1954 paper by calculating the number of deaths from lung cancer that would be expected in each age band separately, irrespective of smoking level, and thence how many deaths there ought to have been among light, average, heavy and non-smokers if the number of deaths were independent of the amount smoked. The results are shown in Table 5.1, and it can be seen that we would have expected four deaths among the non-smokers but in reality there were none. Fourteen deaths would have been expected among the light smokers and only seven among the heavy smokers, but the actual figures were 12 and 13 respectively – many more deaths in the 'heavy smoking' category than would have been expected on the basis of age alone.

As you can see, the data-collection design of a survey like this is relatively simple compared with the design of an experiment – you just send out questionnaires and hope to get a reasonably high proportion back usefully filled in. *After* data collection, however, a lot is done in analysis to try to emulate the logic of comparison which is built into the design of a true experiment. The 'treatment group' is smokers (a self-administered treatment!), and the control or comparison group is non-smokers. An apparent effect of smoking is demonstrated – smokers are much more likely than non-smokers to die of lung cancer, even over the relatively short period of the study (29 months) – and the likelihood of smoking being the causal factor is increased by the fact that the lung-cancer death rate increases with the *amount* smoked. This is only the start of the analysis, however; much remains to be done, to eliminate alternative plausible explanations for the results.

Some of them are eliminated in this study at the design stage, by the choice of respondents. One problem with the retrospective studies discussed earlier was that the possibility that the control group was selected in a biased fashion because the nature of the study was known, and another was the possibility that those who knew they had lung cancer might have exaggerated the amount they smoked in the light of this knowledge. The first of these possibilities is eliminated in the 1954 study by the fact that the control group is not selected by the researchers but given 'in nature': we compare people who smoke with people who have not smoked. The second is eliminated by the prospective nature of the study; at the time when the level of smoking is being reported, none of the deaths has occurred. A third problem with the retrospective study, that likelihood of dying of lung cancer was associated with occupation, is eliminated in this study by using only doctors as respondents, and further distracting possibilities are eliminated by discarding the women and those under the age of 35 from the sample.

Because the allocation to 'experimental' or 'control' group is not under the control of the researcher and not conducted randomly, however, other possibilities arise which have to be eliminated in the analysis. For example, because the groups are not of equal sizes we cannot just compare raw numbers of deaths; we have to express the deaths as rates per thousand or percentages to eliminate the effect of unequal group size. It was also noticed that lung-cancer death rate and level of smoking both varied with age, so age was a possible cause of both (independently of each other). This was eliminated as a plausible alternative explanation, however, by calculating 'expected numbers' on the basis of age alone, irrespective of smoking level, and showing that amount smoked had an effect on the death rate over and above what would be expected on the basis of age alone.

A second point we might reasonably make is that real answers often take more than a single study to produce. We often talk as if the 'unit of research' were the experiment or the survey or the set of interviews, but quite often it makes better sense to talk about a whole *programme* of research. In the case of the lung-cancer research, an initial study confirmed earlier work and showed that there was an apparent association between smoking and lung cancer – in other words, that there *was* a question to answer. It also cleared up one or two of the possible alternative explanations – age and gender, for example. Considering possible objections in terms of the methods of the study – possible reactive effects of the situation on the answers given, or possible unconscious biases in the interviewers – the authors were able to deal with some, but others were inherent in the design of the study. The 1954 paper has a different, prospective design – it collects data on people who do not yet have the cancer, and then waits to see which of them contract it – which avoids many of the methodological problems of the earlier work. Further alternative explanations are dealt with: social class (or rather, something associated with it, such as working conditions) is not the causal factor, because the differences hold up when we consider people who are all in the same profession. A second report of the prospective study (Doll and Hill 1956) confirms the trends, with more certainty because the number of deaths concerned was (obviously) greater after four years than only 29 months. It also deals with whether place of residence is a causal factor (e.g. because of atmospheric pollution) and shows that the effect holds in remote rural areas as well as in the inner cities, so this is eliminated as an alternative explanation of the results. In a final report the analysis is repeated in more detail, with a still larger sample of deaths. The authors had also sent a follow-up questionnaire to surviving doctors in the interim, asking whether their smoking habits had changed, and so they were able to show in the 1960 paper that death rates among those who continued to smoke during the whole period of the study were significantly higher than among those who stopped smoking in the course of it.

This programme is a good example of what we sometimes call quasi-experimental analysis – a comparison like an experiment in form, and following the same logic as an experiment, but not truly experimental because the independent variable (the one which is supposed to have a causal effect) is not under the control of the researcher. In this case the dependent variable is death from lung cancer and the proposed independent (causal) variable is smoking – whether the subject smokes at all, and the *amount* he smokes if so. A connection is easily demonstrated, but there are many possible alternative explanations for it which might be advanced, to do with other variables on which those who died differed from those who did not or to do with the way in which the research was carried out. The papers we have discussed constitute a systematic, careful and painstaking attempt to eliminate each of these alternative explanations in order to show that the smoking was not itself caused by a variable which also caused the cancer. It is this kind of programme which most evidently demonstrates the point we made earlier, that any research report travels from a problem to a conclusion supported by evidence, *via* a series of arguments as to why the evidence should be taken to mean what the researchers say it means.

One more point to note is that in many experiments and quasi-experiments the outcome measure is more trivial, more artificial, less 'real and earnest', than the real thing for which it is taken as proxy. This is not the case in the Doll and Hill research – the dependent variable is death from cancer, not some more trivial substitute. (In general, one advantage of quasi-experimental analysis is that it makes research possible on real-life topics where true experiments could not be carried out for ethical or practical reasons.) However, even so it is not a perfect operationalization of what the authors want to study. Their interests are in what causes cancer; their research, for reasons of accessibility of data, is on *deaths* from cancer, which is not quite the same thing.

(You will find, incidentally, that what this kind of research is *called* varies according to the discipline from which the research emanates. In social research, studies which involve a controlled manipulation by the researcher are called 'experiments', while studies which depend on comparing naturally occurring cases are called 'quasi-experiments' or a kind of 'survey'. In medical and health research the former is often called a 'controlled trial' if it involves the testing of a drug or procedure, while studies comparing, for instance, otherwise similar people who do or do not have a given disease are referred to as 'case-control studies'.)

Summary: points for evaluation

1 Controlled trials, experiments and studies which are like experiments stand or fall by two factors: (a) clear definition and measurement of a dependent variable (the thing to be influenced) and one or more independent variables (the thing(s) doing the influencing); (b) the elimination of all other possible explanations of any obtained changes in the dependent variable.

2 In quasi-experimental analysis ('case-control studies') both of these are likely to be problematic, but the researchers should do their best to convince us that other plausible explanations are ruled out.

3 The major way in which change is demonstrated – and a large class of other explanations eliminated – is by comparison between groups which differ on the independent variable. The comparison is often based on a contrast between an 'experimental' group which receives some treatment and a 'control' group from whom it is withheld. The logic of the argument will work only to the extent that these groups are comparable.

4 In some studies a 'same subjects' design will be used, with the same person participating, sequentially, in the 'experimental' and the 'control' condition. In this case, however, it is important to rule out explanations of observed changes in terms of changes in the people concerned – learning, fatigue, etc.

5 However perfect the design, experimental research very often suffers from a tendency to trivialize or 'artificialize' the real situation which it is seeking to simulate. This should be looked out for in evaluating such studies.

> **Exercise 19**
>
> Now re-read the two papers in the light of our comments.

Further reading

Women and psychiatry

Brown, George and Harris, Tirril (1978) *Social Origins of Depression: A Study of Psychiatric Disorder in Women*. London: Routledge and Kegan Paul.

Busfield, Joan (1991) *Women and Mental Health*. London: Macmillan.

Fulani, Lenora (ed.) (1988) *The Politics of Race and Gender in Therapy*. New York: Haworth Press.

Nairn, K. and Smith, G. (1984) *Dealing with Depression*. London: Women's Press.

Orr, Jean (ed.) (1986) *Women's Health in the Community*. Chichester: Wiley.

Penfold, Susan and Walker, Gillian (1984) *Women and the Psychiatric Paradox*. Milton Keynes: Open University Press.

Smoking and lung cancer

Ashton, Heather and Stepney, Rob (1982) *Smoking: Psychology and Pharmacology*. London: Tavistock.

Graham, Hilary (1993) *When Life's a Drag: Smoking and Disadvantage*. London: HMSO.

Doll, Richard and Peto, Richard (1981) *The Causes of Cancer: Quantitative Estimates of Avoidable Risks of Cancer*. Oxford: Oxford University Press.

READING SURVEY RESEARCH

Research paper 1: Abbott (1997) 'Home helps and district nurses:
   community care in the far South West'
Research paper 2: Abbott and Sapsford (1993) 'Studying policy and
   practice: use of vignettes'
Discussion
Summary: points for evaluation
Further reading

Surveys are about finding out what is there – asking questions or observing, and counting the answers. (This is far too simple a definition to encompass anything like the full range of survey research, as we shall quickly see, but it is a good starting point.) The 'ideal survey' is the 10-yearly **Census** of Population, when squads of interviewers (known as enumerators) receive standardized training and then go out to find every household in the country and get the answers to a range of basic questions about the people living there. Most surveys are smaller in scale than this and cannot hope to reach every member of the population. What they do is to ask questions of a *sample* of the population and hope that this sample is **representative** – that what is true of the sample will be true of the population as a whole. The General Household Survey, for instance, is another large government survey, happening more frequently than the Census, which also asks for household composition and living standards, but of a **randomly** drawn sample of the population – quite a large sample, but only a small percentage of the people who might have been asked. If the sample is random and reasonably large, then we can have every confidence that it is reasonably representative.

Most surveys are smaller still – including the one at which we shall look in this chapter. They share two key issues with larger ones, however. The first is the question of representation: to the extent that a survey sets out to describe a population on the basis of a sample, it has to be able to demonstrate that the sample is likely to be representative of that population. The second is **validity of measurement**: the answers, which are ultimately recorded as numerical codes, have to have been produced by clear, appropriate questions, or 'measuring instruments', which really do measure what the researcher says they measure.

The example examined in this chapter consists of two research papers describing a project carried out in Cornwall into the provision of community care to older and/or disabled people by home helps and district nurses. The first of the two papers may be seen as primarily descriptive – it examines what services are actually provided and by whom – with the intent of making recommendations about the 'skill mix' needed and how it may best be provided. However, many surveys are not just descriptive. They have a **quasi-experimental** element about them: they were set up to test some statement about differences between two or more groups, or the (**causal**) **association** of two variables. The Doll and Hill paper in the last chapter, which we described there as quasi-experimental, was a survey; all quasi-experimental analyses are also survey based.

Exercise 20

You may now like to read the first of the papers, Pamela Abbott (1997) 'Home helps and district nurses: community care in the far South West', in Abbott and Sapsford (eds) *Research into Practice: A Reader for Nurses and the Caring Professions* (2nd edition).

Research paper 1: Abbott (1997)

This is a much shortened summary of a multi-method project carried out in Cornwall in 1992, which examined community care provision in three GP practices – a small market town, a small coastal port and a village. (The port and the village received district nursing services from the same team, which was based in a nearby small town.) Abbott points out that Cornwall is not **typical** of the rest of the country – no county is entirely typical of any other – in that it has a large elderly population (as a 'retirement area') and faces particular problems of service delivery because of geographical isolation leading to high transport costs both for the service providers and for the old people themselves (coupled, for the latter, with low availability). However, Cornwall faces the same problems of policy and practice in delivering care as other areas, so its practices may illuminate those of other areas also.

The first point made in the paper is that 'community care' is not synonymous with 'statutory services'. Other 'literature' shows that only a very small percentage of those aged 65 or older receive help from the state or voluntary agencies: about 7 per cent attend a day centre or lunch club, about 1 per cent receive 'meals on wheels', and around 4 per cent are clients of the home help or district nursing services. (The figures rise, for those aged 75+, to 7 and 5 per cent for day centres and 'meals on wheels', 8 per cent receive district nursing, and about 14 per cent have a home help.) Most care is provided by relatives, with spouses accounting for about two-thirds of it (the other substantial category being daughters or daughters-in-law) – and it is worth remembering from the start that the vast majority of these spouses were themselves old and perhaps frail.

Fieldwork comprised five elements:

1 a 'casing' of the area – talking to social services and health authority staff and GPs and following up contacts, to identify all the statutory and voluntary services offered to older people and those commercial services

which were discounted for older people (e.g. pubs offering a special price on meals for pensioners);

2 structured interviews with carers and those who were cared for, to identify the services they received and how they felt about them, and to collect some basic demographic information (e.g. age, type of residence, distance from nearest family member);

3 a structured **questionnaire** to home helps and district nurses, to ascertain the services they provided formally and informally, and their attitudes to the work;

4 a structured questionnaire was completed by district nurse team leaders and home help organizers which was designed to elicit information on who was responsible for care tasks for clients in different circumstances;

5 home helps and district nurses were accompanied on their rounds by one of the researchers.

The interview with carers and the 'cared-for' was administered to 100 clients in total – 32 men and 68 women – identified by district nursing team leaders and/or senior home helps as users of their services in the three GP practices in October 1991. (All agreed to take part, but not every client answered every question.) A list of care tasks was derived from the home help and district nurse job descriptions and from common-sense analysis of the needs of older people; the interviewer asked which of these were received on a regular basis, and from whom. 'Informal' carers (relatives, friends, neighbours) provided domestic and social rather than personal and nursing care – shopping was the task most frequently mentioned. Sixty-one informants were being seen by a member of the district nursing team, and 54 had home helps. Home helps most often provided general housework and/or social care tasks (e.g. shopping, accompanying to doctor, collecting pension, paying bills) but also carried out some personal care tasks, the most frequent being helping with bathing. District nurses (or auxiliaries) most frequently gave medical/nursing treatment, help or advice and personal care tasks (bathing, washing, help with getting up or going to bed). There were some discrepancies between what clients said they received and what providers said they provided, but on the whole the answers paralleled each other. While the great majority of district nursing patients required nursing care, all the members of the district nursing team except three said they visited patients requiring only personal care – bathing, shaving or getting up/getting to bed.

A majority of users received only one statutory service, but a small number had more than one. Sometimes this was because a very specialized service was being received (e.g. Macmillan nursing), but sometimes both home helps and district nurses visited the same client. Mostly they provided complementary services, but there was overlap in the provision of personal care (e.g. bathing), particularly in the area in which the district nursing team included auxiliaries.

[I]f we examine the cases where clients were visited by both . . . there seems to be a clear division of tasks. In the majority of cases the interview and observation data suggest that the district nurses were carrying out specialised nursing tasks and the home helps personal care tasks. Observation of the district nurses in [two of the practices] suggests they carry out personal care tasks . . . on days or at times when the home help was not visiting. In [the third practice] . . . most personal care, including baths, was done by home helps. However, the district nurses were concerned about the ability of the home helps to do personal care and the home helps felt that they were not recognised as part of the care team by the district nurses.

(Abbott 1997: 89)

Both district nurses and home helps were asked whether they ever performed tasks for clients which were not on the agreed care plan. All except one of the district nurses admitted to doing so, the tasks frequently mentioned being generally related to nursing care – collecting dressings and prescriptions, making tea/coffee, occasionally making breakfast if the patient was unwell. Other tasks mentioned by at least one included advice on forms, changing light bulbs, washing underwear, lighting the fire and putting dirty linen in to soak. However, few tasks overall were performed which were not part of the nursing care plan. Most of the home helps said clients asked them to do tasks additional to their duties – mostly occasional or heavy cleaning tasks – and nearly all said clients telephoned them at home, to do shopping before they next called or occasionally because they required help (for example, after a fall).

Where district nurses visited patients who were also visited by home helps, most regarded themselves as having regular contact with the home helps, though sometimes only on a casual basis. Most of the home helps had clients whose care was shared with district nurses, and all thought that the arrangements worked well. Liaison was sometimes a problem, however:

Ten of the home helps said that they had opportunity to liaise with the district nurse. One other . . . said there was liaison with a senior. The home helps seemed to feel that they had less opportunity to liaise with the district nurses than vice versa. Observation and information obtained from interviewing would indicate that this liaison was ad hoc and opportunistic rather than formalised.

(Abbott 1997: 92)

District nurses receive the standard nursing training and then do a post-qualification course (though the auxiliaries are not trained nurses and are considered to be under the supervision of a qualified nurse at all times). Home helps said they received very little training for the domestic and personal care tasks they undertake. All except two of the informants said they had done the basic three-day home help course on duties and responsibilities, nutrition and hygiene, incontinence, the lifting of clients, and health and safety aspects of the job. The three senior home helps had also done City and Guilds qualifications. The level and status of work seems to be seen as inferior to that of nurses (or even the relatively untrained auxiliaries) by the district nursing team and the clients – which, of course, makes them seen at the same time as more approachable by clients.

Only one home help expressed a negative view of her work . . . 'Some people call us the Community Dogsbodies'. However, while we were accompanying home helps in two of the areas, a number of them

referred to the negative stereotype that they thought home helps had
... and suggested that the district nurses (including auxiliaries) looked
down on them ... One mentioned a meeting ... where the auxiliaries
had said that they would not take on the work home helps did because
it was demeaning ... We were told that clients would not think of
asking nurses to do extra tasks for them or ringing them at home, and
our research appears to bear this out.

(Abbott 1997: 94)

Senior home helps have guaranteed hours of work, but the basic-grade
workers are all employed part-time and have no guaranteed hours of work;
for some, fluctuation in hours was a financial problem. Despite this, and
despite a general feeling that there was too little time to do the job properly
and chat with clients, home helps exhibited a very high level of job satisfaction. In defining their job, most emphasized the caring or helping element, and most felt that the words 'carer' or 'caring' would be appropriate in
the job title. Most said they had joined the service because they wanted to
help people and because it was a job which drew on their skills and experience as carers in the domestic sphere.

Exercise 21

The second paper in this chapter, which you may want to read now, is a
more detailed report on one aspect of this research – Abbott and
Sapsford (1993) 'Studying policy and practice: use of vignettes'. This
was originally published in *Nurse Researcher* (1993) and is reprinted in
Abbott and Sapsford (eds) (1997), *Research into Practice: A Reader for
Nurses and the Caring Professions* (2nd edition).

Research paper 2: Abbott and Sapsford (1993)

This paper picks up one particular aspect of the Cornish research and
examines it in more depth. Part of the questionnaire sent to home help
organizers and district nursing team leaders – the people who actually
made assessments of needs in the real situation and allocated services – was
a series of '**vignettes**' on which notional decisions were to be made. A
vignette is a short description or story – a fictional situation – which can be
discussed in the same kind of way as comparable real situations are discussed. Vignettes have the advantage over real-life situations (a) that they
can be discussed without the ethical and practical implications of discussing real cases, while still being closer to real situations than generalized
questions about policy or practice divorced from actual cases, (b) they
allow a range of cases to be covered which is wider than would probably be
encountered in research observing real cases over some finite time-period,
and (c) that the details can be varied systematically to test ideas about the
decisions people make. They have been widely used in social psychology,
in research on decision-making and moral reasoning, and in social policy

research to examine professionals' use of concepts such as 'child abuse' and to measure attitudes to community care. All the home help organizers and district nursing team leaders were sent the questionnaire, and usable replies were received from 19 team organizers and 28 team leaders.

A typical vignette would be 'Case 1: Mr and Mrs Jones':

> Mr and Mrs Jones, who are in their early 70s, live in a modern bungalow about a mile from local shops and ten miles from the nearest town. They both have occupational pensions in addition to the state's. Mrs Jones can drive, but Mr Jones, who has Parkinson's disease, has severe mobility problems and is no longer able to leave the house without professional assistance. He attends the day hospital one day a week and has regular periods of respite care. Mrs Jones has a heart condition and has had two hip replacements – both of which are now causing her problems. They moved to Cornwall on retirement and have no relatives living locally.

Respondents were asked to say who should be providing help with a range of tasks (e.g. bathing, shaving, treating pressure areas, shopping, housework), from a long list of possible providers (including spouse, friends, neighbours and relatives as well as 'professional' providers). In the paper we consider how the responses have been clustered, in order to examine a 'skills mix' question, into 'district nurse', 'home help', 'both', 'neighbour/friend' and 'relation' – the last category including spouse. The results are summarized in Table 6.1 for six of the tasks.

Even in this small sample of responses some pattern can be seen. Nursing care (exemplified here by 'treating pressure areas') is seen as a nursing

Table 6.1 Responses to Vignette 1 in the Cornish research for six selected tasks (%)

Task	District nurse and home help	District nurse alone	Home help alone	Neigh- bour/ friend	Relative
Home help organizer responses					
Bathing Mr Jones	44	17	28	—	—
Shaving Mr Jones	6	—	88	—	6
Treating pressure areas	17	78	—	—	—
Shopping	—	—	78	6	17
Meal preparation	—	—	44	—	38
Light housework	—	—	28	—	22
District nurse team leader responses					
Bathing Mr Jones	22	48	22	—	—
Shaving Mr Jones	30	7	52	—	11
Treating pressure areas	26	70	4	—	—
Shopping	—	—	79	17	4
Meal preparation	—	—	74	7	11
Light housework	—	—	64	—	18

Note: Percentages in some rows total less than 100 because of missing answers or 'other' responses.

province, as one would expect, though some respondents thought home helps could also administer the treatment, alone or in conjunction with district nurses (only the nursing team leaders suggesting home helps alone). Personal care – bathing, shaving – is seen as the province of both home helps and district nurses; home help organizers were most likely to suggest a combination of the two for bathing, and were relatively unlikely to suggest district nurses on their own. Shaving, however, was seen as overwhelmingly a home help task. Nursing team leaders see a larger role for district nurses in personal care – particularly bathing – but over half relegated shaving to the home helps. Shopping, meal preparation and housework are seen as home help jobs and not appropriate for district nurses, but the spouse is also expected to play a part, particularly by the home help organizers. Other small insights may be gleaned which would be worth following up. For example, although no neighbours are mentioned in the vignette, and indeed it is suggested that the house may be quite isolated, a small proportion of home help organizers thought neighbours should do the shopping (and quite a large proportion of nursing team leaders), and a small proportion of nursing team leaders thought they should help with cooking.

Overall, for a wide range of different kinds of 'case', there was substantial agreement among respondents both within and between respondents that nursing tasks belonged predominantly to district nurses and domestic ones to home helps. Home helps were sometimes seen as appropriate for the former (after training, presumably), but district nurses were never seen as appropriate for the latter. There were some differences as regards personal care, mostly in the direction of district nurse team leaders tending to see this more as a part of nursing than did home help organizers. There were also interesting differences in the extent to which spouses (particularly wives) and relatives living within reasonable reach are seen as responsible for domestic, social and (if female) personal care. Thus in this paper the vignette technique has enabled the researchers to explore a wide range of different kinds of 'community care problem' and obtain detailed information on concrete cases, avoiding the **rhetoric** of generalized questions and the ethical and practical difficulties of scrutiny of real cases.

Discussion

Three points are worth considering about these papers and all others of their kind, points which bear directly on our evaluation of published research. The first is the question of measurement. As we noted earlier, clear measurement of the quantities which are to be counted is quite essential for this kind of research. The structured Cornish research questionnaires, asking for a list of the services which are performed or received, come off quite well in this respect; the questions which were asked were obviously quite clear and 'factual'. However, we should note the discrepancies between professionals' accounts of what they provide and users' accounts of what they receive. These may be due to poor memory, but they may also be due to lack of knowledge – where district nurses claim to be giving far more advice than users claim to be receiving, for example, they may not realize that what the researchers mean by 'advice' includes casual chats and incidental suggestions. If this explains the difference, then we would describe it as being an artefact produced by **reactivity** – produced by differential interpretation of the questions rather than by the practice which the questionnaire is intended to measure, and so a product of the design of the questionnaire rather than of the social situation at which it is aimed. Secondly, on the other hand, the difference may be seen as a real one, between the world-pictures of the professionals and the users – that the professionals (deliberately) proffer advice in forms in which it will not be seen as advice by the users – in which case both could be 'right' about what goes on. A third possibility is that the discrepancy is due simply to faulty memory on the part of one party or the other. This is less likely in this case, where the events and practices under examination are relatively recent. Longer-term questions, about events which have happened in the more distant past, would be more suspect in this respect. Memory of the past is prone to inflation or diminution, depending on what point the informant thinks the survey is trying to prove. In survey research, just as much as in less structured styles, the informant makes sense of the situation and tailors his or her replies accordingly.

Even within these structured questionnaires, however, some of the questions should not be taken as simply factual – those on 'how you feel about . . .' some aspect of the situation. How do you feel about reading this book, at this precise moment? Are you satisfied? Fairly satisfied? Neither satisfied nor unsatisfied? Puzzled about how to answer the question, given that some aspects of the book may be quite useful, but others are clearly tedious or over-simple? Puzzled about how to answer the question before you have finished reading it and had time to think about it and perhaps use it in other contexts?

The vignette measurements certainly need more thought and justification, because they concern not what *is* done but what *should* be done or *would* be done, in a hypothetical situation. This raises a second aspect of reactivity – the artificiality of the situation and the extent to which what is produced by respondents is a reaction to that artificial situation and fails to generalize to 'real' life beyond it. (A frequent criticism of 'scientific' social psychology, for example, is that it has spent over a century working out the rules and laws of social behaviour in artificial small groups, in laboratories, and is still no nearer to explaining what people do in their everyday lives.) The vignette technique is better than just asking 'what is your policy about . . .?', because it directs people's attention to the needs of the case and therefore stands some chance of avoiding some of the general rhetoric surrounding the topic. It gives practitioners an anchor for their deliberations, so that they can try to make realistic estimates of what they would say and do in the real case. The use of the postal questionnaire also gives the technique the strength of this kind of survey research, of being able to reach a large number of people in a relatively short space of time and with relatively low use of resources. However, when all is said and done, the fictional case is *not* a real case, and we cannot be *certain* that the outcome in the real case would be the same. The fictional case does not put the respondent under the same kind of pressure as the real one, because the outcome of decisions taken in the fictional case does not have any real costs, and also the information available to the decision-maker is severely limited. This last problem can be overcome by increasing the realism of the situation; Wasoff (1992), for example, investigated lawyers' advice in marital cases by setting up a 'stooge client' with the lawyers' consent – one of the researchers acted the role of the client, instead of details being provided in written form, and so the situation was very close to that of a real consultation. However, this is resource-intensive and loses the survey's advantage of reaching substantial numbers of respondents cheaply.

A further question, for evaluation, is the question of representation (**sampling**). A real attempt was made to get representative samples of users and patients from the three GP practices and to get responses from *all* the district nursing and home help teams which served them – and from all the organizers and team leaders in the whole county, for one of the questionnaires. We do not know how representative the achieved samples were, however, because the report does not tell us much about non-compliance – about the people who refused to fill in questionnaires or be interviewed. It is always a problem that if people who refuse to answer are very different in some respect from those who did comply with the research, then the **descriptive statistics** may be in error in some respects. (In fact there were no refusals; all the patients/clients on the three GPs' lists who were receiving services agreed to be interviewed, and all the home helps and district nursing team members in these three areas cooperated in the research.) Even if the samples were representative of the GP practices, we still have to ask how representative they were of the county as a whole and of the country as a whole. We have no reason to suppose that they are *un*typical, except that the rurality of the location puts service provision under greater stress than in central urban areas, and the researchers did their best to ensure typicality. However, some caution still needs to be exercised in interpreting the figures.

Summary: points for evaluation

1 In any piece of survey research one important question is how well the things which are being counted have been defined – how good the measurement is. There are four sub-questions which might follow from this:

   (a) Looking logically at the argument of the paper, have the right things been measured? (Are the concepts correctly **operationalized**?)

   (b) Are the factual questions clear and unambiguous, and how likely is it that the respondents have answered them accurately?

   (c) Where what is being asked is being taken as a measure or indicator of something underlying, is it a valid indicator? In other words, what is the proof that it does measure what it is claimed to measure? Questions of the artificiality of 'stimulus situations' may validly be asked here.

   (d) Looking at the interview or recording session as a social situation of which respondents have to make sense, how likely is it that the sense they make of the task will lead to them giving the information which the argument of the paper needs (as opposed, for instance, to something which is specific to the interview situation and is not likely to have any bearing on any other part of their lives)?

2 How typical is the sample of the population to which the results are to be generalized?
   (a) Was the sampling carried out in such a way that it is likely to be representative, or by a method which makes bias likely?
   (b) Were certain parts of the population excluded from consideration, either deliberately or accidentally (e.g. by non-response to self-completion questionnaire), and what difference might that make to the conclusions?

Exercise 22

Now re-read the two papers in the light of our comments.

Further reading

Community care for older people

Arber, Sara and Ginn, Jay (1991) *Gender and Later Life: A Sociological Analysis of Resources and Constraints*. London: Sage.

Davies, Bleddyn, Bebbington, A. and Charnely, Helen (1990) *Resources, Needs and Outcomes in Community-Based Care*. Aldershot: Gower.

Garrett, G. (1990) *Older People: Their Support and Care*. Basingstoke: Macmillan.

Jamieson, A. (ed.) (1991) *Home Care for Older People in Europe*. Oxford: Oxford University Press.

Jefferys, M. (ed.) (1989) *Growing Old in the Twentieth Century*. London: Routledge.

Phillipson, C., Bernard, M. and Strang, P. (eds) (1986) *Dependency and Interdependency in Old Age: Theoretical Perspectives and Policy Alternatives*. Beckenham: Croom Helm.

CHAPTER SEVEN

READING SECONDARY SOURCES

Using secondary sources
Research paper: Abbott and Tyler (1995)
Standardization and comparison
Summary: points for evaluation
Further reading

Using secondary sources

Like most methods courses and textbooks, we have talked so far as if all research were a matter of going out and collecting fresh data. In fact, the most commonly practised kind of research involves illustrating or supporting an argument by reference to data which have already been collected by someone else, generally for some other purpose. This is known as the secondary use of data, and we refer to the sources as **secondary sources**. Most commonly when we use the term we mean published numerical data – 'statistics', in the original meaning of the term, meaning numerical information about something of interest in the population. Possible sources range widely, from the statistics contained in other people's published research, through various kinds of regular **survey** such as the General Household Survey or the **Census**, and statistics collected for governmental research reasons (e.g. the incidence of certain kinds of infectious diseases), to statistics which are purely a by-product of the administrative process (criminal convictions, admissions to hospital, birth and death statistics, etc.). These are very good sources of information in that they can usually offer a degree of coverage which is beyond the resources of the individual researcher or research team. It would not be possible for you, for example, to count every baby born in the country each year, but the government counts them routinely. The use of secondary sources presents special problems, however, precisely because it is a secondary use; we are often trying to use statistics for purposes for which they were not originally intended. We have to be especially careful, therefore, that the ones we use are **reliable** (i.e. an accurate count of what we want to count, collected in a consistent way), and **valid** for the purposes for which we want to use them.

As a case of unreliable statistics, we might briefly consider the statistics on suicide available from the government publication *Statistics of Deaths Reported to Coroners*. This gives a count of the number of cases where a coroner has determined (with or without the aid of a jury) that the cause of an unexplained death shall be recorded as suicide; that is *precisely* what they count – not the 'real' incidence of suicide, whatever that may mean.

1 Not all suicide cases, almost certainly, are reported to coroners in the first place. If the deceased was under the care of a doctor and the doctor certifies the death as being from natural causes, and no other person reports the death as suspicious to the coroner or to the Registrar of Deaths, then the case will never come to the attention of a coroner at all and, therefore, cannot appear in the statistics.
2 The coroner (and probably the police) will investigate cases of suspicious death before the inquest, and they may find sufficient evidence to justify a suicide verdict.
3 When all the evidence is in, the decision as to whether the case is a suicide, an accident or some form of homicide is a subjective one on the part of the coroner (or the jury, if one has been called), and therefore liable to be affected by the personal values of those taking it. This invalidates any sort of class or gender comparison even within one country, because it is all too likely that suicide will seem a more plausible explanation for one class than another, or one gender than another, on a systematic, culturally determined basis. It certainly invalidates comparisons between countries given, for example, the different social consequences of suicide in Catholic and Protestant countries.
4 At a more fundamental level, it is not possible even in principle to have an accurate count of suicides. We cannot ask the suicide whether he or she really meant to die. If we give any credence whatsoever to the concept of suicide attempts as cries for help, and allow that some attempts which if they had failed would be seen as 'not serious attempts' might accidentally succeed in killing the person concerned, then we cannot ever know whether the person in question died by deliberate self-slaughter.
5 Even if it had been possible to ask, or if an explanatory note has been left, we still cannot be quite sure, because one cannot be quite sure (given any idea of unconscious motivation) that even the victims themselves are in a position fully to explain their actions.

By contrast, the Census is a reliable source of information about the population. There are still some areas in which it may fall down. When counting households, for instance, it relies on its enumerators (data collectors) to apply a definition of 'household' consistently, and despite subsequent checking we can never be quite certain that this has been done in the case of non-standard households. The count of the homeless is frankly suspect, being carried out by police officers going round the likely haunts of those who sleep rough and trying to get what information they can. In the last instance, moreover, the accuracy of what is put on the form depends on the honesty and understanding of the individual informants. By and large, however, we would be prepared to accept the Census as one of the most reliable of data sources.

The paper which we shall be considering in this chapter is an illustration of what can be done from census data. It uses just two tables from the 1991 Census to explore some quite complicated questions about the employment of women, and particularly of women from 'minority ethnic groups'.

The aim is to test whether the effects of gender and 'race' are additive – two separate kinds of discrimination, with Black women suffering both of them – or whether they **interact** to produce something which is more or less than the expected effect of adding the two together. The answer which emerges from the figures is 'It's more complicated than that!' and the analysis illustrates both the strengths of quantitative work and the amount of knowledge and imagination which is often needed if the results are to be interpreted correctly.

Research paper: Abbott and Tyler (1995)

Exercise 23

You might now read Abbott and Tyler (1995) 'Ethnic variation in the female labour force' (*British Journal of Sociology*, 46: 339–53, or reprinted in Abbott and Sapsford (eds) (1997) *Research into Practice: A Reader for Nurses and the Caring Professions*, 2nd edition). You should not get too deeply involved in the figures when reading the paper – read it for the main conclusions and look to see how the tables support them.

The article starts from premises well established by other research – that gender and 'race' are important factors contributing to the structure of the labour market and sources of discrimination and exploitation within it. 'Ethnic' disadvantage in the labour market is a well established feature, with Black people discriminated against for jobs and likely to finish up, for a given level of qualification, in a lower and worse-paid occupation than a comparable White person. The effect of gender is also well documented. Women are segregated both vertically in the labour market – to some extent excluded from 'higher' (managerial, professional) occupations and from the label of 'skilled' when they are in manual work – and horizontally in terms of there being distinctive 'female' sectors of the market. Women are secretaries, nurses, 'carers', teachers (particularly in primary schools), social workers, shop workers, personal service workers; but they are relatively rarely engineers, scientists, lawyers, accountants, police, army, drivers, miners, skilled factory workers. Or they are semi- or unskilled manual workers in certain trades but not others. While men are clustered in the managerial, administrative and professional grades or in skilled manual work, women are clustered in routine manual work (secretarial and clerical) – which accounts for some 40 per cent of female employment – and in the service sector. Within any given band of employment, women tend to be located at the bottom and men in the higher reaches. More men are self-employed professionals and more women professionals work for a salary. Men are disproportionately represented as head teachers, senior social workers, professors and managers, even in the 'female' employment sectors – the most obvious case being nursing, where few men are nurses but disproportionately many are senior nurses.

The authors' interest was to examine the way in which these two dis-
criminations – by gender and by ethnic group – interact to shape and constrain the location of Black women in the labour market. Such research had
been well-nigh impossible in the past, because the target group form such a
small proportion of the UK population; in 1991, according to Census data,
only 1.5 per cent of the population were Black (of African or Caribbean
origin), 1.8 per cent were of Asian origin, 0.2 per cent of Chinese origin,
and 0.3 per cent 'others' – a total of less than four per cent of the population, and clearly a much smaller proportion if you count only the women.
Thus sample surveys were not able to look at the position of women from
minority ethnic groups with any degree of accuracy or perceptiveness,
because of the very small numbers involved. However, the 1991 Census
asked a question about ethnic origin which was fairly well answered, so
Census figures give us information about the whole population in terms of
ethnic origin. This paper used the tables of ethic origin by work status and
category.

The headline results were that Black women of Caribbean or African
origin were more likely to be economically active than White women –
more likely, that is, to be in work or to describe themselves as seeking work
– and if employed they were more likely to be in full-time jobs than White
women. All non-White economically active women, however, were more
likely than White women to be currently unemployed or taking a government training scheme offered as a substitute for employment.

We immediately become aware, in looking at these figures, that statistics
do not just 'present the facts' but have to be interpreted through a knowledge of how they are collected. The Census counts people as economically
active if they say they are currently seeking work or currently have a job.
(We may note, incidentally, that there may be cultural differences in
whether a married woman describes herself as 'seeking work' when unemployed, so that there can be more than one explanation for some of the
observed difference between Black and White women.) Other surveys
might count people as unemployed *whether or not* they were seeking work –
counting simply the fact of not having a job, rather than trying to count
just those who are available for work – and come up with a larger figure for
unemployment. On the other hand, another major source of statistics is
the count of those *claiming benefit* and *registered* as seeking work, produced
by the relevant administrative departments of the government. This gives
a smaller figure than the Census, because it excludes those who are seeking
work (or would take it if offered it) but have not registered themselves at
the relevant office – many of whom may be married women. Which figure
you use when assessing unemployment will depend on the purpose for
which you are making the assessment, but it is clearly important to think
about the source of the figures and what is included in or excluded from a
particular source.

A major finding of the analysis presented by Abbott and Tyler is that
'ethnic group' is not a simple, monolithic category when it comes to
looking at labour market position. In particular, women from minority
ethnic groups are *not* uniformly in the 'lower' employment grades. Women
of Pakistani or Chinese origin are overrepresented in managerial and professional grades, compared with women from other ethnic minority

groups or with White women, and there are more Chinese women acting as managers or owners of small businesses than there are Chinese men! Thus the interactions between gender and 'race' are clearly not simple ones, and we cannot predict a person's labour market position by simply 'adding the effects together'.

This paper illustrates the major strength of research using published statistics. Using the Census meant that the authors had access to figures they could not possibly have collected for themselves, and a complex research question could be answered by two people, in a fairly short space of time, mostly from just two tables of data. It also illustrates the weakness of such research, however – that you have to work with what is provided, rather than what you might have collected for yourself. What we have is counts of the ethnic group into which respondents are prepared to assign themselves, and their answers to questions about whether they are currently in employment, on a government training scheme, seeking work or, in various ways, not economically active (retired, permanently sick or disabled, a student, a 'full-time housewife', etc.). Using these figures we find that women from some ethnic backgrounds are more likely than White women to be economically active (but less likely to be actually in employment) and more likely to be working full-time, and that women from others are disproportionately to be found in 'higher' employment categories. From this we could be tempted to argue that some groups do not experience discrimination. However, this takes no account of the position of those groups where the women are *not* as likely to be in employment as men, nor of the women's educational and professional qualifications and whether their current occupations are commensurate with them (areas which could have been explored if the authors had been carrying out their own survey). Further, it accepts the grading system of occupations used by the Registrar General and in the Census and is not able to explore precisely *what* jobs White or minority women carried out within a category. Knowing as we do that the Registrar General's schema puts 'air hostess' and 'cafe waitress' in the same category and consigns a one-person computer engineering concern to the same category as a jobbing gardener who works alone, we must at least *wonder* whether some of the attributions to the higher categories conceal discrimination or disadvantage in terms of the precise *kind* of job carried out. Further, we do not know the precise ways in which patriarchal control is exercised over women in different minority ethnic groups, as influenced by cultural heritage, current experience and current structural position. As the authors say,

> it should be noted that this type of analysis does not permit control for factors such as the relationship between educational qualifications and occupational category, or indeed the 'unpicking' of precise occupational position within the broad occupational categories of the Census, so that significant forms of discrimination must necessarily be invisible to it.
>
> (Abbott and Sapsford 1997: 159)

One thing the paper does do, covertly and implicitly, is to question an **ideological** 'taken-for-granted' of research and social practice. 'Black', or 'ethnic minority', are in many ways not descriptive categories but ideological objects – very different people are classed together in the one group, for political reasons rather than because they necessarily have much in common. (It is worth thinking, in this context, about the different uses of 'Black' in French research – where it may often mean someone of Algerian or other North African origin – and in German research, where it may often mean a Turk.) The paper demonstrates just how little the women of different ethnic groups have in common in terms of their labour market position. However, at another level the paper also perpetuates the ideological category. To select people of African, Caribbean, Chinese and other Asian origin as the 'minority ethnic groups' to be considered, and leave out people of Polish, Irish or North American origin, is in itself to perpetuate the notion that these people form a bounded group somehow different from White people of European or North American (but non-British) origin.

> **Exercise 24**
>
> Now re-read the paper in the light of our comments.

Standardization and comparison

One concept which you need when tackling any kind of quantitative research report is that of 'comparing like with like' by **standardizing** the figures – which sounds difficult and abstract but is actually often a very simple process indeed. If you have two sets of figures which are in some way unlike each other, you standardize when you do some simple (or sometimes not so simple!) arithmetic on them to make them easier to compare with each other. The simplest form of standardization is the familiar operation of expressing figures as percentages. If for example you were given the figures on the left of Table 7.1, which group of boys would you say was the greediest? Those in the first column ate more cakes, but there were also more of them. By percentaging, we eliminate (control for) the difference in number of boys, so that we can see clearly that it is Group B which ate proportionately more of their cakes – the figures on the right of the table. Then, in the final line of the table, another form of standardization is demonstrated – reducing the figures to a common base of cakes per boy, again showing that Group B were the greedier. Putting it another way, Group B's boys ate more cakes each, on average, than we would expect if we took Group A as typical.

More complex transformations are necessary when you want to look at underlying causes of a complex phenomenon which are obscured by other, related differences. Take the case of mortality statistics, for example, and the **standardized mortality ratio** (**SMR**). The SMR, as its name suggests, is a form of standardization, and it is similar in essence to the notion of cakes per boy in Table 7.1. Eastbourne has a much higher death rate than the country as a whole – per thousand of population, more people die there in

Table 7.1 Two illustrations of standardization
Each boy in two groups was given ten cakes and told to save as many as he could, but to eat if he was very hungry.

	Actual numbers		Percentages	
Group	A	B	A	B
Number of boys in group	5	2		
Number of cakes available	50	20		
Cakes eaten	15	8	30%	40%
Cakes eaten per boy	3	4		

the course of a year than we would expect from looking at the death rate for the population as a whole. On the other hand, it also has a larger than average population of pensionable age, so on the whole you would expect there to be more deaths. It is also well known that women are hardier than men at all stages of the life-cycle – less likely to die by any given age, and more likely to 'make old bones'. So if we wanted to look at how different Eastbourne's medical services are, using death rates as a basis of comparison, it would hardly be fair to Eastbourne just to take crude death rate as our measure. What we do is to say arbitrarily that the SMR for the population as a whole is 100. Then we look at the area we want to analyse (Eastbourne) and see how its population compares with the country as a whole in terms of age and sex. For each age band in each sex we work out a separate *age- and gender-specific death rate* for the population as a whole – what proportion of men aged 30–39 died in the population as a whole, for instance, what proportion of women aged 30–39, and so on. Then we apply these specific death rates to the numbers in the population of Eastbourne to find out how many deaths we would expect if the age and gender structure of Eastbourne were the same as that of the whole population. We can then compare this **expected figure** with the number who actually died, dividing the one by the other and then multiplying by 100. If the result is less than 100, then Eastbourne has fewer deaths than might have been expected. If it is larger than expected, then it has more deaths than might be expected. We can even say how much less or more: an SMR of 80 would mean that Eastbourne had only 80 per cent of the deaths we would expect if it were similar to the rest of the country in terms of age and sex balance; an SMR of 120 would mean it had 20 per cent more deaths than expected. (Eastbourne actually has a relatively low SMR: its hospital and community practitioners have considerable competence in geriatric medicine.) So the calculation of SMR may be difficult, but the basic idea is a simple one: find out if we have more or less deaths than we would expect after *controlling for* the effects of age and sex.

One thing that standardization does is to allow us to say something quite complicated in one or two figures. For example, instead of saying 'Compare "one out of ten" with "17 out of 340"', we can say 'Compare 10 per cent with 5 per cent', which is much easier to understand. Many complex statistics are used for this reason – to allow us to make precise statements about relationships in a simple manner, as in the case of the standardized mortality ratio.

Another statistical tool of this kind is the correlation coefficient (r), which allows us to express a relationship between two variables as a single figure. Two variables are said to be *associated* or **correlated** if there is a relationship between them such that extreme values on one predict extreme values on the other and a middling value on one predicts a middling value on the other. So height and weight are correlated: all things being equal, taller people weigh more. This is called *positive correlation*, with high values on one variable predicting high values on the other. *Negative correlation* occurs where high values on one variable predict low values on another: an example might be fitness and blood pressure – all things being equal, the less fit you are, the higher your blood pressure. *Perfect* correlation (positive or negative) is said to occur when the values of one variable exactly predict the values of the other – distance covered in a given time is perfectly correlated with speed of running (by definition). Perfect correlation is seldom found in social research, however. When we say that height and weight are correlated, we do not mean that all tall people are heavier than all people shorter than them, but that on the whole the heaviest people will be among the tallest.

The *correlation coefficient* is a mathematical way of expressing the degree to which two variables are correlated – tedious to calculate, but quite easy to understand. A coefficient of correlation carries the value of +1.0 if there is perfect positive correlation between the two variables, –1.0 if there is perfect negative correlation, and zero if there is no correlation at all. The values in between express the degree and direction of correlation, so +0.7 is a reasonably high degree of positive correlation, and –0.2 a reasonably low degree of negative correlation. For those who like playing with their calculators, if you square the correlation coefficient (i.e. multiply it by itself) and multiply the answer by 100, you get *percentage of variance explained*. (The variance is the amount the figures differ among each other.) A perfect correlation of 1.0 or –1.0 explains 100 per cent of the variance. A correlation coefficient of zero explains none. The correlation of 0.7 above explains 49 per cent of the variance, and the one of 0.2 only 4 per cent.

Summary: points for evaluation

1 With secondary-source material, as with any other data, it is very important to understand just how the 'facts' have been collected and to be able to assess the reliability of the source – whether it works accurately and consistently in its data collection.

2 With secondary sources even more than other forms of data the question of validity arises – whether the data collected quite correspond to what the researcher wants to use them for.

3 With secondary-sources data as with other survey-based sources, we should note that the argument which is put forward tends to be based on correlational or **quasi-experimental** logic. Arguments of this kind can

be very strongly suggestive, but they do not, strictly, establish **causation** beyond doubt.

4 However, it is quite possible for an argument of this form to be so strongly suggestive that it may be worth altering social policy and spending social resources on the basis of it. We should always ask ourselves what we can do on the basis of findings as well as what we can conclude.

Further reading

Vital statistics and statistics on health

A basic source of statistics on birth, death, disease, marriage, etc. is the *OPCS Monitor* series, of which specific annual issues deal with specific topics:

DH2 Deaths, by cause
DH4 Deaths from accidents and violence
DH5 Infant and perinatal death statistics
MB2 Infectious diseases
FM1 Birth statistics
FM2 Marriage and divorce statistics

Birth and death statistics may also be found in the *Social Trends* and *Population Trends* (or, for Northern Ireland, *Health and Personal Social Services Statistics for Northern Ireland* and the *Annual Report of the Registrar General for Northern Ireland*). Statistics on illness may be found in *Health and Personal Social Services Statistics*. For figures on health inequalities by class and region see Peter Townsend *et al.* (1990) *Inequalities in Health*. Harmondsworth: Penguin. This volume contains both *The Black Report* and *The Health Divide*, government-funded reports on health a decade apart.

DOING RESEARCH

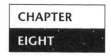

USING SECONDARY SOURCES

Using libraries – review of literature

Most research reports begin with a section (or sections) which outlines the area of research, explains why it is interesting and/or important, and probably summarizes what is known so far and what the research which is reported has to offer which is new or different. Readers need to know what you can take for granted and build on, and why you choose to look at the problem in the way that you do. For the construction of this section of a report you will have to use the resources of libraries. In fact, you would almost certainly want to do so at a much earlier stage of the research. Reading past research reports and descriptive papers, and more theoretical articles and books, is an important part of the process of refining the research problem and forming ideas about how to carry out the research.

From your point of view, libraries come in two kinds – public and academic. The libraries of universities, colleges and schools of nursing are the better stocked from the point of view of carrying out a search through the 'literature', and if you are a registered student you will have automatic rights to use them. If you are not, however, your access will be limited. Most will allow you reading rights – to look at books and journals on the premises – and some will allow you to borrow books. Many will charge for the privilege. You will have to ask the librarian what is allowed in the particular library which is convenient for you. Public libraries are more accessible, and the larger branches will have some of what you need, but you are unlikely to find that they carry a large stock of publications of the kind you are looking for.

In both kinds of library you will find:

- books, generally arranged according to a subject-based cataloguing system;
- journals, newspapers and other periodicals;
- the catalogue, which lists what the library stocks, by author, title and often subject area;
- abstracts (volumes which contain a complete year-by-year list of publications in a certain area, by author and title, with a brief summary of contents, and generally an index classified by subject-matter to help you locate useful works); for example, *Nursing Abstracts* lists and describes a wide range of research on nursing;
- Annual review journals – for example, *Research in Nursing and Health*;
- other bibliographic instruments – e.g. lists of published works such as *British Books in Print*.

There is a national borrowing network based on the British Library, a copyright library that receives copies of everything published in this country, which also acquires quite a range of works published abroad. Books can be borrowed, and photocopies of journal articles obtained, by what is called 'inter-library loan', and you should talk to the librarian if you need this. Be warned, however, that it can often take quite a lot of time to obtain books or articles by this means, and that there may often be a quite substantial fee for the service unless you are a registered student.

The library of the Royal College of Nursing, in London, has a very large collection of relevant publications. People doing research on health and nursing should contact them if their local facilities are meagre or their subject-area is a very specialized one.

In general, the most useful resource of all in a library is the librarians, who are generally very willing to help the student or researcher.

There are four main 'tricks' for homing in on relevant books and articles reasonably quickly:

1 Identify the catalogue reference which most closely fits the subject-matter of your enquiry (asking the librarian's help if necessary) and just look along the shelves at this point to see what the library has. You will be interested in anything which is fairly recent and/or which obviously bears closely on the question which underlies your research.
2 Browse through the last couple of years' issues of relevant journals for ones which are obviously, by their title, relevant to your work, and ones which you have noticed crop up quite often in the reference lists of other papers and books which you have been reading. (Don't neglect the book reviews, nor publishers' advertisements for books about to be published.)
3 Starting from papers which you have read and found useful, look in the reference lists to identify other articles or books which may be relevant. If they are, when you read them, look in their reference lists in turn for other works. Then look through current journals or abstracts (see below) for the most recent work by the same authors.
4 Use the subject index of the major series of abstracts in your field (ask the librarian if you are not sure) to identify further relevant references. This is the most comprehensive stratagem, but the riskiest in the short term, because you may put in a lot of work locating papers or books which turn

out not to be of immediate relevance. It is a relevant way to proceed if you are writing a book or thesis, or if you are stuck for any references whatsoever, but on the whole it is not a good way to start.

Exercise 25: Literature search

If you have access to a reasonably large library, try your hand at an embryonic literature search. Take one of the papers you read in Section 2 which interested you, and try to identify and locate further articles or books which bear on the same topic.

Finding statistics

A part of the 'literature review' of any research paper will generally comprise an attempt to set the object of study in its context – to say how many of the people concerned there are, what proportion of the population they form, and in general how big the problem is. For this we need the figures which are collected by governmental and other bodies, published and made available in libraries: annual reports of government departments, figures routinely presented to Parliament, regular governmental **surveys** of the population or the economy or the institutions for which government is responsible. We may also need such figures to show how **typical** or **representative** our research samples are of the population which they purport to represent. Indeed, as we saw in the last chapter, it is quite possible to conduct an entire research project on such secondary data. Often it will be the case that using already available statistics is the best way of tackling a research problem; the figures generally give a breadth of coverage that would not be available to the individual researcher without the expenditure of very large amounts of money and time.

Very often the figures you need will be in one or other of the regular annual summary publications. *Social Trends* produces annual 'headline' figures from a wide range of statistical sources and gives an overall picture of the state of the nation. Detailed figures on births, marriages, deaths, family formation and so on can be found in the monthly *Population Trends*, and more localized figures are available in *Regional Trends*. These often include articles analysing and commenting on trends. For the audience of this book, the annually published *Health and Personal Social Services Statistics* is also likely to be an important source.

For more detailed work and for statistics which are harder to find, the 'bible' of the secondary-source researcher is the *Guide to Official Statistics* published from time to time by the Central Statistical Office (CSO). This gives an annotated list of virtually all sets of published official statistics, and some statistics published by non-governmental bodies. Consulting the CSO *Guide* is a normal first step in any secondary-source research, unless you already know your sources very well.

Population and vital statistics

The major source of statistics on the population and its demographic characteristics is the **Census**, held every ten years. (We have already looked at this briefly in the last chapter.) The Census asks every household questions about who is present on Census night, who is usually present, their age, marital status, country of birth, employment, means of transport to work, educational qualifications, where they used to live, the details and amenities of their living accommodation, etc. It is the best source for reliable and authoritative information on the population and their housing in a given area. Results are presented on a regional basis and by county, as well as in national terms (for some of the analyses), and statistics of smaller areas are available on request, in tabular form or in a form amenable to computer analysis. (Some of the more complex analyses are carried out not on the full returns, but on a sample of them.) A limited range of statistics are also available for local authority areas, urban areas, political constituencies, and even wards and parishes.

Happening every ten years, the Census is inevitably out of date for large parts of a decade. More recent information (though generally based on samples rather than the whole population) may be obtained from the monthly Office of Population Censuses and Surveys (OPCS) publication *Population Trends*, from *Regional Trends* if geographically more specific information is required, and from the annual *Social Trends* if all that is required is a broad overview. The other main source of descriptive population statistics, also carried out by OPCS, is the *General Household Survey*, a sample survey of a **panel** of households which asks some of the questions covered in the Census, but also more detailed ones on household amenities and income. A report of the survey is published annually.

There is a strict legal requirement for births and deaths to be reported, so these are among the most **reliable** of the published statistics. *Population Trends* gives numbers of births and deaths by age and gender, noting also numbers of stillbirths and of illegitimate births, and broad summary figures are also given in the annual *Social Trends*. More detailed figures are given in various of the *OPCS Monitors*; you should consult the CSO *Guide* for a list of these. Figures are often given as rates per thousand or ten thousand of the population (or of women of child-bearing age, in the case of births), a more useful way of representing them than simple raw numbers. Death rates may be further adjusted to take account of the age and sex structure of the population under examination – the **standardized mortality ratio**, discussed in the previous chapter, is set at 100 if the group or region's adjusted death rate is identical to the national average. Some statistics for Scotland and Northern Ireland will be found in *Population Trends*, but the major sources here are the *Annual Report of the Registrar General, Scotland* and the *Annual Report of the Registrar General (Northern Ireland)*.

Health and the National Health Service

There are no systematic statistics on the health or disease of the population, but only records of particular illnesses or causes of death. A variety of death figures are available – childhood deaths at various stages around and before birth, causes of death as recorded on death certificates, deaths from accident or violence, occupational mortality, etc. These are reported in *OPCS Monitors* and in a variety of other publications (see the list at the end of the previous chapter, and the CSO *Guide* for more detailed and up-to-date information). Certain infectious diseases have to be reported, and figures for these are given in *Health and Personal Social Services Statistics for England* (or comparable publications for the other countries of Great Britain – see the CSO *Guide*), as are reported cases of sexually transmitted diseases, registered cases of cancer and notifications of congenital malformation. This source also gives numbers of reported pregnancies and numbers of abortions carried out. The *General Household Survey* asks questions on smoking in even-numbered years and publishes the results, and the 1980 and 1982 volumes include data on drinking (which is also covered in summary form in *Social Trends*). Again there are more detailed sources of information which offer a range of analyses, and you should consult the CSO *Guide* for a list of them.

Statistics on the working of the health service are somewhat more comprehensive. Numbers of personnel in the hospital, family practitioner committee and community health branches of the service, and local authority social service, are given in *Health and Personal Social Services Statistics*, as are costs, sources of finance and charges to patients or clients, and a breakdown of hospital beds by location and department. This volume also gives figures on use of hospital treatments, and the age and gender of patients, numbers of general practitioners, the number and cost of prescriptions dispensed, numbers of dentists and incidence of dental treatment, numbers of ophthalmic practitioners and the use (and cost) of their services, the numbers and usage in the ambulance service, and numbers in the school health service and the number of pupils inspected. There are cognate publications for Scotland, Wales and Northern Ireland, and many more specialized sources dealing with particular aspects of the service – again, see the CSO *Guide*.

Social services statistics

The major source here is *Health and Personal Social Services Statistics for England* (and comparable sources for the other countries of the British Isles – see the CSO *Guide*). This gives details of personnel and all the services which have been provided – domiciliary services, residential services, children and young persons in local authority care, housing and homelessness, etc. It also gives numbers of adoptions of children. *Local Government Financial Statistics* gives financial data on the personal social services. Again there are more detailed sources, for which you should consult the CSO *Guide*.

> **Exercise 26: Exploring secondary data**
>
> If you have an adequate library available, why not spend a few hours seeing what you can get out of available statistics. Pick some limited area of enquiry, look for relevant figures in the overall summary volumes such as *Social Trends*, look in the CSO *Guide* to see what else might be available and follow it up.

Problems with published statistics

Published statistics are a very strong source of information – the only available one for making comparisons over extended periods of time, unless you have a very long time in which to conduct your research, and with a 'sample size' that you are very unlikely to be able to match. There are problems, however, connected with the ways in which they are assembled and the purposes for which they are collected, which mean they have to be treated with even more caution than other sources of information.

The first problem is the question of **reliability**: are the statistics collected in a consistent way, so that one year's figures are comparable with another's? There may be several stages in a statistic's 'history' at which an individual's discretion comes into play, and this could be exercised in different ways from year to year, from place to place and from person to person. There are also gross changes of law, practice and the state of knowledge to contend with. Diagnosis of disease or handicap, for example, depends on someone presenting himself or herself to a doctor, who then exercises medical judgement as to whether a diagnosable condition is present and, if so, what it is. There are advances of medical knowledge which will change particular diagnostic practice from time to time. Reliability may also be influenced by more social factors. For example, now that there are incentives to doctors for screening of women for cervical cancer, cases will be diagnosed earlier and there will be a temporary rise in the statistics – fewer cases will wait for the diagnosis until the condition becomes acute. The government statistics on numbers of deaths are reliable, being taken from counts of death certificates. The statistics on cause of death are also taken from death certificates, however, and these are not reliable: they depend on the potentially fallible diagnosis of doctors, plus an additional level of 'clerical discretion', where more than one cause is recorded and a clerk will have to decide which to take as the primary one. All survey questions – even apparently simple ones such as 'How would you describe your ethnic origin?' Or 'Have you ever been raped?' – have to be scrutinized to see whether fashions in avowal or differential pay-offs for answering one way or the other might change the pattern of answers over time, even if the underlying 'facts' had not changed. Information collected by some government department, often for quite different purposes, needs to be scrutinized even more carefully.

This leads into the question of **validity** – do the statistics measure what they purport to measure? Putting it another way, is what they measure what you want to consider in your research? Diagnostic statistics, for example, measure not the extent of a given disease, but the extent to which it has been diagnosed, and diagnosis is not an automatic process, but one involving human decision-making. The statistics are very likely to be correlated with the real extent of disease – to go up when it goes up and down when it goes down – but the relationship could be quite a loose one, and small changes are as likely as not to be the result of a change in reporting or recording practice. So we need to remember that what we are measuring is, in part, a social construction, not a 'fact', and that there is error in the figures.

Another aspect of the validity question concerns the way that we tend to use what is available, even if it does not quite match up to what we need. In the Abbott and Tyler paper discussed in the last chapter the authors had to use the Census occupational categories simply because they were available. Abbott and Tyler were well aware, however, that these are not well designed for discriminating between women's jobs and tend to 'lump together' occupational positions which are in some ways very different, so that there could be differences between Black and White women which are concealed by their aggregation into the same set of categories. As another example, we might assess the efficiency of hospitals by their throughput of patients and/or the number of patients treated for a given cost, but this would take no account of the quality of treatment. It is very easy to distort the original research question in the interests of using available statistics, or even to miss the core of it altogether.

The moral is that we must always scrutinize the secondary statistics which we are considering with at least as much care as we would scrutinize methods of data collection we intend to use ourselves first-hand. Are the figures likely to be consistently and reliably collected? Do they measure what they purport to measure? Do they measure what *we* want to measure? Will the use of them in any way distort or prejudice the analysis of the original question? If so, what other figures can we use to overcome this, or what research ought we to go on and do to supplement what we can learn from the figures?

'Qualitative' sources

We have talked so far as if all secondary analysis is carried out on published statistics. It is also possible, however, to do qualitative secondary analysis, looking at what people have written or what has been written about them. Studying social policy, for example, government reports and White Papers can be a rich source of information, and for more detailed work one can go to *Hansard*, the daily record of what is said in Parliament, or to the newspapers (*The Times* and *The Guardian* have an annual index which makes it relatively easy to track down the date of 'policy events' – or you may be able to access a CD-ROM version, in which case you can use computerized search facilities). Professional journals can also be very useful in this respect. One should remember that what is presented is what the policy-makers say – how they justify what they are doing – and the criticisms that have been made from a range of entrenched positions; such work is seldom to be taken as a purely factual source of information. In this, however, they differ little from any other qualitative source; it is always necessary to remember that people give *accounts* of their lives and actions, not straight factual reports.

With this same qualification, people's own personal accounts can also help to 'flesh out' figures or can be used as a source in their own right: auto-biographies, published collections of letters, diaries, even novels can help to give some feel for what a situation or condition is like 'from the inside' in circumstances where interviewing is not possible. One may also go to reports of ethnographic research for summarized accounts of other people's interviewing. Thus the literature review can also be a form of data collection.

Exercise 27: Exploring qualitative sources

Taking the topic which you explored in Exercise 25, spend a few hours in a large library looking for anything qualitative which bears on it – diaries, letters, autobiographies, ethnographic research reports, official pronouncements. (In other words, get started on a literature review.) See what these add to the quantitative material you have developed.

Summary

1 A fair amount of research analysis can be done without carrying out research fieldwork – through examination of the research of others and by analysis of figures collected and published by government and other agencies.

2 When using these figures – particularly those collected as a by-product of administration rather than by specifically designed surveys – care has to be taken to ensure that the figures are reliable over time and as measures of what they purport to measure. To ensure this, a fair amount has to be known about how the figures are collected.

3 Even where figures are reliable measures of what they claim to measure, care must still be taken that they are valid for the *researcher's* purpose.

4 Sources other than figures – diaries, letters, newspaper articles, speeches, even novels – can also cast useful light on research questions.

Further reading

Hakim, Catherine (1987) *Research Design: Strategies and Choices in the Design of Social Research*. London: Routledge (Chapters 2 and 4).

Hindess, Barry (1973) *The Use of Official Statistics in Sociology*. London: Macmillan.

Irvine, John, Miles, Ian and Evans, Jeff (eds) (1979) *Demystifying Social Statistics*. London: Pluto Press.

McLeod, C.J. and Slodatski, A.N. (1978) How to find out: a guide to searching the nursing literature, *Nursing Times*, 74(6): 21–3.

Plummer, Kenneth (1983) *Documents of Life*. London: Allen and Unwin.

Useful journals for reports of nursing research

Nursing Standard
Nursing Times

British Journal of Midwifery
British Journal of Nursing
Health Visiting Journal
Journal of Advanced Nursing
Nurse Education Today
Nurse Researcher
Surgical Nurse

Social Science and Medicine
Social Sciences in Health
Sociology of Health and Illness

See also, for summaries of research studies, *Nursing Abstracts*.

SURVEY RESEARCH: DESIGN AND SAMPLING

In this chapter we have in mind the sort of research that a practitioner might do in his or her own institution:

1 **surveying** the attitudes of the client population to a service;
2 comparing two groups of clients to see, for example, whether the medical and care needs of elderly men are different from those of elderly women, or whether Black families have different social-work needs from White ones (a sort of **case-control study** of social needs);
3 trying to predict outcomes or looking for **causal** links (e.g. whether some forms of nursing care are more effective than others at achieving a desired end, or whether clients who make repeated use of a counselling service differ systematically from those who come once and then drop out).

We shall also look at how respondents are selected, how **observation/interview schedules** are constructed (including the construction of attitude and personality scales), what problems for the interpretation of the data can usefully be anticipated at the design stage and the eventual use of **questionnaires** in the field.

The usual stages of survey design are:

1 Formulating the 'problem' or area of study as precisely as possible, probably after:
  (a) reviewing the literature;
  (b) a first **pilot** stage of talking to potential respondents in a fairly open

and unstructured way about the topic(s) of the survey, to get their ideas and some notion of the terminology they use;

(c) where the research is to be carried out in a limited number of settings (e.g. one or a few institutions), spending some time there familiarizing yourself with what goes on.

2 Selecting the sample of respondents or settings, or devising rules for how a sample is to be picked.

3 Deciding on the best mode of 'delivery' – whether you are going to observe behaviour in a systematic way or ask questions; and, if you decide on a questionnaire, whether it will be administered by an interviewer or sent by post for self-completion or delivered by some other means. At this time you would plan what to do about refusals and non-response – whether and when to send follow-up letters, for instance, and whether it is possible to collect any descriptive information about people who refuse to cooperate.

4 Thinking carefully about what descriptive ('demographic') information might be necessary or useful – age, gender, social class, etc. – and precisely how to record it.

5 Thinking what alternative explanations might be offered for any results you obtain, and what extra information you need to collect to explore them.

6 Designing the questionnaire or observation schedule. If this includes measurement scales not in common use, a second stage of pilot work would be needed, to check on the *validity* of the measures (looking for evidence that they do measure what you want) and their *reliability* (that they produce fairly stable and consistent results).

7 In a final pilot stage you would try out the questionnaire or schedule, to identify and deal with problems in its administration. You would also, at this stage, think about how the results are to be analysed, to make sure the data will be recorded in a suitable form.

These stages are described with the usual **cross-sectional** survey in mind, wanting to know what is the case at present and asking a sample of people about it in a **one-shot survey** design. When looking, for example, at changes over time, more sophisticated designs may be required, because of problems of memory and how the present tends to reconstruct the past (see Chapter 6). The two classic ways round this kind of problem are:

1 repeated cross-sections – drawing fresh samples at each time-period, and asking about the present, e.g. sampling a population before broadcast television is introduced to an area, sampling it again afterwards, and comparing the two sets of results;

2 **panel** or **cohort** designs – taking a group of people and asking them questions at designated time-periods, e.g. taking a sample before broadcast television is introduced to an area and questioning the same people again afterwards.

(We tend to talk of 'cohort studies' where the sample purports to be representative of an age group, and otherwise of 'panel studies'.) The panel or cohort study is superior in design terms, but more difficult to set up and maintain.

Most of this chapter will be about questionnaires – asking people questions about themselves and what they think and believe. We should start off by pointing out, however, that surveys do not *have* to ask people questions. The systematic observation of behaviour is an equally important survey technique, and where it is applicable it may be a stronger approach than verbal questioning, because you do not have the difficulty of interpreting the sense which respondents have made of the questions and what they meant by their answers. As a survey technique, observation must be systematic – it must entail counting or measuring behaviours in some consistent and **reliable** fashion. If you have to construct a classification system for yourself, your research would be preceded by a period of more general observation, to obtain a list of the behaviours which can be observed and to work out ways of defining them tightly. Often one researcher will devise a coding system and have it tried out by other researchers; if they can also apply it consistently, then the system is a reasonably reliable one and not just the exteriorization of its author's fancies and prejudices. A further period of observation would then follow, in which all those who were destined to use the system practised it, preferably together and on the same 'cases', until a consistent level of performance emerged; this stage of training and practice would be equally necessary even if you were using another researcher's classification system. A better stratagem is to video the behaviour and do the classification afterwards. This lets you work over the same scene several times, with colleagues, until you reach agreement about what is going on.

Selecting respondents

The ideal 'sample survey' is a **census** – questioning every member of a population (every nurse or patient in a hospital, every client on the caseload, every household in an area). This is seldom practical, however, and so researchers have to **sample** their populations. Very many of the surveys of opinion with whose results we are bombarded by newspapers and manufacturers, however, are grounded in quite inadequate samples. **Market researchers**, for example, may ask their questions of people who pass in the city street, generally during the day. Such people are not typical of the population as a whole: they are those who happen to be on the street at the time, and probably underrepresent people in full-time employment, people at schools or colleges, people who shop locally rather than in the city centre, and so on. Alternatively, they sometimes go from house to house in selected streets. This is a better stratagem, provided that all times of the day and days of the week are covered, but if not, then they are again unlikely to draw **representative** samples, because they will exclude those who are not present at the time in question. Newspaper 'surveys' are often based on even less representative 'volunteer' samples – those who bother to answer a request for information, or those who write spontaneously about something that excites or annoys them. There are better ways of working than these – methods more likely to generate samples which are representative of their populations.

Random sampling

The best kind of sample for survey work is the **random** sample – one drawn from a complete list of the population (i.e. of those to whom we want the results to generalize) in such a way that every member of it has an equal chance of being represented and it is chance that determines which particular members are selected. A sample drawn in this way cannot be seen as influenced by the views and expectations of the researcher – you cannot pick a random sample deliberately in such a way as to prove your own views – and, provided it is fairly large, it stands a good chance of resembling the population from which it is drawn. So if you were looking at some characteristics of your clients, a very good way to proceed would be to obtain a complete list of the current population of clients or of people who have come in over the past months or years and, if the population is small, put all the names in a box, shake it well and draw out as many cases as you want for your sample. If the population is larger than that, you might want to take every nth name, from a randomly chosen starting point – for example, every tenth name, if you wanted a sample of 100 from a population of 1000.

Better still is to resort to a table of random numbers. These are published in all sets of statistical tables and most statistics textbooks, and they consist essentially of a string of numbers with no discernible pattern to them – e.g. 31415873920408279 . . . They may be arranged in sets of five or ten, in columns down the page. All you need to know, to pick a sample using them, is the size of your population and the desired size of sample. Say your population was 10,000, and you wanted a sample of 100. If you picked every hundredth case (as 10,000/100 = 100) you would get the right size of sample, but there might be some pattern to which cases came up a hundred apart; and if the population were actually 10,030, the last 30 cases would stand no chance at all of being selected. So you can use the first four numbers in the table to determine a random starting point: if they were 0001, you would start with the first case, but in this case they are 3141, so you start with the 3141st. Now you could take every hundredth case. Cleverer still is to divide up the population into hundreds and take the nth case from each hundred according to the next pair of random numbers – the 58th from the first hundred, the 73rd from the next hundred, and so on. (When you get to the last case on the list, you carry on counting from the beginning again, as if the cases were arranged in a circle.) This kind of procedure gives you absolutely the least chance of picking a sample which is in any way systematically biased.

If there is no complete list of the population, you might be able to draw a sample by taking the next n cases to come in (e.g. the next 50 cases, if you want a sample of 50), provided cases come in randomly and there is no systematic pattern to the order in which they are received. This last point is crucial, however, and you need to think very carefully about the possibility of patterns occurring – to use your researcher's imagination to think what might be happening. If you took the next 50 cases to come in to the casualty department of a hospital, for example, and you picked the period just after a disputed football match, you would get a very different sample from one drawn in the days immediately preceding Christmas (more victims of fights in the former case, and more victims of drunken driving in the latter). Different kinds of cases come in at night than during the day. It would clearly be best, if you want a representative sample, to preselect times of the day, days of the week and weeks of the year, randomly, and use these as your 'collection points'. Wherever there is any possibility of patterns occurring in a population list or a series of admissions, you should make sure that your selection procedures are random enough to overcome it, and there is no single and simple way of doing so.

Because the random sample *is* random, drawn by chance, it is reasonably likely to be roughly representative of the population, but only roughly. It is possible to improve the representation by a process known as **stratification** – separately sampling the strata or layers of the population, using a variable known to be of some importance. If you draw a random sample of a year's hospital admissions, for example, there is every likelihood that your sample will be roughly representative of the population in terms of numbers of males and females, but only roughly. If you know that gender is an important variable in terms of your research question, you can improve the representative nature of your sample in this respect by drawing separate samples of males and females, in numbers proportionate to the numbers of the two in the population.

Cluster sampling

Frequently, when drawing samples from 'the world at large', rather than a particular institution or setting, a random sample is not appropriate because there is no list of the population from which to draw it, or because the geographical spread of a true random sample would be too great for any researcher to handle. A random sample of 500 housewives scattered across the British Isles would not give more than one or two in each town, and a national random sample of schoolchildren or hospital patients would not be much more accessible. Here we often resort to a process called **cluster sampling** – picking geographical clusters, then sampling within them. If you wanted a national sample of hospital patients, for example, you might pick five or ten hospitals at random and then take a sample of patients within the sampled hospitals. If you wanted a sample of the people in a town, you might pick three or four districts at random, and within them three or four streets, and within them three or four houses, and then interview all the people in the designated houses. There is a risk that your sample will be unrepresentative because the range is constricted – if certain sorts of people occur according to some geographical pattern, then you may oversample those sorts of people and undersample others. However, you can apply the principle of stratification to overcome this risk by selecting your clusters according to some sensible system. If you were sampling within a town, for example, you would make sure to pick some inner-urban areas and some suburban ones, and to select a mix of working-class areas and middle-class ones. If you were sampling hospitals, you would make sure that all types of hospital were represented.

Quota sampling

When nothing else is practicable we tend to resort to **quota sampling**. This is a procedure where we seek to obtain a representative sample of the population by setting up 'quotas', by sets of important variables, which match the population. We might set out, for example, to interview so many elderly middle-class women, so many elderly middle-class men, so many middle-aged middle-class women, and so on. This procedure will guarantee that the sample is representative with respect to the variables which are used to form the quotas. However, there is no control over other variables – interviewers may select whom they like to fill the quotas provided that the quota design is adhered to. Quite serious biases can, therefore, creep into the sampling. For example, in an Open University student survey (see Abbott and Sapsford 1987a) the student interviewers were set a quota design by age, social class and gender, and they matched it fairly exactly. However, the respondents whom they interviewed turned out overall to be better educated than the average, there were substantially more women in full-time employment than one would expect, and women in routine non-manual work were somewhat underrepresented. This pattern undoubtedly reflects the kinds of people Open University students find easy to locate and interview.

There are a number of ways in which quota sampling can be improved, if the interviewer is prepared to expend the effort. For example, an additional element of stratification may be introduced into samples of households by sampling from a variety of areas rather than allowing the quota to be filled from a single area. Time-periods can be randomized or systematically sampled, to minimize the risk of missing certain kinds of people because of their hours of work. A random element can be introduced – picking streets or postcodes at random as starting points. Nevertheless, and with all these improvements, quota sampling remains inherently inferior to random sampling as a way of guaranteeing a sample representative of its population.

It remains a widely used procedure in market research, however, because of its comparative ease and cheapness: there is no need for a complete list of the population to act as a sampling frame, and interviewers do not need to call back if they find a given respondent not at home but can replace him or her with someone else of the right characteristics. In political opinion research, quota sampling has almost entirely replaced more random methods because it has been found that the improvement of prediction given by the latter is too slight in this area of research to justify the extra cost (see McKee 1981).

Exercise 28: Sampling

The first six pages of the 'residential' section of your telephone directory will be the population for this exercise (or some other list with at least 200 names and addresses on it). Count the number of names overall, and also (a) how many of the names have the letter 'a' as the second or

> third letter of the main surname of the entry, and (b) how many of the
> addresses list a house *name* of some sort instead of a house *number*.
> Then take two types of sample:
>
> 1 do the same counts for the first 50 names in the list;
> 2 do the same counts for a random sample of 50 drawn using a table of
>   random numbers.
>
> Compare the results. Which type of sample comes closest to matching
> the population?

Devising the questions

If you are asking questions rather than observing behaviour, you need a
questionnaire. (This holds even if you are interrogating not people, but
files or documents; you still need a consistent list of questions to ask about
them and a consistent way of recording the answers.) This will contain,
broadly, three sorts of questions:

1 There will be demographic questions – age, gender, occupational details
   (for coding social class), and other explanatory or descriptive variables
   about people's lives that you are going to need at the analysis stage, such
   as where they live, the level of their education, etc. You will probably *pre-
   code* these – work out the possible range of answers and set up categories
   with the question, so that all that has to be done is to ring a number or
   tick a box. Be careful, however, to ensure:
   (a) that all possible answers are covered (you may need categories for
        'don't know' and/or 'refused to answer');
   (b) that categories do not overlap (age is coded, e.g. as 20–29, 30–39, etc.,
        not 20–30, 30–40, etc., because in the latter coding scheme the code
        for someone aged 30 is ambiguous); and
   (c) that you will get a reasonably even distribution of responses between
        the categories of a variable.
   If you do not know the age distribution of your population in advance,
   for example, it is better to record the actual age in years (or even years
   and months, for children) and work out categories afterwards.
2 There will be factual questions about people's past histories: whether
   they have been burgled in the past, when and for what they have been in
   hospital, their work histories, or whatever. The two problems here, both
   aspects of validity of measurement, are (a) definition and (b) memory. It
   is of paramount importance that you define precisely what you mean by
   the event or happening on which your respondents are to report; otherwise, differences between groups may be due to differences of interpretation, not differences of experience. Secondly, memory for the past is
   unreliable; people usually remember what has happened to them, but
   often not precisely when. So it is unwise to ask how many times x has
   happened 'in the last year'; precisely anchored time-periods such as
   'since Christmas' are to be preferred.

3 Questions about attitudes and beliefs – these are more complex than they may at first appear, and there are several ways of proceeding. We shall talk about them in the next section.

Measuring attitudes

Much survey research is concerned with the measurement of attitudes, beliefs, opinions, intentions, etc. If you think of attitudes as something a person has and can report on, then the best way of getting at them is quite simply to ask about them. Much market research takes this stance: 'Which of these two coffees do you prefer?', 'Which would you buy, if they were the same price?' Much political research does likewise: 'How would you vote if there were a general election tomorrow?' The Cornish survey which we examined in Section 2 asked straightforwardly for people's opinions about service provision, as well as about their factual experiences. The only technical problem, in this approach, is to phrase the questions clearly, unambiguously and in such a way that the answers can readily be understood by the researcher.

Another view of the area of attitudes/beliefs/intentions would be to regard an attitude as something that a person has, but is not necessarily able to report – a complex of beliefs and tendencies to behave in certain ways, bound together from an outsider's point of view, but not necessarily apparent to the insider's conscious thought-processes. In that case you would want to find or construct some sort of 'measuring instrument'. You would administer a list of questions which can be shown to be 'symptomatic' of the attitude in question in a number of people, and add the answers together in some way to give a score. Many clinical scales are of this kind: they seek to measure a mental state (e.g. depression) by asking a number of relatively innocuous questions which people who have that particular state typically answer in one way – e.g. 'Do you often feel unhappy?', 'Do you often cry for no reason?', 'Do you have difficulty in sleeping?' You might want to adopt this tactic if the question which underlies your scale is a sensitive one which might offend the respondent, or if there are very strong social norms prompting the respondent to answer in a particular direction.

One way of constructing such a scale is to get a panel of experts in the area to generate a pool of statements which they would see as symptomatic of the attitude or mental state, and use the ones on which the experts appeared to agree. A second and more common way of proceeding is to generate a large pool of items which have 'face validity' – they look at least as if they ought to measure what is required. You then go through at least four stages of pilot work.

1 You administer the items to a group of people (about 20?), getting them to score them on a seven-point scale from, for example, 'very true of me' to 'not at all true of me'. You throw out all those items which tend to attract scores in the middle of the scale from everyone, because they will not help to discriminate any group from any other.

2 You administer the remaining items to two separate groups who can be guaranteed to differ from each other on the variable which the scale is measuring – for example, if you were measuring 'satisfaction with the service we provide' you might pick ten people who have taken the trouble to come and tell you afterwards how good the service was and the ten people who had complained most virulently. You would keep the items which are consistently, on average, answered one way by one group and the other by the other, throwing out those items which did not discriminate.

3 You would retest your original group, a little time afterwards, to see if they gave similar answers (a test of reliability).

4 You would validate the final scale by finding two more groups who undoubtedly differed on the variable in question and seeing if the scale differentiated between them (to ensure that you are not just capitalizing on a chance set of differences in the first pair of groups).

If you had professional resources at your disposal there are two more things you might well do:

5 You might get scores from a large sample of the normal population and from large samples of people who would be expected to score particularly high or low, to establish the normal range of scores and what might be expected of extreme groups.

6 Taking this fairly large data-set, you might subject it to *factor analysis*, a statistical procedure which tests whether all the items **correlate** together (the extent to which they are measuring the same thing) or whether one can distinguish groups of items which correlate with others within the group, but less so with items outside the group (in which case your scale may be measuring more than one variable).

The final scale is demonstrably **valid** and **reliable**. To the extent that these stages have not been undertaken, this cannot be asserted.

Yet another way of looking at attitudes, beliefs and intentions is to see them as products of how the respondent sees the world – what sort of a world he or she thinks we live in, with reference to your area of interest. One can get at people's ways of classifying their world, their 'constructs', by a technique devised by the American psychologist George Kelly (e.g. 1955), known as the Role Repertory Grid. This was originally devised for therapeutic interviews, but has since been widely used for a range of psychological studies of people and how they see the world, and even in market research (to explore 'brand images'). For an introduction to Kelly's theories and to uses of the Grid, see Bannister and Fransella (1980). A related technique is the semantic differential scale pioneered by Osgood *et al.* (1967), where sets of *supplied* adjectives form the scales on which people, groups or objects of interest are to be rated. The adjectives typically include some of very general reference (e.g. warm/cold, strong/weak) and perhaps some more specific to the particular research topic.

Finally, a useful way of getting at difficult concepts unobtrusively is by the use of what are known as 'projective techniques' – segments of 'verbal behaviour' into which respondents may be seen as projecting or expressing some aspect of mentality. One classic, for example, is the TAT (Thematic

Apperception Test), which consists of a series of ambiguous pictures looking something like magazine illustrations. The respondent is asked to write or narrate the story illustrated by each picture, and it is argued that what appears in the story (not being supplied by the pictures, which are as near neutral in content as possible) expresses something about the respondent. For example, a picture of two men in a room might be seen as brothers at home, or as two colleagues conspiring, or as a homosexual affair, or two people planning to start a successful small business, or . . . The original use of this test was to measure 'achievement motivation' by the amount of achievement-oriented imagery that was produced (McClelland *et al.* 1953). Another example would be the use of photographs to measure affective flattening – getting people to describe what they saw in pairs of photographs of people and seeing the extent to which they did or did not impute emotions to the subjects of them (Dixon 1967; Sapsford 1983).

Anticipating problems

Non-response

Nearly all surveys have a problem of non-response: people refuse to answer, or randomly chosen respondents cannot be contacted, or if you left questionnaires to be filled in by the respondents some of them will not bother to do so. It would be very destructive of a survey's claims to represent the views of a population if the non-response rate were very large, and particularly if the non-respondents were not a random subset of the sample – if particular kinds of people tended not to respond. There is a certain amount you can do about this problem at the fieldwork stage and we shall discuss this later. Two precautions can be taken at the design stage, however. First, it may be possible to anticipate which kinds of people may not respond and to oversample them: in a questionnaire about the banning of smoking at work, for example, you might deliberately set out to question more smokers than would be needed to represent their proportion of the population, anticipating that many smokers will be hostile to the purpose of the questionnaire. (This assumes, of course, that you know the population distribution and that you can reliably identify smokers and non-smokers beforehand.) This kind of *disproportionate stratification* is also useful for making sure that rare groups in the population are adequately represented. The second tactic is to try to find out at least basic demographic characteristics even of the non-responders, so that you can compare them with the respondents and see if they differ in any significant way. If you are interviewing face to face it should be possible to note gender and estimate age and even rough social class. If you are sending out questionnaires and ensuring confidentiality by *not* asking for names and addresses to be sent in, you might still get the postcode or area of town on the respondents' questionnaires, and if you kept a note of how many you dispatched to each postcode or area of town then you can at least see if there is any geographical inequality in the response. (A directory of postcodes is kept in every central post office.)

Reactivity

A second problem which must be anticipated at the design stage is **reactivity**, the risk that some of the answers will be prompted by the way the questionnaire is designed or delivered. You will take great pains at the design stage, for example, to avoid social desirability effects – the tendency of people to 'be in favour of honour and virtue' and to give answers that will represent them as respectable and socially conforming in the eyes of the researcher – by finding ways of phrasing questions which allow the socially less unacceptable responses to seem acceptable. You will avoid too many questions which could naturally be answered 'yes' or 'no'. You would be very sure not to suggest in your question-wording what answer you expect the informant to give. You would also be careful of the order of questions, so that the answer to one question is not suggested by the answer to a previous one.

Alternative explanations

Finally, you need to collect a certain number of demographic variables to test for whether they provide alternative explanations for your results to the explanation which you propose to put forward. If you were examining the relationship between unemployment and certain kinds of 'health behaviour', for example, it might be that poverty provided a more comprehensive explanation than unemployment – that all people in poverty showed the behaviour in question, whether or not they were registered as unemployed. You would, therefore, need to collect some kind of measure of household income, to check whether this was the case. You would also want to collect the obvious demographic characteristics – age, gender, social class, etc. – in order to be able to check that your sample is typical of the population.

Exercise 29: Questionnaire design

Try your hand at designing a questionnaire. Imagine you are commissioned to examine clients'/patients'/customers' satisfaction with the service your agency or firm provides (if you work for an agency or firm), or with a service which you or your family receive (e.g. the service provided by your local primary school). Think carefully what this 'service' is – how many different things the agency or firm does, and the different goals which the clients, etc. might have. (You may need to talk to some people before you start.) Think also who the clients actually are – in the case of a school, for example, are the clients children, or parents, or the education authority, or all of these? Then work out what questions you need to ask, including demographic variables for describing the population, checking on the quality of the sampling and looking for patterns in the results. (You may need different questionnaires for the different kinds of 'client', if their interests are different.) Think carefully how you would ask the questions, for maximum acceptability to the respondents and maximum clarity when you come to analyse the results. If you are able, try your draft out on three or four appropriate people, and see what changes you want to make to it after you have seen their responses.

Doing the research

An essential element of research design which we have not yet discussed (because it affects fieldwork even more than design) is the notional 'research contract' between you and your respondents. You will, of course, have ensured that your research procedures will not cause pain or distress to informants, but what are you going to tell them about the research? Are you asking questions to collect data, regarding what you do with the data as in a sense none of their business? Or are you adopting a fully collaborative stance, taking them fully into your confidence, carrying out the work as much to further their interests as your own and regarding the work as in some sense joint property? If the latter, have you worked out what form the collaboration will take? Will they be collaborating in the writing of the report? Will they have free access to each other's data (see 'confidentiality', below)? If they disagree with your interpretation of the data, do they have the right to change what is reported, or to have their disagreement registered, or are their comments to be only advisory? If you enter into a collaboration, the rules must be clear to all parties.

It is general practice to promise respondents *confidentiality* – that only you will be able to match up names and questionnaires, and that the information will never be used in such a way that the respondent can be identified. You will need to think carefully about building in procedures which ensure that this is the case – for example, sampling widely enough that no individual is unique. Confidentiality is particularly important if the respondents stand to lose by being identified – if, for example, they are patients or clients of your agency, or working colleagues, and their views could be held against them by 'management'. (Sometimes respondents will not *want* confidentiality – when they want their specific complaints to be dealt with, for example.)

Also a design matter, as well as an aspect of fieldwork, is precisely how you intend to deliver the questionnaire. Will you take it round to respondents yourself and ask them the questions, filling in the answers yourself? Will you use other (perhaps paid) people as interviewers? Will you hand it out personally, but ask them to fill it in for themselves and return it to you? Or will you post it to them and ask them to return it? Each of these methods has advantages as well as disadvantages. If you are your own interviewer, you can have maximal confidence in the data. You will also probably get a fairly low refusal rate. On the other hand, you cannot cover very many cases. Postal delivery is the best method for reaching a wide target population, but the refusal/non-response rate is generally very high; 50 per cent response would be considered quite high for a postal survey. You will, therefore, do everything you can to increase response rate if you adopt the postal strategy: including a stamped addressed envelope for the return of the form, and writing again, perhaps two or three times, to people who do not respond to the first letter. (This is, of course, impossible unless you are sending the questionnaire to preselected named individuals.) Delivering the questionnaire yourself improves the response rate, but there are still problems. Finally, using others as your interviewers can give you the advantages of personal interviewing but allow you to cover more cases than you could manage by yourself. It may, indeed, be the only way to obtain face-to-face interviews if you are not an appropriate person to be carrying out the interviews yourself. For example, it is better to have a Black interviewer when approaching Black people and a young interviewer when approaching young people – respondents are more at their ease and less likely to give an 'official response'. On the other hand, it is very important that the interviewers be trained to use the questionnaire all in the same way; otherwise differences might be due to characteristics of the interviewers' behaviour rather than characteristics of the respondents.

This question of training also applies to you yourself, if you are administering your own questionnaire. The whole point of this approach is that data shall be collected in a uniform manner from all respondents – that they all answered the same questionnaire, administered in the same fashion. (This is another argument against postal delivery – that you cannot control the conditions under which the questionnaire is filled in.) It is quite vital that all who are to administer the questionnaire know exactly what to do with each question, including the extent to which it is legitimate to explain what is meant and the extent to which they may be required to prompt respondents for more information. The questionnaire must be as standardized a measuring instrument as a thermometer, if we are to put complete confidence in its results.

Finally, we cannot overstress the importance of pilot work. All questionnaires should be tried out, to see what could go wrong, before being administered to the sample at large. It is particularly important to pilot questions, scales, etc. which are intended to measure aspects of attitude, intention or personality. These are of little value as evidence if you cannot demonstrate they are reliable (answered the same way by the same informants over a period of time short enough that change would not be expected) and valid as measures of what you claim that they measure.

Summary

1 If a census (survey of 100 per cent of potential respondents) is not feasible, then surveys have to be based on a sample of the population. A *random* sample drawn from a complete list of the population yields results which are most likely to be representative of the population. *Stratification* may be used to improve the precision of the sampling, where a variable is known to be of importance to the research.

2 When true random sampling is not possible, *cluster* sampling – selecting geographical clusters and sampling within them – may be substituted, but at the risk of some loss of the ability to cover the full range of variation in the population. Alternatively, a *quota* sample may be selected to be representative of the population in terms of variables known to be important – but there is a strong risk that it will be unrepresentative in other respects because the selection of cases to fill the quotas is left to the interviewers.

3 However good the sampling, non-response may render the achieved sample unrepresentative of the population. It is essential to take all possible steps to minimize non-response and to try to record at least basic demographic characteristics of those who refuse to cooperate or cannot be located, to the extent that this is possible.

4 Survey questions may vary from very direct and open enquiries – demographic questions about age, gender, etc., or straightforward questions about behaviours or beliefs – to complex scales made up of items known to correlate with some aspect of personality or attitude. Even with the straightforward questions it is necessary to think carefully about how they will be understood by the respondents and what effect they will have on them. A pilot stage is also desirable to try out the questions, validate their use (i.e. check that they *do* measure what is wanted) and test whether they are answered reliably (i.e. that they produce the same answers when asked more than once). An important factor in question naire design is the avoidance of reactivity – the tendency for the pattern of the answers to be produced by the way the questions are asked rather than by genuine differences among informants. With more complex measuring scales pilot work is essential.

5 Surveys usually involve asking identical questions across a population, but more personalized explorations are also possible. Kelly's Role Repertory Grid is an example of an instrument designed for personalized exploration of beliefs and attitudes.

Further reading

Survey design

Hakim, Catherine (1987) *Research Design: Strategies and Choices in the Design of Social Research*. London: Routledge (Chapters 5, 7 and 8).

Oppenheim, A.N. (1992) *Questionnaire Design, Interviewing and Attitude Measurement*. London: Pinter (Chapters 1–4, 7–8).

Polgar, Stephen and Thomas, Shane (1988) *Introduction to Research in the Health Sciences*. London: Churchill Livingstone.

Witts, L.J. (ed.) (1964) *Medical Surveys and Clinical Trials*. London: Oxford University Press.

Measurement scales and psychological/attitude tests

Anastasi, Anne (1982) *Psychological Testing*. London: Macmillan.
Hollander, Edwin (1981) *Principles and Methods of Social Psychology*. Oxford: Oxford University Press (Chapter 3).
Jensen, Arthur (1981) *Straight Talk about Mental Tests*. London: Macmillan.
Newmark, Charles (1985) *Major Psychological Assessment Instruments*. Boston, MA: Allyn and Bacon.
Oppenheim, A.N. (1992) *Questionnaire Design, Interviewing and Attitude Measurement*. London: Pinter (Chapters 9–12).
Osgood, Charles, Sui, George and Tannenbaum, Percy (1967) *The Measurement of Meaning*. Urbana, IL: University of Illinois Press.

Role Repertory Grids and George Kelly's approach

Bannister, Don and Fransella, Fay (1980) *Inquiring Man*. Harmondsworth: Penguin.
Kelly, George (1955) *The Psychology of Personal Constructs*. New York: Norton.
Smith, Jonathan, Harre, Rom and Van Langenhove, Luk (1995) *Rethinking Methods in Social Psychology*. London: Sage (Chapter 11).

Quantitative (statistical) analysis

To teach statistics is beyond the scope of this book, but there are many good texts on the market. Two books are particularly recommended. The first is the best for the beginner, a very good introductory text; it was recommended to us by our students. The other is also good, and does not assume any prior knowledge of statistics, but it is pitched more at good third-year students and postgraduates.

Clegg, Frances (1982) *Simple Statistics*. Cambridge: Cambridge University Press.
Marsh, Catherine (1988) *Exploring Data*. Cambridge: Polity.

EXPERIMENTAL PRACTICE

In this chapter we shall assume that any **experiment** you want to carry out will be a 'field experiment', set in the real world. We shall look mainly at how you would go about evaluating some aspect of your own potential practice – how you would try out a new treatment technique or style of working. The same techniques would also be appropriate for wider-scale testing of new practices – for assessing the effects of a new management structure or a general change in practice imposed from outside, or for comparing wards or wings of an institution in which different regimes were in force. (You should note, however, that this kind of **controlled trial** is by no means the only way in which practices can be evaluated. Most of the rest of this book will be about evaluation, offering a wide range of styles of working. This chapter is firmly set within a positivist epistemology and is concerned more with demonstrating **causal** influences than with understanding the nature of phenomena.)

Uncontrolled trials

The simplest kind of 'experimental' research you can do is just 'trying things out' in its crudest form – making a change and seeing what happens. Though by no means the best design for the purpose, this is a very common form of research into practice, often used in circumstances where nothing more elaborate is possible or where insufficient preparation rules out better designs. Here we have termed it 'the *un*controlled trial' to distinguish it from more rigorously designed research. To obtain interpretable results, careful and **reliable** measurement and exhaustive documentation are essential. We need a clear and reliable measurement or description of what the treatment procedure or programme of change is, so that we know what it is that is causing any change that may occur. We need a clearly defined set of outcome measures, so that we can see what change is brought about. We need also to measure anything in the environment which might function as an alternative explanation of the results.

Measurement of the treatment and the outcome are not as simple as might at first appear. We need to have thought very carefully about what it is we are trying to achieve and what will count as having achieved it. In psychiatric and counselling research, for example, it is seldom possible to produce definitive proof of 'cure' following treatment – something that would be accepted by others, rather than just the researcher's/therapist's personal judgement. One tends, therefore, to ask the clients/patients what they *thought* of the therapy and whether they were satisfied with it; at least this is something more concrete than the therapist's judgement of his or her own cases. However, whether a feeling of satisfaction in the patient or client is what the therapist was trying to achieve is open to question: would he or she not be better satisfied with an amelioration of the condition, whether or not the patient felt good about the therapy. There is a great tendency in experimental research to substitute something measurable but not totally appropriate for the outcome which we really want to assess. If you were carrying out the research for someone else, you would need to think even more carefully about what outcome is desired and not necessarily to accept what the client said was the outcome. A declared aim of a hospital administration, for example, might be to improve the care of certain patients, as measured perhaps by whether they had to be readmitted for the same condition within a specified time period. However, it is a reasonable bet that they would not implement a recommendation to increase staffing levels unless it could be shown that the costs of readmission were higher than those of increasing the intensity of nursing care.

Reactivity is the second problem. Inevitably, your ideas about the measurement of effectiveness have an effect on your practice – you do such and such because it appears to be working. We have hinted at this already, talking about problems in defining output measures: it is essential that you define what shall count as a success *before* starting to measure. Otherwise you are in the position of the punter who placed his bet after the race was won: you are claiming to predict what you have, in fact, observed happening. The nature of the treatment itself is even more prone to reactive effects in this kind of research. To the extent that you are not able to define precisely what your treatment will be *before* starting to measure its effects, your results will always be suspect: you may always have modified what you are doing to fit in with changes which you have observed (unconsciously, even). There will also be **confounded variables** – factors associated with your treatment which might provide alternative explanations of the outcome. In the earlier part of this century, great claims were made for the efficacy of insulin injections as a cure for certain kinds of mental disorder. These claims were dispelled by later analysis of what the process entailed – extreme physical debilitation, followed during the recovery period by constant and sympathetic attention from nurses. The subsequent discovery that the attention and sympathy were equally effective when *not* accompanied by the insulin injection more or less put paid to this therapy's claims.

The problem is in three parts:

1 There will be aspects to what you are doing of which you are not aware, probably aspects of your own behaviour and the way you budget your time.
2 These may as easily explain any changes which you observe as the deliberate manipulation of treatment which you are instituting.
3 There may be no way, within the crude design of this kind of research, of separating out these effects: doing a certain kind of therapy or social work or nursing care may inevitably mean spending more time with the 'experimental' subjects or behaving to them in a certain kind of way, and it may always be this rather than the deliberate manipulation which is producing the effect.

The best you can do is to try to note all these confounded influences, perhaps, if possible, getting someone else to watch you at work and examine your practice – and note them in your report as areas for further study.

Exercise 30: Critique of uncontrolled trials

Imagine you have just joined the staff of a ward or office where a new procedure has been introduced. What steps would you take to monitor its progress? (Assume that back records, etc. are not available.) More important, what could you *not* conclude from your results? (Think of this as a logical problem, not a practical one.)

However well you design this kind of study, it has certain logical flaws which inevitably mean that what can be concluded from it is strictly limited. You may institute a change and observe a result. However:

1 you can never be quite sure what produced the result – all manner of things will have been changed by the fact of your instituting an 'experiment', apart from your nominated treatment or experimental manipulation;
2 there may have been differences between people which are equally responsible for who showed the 'effect', and while you may have collected information about these, your 'sample' will lack sufficient structure for you to be able to disentangle or disprove such effects by statistical means;
3 you will not be able to say whether the effect would have occurred even without the treatment;
4 worst of all, you will not even be able to specify what the effect is – you will have measurements on how people perform after the treatment, but in the design discussed so far you have nothing with which to compare them.

Towards the controlled trial

The easiest of the faults to remedy in this very crude research design is the problem of knowing whether a change has occurred or not. The first and most basic element in any experimental design is that measurement of the **dependent variable**(s) shall be undertaken *before* the manipulation/treatment is undertaken as well as afterwards. Indeed, to do so would be characteristic of any decently planned **action research**. Your basic data, in looking for causal influences, are not measurements, but differences between measurements: we are looking, not for some absolute value of a dependent variable, but for a change in it. You might, indeed, go further: if what you have achieved is a lasting change, not just a temporary one, then you will need post-treatment measurements after a period of time to demonstrate the fact.

However, a series of measurements on one group which has received a treatment are not in themselves logically convincing. Certainly, you can demonstrate that a change has occurred, but you cannot demonstrate *why* it occurred. Specifically, you cannot demonstrate that it occurred as a result of the treatment which was applied; it may be due to any number of other things which occurred to the group being treated during the same time as the treatment. The other essential of experimental design, therefore, is a **control** or **comparison group** – one which is alike in every respect to the treatment group, and undergoes as similar as possible a set of experiences, but does not actually receive the treatment. (In drug research they would typically receive a placebo or dummy – a pill or injection which looked like the experimental drug but was in fact chemically inert.) One basic stratagem for making sure that the two groups are alike is to assign people randomly to treatment and control groups, as we have seen: provided your groups are reasonably large, this should 'even out' any chance differences. Guaranteeing similarity of experience is more difficult, outside the laboratory, but you would want to document their lives in as much detail as possible during the period of the experiment, looking for any possibly significant differences.

As we pointed out in Chapter 5, there are other ways of picking control/comparison groups which may be more effective for some purposes. With small numbers you probably need to institute some kind of **matching** procedure, picking pairs of subjects who are comparable on variables which you know might well be important (age, class, gender, medical condition, social circumstances, or whatever) and allocating one of the pair at random to each group. This absolutely guarantees comparability at least on these variables. Indeed, where you are trying to control for some well known alternative explanation at the design stage, matching is perhaps the best stratagem; like **stratification** in **random sampling** (see Chapter 9), it may improve on the simple random procedures in ways which are important to you. Best of all, if your design lends itself to it, is to use the same subjects as both 'experimentals' and 'controls': then you are certain that those in the two groups have the same history, the same physical and mental constitution, etc. This is seldom possible in practice, however, because the administration of the treatment alters the subjects to the point where they are no longer comparable with their past selves with regard to the manipulation which you want to test.

The allocation of subjects to treatment and control groups raises an important point about the conduct of experiments. It is for each researcher to decide whether the purity of including an untreated control group is worth the ethical dilemma of leaving some people deliberately untreated, but on the whole many researchers and professionals would regard doing so as unethical in a wide range of circumstances. A way round may be to compare a new treatment with people undergoing the best of what was previously available: then at least no one has deliberately been debarred from treatment. It is often difficult to reconcile the needs of the research – including the benefit to future sufferers if a treatment can be shown unambiguously to 'work' – with the deliberate mis- or non-treatment of a proportion of sufferers.

A final point to watch is what is known as the Hawthorne Effect (a form of reactivity). The name derives from a famous series of studies at the Hawthorne Works in Chicago in the 1920s (Roethlisberger and Dickson 1939). The researchers were commissioned to seek ways of changing environment and working conditions to improve output, and they tried out a range of possible modifications, each of which did, indeed, improve output – improving lighting and physical comfort, introducing coffee breaks, shortening the working day, etc. However, when as the last stage of the experiment (using a 'same-subjects' design) they returned everything to its original state, output went up again. It was concluded that the major (and confounded) variable, which might have been responsible for any of the results, was the subjects' awareness that they were taking part in an experiment. To the extent that the subjects of your treatment know that it is a new treatment, their reactions may be conditioned by this knowledge as much as by the treatment itself. Even your own knowledge that your treatment is experimental may change your behaviour in unconscious ways: how you behave may not be how you would behave if the new procedure had been accepted and you were applying it routinely. Drug researchers commonly adopt what is called a **double-blind** technique, where neither the recipient of the drug nor the person handing it out in conformity with a prearranged administration schedule knows whether what is received is the active drug or an inactive placebo. The ethics of this kind of procedure in social research may again be open to question, however.

> ### Exercise 31: Experiment
>
> Try making some small change in your own practice: a change of procedures or the ordering of jobs, aimed at getting patients to talk to each other more, or a different way of arranging your interviews with people to set them apparently more at their ease, or a different way of budgeting your time to allow more time for study or to get the household chores over faster. Think carefully, before you start, what precisely your manipulation or treatment is to be – write it out as a set of instructions for yourself – and what is to count as having achieved your desired outcome (in measurable terms). Think what other changes might occur as a result of your changed behaviour, which might affect the outcome, and think about ways of measuring these and controlling for them either in the design or by **statistical control** at the stage of

analysis. Start your measurements before you start your 'treatment', to give yourself a baseline 'before' measure with which your outcome can be compared. Think carefully also about the extent to which the fact that it is your own practice which you are examining may contaminate the results. For example, to what extent might the awareness of an impending experimental change affect your behaviour during the period of measurement before the experiment started?

Single-case experimental designs

Schematically, this kind of design can be represented as ABA or perhaps ABlB2B3A – untreated state (A) followed by treatment (B) followed by a period of untreated observation (A), or perhaps untreated state (A) followed by a series of treatments until one appears to work (B1, B2, B3 . . .), followed by a period of observation without treatment (A). The problem is in establishing the **validity** of the conclusion that it is the treatment (or something associated with it) which produces the effect. As a logical argument this form of study is obviously weak: it lacks the evidence of the same procedure working on several different people, and it lacks any element of **replication** – repeating it to see if it works twice (with the inference that if it does not work the second time then the first effect may have been a fluke). The basic form of any superstitious argument lies in an appeal to this kind of experience (I crossed my fingers and the terrible thing failed to happen, so it must not have happened because I crossed my fingers – ignoring the many times when one has crossed one's fingers without effect, and the many times that something terrible has happened and might well have happened even if one did cross one's fingers).

A basic element of the single-case experimental design is measurement over time and the comparison of treatment with the state of the subject while untreated. Thus the simplest kind of project would establish baseline measurements before treatment and then alternate application and withdrawal of treatment – ABABABA . . . In this way the subject acts as 'control' as well as 'treatment' condition – the state when untreated repeatedly acts as a comparison point for the state after treatment. There is variability within subjects as well as between them – people differ across time – but by alternating treatments one effectively controls for within-subject variability. It is possible to evaluate different treatments against each other by this means as well, comparing each with the untreated state – ABlAB2AB3 . . . (Because the person changes in the course of the treatment series, it would actually be necessary to apply each several times in alternation – ABlAB2ABlAB2 . . .) The argument always rests on the stability of Condition A, the untreated condition, however; the subject may show variation, but this must average out. The basic 'resting state' against which all else is compared must broadly resemble itself from one period of measurement to another (or any trends must be calculable, so that allowance can be made for them).

A second way of overcoming the variability of the individual subject is by frequently repeated measurement. If you were working with a group of subjects you would take a measurement from each of them and average them to get a stable estimate of how the group was proceeding. With the single subject this is not possible, so one has to average over time, which means measurement at more frequent intervals than would be normal in group research. The measurements can then be added together and averaged to give a single reading for a designated time-period; this is to some extent free of chance variation because several different readings have gone into it, any of which could by chance have varied in either direction from the average. Repeated measurement over a reasonably long time-period is particularly important at the diagnostic stage, to establish with some reliability the baseline against which the results of treatment(s) are to be judged.

The problem with single-case designs, quite clearly, is establishing validity, reliability and generality without the power to average between subjects to eliminate chance fluctuations and unique events. Repeated and frequent measurement may answer the problem of reliability – the extent to which the measures taken are stable ones – by the direct test of repeating them. Validity may be established by a number of means: validity of measurement by using already validated tests, or by using more than one observer or more than one kind of measure and checking that all show similar trends; validity of design by careful specification of the treatment and careful definition of goals, and by putting great care into establishing that the initial baseline measurements are stable. The question of generalizability is more difficult; it is difficult to generalize from the single subject to a population. Sometimes, where the aim is assessing the results of a particular therapy on the single patient, this may not matter. Often, however, one wishes to be able to say whether a treatment that has succeeded in this case would succeed in others, and if so, then which others. The best we can do here is to argue that what works for one subject stands a reasonable chance of working with other 'similar' subjects. Single-case research may be a good way of building techniques, but research on groups may be needed to test them.

We have stressed the disadvantages of single-case studies, in terms of generalizability. One should realize, however, that there are countervailing disadvantages to studies of groups. The need in **applied research** to work with what is available may lead to very unrepresentative group results; where a 'problem' is not randomly spread through the population, and where a non-random subsection of those coming forward with it actually reaches research attention, there is no reason to suppose that an available group is any more **representative** of the population than a single case. Indeed, because of the depth in which single cases are studied and the effort which is put into specifying the population of which they may be **typical**, it can in practice be true that single-case research is more readily generalizable than more conventional research carried out on groups.

The generality of results from single-case research is . . . a major issue. Concerns often have been voiced about the fact that only one or two subjects are studied at a time and the extent to which findings extend

to other persons is not known. Actually, there is no evidence that findings from single-case research are any less generalisable than findings
from between-group research. In fact, because of the type of interven-
tions studied in single-case research, the case is sometimes made that
the results may be more generalisable than those obtained in between-
group research.

(Kazdin 1982: 288)

A major check on results, in single-case research as in any other, is replication – doing the job again. In probability terms, if the probability of a
chance result is low when you do the research once, then the chances multiply when you do it twice and get the same result. The chance of drawing
the King of Spades from the pack once is 1 in 52. The chances of doing so
twice are 1 in $52 \times 52 = 2704$ – vanishingly small. Where there are doubts of
generalizability and of control of sporadic variation, as in single-case
designs, replication becomes particularly important. It is for this reason
that the ABAB design is seen as basic to single-case research – it builds in
one automatic replication on the same case. Partial and systematic replication may be used to explore conceptually distinct aspects of the original
successful treatment, by varying aspects of the original 'package' systematically in subsequent cases.

Replication can be accomplished in different ways depending on the
precise aspect of generality in which the investigator is interested. To
investigate generality across subjects, the investigator can conduct a
direct replication . . . applying the same procedures across a number of
different subjects. To evaluate the generality of findings across a
variety of different conditions . . . the investigator can conduct a systematic replication . . . purposely allowing features of the original
experiment to vary . . . Actually, direct and systematic replications are
not qualitatively different. An exact replication is not possible in principle since repetition of the experiment involves new subjects tested at
different points of time and perhaps by different investigators . . . all
replications necessarily allow some factors to vary.

(Kazdin 1982: 284)

Exercise 32: Planning a single-case experimental design

Develop a plan for research into the treatment of obesity in a single
patient. How would you demonstrate validity, reliability and
generalizability? What modifications might you need to make to render
your design ethically acceptable as research?
   There are no right answers to these questions, but our attempts at
them may be found at the end of the chapter.

Quasi-experimental logic

A sure way of getting over most ethical problems with experimental research is the **natural experiment** or **quasi-experimental** comparison (the **case-control study** of medical research). Here what you do is to take a change which is being imposed anyway and collect or obtain statistics from before the change, during it and after it. These are treated as the 'pre-test' and 'post-test' statistics of the true experiment. You can generally organize some kind of control or comparison group as well: a similar area in which the change is not occurring, for example. A classic example is the Connecticut Crackdown, a change in motoring laws in one American state which was aimed at decreasing traffic fatalities. A team of researchers looked at the changes it made to fatality statistics by comparing figures from before the changes of law and practice to figures from after it (Campbell and Ross 1968; Ross and Campbell 1968; Campbell 1969). They controlled for extraneous events by comparing surrounding states, where these changes had not been made, and found that fatalities did not decrease similarly over the same period. The argument that it was the changes in law and practice which brought about the change in death-rate is, therefore, fairly convincing, and the logic of the argument follows the argument of an experiment. Its weakness, however, is that the design is not experimental in that there is no control over allocation to experimental and control groups. However carefully the two are matched, it is always possible to argue that there may be some unobserved difference between the two which is responsible for the results.

Finally, two points which we have made earlier in the book are worth repeating here, because they have implications for your own design of research:

1 The basic purpose of many pieces of **survey** research is quasi-experimental comparison – looking for the association of one variable with another, with the intention of arguing about causal influence. This is why it is so important to pre-guess alternative explanations and collect variables relevant to them, to be able to eliminate them by statistical control at the analysis stage.

2 On the other hand, many studies which masquerade as true experiments are at best quasi-experimental, because there is no true control over allocation to groups. Experiments comparing males and females, for example, are at best quasi-experimental: there may be characteristics contingently associated with gender but not central to its definition – such as experience of early socialization, for example, or outright discrimination and stereotyping in adult life – which are confounded with gender itself and cannot be eliminated by any kind of random allocation. The same holds true for experiments comparing clinical types, or different types of offender, or any experiments where the allocation to groups rests in essence on a 'naturally' occurring difference.

Summary

1 The simplest kind of 'experimental' research which you can do, which we have called 'the uncontrolled trial' involves making a change and looking to see what follows. This is badly flawed as a design, because it does not compare the outcome with the 'state of play' *before* the change was made, so it is not possible to say with certainty that any change *did* occur.

2 A true experiment (or 'controlled trial') involves measurement before the change, the imposition of a change on one group but not another, measurement after the change, and so a demonstration that a difference occurred as a result of the change in the group which was 'treated' but not in the other group. If the two groups differed in nothing except the experimental treatment, then this design is a very strong demonstration of the causal effect of the treatment.

3 Clear and unambiguous measurement of **independent variable** (treatment), **dependent variables** (effects) and other variables on which the groups might have differed before or during treatment is essential for this kind of research.

4 It is possible to run experiments on single cases. They generally involve repeated measurements and the imposition of one or more treatments according to a controlled and logical pattern.

5 There are often very serious ethical problems involved in experimental research, to do with the manipulation of subjects against their interests or the withholding of treatment from some subjects in order to form a control group.

6 Quasi-experimental analysis can be carried out with a similar degree of rigour in logic and measurement on changes which are occurring 'naturally' in the world. This avoids many of the ethical problems of the experiment. It is never possible, however, to demonstrate with rigour that it was the treatment and not something else which produced the effect.

Further reading

Breakwell, Glynnis, Foot, Hugh and Gilmour, Robin (eds) (1982) *Social Psychology: A Practical Manual*. London: Macmillan/British Psychological Society.

Hakim, Catherine (1987) *Research Design: Strategies and Choices in the Design of Social Research*. London: Routledge (Chapter 9).

Hersen, Michael and Barlow, David (1976) *Single-case Experimental Designs*. Oxford: Pergamon.

Kazdin, Alan (1982) *Single-case Research Designs*. Oxford: Oxford University Press.

Polgar, Stephen and Thomas, Shane (1988) *Introduction to Research in the Health Sciences*. London: Churchill Livingstone.

Witts, L.J. (ed.) (1964) *Medical Surveys and Clinical Trials*. London: Oxford University Press.

Answer to Exercise 32

What you would do here depends crucially on your theoretical stance. If you are taking a behavioural stance to the problem, you would be focusing on overeating as a set of habits and looking for weight reduction via control of eating or control of circumstances in which eating takes place. Your 'treatment' might involve making the person aware of how much he or she eats, and how often, by getting him or her to keep a 'food diary' and even perhaps to weigh all food before eating. It might involve a controlled diet, to reaccustom the stomach to being less distended. It might involve identifying the circumstances under which the person 'snacks' and getting him or her to avoid those circumstances, or substituting another activity – walking, listening to music – for the snacking. If you take a more **holistic** stance you might be looking more to underlying factors which initiate the overeating – depression or over-strain or some idea of making oneself more or less attractive for some at most half-admitted purpose. Then your treatment might involve counselling – to attack the feelings and self-judgements directly – and an attempt to rearrange the person's life to make it more rewarding or to substitute other rewards for the rewards of eating.

Whichever, the first stage would have to be a very thorough investigation of the existing situation – how heavy the person is and how the weight fluctuates, what is eaten and when, what the person does during the day, with whom (and with what success) he or she interacts, what demands are placed on him or her, perhaps his or her self-image and beliefs about the self, and his or her feelings and beliefs about food and eating. A goal would be formulated in terms of weight loss and perhaps a change in patterns of social interaction. (The goals would have to be formulated in collaboration with the client – ethically because it is his or her body and his or her life, and practically because the client would be the one actually to 'apply the treatment'.) You would arrange for the client to keep records during the treatment, and times would be assigned for you to visit again to collect information yourself. At regular intervals you would monitor the achievement of the goals and decide whether to discontinue the 'treatment', to continue with it or to change it, and to see whether other problems emerged apart from the one you were 'treating'. At the end, after treatment is discontinued, you would continue to monitor for a while, to ensure that progress was maintained.

You would deliberately alternate periods of treatment and non-treatment – return to previous behaviour – to establish convincingly that it was the treatment that produced the effect. You might well feel that this kind of experiment, with its deliberate reversions to the untreated condition, was not an ethically justified way of proceeding against any problem which really mattered to the client, whether or not consent and collaboration was achieved.

OPEN INTERVIEWING

This chapter deals with the conduct of 'open' or 'unstructured' interviews with groups of people. You might be interviewing simply to find out people's views on a topic or a service, not knowing enough in advance to put together a structured **questionnaire**. (Indeed, a short phase of open interviewing is a normal precursor to constructing a questionnaire – 'mapping the ground', finding out the range of views and topics which should be covered, learning the language in which informants are likely to express themselves.) You might be exploring a topic where it is desirable not to introduce previous theory, but to 'let the participants speak for themselves'. Much feminist work is of this kind, trying not to apply preconceived (and male-conceived) categories to women's lives, but talking to them to see what they think is important and how they understand their world. You might be carrying out an evaluation of a setting or of a service you have been providing, and need to get at how the clients and staff have experienced it without letting your own or management's preconceptions intrude. You might be doing something much less structured – talking to groups of people in categories of interest, just to understand their lives and how they make sense of them.

'Open interviewing' is not one method, but our term for a range of different ways of proceeding. They have in common:

1 the aim of eliciting the informants' views in the informants' own terms;
2 the attempt to make the interviews resemble natural conversations as far as possible;
3 the desire to impose as little as possible of the researchers' ideas on the conversation.

While agreeing on these aims, however, interviewers have differed a great deal over how to pursue them. Some interviews are virtually undirected by the researcher, with the informant controlling most of the direction of the conversation. In others the interviewers take more control, trying to cut through 'irrelevance' and 'keeping the informant to the point'. Most interviewers go in with an outline 'agenda', but for some this consists only of a list of topic areas to cover and a few 'stock questions' to get things started and bridge gaps in the conversation. In other cases, however, the researcher may have a quite detailed list of questions to ask of all informants and may even try to determine the order in which they are answered. Mostly, we adopt a 'neutrally sympathetic' manner when interviewing, but in some research (e.g. on managers of large corporations) the researchers have thought it appropriate to adopt an adversarial style and provoke an argument in order to test the informants' beliefs. All of these are valid ways of doing interview research, and each has its strengths and corresponding weaknesses. On the whole, the more structured the approach, the less the **naturalism** and the more the danger of attributing the researchers' ideas to the informants. On the other hand, structure makes for uniformity of coverage and so for more interpretable data.

After an initial section on kinds of design for interview projects we work backwards in this chapter, from the nature of the work to the ways in which it is conducted. What kind of an exercise you think you are undertaking – what model you hold of the informants and their social world – shapes not only the analysis of the data, but also the conduct of the interviews and the way the study is initially planned, so this is considered first. Thereafter, we talk about the conduct of interviews, about gaining access to informants and about the selection of informants.

Life-history interviews and comparative interviewing

One form of open interviewing is the 'life-history interview', where you pick a single informant and interview repeatedly, exploring the whole of his or her life. You would start off in a comparatively non-directive fashion – perhaps making sure that each segment of the life was covered, and redirecting the informant from what were obviously long and non-productive detours, but otherwise asking little except 'What happened next?' In later interviews you might want to clarify the earlier ones – we are all sometimes inconsistent and even inaccurate in detailing our past lives, and the 'outside eye' of an interviewer can often help to clarify chronology – and to feed back reports of later judgements which are formally inconsistent with reports of earlier ones (as where a particular person is reported as untrustworthy in describing an early stage of life but as a friend in a later one or vice versa). In still later interviews you will be questioning expressed value judgements, to make sure you understand them and their limitations, and posing formal inconsistencies as questions for the informant to rethink. In later interviews again you might be posing the questions which matter to you as a researcher/practitioner.

Life-history interviewing allows a considerable penetration into informants' lives as they see them and gives access to the unobservable past (though necessarily refocused through the lens of the present – present views and concerns shape our memories and our understanding of our own past lives). Most open interviewing contains some element of life-history work; it is a very good technique for getting people talking about their lives in their own words and concepts, without imposing the views and concepts of the researcher. However, a single informant is a limited field for generalization, and most open interviewing involves interviews with a larger number – perhaps ten or 20 informants. With larger numbers it is possible to introduce a comparative element, comparing the views of women with men, for example, or practitioners with patients, or those to whom some event has happened with otherwise similar people to whom it has not. This kind of comparison draws on the same logic as that of the **experiment** and is essential for bounded generalization. You cannot, for example, say what is true of women as opposed to men – how the genders differ – from interviews with women alone; you need a basis of comparison.

Open interviewing of one informant or groups of informants is the approach which you would undoubtedly use if your field of study were not already well researched, or if you were unhappy with the research and theorization which dominated the field so far. It allows you to carry out research which is **holistic** and comparatively unfocused. That is, it does not focus in on variables, but tries for a complete description of the person's life and how he or she sees the social world. Within this description you hope to find your 'problem' – health attitudes, or growing old and coping, or dealing with heart disease in the family – located and intermeshed with all the other aspects of life and relationship. (If not, a bit of judicious probing will undoubtedly allow you to trace out the relationships.) Even if you propose a **survey** or **experiment** at a later date, in an ill-explored field you would undoubtedly start with some form of open, qualitative interviewing, and life-history interviewing is the form which imposes least structure and preconception on the informant.

It may also be a relevant way of conducting research into practice. What we have talked about so far are treatment-oriented techniques of differing degrees of **reductionism** and quantitative complexity. Another kind of evaluation of the service you are providing, however, stands back from immediate detail and tries to understand the client's or patient's life as a whole, with your treatment-oriented concerns fading to become just one part, and perhaps not a very large part. Understanding maternity, or old age, or chronic disability or the problems of those caring for sick or disabled dependants might best be approached by this means. It might also give you a better perspective than more focused evaluation on whether the service you provide is effective, or relevant, or even noticed particularly by the informant. More focused evaluation techniques can explore treatment packages and service provision in the terms in which you conceive them, but to explore their place in the informant's life you need the more open and less prestructured approach which open interviewing can offer.

The disadvantage – or indeed, perhaps the advantage – of this approach to understanding the informant's life is that it is almost entirely retrospective. You are asking the informant to tell the story of his or her life from now backwards, or from the beginning until now, but in either case it will be told as it makes sense now. It will be an account from the point of view of the present, weighted according to present concerns and structured to make sense of the present. The informant may on occasion be able to report that 'things seemed different then', but even this is an account of past feeling structured from the point of view of the present. The disadvantage, as with all accounts, is that the past will be 'constructed' to make sense. (This is not because it is the past, but because what we have is an account; an account of the present would be similarly constructed to make sense.) The advantage is that what we learn is not an array of dispassionate 'facts', but that way of structuring the informant's past which demonstrates (or conceals, but makes available for discovery) its impact on present life and attitudes.

Exercise 33: Life history and comparative interviewing

If you were exploring the theme of obesity, how would you go about conducting a life-history interview to cast light on the topic? What sort of person would you want as informant? How would you approach the task and structure the series of interviews? Under what circumstances might the outcome be relevant for professional practice?

What could a series of comparative interviews tell you that life-history interviewing of a single informant could not? Where might the life-history interviews be *more* informative?

Our attempts at answers are at the end of the chapter.

The nature of the data

At its simplest, the open interview is a way of finding out what people *think* about a situation. With the minimum of imposed structure necessary to keep the focus of the interview within bounds and save ourselves the time involved in listening to totally extraneous material, we let people talk about the situation and what matters to them about it. This is by far the best way of finding out what is *salient* to them about it – what most readily springs to their lips. With a little probing to get them to assess which ideas matter and which are just 'tried on' to see how well they hold together in the interview situation, we can assess what is *central* – what they see as the irreducible core of their beliefs. We would probably impose an agenda of areas to be covered, so that we can be sure all informants have covered the same ground. We should be careful how we used such an agenda, however, or our introduction of particular topics could obscure whether they were, in fact, salient for the particular informant; once we have introduced a topic, we can no longer tell whether it would have cropped up spontaneously in the course of the interview.

An alternative view of how people work and make sense of their world is to see them as not always aware of what is important to them. If we want to know what the informant *feels* – what motivates his or her behaviour, whether or not he or she is aware of it or able (or willing) to mobilize it in conversation – then we must see our task in a rather different way. People may well have a set of well articulated views – a 'rhetoric' – which are strongly held and firmly believed, but their actual behaviour and the decisions they make may sometimes suggest to the outsider a quite different set

of norms and values. For example, the more educated respondents generally have a clear and consistent set of beliefs to enunciate about social class,
the structure of society and their place in it. When it comes to asking them
about the detail of their lives, however – which schools their children go to
and why they are 'good' or 'bad', which areas they see as good or bad ones
to live in and why, what kinds of job they wish for their children and why –
an equally clear set of implicit beliefs often emerges, but one which is not
consistent with their declared 'rhetorical' position. This matter of rhetoric
is an important one for open interviewing: whether we accept what the
informant says at face value, or allow that we may all have sets of verbal
beliefs which are sincerely held but which may not be the unifying principles behind our practical actions.

If you hold this view of how people work in the social world, then you
will be imposing a little more structure on the occasion than if you just
accept what informants say at face value. You will be introducing questions, and areas of discussion, precisely in order to 'get underneath' the
rhetoric and see what you can elicit about the less formally organized and
recognized structuring principles which people apply to the social world
when making their practical decisions. Doing so, however, will face you
with the ethical question of the extent to which you are prepared to 'lead
informants on' in order to elicit from them material which it is your intention to interpret in ways which might well offend them.

Now suppose that what you are trying to find out is what the informants
want done about a situation – how to solve a problem which has occurred, or
how to improve an institutional setting, say. A mixture of these two models
would undoubtedly be what is appropriate. You would be required and
require yourself to represent faithfully the views which the participants
had expressed. At the same time you might suspect that the immediate
focus of complaint was not really 'what was wrong', and so you would be
looking beyond and underneath their 'rhetoric' for more nebulous features
of their situation which might be at fault. If you were playing your research
to any extent **collaboratively** – as seems wise and reasonable, if there were
any chance of your 'solution' being foisted on the informants – then you
would want to discuss your eventual conclusions with them and reshape
them to reflect their reactions (perhaps several times, until you found a set
of recommendations and a form of words for expressing them which was
acceptable to all parties). Given courage, you might even discuss your conclusions about particular interviews with the individual participants,
before coming to a public set of general conclusions. This would take
courage, however, if you had presumed to any extent to 'see behind the
words' and draw conclusions on the basis of knowing better than the
informant what was important in his or her life.

Doing the interviews

The core of the open style of interviewing is a very lively appreciation of how
you are trying to present yourself and the task, and the way in which the
informant is making sense of the task and of you (in a word, **reflexivity**).

Right from the start of any such project you would be watching carefully whether you 'came across' in your professional identity (social worker, nurse, doctor), or as a student, or as a researcher perhaps associated with an academic institution, or as someone writing a book, or whatever. You will be monitoring carefully the impression you give of the task – whether it is a student exercise, or the gratification of your own curiosity, or an academic investigation, or a study of shortcomings that might perhaps be put right as a result of it. Who you are and what the task is seen to be is all the informants have out of which to make sense of the exercise, and what sense they make will crucially determine what kind of an account they give of the phenomena in which you are interested.

Your choice of location for the interview (if you have a choice!) will be governed by the principle of naturalism: you will try to put yourself and the interview in a 'frame' which might be a natural one for the informant. For many purposes the informant's own home may be the best setting – putting oneself in the territory of the other – but there are circumstances where the home might be the wrong context. Talking to people about their work, for instance, it may be better to talk at the workplace or, better still, wherever they go to relax after work sessions – the canteen, the staff room, the local public house. There may be circumstances where the interview is best conducted on your own territory – in your office, or at the hospital bedside – but this will generally be appropriate only if you normally ask questions or have conversations with that informant in that setting. Best of all, if you are doing more than one interview with the same person, may be to vary the setting and take note of the different shades of perspective which are expressed in the different settings.

In the interview itself you will be trying to present yourself as friendly but neutral, as someone not intimately involved in any disputes or differences of interest which may be mentioned. If the conversation is to be at all natural and relaxed you will have to say a bit about yourself and to contribute opinions to the flow of the occasion. To the extent that it is possible, however, you will avoid doing so – even if you are adopting a collaborative stance and interviewing for a declared and agreed purpose. It is all too easy, reading the transcript of an interview after the event, to see where opinions or categorizations of your own have been taken up and incorporated by the informant, so that you cannot tell whether they are part of the way in which the informant sees the world or on loan from the interviewer. It is regrettably all too easy to express your own attitude to a situation and have the respondent agree with you – perhaps out of conviction, but perhaps out of politeness or a desire to adopt a 'socially desirable point of view'. Insofar as is possible, in a situation which can only be what it is because of your participation in it, you must avoid these forms of **reactivity** by contributing as little as you can; it is the informant whose views and feelings you want to collect, not your own. To the extent that detachment is not possible, you must try to be aware of your own contribution, take notes on it immediately afterwards, and if necessary report on it in your account of the findings.

Before entering the field you will have taken the opportunity to read as much as you can about the background and circumstances of the people whom you will be interviewing. If you are to be working in a hospital, you will read anything that has been written on that hospital or that class of hospitals, including what is said about it in Parliament and in the newspapers, to get a feel for the 'working rules' and the declared aims, and to be aware of any outstanding problems (e.g. financial). If you are interviewing a particular class of professional staff, you will scan their professional journals for articles expressing their problems and discontents and for what you can find on the letter page. If you are talking to a group of people who have a given medical condition, you will familiarize yourself with the literature on that condition. If you are talking to people who fall in a 'social problem' category, you will make sure you are familiar with the benefits and services available to such a group. When you go into the field you will want to be as well informed as possible, so that you do not miss veiled allusions to common features of the situation and so that you are aware of any glaring omissions in participants' accounts.

On the other hand, you will want to conceal your knowledge as far as possible. The correct role for the qualitative researcher has often been described as that of the 'amiable incompetent' – someone friendly and intelligent but lacking knowledge, someone who has to be *told* things. (This may pose ethical problems, when for instance you know of some benefit or service to which the informant is entitled, but which he or she has not claimed. Try to restrict the information which you yourself communicate to the end of interviews, so as not to contaminate the material you collect or to 'break role' more than is necessary.)

Two particular problems arise when you are yourself a known 'expert', e.g. a health visitor interviewing other health visitors. The first is that it is difficult to get your informants to 'spell things out', because they assume you must know all about it already. The other and more serious is that you will find it difficult to put aside your professional socialization and 'make the familiar strange' – to ask your informants to spell out what they mean rather than filling in the gaps from your own knowledge. This matters because your knowledge may, in fact, be faulty: informants may not mean what you take for granted that they mean, and they may not have shared precisely your professional experience.

How much you ask direct questions will depend on the time available and the subject of the interview. To get the best out of this approach you will want at least some early portion of the interview to be conducted in a fairly undirected fashion, letting the informant develop things at his or her pace and seeing what crops up without prompting. To be sure you have covered the topic which is of interest to you in enough detail that you can be sure of doing justice to your informant's views, however, you may have to resort to direct prompting, to explore topic areas that have not come up by themselves. Remember, however, that once a topic has been introduced by you, you can never know whether it would have come up spontaneously. Best practice if time permits might be to have more than one interview with each informant and to save direct prompts for later ones; then you could also introduce questions on views and topic areas which had not come up in the particular interview but *had* been raised by another informant.

much detail as possible and 'surface' any possible contradictions in the informant's map of the world. This has the strengths of detail and thoroughness, but the weakness that it is restricted to one or a few informants and therefore difficult to generalize.

3 Similar methods may be used, with larger numbers, to compare groups and learn from the comparisons.

4 The purpose of such interviews is to get as close to a natural situation as can be achieved in what is patently a research situation, and this guides the manner in which the interviews are conducted.

5 The interpretation of open interview data is not simple but depends on taking a theoretical stance as to the relationship between what people say – in particular situations, in response to particular questions – and what they know, believe, feel and have experienced.

Further reading

Burgess, Robert (1984) *In the Field*. London: Allen and Unwin.

Hammersley, Martyn and Atkinson, Paul (1995) *Ethnography: Principles in Practice* (2nd edition). London: Routledge.

McCracken, Grant (1988) *The Long Interview*. Beverly Hills, CA: Sage.

Patton, Michael (1987) *How to Use Qualitative Methods in Evaluation*. Beverly Hills, CA: Sage.

Answers to Exercises

Exercise 33

Here you would be trying for a broad descriptive focus on the person's life. You would not be working towards 'treatment' at this time – except insofar as the mere act of researching a problem and taking an interest in those who suffer from it has a therapeutic effect in itself, something which has often been found. You would start by getting the informant talking about his or her childhood in general terms, probably, and lead steadily up to the present day and plans for the future. On the way through you would be taking note of anything that emerged about food, meals, poverty, attractiveness or other potentially related topics, but you would probably leave it fairly late in the series of interviews to introduce these deliberately as topics for discussion. At the end you might well find clues as to treatment for this informant or similar informants, in general. For example, using the more structured approach of the Role Repertory Grid, Fay Fransella has examined groups of obese people and also groups of stutterers, eliciting their pictures of themselves and key others in their lives, and also their picture of people who are obese or who stutter (the work is described in Bannister and Fransella 1980). The most interesting thing is that the people with the 'problem' had a quite clear picture of the kind of person who had that problem, but they did not describe themselves in those terms. It was as though, for example, the world were divided into obese people and others, and some of the 'others' (including the informant) happened to eat rather a lot.

The major drawback of the single-case life history is obviously that it *is* based on a single case. However **typical** you may suppose the informant to be, you cannot generalize from one case to a population except very tentatively. You cannot tell from the single case, for example, whether there is a single basis to obesity or whether a typology of different reasons for being obese or different roles of eating in people's lives might be more appropriate. Moreover, you do not have the power which a comparative design offers of learning from comparisons – comparing obese people with others who are not, comparing both with people who used to be obese but have lost weight, and so on. (You can do a little comparative work on the single case, however, by comparing current views with what they say about the time before they became obese – bearing in mind that the past is reconstructed here in the light of the present, and in the light of the 'demand characteristics' of the interview.)

The *strength* of the life-history approach is its sheer detail and the exhaustive nature of the interviewing. You have time, when dealing with a single case or a very small number of cases, to get as much detail as is available about everything which is of interest to you. Further, you go on interviewing till all the possible contradictions have emerged and been resolved or at least discussed, and until nothing further of use appears to be emerging ('theoretical saturation').

Exercise 34

When one of us (Abbott) undertook this kind of research, she conceptualized the purpose as 'to see how health visitors made sense of their professional role', in the light of literature which suggested that they themselves were uncertain about their role and its relationship to social work on the one hand and nursing on the other. She discussed what she intended with the Senior Lecturer in Health Studies responsible for health visiting courses in the institution where she worked as a lecturer. The Senior Lecturer gave her the names of the nurse managers in charge of health visiting in the three health districts for which training in health visiting was provided by the institution. Abbott wrote to each of these, enclosing a copy of her research proposal and asking if they would be willing to give her access to the health visitors working under them. Each of them wrote back and suggested that she went to see them; she did so, and each agreed to her request. In each district the nurse manager provided her with the names and telephone numbers of health visitors working in different settings (rural, urban, working-class or middle-class areas) and with greater or less professional experience. She contacted selected ones and explained what she wanted, and all agreed to participate.

She carried out interviews with health visitors at their place of work. Each interview lasted between 1 and $1\frac{1}{2}$ hours. Beforehand, she prepared a list of topic areas she wanted to cover, to act as an *aide mémoire*, but the basic approach was life-history interviewing: she started by asking each informant why she had decided to train as a health visitor, and from this got them talking generally about their work and their professional careers. After each of the interviews she went out with each health visitor for a half or a whole day, **observing** what they did with 'cases' and talking to them further. This was to give her a greater familiarity with what health visitors actually do and an opportunity to chart their day-to-day work.

This research was very much centred on health visitors' conceptions of their own roles. If the researcher had been more interested in organizational constraints and/or official goals, she would have interviewed more senior staff. If the focus had been organization at the local level, a better approach might have been to concentrate on certain 'patches' and try to interview doctors, practice nurses, midwives, etc., as well as health visitors (and perhaps social workers – particularly if she had wanted to explore questions of the mistreatment of children). With a focus on whether health visitors deliver what their clients want, interviews with the clients themselves would have been indispensable.

ANALYSING TEXT

This chapter is concerned mostly with the analysis of qualitative data: **field notes** from **participant observation**, notes on qualitative interviews, audio tapes or secondary textual sources – diaries, newspapers, articles, historical documents and so on. All of these may be seen in some sense as 'text' – verbal material not structured for the purposes of the research as is the output of a **survey** or an **experiment**, but awaiting such structure as you can impose on it or draw out of it. Qualitative data, even more than quantitative, do not speak for themselves, however much they may appear to do so; they need to be analysed. (Text may also be analysed by quantitative methods – measuring the frequency of occurrence of a topic or a concept or a word, or the space given to it in a report, or in some other way reducing the complexity of the material to analysable numbers.) In this chapter we shall talk about the descriptive use of qualitative materials, about **holistic** analysis in terms of 'cases', and about analyses in terms of the detailed content of interviews or documents. These forms of analysis blur into each other, as we shall see, but it is useful to separate them out and consider them separately here.

The first step is to get the material into a form in which it can be ordered and analysed. Tapes need to be transcribed, for example – or if you do not have the time for this (an hour's interview takes several hours to transcribe) then you at least need to take detailed notes from the tapes, plus an index of what is where (by noting the counter reading on your tape recorder which corresponds with each topic). You will need to work out a system for locating material – perhaps case numbers or day records, page numbers within them, and line numbers within the pages – so that it is possible to locate particular references easily at a later stage. You will need to read all the material you have collected, to familiarize yourself fully with it and form a tentative overall impression of it. You need also to establish a filing system. This may be physical: storing relevant material together in one place, such as a series of clearly labelled envelopes or wallet files. In this case you will need multiple copies of all your material, as some of it may well need to be stored under a number of different headings. Alternatively, your filing system may be indexical – you may 'store' references in the form of location indicators, on file cards or on the computer. (Indexical 'storage' is easier in the early stages, involving less physical transfer of material, but physical means of storage are far less trouble when it comes time to write up, as you have your source material already segmented and organized into 'sets'. However, some computerized analysis packages – for example, NUD.IST – offer the advantages of both approaches.)

The amount of data that you will have collected may well be vast, and you may feel that it is a daunting task that faces you. The first thing to do is to focus down and remind yourself <u>what the purpose of your inquiry was</u>, <u>what you were interested in finding out</u>. You will then realize that quite a lot of the material you have collected is not relevant to this. It may be interesting in its own right, and you may want to keep it to analyse at some time in the future, but it is not needed for your immediate purposes. When we interviewed mothers whose children had learning difficulties, for example, one copy of the transcribed interviews filled six or eight box files. A relatively small amount of that was relevant to what we were originally investigating: the load on the mother as compared with mothers of 'unlabelled' children, and the social and self-stigmatizing that occurred (Abbott and Sapsford 1987b, among other reports). More detailed material from a few particularly interesting 'cases' yielded another paper, on the *diversity* of mothers' experiences (Abbott and Sapsford 1986). The rest sits in the cupboard, brought out only for teaching examples, until such time as one of us wants to use it for another purpose, perhaps some kind of analysis of socialization and growing up, as we elicited the women's life histories as well as their current circumstances.

Qualitative description

Much of your material will be descriptive – describing situations and events – and you will want to use it in writing a descriptive account in your final report. <u>Description could be a main purpose of your research</u>. For example, in some research on evaluating Enterprise in Higher Education (EHE) which one of us (Abbott) carried out, the report on qualitative evaluation of individual enterprise programmes requires that there be a description of the programme, including the aims and objectives of its leaders, what they did and what the outcomes were. The descriptive material may itself begin the analysis by the way it is ordered under headings – e.g. in the EHE example, the programme as a whole and individual programmes as broad headings, and relevant sub-headings within each broad category. <u>(You will find that much of the work of qualitative analysis involves sorting into hierarchical categories, in one way or another.)</u> Careful reading of your data and thinking about what 'story' your report is to tell will enable you to decide on relevant sub-headings. All of the material for the descriptive account can be collected together and put in a file or series of envelopes labelled 'descriptive material'.

Under some circumstances it may be relevant to work through each case or setting or visit or whatever in some detail, organizing the material under relevant sub-headings. For example, if you had life-history data on a person, you could separate the purely descriptive material from the rest and organize it chronologically and under separate headings – e.g. 'childhood relations with parents', 'education' . . . Even where this is not a relevant way of proceeding, however, it is good practice to write brief notes telling the story of each case – summarizing in a few sentences what the informant has to say about himself or herself, his or her life and the topics which are of particular interest to you, or what the significance of the setting or programme appeared to be to you and to the participants. (This may also allow your **reflexive** notes about particular data-collection sessions to have some impact on the analysis.) You may never use these overall summary accounts in your written report, but they will help to shape your analysis, and comparing them across cases may allow interesting patterns to emerge. They are also a good early point of the analysis at which to think about the informant as a whole person. (Note, however, that a proportion of published research on medicine, psychotherapy, counselling and social work draws on this kind of impressionistic material – 'case notes' – as a prime source, treating it as factual rather than as field notes of a process of participant observation and failing to acknowledge the role of the researcher/practitioner in the construction of the data.)

Case analysis

Qualitative analysis which goes beyond description consists essentially of the processes of sorting, comparing/contrasting and consolidating. Most of what follows involves, in one way or another, sorting cases or propositions or utterances or words into categories such that the members resemble each other and differ from other categories in ways which are of interest to the researcher.

The simplest form of such analysis is 'impressionistic' case analysis, sorting cases into 'heaps' which have something in common which they do not share with other cases. This is what we did at one stage of the analysis of the interviews with mothers of children with learning difficulties. We read through the transcripts of interviews and formed impressions about the mothers who were speaking, holistically rather than on the basis of any particular detailed feature of what was said. On this basis we sorted mothers (families) into those who effectively denied that a problem existed, those who acknowledged that a problem existed and were trying to cope with it (distinguishing between those who had some expressed long-term strategy and those who appeared to be keeping their heads above water on a more day-to-day basis), and those who had managed to reconstruct the situation as one with positive advantages. This kind of analysis is faithful to the data in the sense that it draws on the interview material and uses it as a basis for classification. It is obviously also open, however, to being very strongly influenced by the researchers' previous ideas, because there are no rigorous criteria for determining what the categories shall be, other than the impressions of the researchers.

More rigorous analysis involves more detailed examination of categories within interviews, rather than just comparison between cases, as we shall see. Even so, however, you ought to return to the holistic consideration of cases at some point of the analysis. In writing up your analysis you will want to give more detailed accounts of a subset of cases – possibly to illustrate different categories or types that you have 'discovered' in your research. For example, in the EHE research the final report could include a detailed analysis of a small number of programmes as examples illustrating the range and the kinds of enterprise they represent. Alternatively, the cases could be selected to illustrate successful and unsuccessful programmes or to illustrate the types of problems encountered by programme leaders in implementing the programmes, and/or students, and/or collaborating employers. All the material relevant to each of the cases needs to be collected together – one file or envelope per case or one index entry.

Content analysis

In your subsequent analysis and write-up of these cases you would look for similarities and differences between them. This is the main process of bringing order to the material, organizing it into patterns, categories and descriptive units. It is now possible to purchase computer programs that can assist in the content analysis of qualitative data, but most of us still have to do some or all of it by hand. Content analysis needs to be done on all the data, including material which you have already sorted out to use for description or as illustrative cases.

The first step is to look for all concepts and make an index of them. A computer qualitative analysis program will do this for you, as indeed will some word-processing packages. Using such a program, you would need to look at its output, eliminate the very rare concepts (after looking to see where they occurred, in case they were important) and grouping others together because they clearly expressed similar ideas even if different words were used. If you have to do it by hand you need to re-read every bit of the data, noting down all the categories that are relevant to the purpose of your analysis – and probably some that do not seem relevant at present, but might seem so at a later stage. First you would look across the paragraphs to see what overall topic areas came up – work, home, geographical area and its significance, the children and so on. Each of these may want breaking down further: children's health, the children's school as a place, the children's school performance as a measure of their worth, sports activities and so on. Finally, you might still want or need to do a full textual analysis, looking for every descriptive category the informant uses (in which case you might seriously consider whether you can get hold of computer assistance).

As a brief example of this kind of content analysis, consider the following short extract from one of our interviews with a mother whose child had learning difficulties:

RJS: What was Wyvern like when you first came here?

Mrs Weaver: It's built up a lot since we first came here. It used very, very quiet, very quiet.

RJS: Did you have this house then?

Mrs Weaver: No we lived in Dunstone Estate when we first mo here . . . and then we moved up here. A very frien place, I think, Wyvern . . . It's nice. And everybody accepted Carl [mentally handicapped son], that's wha we like. In a normal way.

In this brief extract we can see a number of 'place' references qualified by adjectives – 'quiet' (as a term of approval), 'friendly', 'nice'. The topic of the mentally handicapped son has also come up, leading to concepts of 'accepting' (by people around) and 'in a *normal* way'. Another person might characterize the same place as 'quiet' (in a pejorative sense), 'nosy', 'dull'. Contrasting people who look at it in the one light or the other, we might find other differences between them – in demographic characteristics, or in the way they see their mentally handicapped children as fitting into the life of the area – and we would be on the way towards model-building. Analysis proceeds by constantly comparing and contrasting interview scripts, looking for similarities and differences, and trying to find which characteristics seem to vary systematically together.

Note that there are two levels at which this kind of analysis can be carried out. On the one hand, you can categorize the material in terms of your own previous interests. In the EHE example, for instance, the categories which are likely to emerge are very likely to be conditioned by the focus of the research. If your enquiry had a wider and less directed focus – e.g. 'What is it like being a prisoner, or a patient or a mother' – then you would want to start further back, by trying to list *all* the descriptive nouns, adjectives and phrases that look even vaguely relevant to the enquiry, clustering them by similarity, and looking further at ones that are at all common or appear to express strong feeling, *before* focusing on particular questions that may be of concern to the researcher. Except where the focus of the research is very narrow and/or the interviews were very directive, the latter is probably a better procedure than the former.

When you have a list of categories you can group them into sets of similar relevance and begin to map their relationships. For example, in our research into community care for children with special learning difficulties we grouped all the concepts relating to 'husband', 'children', 'mother', 'other kin', the ones relating to 'neighbours', to 'schools' and so on. These were clusters which appeared to make sense to the informants and which made sense to us. There is no magic formula for how concepts are to be clustered – you are just looking for ones that appear to go together, express the same underlying idea or are related to the same topic sub-area. The clusters can again be grouped more broadly in further analysis – 'husband' and 'children' go together as 'nuclear family', 'mother' and 'other kin' go together as 'kin network'. At this stage, as far as is possible, the themes and categories should come from the data rather than from previous ideas – they should reflect patterns found more than patterns looked for.

Another problem even with 'open' participant research is encountered where any kind of power relationship is involved – where the setting in which the research is being carried out involves clients or patients or pupils or inmates. Not infrequently when researchers say that they were open participants in a setting they mean that their identity was known to the professionals in it – the doctors, nurses, social workers, health visitors, teachers, prison staff. Rather less often is their presence as researchers explained or even made obvious to the patients, clients, pupils or inmates. Intimate or private aspects of clients' or pupils' lives may be reported in research which did not ask for their consent to this. It is not entirely clear, in all situations, whether asking consent would be in the patients' interests: it could distort the relationship with the professionals and interfere with the effectiveness of the service they require, if they were aware that they were under research scrutiny. However, whether participant research is ethical under such circumstances must therefore be a matter for debate. Furthermore, even where consent is given by clients or pupils or patients, it is not clear how free that consent is: where someone requires a service from a professional (as in health care) or is under a professional's authority (as in schools), it is difficult to refuse such requests.

Another problem (which applies to 'open' interviewing as well) is that the informants may not have realized the 'rules of the game' as seen by the researcher. In interviews, the informant is well aware that what is said to the tape recorder will be used for the research. He or she may not be aware that what is said 'off-stage' during coffee breaks or casual meetings will also be used. (The researcher may agree not to use material which is declared to be 'not for the tape recorder', but there is no way that he or she can *avoid* using it; it is *there*, in the researcher's mind, during the analysis, and it must necessarily shape how the formally recorded material is interpreted.) Similarly, a teacher may quite happily allow a researcher to participate in classroom sessions. He or she may not feel, however, that the contract stretches to the (inevitable) use of remarks and conversations overheard in the staffroom or even the toilets.

The overarching methodological problem with reports based on participant observation data, whether covert or overt, is the problem of **validity**: why anyone should take your word that what you claim to have seen and heard is what any other reasonable person would have extracted from the situation. Inevitably, however much you illustrate your report with quotations and extracts from field notes, the reader has to trust you to have interpreted what you saw, heard and experienced in the same way that he or she would have interpreted it. The two guarantors of validity to which you may make appeal are **triangulation** and **reflexivity.** Triangulation, a metaphor drawn from navigation, means taking more than one bearing on a point in order to locate it uniquely. In research terms it means being able to show that more than one source has been used, each with its own bias, but not necessarily the same in each case. Thus observation is supplemented with interviews, to show that what you conclude from observing behaviour is what the participants also understand by it, or at least that what you conclude makes sense to the participants. One may draw on informal conversations overheard in staffrooms, toilets, etc. to supplement formal interviews. One may look for diaries, letters, articles which participants have written for the newspapers, etc. in order to extend the range of per-spectives. Ideally, one may have more than one observer, perhaps located in different parts of the 'research field', to elicit different viewpoints and different interpretations. Each of these sources leads to an account, and no account is necessarily privileged over other accounts, but to the extent that differently based accounts appear to agree we may have more faith in the result. To the extent that they do not agree, further research may be needed before you are in a position to report.

Reflexivity is of even more importance. At every stage of the research, right from the initial introductions, you must be thinking about how the participants are making sense of you and your presence, what you are taking for granted or learning as new about them, and how what you are doing may be shaping particular pieces of data or the whole relationship between you and participants. This is important for three reasons. It acts as a form of self-monitoring, so that you can spot something going wrong and be at pains to correct it. It is, itself, a form of data analysis, one way in which you find your way through the morass of material towards the underlying model which simplifies and makes sense of what is going on. Finally, it is the basis of your self-justification in the eventual report, your way of showing that others should believe that your interpretations are reason-able ones.

Observation in the workplace

There are obvious advantages in being a 'participant observer' in your own workplace, but equally obvious disadvantages, given what we have said above. The major advantage is that you already have a natural role, the one you are carrying out in your job. There is no question of 'joining' or 'passing': you are already *in*. Equally important, at a practical level, you have no need to find your way through a maze of 'gatekeepers': you are already in the situation and can take whatever notes it pleases you to take with no need for anyone's permission. (You may find your superiors feel they should have been consulted if you ever decide to publish anything from your notes, but if what is at stake is a piece of 'internal research', examining and drawing conclusions from the practice and ethos of your unit, then no one can restrain you from doing it.) The overwhelming problem, however, is that you are a part of what you are examining. It is very difficult indeed to stand back from your normal practices and see them as anything other than the only or best way of coping with the situa-tion. It is very difficult to stand back from the normal assumptions and typifications of your trade, and see them as anything other than inevitable and sensible. (Sensible they may be, but it is a necessary part of taking the research stance that you do not regard them as inevitable but try to see them as what *happens* to be there, among the wide range of what *might* have been there.) All this may require you to put aside your own values and goals and your professional socialization; you work in a situation you may have struggled for years to make familiar, but the research requires that you stand back from it and make it strange to yourself. Most difficult of all is to put down your own automatic assumptions about what is normal, sensible, right in any given situation and ask yourself, first, whether others hold the same values and, secondly, whether what you all do may also (or instead) serve some other purpose.

A good starting-point for such research is autobiography. Spend a good period of time trying to describe your own life and values on paper, from before you ever joined the given line of work to the present day, covering what you think the job is for, what you want out of it (not necessarily the same question), where you would like to go next, what you think brings others into the job, what you think motivates them, whether it motivates you. Study this record as if it were a set of life-history interviews conducted with someone else, and analyse it for major themes; learn from these themes what your own preconceptions are likely to be. Better still – because diary-writing of this kind is still shaped by the presence of an 'other in the head', an other who looks for socially acceptable positions – get someone else to interview you and ask the questions; others can push you to clarify ideas which might seem to you self-evidently clear when you write them down. Best of all, do both – but write the autobiography before undergoing the interview, because both are fallible accounts and the power of an interviewer to make you clarify what you might otherwise have passed over is likely to affect any subsequent account that you write.

Whether working covertly or overtly, you have to be very careful about your working relationships when researching your own work setting. A clear distinction must be made here between 'research' – activities leading to a publication or a report to management or even a set of conclusions announced in public – and the monitoring of your own daily practice, and the practice of staff for whom you are responsible, which is a necessary part of most professional jobs and can benefit from the application of research techniques and the research imagination. Monitoring must be done and, therefore, should be done well. 'Research' is something undertaken additionally, and faces the ethical problems of participant research which have been discussed earlier in the chapter – problems of interfering in the working lives of colleagues and clients/patients, with or without their consent. You will necessarily find yourself asking questions which probe into a level of intimacy which may not be appropriate for the stage of acquaintanceship which you have reached. Even if you do not find people 'cooling' to your inquisitiveness, you will find yourself in possession of information which would normally be appropriate to a much closer level of intimacy than you have so far reached, because you will have paid attention to people in a way that you would not normally as part of your everyday working life. Handling this at the personal level can be a problem. In open research – or even more, in covert research when your cover is blown and people realize that you are taking notes on them – you can become labelled as a spy or a reporter, someone with whom interaction has to be very guarded.

Perhaps more difficult still is the effect of researching your own working milieu and its 'normal rules' on your relationship to your own professional practice. Our professional lives depend in large part on the values which we have incorporated, and on a set of working practices and priorities which have become largely unconscious by the time that we have become competent at our trades. To stand back and question these can be like the priest questioning his faith and his commitment to the church – once we 'make the familiar strange', it may *remain* strange, and we may not be able to find our way back to professional commitment. The methodological imagination involves a great degree of self-questioning, and those (which is most of us) who are unsure of themselves should be careful how deeply they question something as crucial to their public and private identities as their professional roles and practices.

A way round some of these problems is the **collaborative** approach. If a whole group of you get together to assess and evaluate how you do your job together, then the loneliness is dispelled, you are not faced with taking the role of the spy, and there are others with whom you can talk out personal problems that may arise in the course of the research. Three warnings, however:

1 There is no 'natural situation' for you to explore: what you have is the contrived situation of a group of people who are all committed to a programme of research and improvement, and who are all watching themselves and each other. The 'autobiography' stage, or prior interviewing of each other, is particularly important here.
2 A Hawthorne Effect, or something akin, is inevitable: what you will be exploring is not normal practice, but how practice can be improved by and during collaborative evaluation.
3 Once started, such an undertaking is difficult to stop, and the atmosphere of the unit can become very intense and critical.

Summary

1 Participant observation may be *overt* or *covert*. In the latter the researcher takes a position in the field and conceals the fact that research is going on. In the former he or she is a declared researcher but still tries to become a part of the natural life which is being observed.

2 The major advantage of covert observation is its naturalism – it disturbs the context as little as possible. It is not always easy to find a plausible role, however; there is always the danger of 'breaking cover', and data collection may be physically difficult to arrange if it is to remain concealed. There are also substantial ethical problems in invading people's lives without their knowledge or permission.

3 Overt observation avoids these problems, and it is easier for the researcher to 'move around the field' and vary methods, thereby obtaining greater coverage. However, the known presence of the researcher must have some distorting effect.

4 Observation research is not just intuitive description. The researcher builds models of what is going on and what it means to participants, and tests them through **theoretical sampling**.

5 Reflexivity is extremely important in all observation research. The researcher must be alive to all possible reactive effects, including how he

or she is received by the participants and what the nature of the research (if overt) is considered to be.

6 The observer needs to be able to 'make the familiar strange'. That is, he or she must be enough immersed in the situation and its meanings to understand it at least to some extent in the same way as the participants understand it, but sufficiently detached not to take for granted what the participants take for granted.

7 This is a particularly difficult stance to maintain when trying to carry out observation research in a setting where one is a natural participant, because one already has a role in the situation and a stake in the outcomes.

8 There are again substantial problems – both personal and ethical – with carrying out research into a context which forms part of your own life. There is great danger of violating trust, and your own relationships and taken-for-granted participation may be disturbed or fragmented.

Further reading

Burgess, Robert (1984) *In the Field*. London: Allen and Unwin.

Hammersley, Martyn and Atkinson, Paul (1995) *Ethnography: Principles in Practice* (2nd edition). London: Routledge.

Patton, Michael (1987) *How to Use Qualitative Methods in Evaluation*. Beverly Hills, CA: Sage.

Taylor, S.J. and Bogden, R. (1984) *An Introduction to Qualitative Research Methods*. Chichester: Wiley.

For a straightforward account of a piece of participant work, see:

Cavendish, Ruth (1982) *Women on the Line*. London: Routledge and Kegan Paul.

IN CONCLUSION

CIVIL HISTORIES

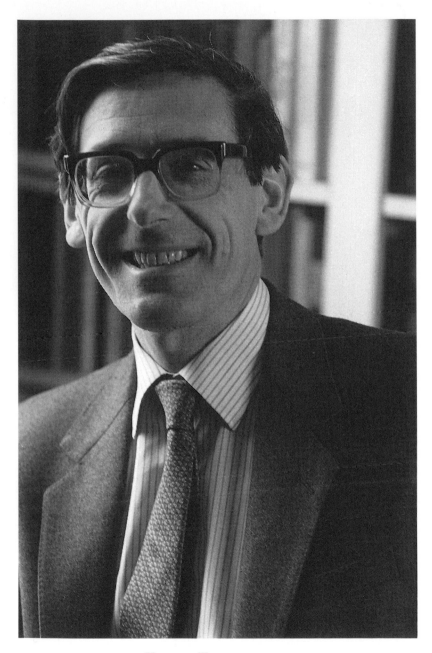

KEITH THOMAS

CIVIL HISTORIES

ESSAYS PRESENTED TO
SIR KEITH THOMAS

EDITED BY

PETER BURKE

BRIAN HARRISON

AND

PAUL SLACK

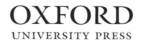

OXFORD

UNIVERSITY PRESS

OXFORD

UNIVERSITY PRESS

Great Clarendon Street, Oxford OX2 6DP

Oxford University Press is a department of the University of Oxford.
It furthers the University's objective of excellence in research, scholarship,
and education by publishing worldwide in

Oxford New York

Athens Auckland Bangkok Bogotá Buenos Aires Cape Town
Chennai Dar es Salaam Delhi Florence Hong Kong Istanbul Karachi
Kolkata Kuala Lumpur Madrid Melbourne Mexico City Mumbai Nairobi
Paris São Paulo Shanghai Singapore Taipei Tokyo Toronto Warsaw

with associated companies in Berlin Ibadan

Oxford is a registered trade mark of Oxford University Press
in the UK and in certain other countries

Published in the United States
by Oxford University Press Inc., New York

British Library Cataloguing in Publication Data

Data available

Library of Congress Cataloging in Publication Data

Civil histories: essays presented to Sir Keith Thomas / edited by
Peter Burke, Brian Harrison, and Paul Slack.
Includes index.
1. Great Britain—History—Tudors, 1485–1603. 2. Great Britain—History—Stuarts, 1603–1714.
3. Great Britain—History. I. Burke, Peter. II. Harrison, Brian Howard. III. Slack, Paul.
IV. Thomas, Keith, 1933–
DA300.C55 2000 306'.0942'09031—dc21 99–42631
ISBN 0–19–820710–7

3 5 7 9 10 8 6 4 2

Typeset by Best-set Typesetter Ltd., Hong Kong
Printed in Great Britain
on acid-free paper by
Biddles Ltd,
Guildford and King's Lynn

PREFACE

For the past forty years Keith Thomas has been one of the most innovative and influential of English historians, and his interest in manners and behaviour has been continuous. A volume of essays concerned with changing notions of civility in the past seems an appropriate way to honour him, and to mark his retirement as President of Corpus Christi College, Oxford. Although it covers only one small sector of his interests, the theme allows us to assemble chapters that have an internal coherence, and that at the same time reflect the range of his influence.

The term 'civility' (unlike 'civilization') was already in use in early modern England, and it was already diverse in its meanings. It was commonly used to denote models of social behaviour. A 'civil' person was someone who was well bred, courteous, or 'gentle'. In this sense, it was associated with the upper classes: gentlemen and gentlewomen who were of good family and at home in courts. To be civil was to be the opposite of 'wild', 'rude', or 'barbarous'. In this context, however, civility was also associated with peace, order, obedience, or 'quietness', and therefore could be widely applied. When Spenser wrote of Ireland as 'reduced to perpetual civility', he probably meant that the Irish would not rebel against their English masters. At the same time, one synonym for civility was 'policy', the two terms being derived respectively from the Latin and Greek words for 'city', with the clear implication that townspeople were better behaved, more capable of political participation, and so more human than country folk. The language of civility also implied a theory of history. Following Cicero, it was argued that humanity had once been completely wild and that it was gradually 'civilized'.

Civility was thus a flexible term, and its normative connotations have changed over time, most radically since the early nineteenth century. Some of its 'civic' content drained away and came to seem anachronistic, as the frontier between town and country disappeared. Civil behaviour became more difficult to define, as forms of political and economic association grew more complicated and more impersonal, although there was a notable reaction in the late twentieth century with the revival of interest in the 'little platoons' that form the building blocks of 'civil society'. Confidence in the distinction between civilized and savage, which underlay the pretensions of imperial expansion, waned with Romanticism and the relativism that came from social anthropology and the social sciences. Civility seems often now to denote little more than the locally defined conventions of a superficial politeness. The essays below explore some of these later shifts of meaning, as well as civility's wider implications in the early modern period.

Many scholars, in several disciplines and from all parts of the world, would have wished to participate in a volume of this kind, and would have been well qualified to do so. The book had to be kept within bounds, however, and one way of achieving this was to draw its contributors exclusively from historians who were Keith's undergraduate or graduate pupils. It is somewhat intimidating for the authors once more to be presenting essays to their mentor. Some of us still write with an imagined Keith Thomas looking over our shoulder, on the look-out for mistakes (though we take some comfort from the fact that Keith himself once confessed to writing with an imagined John Cooper looking over *his* shoulder). He will doubtless reach for his pencil while reading this volume, whether to mark typographical errors or to make penetratingly critical marginalia. All the same, we hope he will enjoy as well as appreciate our civil tribute to a remarkable historian.

U.P.B.
B.H.H.
P.A.S.

CONTENTS

LIST OF ILLUSTRATIONS

LIST OF CONTRIBUTORS

JONATHAN BARRY is Senior Lecturer in History at the University of Exeter. He has edited *The Tudor and Stuart Town* (1990), *Culture in History* (1992), *The Middling Sort of People* (1994), and *Witchcraft in Early Modern Europe* (1996), and published essays on religion, culture, and urban society in early modern England. He is completing books on Bristol and on witchcraft and demonology in the south-west.

IAN BOSTRIDGE was a British Academy Postdoctoral Research Fellow at Corpus Christi College, Oxford, where he completed his book *Witchcraft and its Transformations 1650–1750* (1997). Since 1995 he has been an opera and concert singer.

ROBIN BRIGGS is a Senior Research Fellow of All Souls College, Oxford. He is the author of *Early Modern France, 1560–1715* (1977), *Communities of Belief: Cultural and Social Tensions in Early Modern France* (1989), and *Witches and Neighbours: The Social and Cultural Context of European Witchcraft* (1996).

PETER BURKE is Professor of Cultural History, University of Cambridge, and Fellow of Emmanuel College. His books include *The Renaissance Sense of the Past* (1969), *Popular Culture in Early Modern Europe* (1978), *The Fabrication of Louis XIV* (1992), and *The European Renaissance* (1998).

EUAN CAMERON is Professor of Early Modern History in the University of Newcastle upon Tyne. He is the author of *The Reformation of the Heretics: The Waldenses of the Alps 1480–1580* (1984) and *The European Reformation* (1991), and editor of *Early Modern Europe* (1999).

BERNARD CAPP is Professor of History at the University of Warwick, and author of *The Fifth Monarchy Men* (1972), *Astrology and the Popular Press* (1979), *Cromwell's Navy* (1989), and *The World of John Taylor the Water-Poet* (1994). He is currently writing *When Gossips Meet: Women, Family and Community in Early Modern England*.

JOHN DARWIN is Beit Lecturer in the History of the British Commonwealth, University of Oxford, and Fellow of Nuffield College. He is the author of *Britain, Egypt and the Middle East: Imperial Policy in the Aftermath of War, 1918–1922* (1981), *Britain and Decolonization* (1988), and *The End of the British Empire: The Historical Debate* (1991).

LESLIE HANNAH has held posts at Oxford, Essex, Cambridge, Harvard, and the London School of Economics. His publications include *The Rise of the Corporate Economy* (1976), *Electricity before Nationalisation* (1979), *Engineers, Managers and Politicians* (1982), and *Inventing Retirement* (1986). Since 1997 he has been Dean of the City University Business School in London.

BRIAN HARRISON is Professor of Modern British History at Oxford University, and a Fellow of Corpus Christi College. His first book was *Drink and the Victorians: The Temperance Question in England 1815–1872* (1971); his latest was *The Transformation of*

British Politics 1860–1995 (1996). Editor of the *New Dictionary of National Biography*, he is also writing The New Oxford History of England's final volume (1951–90).

RALPH HOULBROOKE is Professor of Early Modern History at the University of Reading. He is the author of *Church Courts and the People during the English Reformation 1520–1570* (1979), *The English Family 1450–1700* (1984), *The English Family in Diaries 1576–1716* (1988), and *Death, Religion and the Family in England 1480–1750* (1998).

MARTIN INGRAM is Fellow, Tutor and University Lecturer in Modern History at Brasenose College, Oxford. His publications include *Church Courts, Sex and Marriage in England, 1570–1640* (1987), and articles on crime and the law, sex and marriage, religion, and popular customs. He has also published on the history of climate.

MARK S. R. JENNER is Lecturer in History at the University of York. The author of articles on various aspects of the social and cultural history of early modern England, he is completing a book on English conceptions of 'cleanliness' and 'dirt' as reflected in the environmental regulations of London *c.*1530–*c.*1700.

PAUL JOHNSON is Professor of Economic History at the London School of Economics. His research interests include the history of savings and welfare, the economics of old age and pensions, and the relationship between laws and markets in Victorian England. He is the author of *Saving and Spending* (1985) and *Ageing and Economic Welfare* (1992).

ALAN MACFARLANE is Professor of Anthropological Science at Cambridge University and Fellow of King's College. His publications include *Witchcraft in Tudor and Stuart England* (1970), *The Origins of English Individualism* (1978), *Marriage and Love in England 1300–1840* (1986), *The Culture of Capitalism* (1987), and *The Savage Wars of Peace* (1997).

GILES MANDELBROTE is a Curator, British Collections 1501–1800, at the British Library. He is co-editor of *The Book Trade and its Customers, 1450–1900* (1997) and of *A Radical's Books: The Library Catalogue of Samuel Jeake of Rye, 1623–1690* (1999).

SARA MENDELSON is Associate Professor in the Arts and Science Programme at McMaster University in Hamilton, Ontario. She is the author of *The Mental World of Stuart Women: Three Studies* (1987), *Women in Early Modern England 1550–1720*(1998) (with Patricia Crawford), and *Paper Bodies: A Margaret Cavendish Reader* (1999) (with Sylvia Bowerbank).

PRYS MORGAN is Reader in History at the University of Wales, Swansea. Among his books are a biography of Iolo Morganwg (1975); *The Eighteenth-Century Renaissance* (1981); *Wales: The Shaping of a Nation* (1984) (with D. Thomas); *Welsh Surnames* (1985) (with T. J. Morgan); and *The University of Wales Centenary History*, iii. *The University 1939–1993* (1997). He is working on *The Oxford History of Wales: Wales 1780 to 1880*.

J. A. SHARPE is Professor of History at the University of York. He has published extensively on the history of crime and punishment in early modern England, and is also the author of *Early Modern England: A Social History 1550–1760* (1987) and *Instruments of Darkness: Witchcraft in England* c.*1550–1750* (1996).

PAUL SLACK is Principal of Linacre College and Professor of Early Modern Social History, University of Oxford. His books include *The Impact of Plague in Tudor and Stuart England* (1985), *Poverty and Policy in Tudor and Stuart England* (1988), and *From Reformation to Improvement: Public Welfare in Early Modern England* (1999).

ABBREVIATIONS

BIHR   *Bulletin of the Institute of Historical Research*
BL   British Library
Bodl.   Bodleian Library
CSPD   *Calendar of State Papers, Domestic Series*
DNB   *Dictionary of National Biography*
EHR   *English Historical Review*
EcHR   *Economic History Review*
HMC   Historical Manuscripts Commission, Reports
P&P   *Past and Present*
PRO   Public Record Office
RO   Record Office
TRHS   *Transactions of the Royal Historical Society*

Unless otherwise stated, all works cited were published in London.

1

Keith Thomas

PETER BURKE, BRIAN HARRISON, and PAUL SLACK

I

Born in 1933, the elder son of a Welsh tenant farmer with 250 acres, Keith Thomas might have been expected to spend a lifetime in rural Wales. Yet he has been knighted, became head of an Oxford college, President of the British Academy, and one of twentieth-century Britain's most innovative historians. He knows well enough how frequently chance determined the outcome. The Vale of Glamorgan, where he grew up, was an Anglicized part of Wales; at first he knew only English, and learned Welsh at his primary school rather as one learns a foreign language. His mother, a schoolmaster's daughter who read English at Cardiff University, was alert to the nuances of social status, confidently identifying conduct that she deemed 'common'; she discouraged him from speaking even English with a Welsh accent, let alone from speaking Welsh. The family was Conservative and Anglican, with no trace of Welsh dissent. Keith's father was a churchwarden and chairman of the Rural District Council; he was interested in politics and economics, and often gave well-prepared speeches at local gatherings of farmers. Churchill's wartime speeches were closely followed, and gloom pervaded the farmhouse kitchen when the general-election results came through on the radio in 1945.

Keith's was a happy and by present-day standards remarkably liberated childhood: roaming the surrounding countryside, doing odd jobs on the farm, sometimes driving the tractor, and occasionally rounding up sheep and cattle with his father. His mother was an efficient housekeeper, cooking for a large household that included farmhands living in, and occasionally warming up frail newborn lambs in her oven. Hams hung from her high-ceilinged kitchen, and food was abundant even in wartime. Books, too, were abundant. His father had left school at 14, but had educated himself in the English classics. Keith's mother frequently gave books as presents, and family outings to Bridgend or Cardiff usually included book-buying at Smith's or Lear's. This 'very conscientious, law-abiding, docile, biddable child'[1] could read before

---

[1] All unidentified quotations come from Brian Harrison's tape-recorded interviews with Sir Keith on 18 May, 29 June, and 28 Sept. 1998. We also owe some details to the interview kindly

attending Llancarfan village school. His childhood reading—not unusual at the time for including *Our Island Story* and *The Boys' Book of Heroes*—assumed the continued existence of the British Empire; nor did he think of contesting that idea when competing successfully as a teenager for a national essay prize organized by the Royal Empire Society. Given his mother's background and aspirations, and the family's high status in this small community, much was expected of him. At 11, he duly came top of the county in the scholarship examination.

Should he go to Barry County Grammar School or to the nearest grammar school, four miles away at Cowbridge? Barry was decided upon, though Keith stood out there as 'a country boy', leaving classes early to catch the bus home. In Llancarfan he knew everybody, and can to this day send himself pleasantly to sleep by recalling who lived in each house as he mentally travels downhill through the village. The very thought of school in Barry was traumatic, and even before arriving he acquired a stammer—now scarcely perceptible, but never completely shaken off. In two senses the new school opened up a new world. An urban school, recruiting from a wide social span that included some quite rough elements, it encouraged strenuous meritocratic achievement; earlier pupils included the historian Sir John Habakkuk and the archaeologist Glyn Daniel. The names of distinguished old boys featured on the honours board; their photographs were on the walls. 'Education was the ladder which got people out of the valleys'; through examination success came social ascent, whether one stayed in Wales or took the high road to England. Keith was soon embattled on two fronts: learning to survive in his new school, yet also defending his educational priorities at home. Whereas his younger brother Tony (now a prominent local farmer) took to farming, Keith's mother encouraged him into what she saw as the relatively refined life of books. When it came to School Certificate 'there ensued many battles' to protect his reading time against the harvest's claims; his father understandably wondered whether Keith, sitting in a deckchair in the garden reading a book for examinations, could really be classified as working.[2] When accompanying his father to farming occasions, 'as soon as they shook hands they'd say "oh, I can tell by your hands you're not a farmer"'. He knew that in distancing himself from farming he disappointed his father, but Tony and his mother were happy enough. Keith's competitive instincts, well developed then and since, ensured such success at Barry that the option of a farming life gradually faded away.

Moving on from farmer's boy to studious teenager was the first of four occasions in his life when Keith unobtrusively and perhaps unconsciously

made available by Maria Lúcia Pallares-Burke with Sir Keith on 28 July 1998, and gratefully acknowledge here the many helpful comments received on an earlier draft from contributors and others.

   [2] K. Thomas (ed.), *The Oxford Book of Work* (Oxford, 1999), p. xvi.

reinvented himself. He was urged on in his studies by a young, leftish, and widely read history teacher Teifion Phillips, whose classes encouraged discussion and intellectual self-reliance. Phillips was crucial in holding Keith to history. Drifting for no particular reason into selecting English, French, and Latin for Higher Certificate, Keith recalls meeting Phillips by chance when crossing the playground to the room where his selection would be registered: ' "You are doing history, aren't you?" and I said "no, actually", so he said "you must", so of course I always did whatever the last person who spoke to me told me to.' Priming him with M. M. Reese's textbook on the Tudors and Stuarts and Tawney's *Religion and the Rise of Capitalism*, Phillips encouraged him towards Balliol's entrance examination. Though he had been abroad twice on school expeditions and twice with the family to London, Keith had never been to Oxford before arriving for the examination in January 1950; standing outside Balliol, he had to ask a puzzled passer-by where to find the College.

Essays written on Luther and Calvin paid dividends, and Phillips had shrewdly advised him to read a book that he could discuss at interview: D. B. Quinn's biography of Walter Raleigh. He also knew something about Marxist approaches to the English revolution. A Phillips pupil had won an exhibition at Balliol the previous year, and Keith just after his seventeenth birthday found himself Brackenbury scholar in history. He was then thinking of becoming a lawyer, and wanted to read Law at Oxford, but this turned out to be no more than 'a momentary impulse'. For at this point Christopher Hill, who had asked most questions at his interview, retained him for history and, with his attractively informal manner, reinforced Keith's seventeenth-century enthusiasms. Balliol's historians wanted him to read history: he could still become a lawyer afterwards anyway. Turning up at Keith's room after the result was announced, Hill said 'you don't need to do that bloody Higher', and urged him instead to read more widely and improve his languages. So school examinations were at an end, and Keith spent the next few months acting on Hill's advice, as well as teaching himself to type.

He would have preferred to go straight up to Oxford, but Balliol encouraged non-scientists to get their National Service over first. Keith's first two weeks in the barrack room at Brecon in the Royal Welch Fusiliers during September 1950 were, he recalls, 'the low point in my life'. He had not been away from home before, and now thinks that he 'must have led a very sheltered life' because he found 'the torrent of obscenity and so on . . . quite new . . . it was just news to me that people spoke like that'. However, he 'gradually surfaced' and had the good luck to go to Jamaica for what was called 'internal security', thereby averting a possibly fatal posting to Korea. He set off from barracks in Chester, so the train passed tantalizingly through Oxford, bound for the troopship in Southampton: 'I remember seeing the view of all the spires and there was I, heading off.' Yet he was thrilled at what then seemed an exotic posting, and was now adjusting more readily to rapidly changing social and cultural situations. Does Jamaica lie at the root of his later interest in social anthropology? He was eager for travel at this time, the island's history interested him, he travelled widely there, and took some leave in Cuba. But social anthropology did not become important till later, and Jamaica's contribution to his career lay elsewhere: it gave him self-confidence and experience in administration and at organizing his time. As the corporal who helped to run the Orderly Room at Up Park in Kingston, he became adept at keeping records; he was the essential person who understood how everything worked and knew all the rules. So successfully, in fact, that the Adjutant wanted him to become a professional soldier with a commission. That was not what Keith wanted, but, with full-time National Service completed, he fulfilled his three-year part-time commitments in Britain as a Lieutenant in the Royal Engineers. In September 1952 he was lucky to return at all; a fortnight after his own flight, the Avro-York bringing home the next batch of conscripts from Jamaica disappeared over the Atlantic.

Oxford seemed 'immensely liberating' after this: 'I was able to do the things I wanted to do and I was surrounded by the people I wanted to be with, and it was just marvellous.' As for his College, 'I adored Balliol from the very first day.' The historians were Balliol's largest subject group, fifty-two out of its 264 undergraduates reading for Honours Schools in 1952.[3] He later complained forcibly and publicly that Oxford's history syllabus was narrow, yet as an undergraduate he felt liberated by Oxford's self-directed sink-or-swim system of instruction, and found ample variety in the first-year course: Adam Smith with Paul Streeten, Tocqueville with John Bowle, Bede with Richard Southern, and historical geography with Hill. 'Greatly to my amazement', he won a distinction in the Prelims examination at the end of his second term. Thereafter it was invigorating to plunge into medieval history at the deep end with four first-year essays for Southern on rather recondite topics. There followed eighteenth-century English history with the somewhat uninspiring A. B. Rodger, moving on to the nineteenth century with the exceptionally clever and subtle Hugh Stretton. Keith took constitutional documents (Prothero and Gardiner) with Sir David Lindsay Keir, Master of Balliol and 'an extremely acute and intelligent tutor'. Political Thought he studied with Colin Leys, a charming Marxist pupil of T. D. Weldon, the iconoclastic Magdalen PPE tutor who infused political studies with the precise verbal and logical analysis for which Oxford philosophers were then renowned: 'so . . . I became a sort of philosopher manqué . . . that's what we all were, really, in those days.' None the less, Hill was 'the *key* figure, far and away', with tutorials on English history and the Cromwell special subject. Alarmingly silent in tutorials, and leaving pupils to choose their own essay topics, Hill was not a didactic

---

[3] *Balliol College Record* (1952), 4.

tutor, yet 'at the same time he managed to instil a sense that only the best would do'.

Term was not all work and no play. Keith 'almost never worked after dinner, and . . . never worked between lunch and tea'. He played cricket, was Treasurer of the JCR, and enjoyed Balliol's rich cosmopolitan social, political, and intellectual mix: 'it was a wonderful melting-pot.' Of 261 junior members in residence during Trinity Term 1952, forty-one came from the Commonwealth, eighteen from the USA, and one each from Eire, France, Germany, and Spain.[4] There seemed 'endless interesting people' in Oxford, senior members and junior. His Balliol contemporaries included the President of the Oxford Union and future Conservative politician Peter Brooke, the then-Communist social historian Raphael Samuel, and the distinguished philosopher Charles Taylor. People who knew Keith in those years recall a provincial, even raw manner, very different from his later polished civility. Nor had a left-wing history schoolteacher and two years' National Service yet shaken his conservatism. But he was learning fast, and 'when I came to Oxford I changed my views on lots of things in my first year'. To him, as to many grammar-school undergraduates in Oxford in the 1950s, a meritocratic and anti-snobbish radicalism came naturally, but his radicalism was neither indiscriminate nor uncompromising. He had friends among all groups within Balliol: 'I was always a sort of "vote with the left, dine with the right" sort of person.' He even occasionally attended Chapel until 1955, and does not recall having felt strongly about Suez in the following year. Yet he remained in Balliol's Arnold debating society, whereas a somewhat raffish group who looked down on 'trogs' working in the library seceded into a refounded Brackenbury Society, and at St John's later in the decade he recalls rebuking the prominent politician Michael Stewart because Labour proposed to leave the public schools intact.

Keith's contemporaries at Barry began to notice the fading of his Welsh accent, which his brother and sister still retain, and which he unconsciously resumes when visiting them. The change was not deliberate, but he had never favoured Welsh nationalism, whose narrow perspective affronted his liberal internationalism. Balliol, like Barry Grammar School, encouraged emulation of distinguished predecessors, and Balliol's college magazine boasted lists of prizewinners, first classes, honours, and elections to Parliament. Keith worked hard as an undergraduate, especially in the vacations, when he often exploited the scholar's right to stay up. In 1954, jointly with the Anglo-Saxon historian James Campbell, he won the Gibbs Scholarship, awarded after a special university examination. In the same year came the Stanhope Historical Essay Prize for an essay on the seventeenth-century antiquary Anthony Wood, whose manuscripts were in the Bodleian Library. University prizes were then stepping stones to an academic career, and the Stanhope nourished a zest for

[4] Ibid.

research: 'I had a *lovely* time in Duke Humfrey doing that.' His love of books extends well beyond their contents: he likes the sight, smell, and feel of them, foraging in the most out-of-the-way places to buy them. There had always been books in his locker in Jamaica, and his undergraduate prizes laid the basis for what is now a huge collection. He became a regular in the back room of Thornton's bookshop in Oxford, where a select few were admitted before the books were priced, and his *Who's Who* entry has long listed 'visiting second-hand bookshops' as his recreation. The Bodleian Library was one Oxford influence that deterred him from accepting otherwise tempting job opportunities elsewhere. From 1968 to 1995 he was on the Council of Management of the Friends of the Bodleian, and chaired it from 1986 to 1993.

In his third year, even before taking Schools, he was offered a Senior Lectureship in Adelaide by Hugh Stretton, who had gone there the previous year. Keith took the offer seriously, but 'I went to South Australia House and I looked at the newspapers, and decided not to go.' Unlucky with some questions in his final examinations, he was surprised and relieved to win a congratulatory First, and went to St Antony's College for graduate work. He then took the formidable examination for a Prize Fellowship at All Souls, which in 1955 included a three-hour essay on 'sin'. His triumph, jointly with George Huxley, was announced on the Saturday, and the next night he was dining in a College whose influence upon him was to be profound. He liked its traditions, enjoyed signing the library register whose first signatory was Blackstone, and proudly inherited L. S. Amery's key to the Codrington Library. All Souls then seemed more central to public life than now, and Keith was fascinated by its unusual combination of country-house living and by an internally egalitarian tone that made new Fellows feel welcome. Significant conversations between important people were regularly overheard, and 'you had a sense, which I suppose I hadn't had till then, of there being a much larger world beyond Oxford'. Well-known historians—Cole, Habakkuk, Pares, Rowse—also regularly gathered, 'and they would talk and I would just sort of sit silently and listen to these great men, and I loved it'.

II

A postgraduate degree was not then essential for anyone choosing to make a career in history at Oxford, least of all for someone with Keith's undergraduate record, yet it was between the mid-1950s and the mid-1960s that he acquired the ideas and insights that were to prove crucial. His earliest research proposals, rapidly taken up and discarded, were no more adventurous than his undergraduate course: a biography of Robert Cecil, James I's court, seventeenth-century antiquarianism, and office-holding. What he now regards as 'the big turning point' was his paper on 'Women and the

Civil War Sects'—as much about the sects as about the women—and in its earlier and longer format entitled 'The Family and the Civil War Sects'. His interest in religious toleration had led him to Thomas Edwards's *Gangraena* (1646), which attacked the sectaries for subverting wifely obedience. He then moved into women's history—impressed by, among other books, Simone de Beauvoir's *Second Sex*. Keith's first lectures in Oxford, in Michaelmas Term 1957, were on 'The relations between the sexes in England from the Reformation to the First World War'. Few came—less because Oxford was consciously anti-feminist, or because Keith was then relatively unknown, than because the subject was peripheral to the syllabus. By contrast, his lectures on 'Aristotle, Hobbes and Rousseau' (first delivered in Trinity Term 1959, and oft-repeated) were so crowded as to require a move to a larger hall. Their appeal lay not just in quality of content and delivery, but in the fact that they catered for a compulsory Final Honours School paper; delivered shortly before the examination, they were a timely pick-me-up for undergraduates.[5]

Keith's paper on 'Women and the Civil War Sects' emerged not from the austerely professional world of the graduate seminar but, as so often with his early published work, from the less formal and predominantly male world of the after-dinner discussion group—more central to Oxford life then than now. Hill encouraged him to write it and then urged him to publish it in *Past and Present*, where it appeared in 1958. Research on women's history was then no help towards getting an Oxford fellowship, and Keith acted on advice not to advertise this preoccupation when applying (successfully) for the tutorial fellowship at St John's, which he held from 1957 to 1985. But his first published paper led him on to studying women's history more generally, and to write his article on 'The Double Standard' after delivering it as a paper to St Catherine's College history society. He knew there was no hope for such a topic with the *English Historical Review*, so sent it across the Atlantic to the *Journal of the History of Ideas*, where it appeared in 1959. He was a pioneer: it was several years before American feminism reinvigorated the British interwar tradition of historical writing on women, though by then Keith's interests had moved on.

In the 1950s his feminism was more than purely academic. In June 1958, when *The Times* published what now seem extraordinarily obscurantist letters against admitting more women to Oxford, he wrote a robust rejoinder.[6] This evoked 'a torrent of sort of hate-mail from readers', and his response was to draft another letter, which *The Times* set up but did not publish, arguing that mixed colleges would increase Oxford's proportion of women. This idea did not get seriously discussed till the mid-1960s; gradually implemented after

---

[5] Cf. Fiona MacCarthy's somewhat different interpretation in *New York Review of Books*, 6 Feb. 1997, 4.

[6] *The Times*, 27 June 1958, 11.

1974, it soon gained almost universal acceptance. In 1961 Keith married Valerie Little, who has subsequently acted as 'sounding-board or critic' for everything he has written; in the preface to his anthology on work, he describes her as 'the virtual co-editor of this book'.[7] Although dons' wives then rarely had careers of their own, she continued teaching in Faringdon, moving on (initially on a part-time basis) in 1967 to Oxford High School, where she taught English literature for thirty years. In a remarkable review article of 1966 Keith wanted British feminism to move on, urging 'a more conscious effort' to render paid work feasible for married women: more training, more nursery schools, more allowance for career breaks. By then Emily and Edmund Thomas had been born, and there is a note of personal urgency in Keith's plea that 'it should be made easier to carry small children about', as 'anyone who has tried to lift a child plus push-chair on or off a bus, or up the steps of a large store, will know'.[8]

Keith's next breakthrough was to recognize social anthropology's potential as stimulus to the historical imagination. Although E. E. Evans-Pritchard was a Fellow of All Souls, Keith had seldom seen him there. What prompted the breakthrough was the arrival on his desk in 1961, when editing the *Oxford Magazine*, of 'a pamphlet which no historian should miss':[9] Evans-Pritchard's lecture *Anthropology and History*. Directed mainly at ahistorical social anthropologists, this was no trumpet call to historians ignorant of social anthropology, and hardly needed reviewing at all; Keith's mind must already have been prepared for it, and it was he (not Evans-Pritchard) who enthused about the new opportunities for historians. He claimed that in Oxford 'a narrow syllabus based primarily on old-fashioned political history has to a great extent succeeded in insulating the study of history from the progress of modern knowledge in such allied disciplines as psychology, sociology, anthropology and economics'. Oxford's Modern History School produced undergraduates 'whose understanding and self-awareness in everyday matters is seldom enhanced by their historical studies' and its constraints on history's agenda were 'educationally a tragedy'.[10] These phrases reappeared almost unchanged, after the review had been refracted through an informal seminar organized by Lawrence Stone, in an article (encrusted with five pages of footnotes) that *Past and Present* published in 1963. Readers of the *Oxford Magazine*, a rather obscure dons' periodical, needed to hang on tight during Keith's lively year as editor, for he trenchantly backed many causes that then seemed radical: dons' salaries must be made public; classical languages and literature must become a Final Honours School; dons must join the Association for University Teachers but give less time to the WEA; and Oxford should admit people

---

[7] Thomas (ed.), *Work*, p. vii.
[8] K. Thomas, 'Women in Adversity', *New Statesman*, 13 May 1966, 691.
[9] K. Thomas, 'Should Historians be Anthropologists?', *Oxford Magazine*, 1 June 1961, 387.
[10] Ibid. 387–8; cf. his 'History and Anthropology', *P&P* 24 (Apr. 1963), 18.

on merit alone.[11] Perhaps unsurprisingly, his review article on Evans-Pritchard evoked no correspondence; radical opinions were all too predictable from this angry young man.

From the early 1960s Keith's writings frequently mention social anthropologists, especially British ones working on Africa—from Evans-Pritchard, who inspired his ethnographic approach, to Meyer Fortes, Max Gluckman, Audrey Richards, Max Marwick, Mary Douglas, and Robin Horton. Nor did he neglect Americans such as Ruth Benedict, Clyde Kluckhohn, George Foster, and (before he became internationally famous) Clifford Geertz. Marxism had attracted Keith the undergraduate for intellectual not political reasons: 'I was just looking for something which enabled one to make sense of things by relating them to each other,' he recalls, and in the 1950s 'Marxism was the only form of sociology or anthropology on offer.' In studying history Keith has consistently preferred analysis and explanation to narrative and description, comprehensiveness and catholicity to fragmentation and specialization. If Marxism soon came to seem unduly limiting, perhaps social anthropology could offer organizing principles, ways of connecting and explaining what would otherwise seem random facts. It is no surprise that one of the few British historians to make a similar move was the Marxist Eric Hobsbawm in his *Primitive Rebels* (1959). Furthermore, social anthropology helped to prise open attitudes in the past that later generations found unfamiliar and even uncongenial. Despite his reputation in Oxford for lecturing on political thought, Keith's main research concern was less with formal theories than with what Crick has called 'the theories of the untheoretical . . . the general prejudices or principles by which even the most practical men, consciously or unconsciously, select from the infinity of possible facts to make some order out of their environment'.[12]

While social anthropology can illuminate attitudes outside the élite in ill-documented societies, Keith thinks it can also help historians 'to recognize the strangeness of very recent times'.[13] He was puzzled to find histories of recent periods so preoccupied with politics and diplomacy; ample sources should, he thought, make it easier for them to embrace social history and acknowledge (in that now hackneyed phrase) how even the recent past is a foreign country where they do things differently. Social anthropology could greatly enlarge the historian's agenda. It could highlight family and community relationships; and 'where are the serious historical studies of popular hysteria, witchcraft and superstition,' he asked, 'of suicide and of attitudes to birth

---

[11] See *Oxford Magazine*, 2 Feb. 1961, 183 (AUT), 185 (meritocratic entry); 11 May 1961, 331 (classics FHS); 18 May 1961, 347 (management studies); 25 May 1961, 363 (WEA); 26 Oct. 1961, 25 (salaries).

[12] B. Crick, Foreword to D. P. Crook, *American Democracy in English Politics 1815–50* (Oxford, 1965), p. x.

[13] Interview with Peer Vries, *Leidschrift*, 6 (1990), 104.

and death, of neurosis and mental health, of adolescence, love and parent-hood?'[14] English family history had 'simply not begun'. Children's education 'has never been properly studied'; indeed, 'whole areas of human experience have either not been studied historically at all or never interwoven with the fabric of social history'. The history of clothes, for instance, 'has a chronology of its own', and there is a history of art 'as a reflection of fundamental changes in human perception'.[15] Already in the 1960s he was thinking about the history of duelling, 'attitudes to pain, suicide, the treatment of animals, drunkenness and the changing conceptions of sanity and insanity'.[16] It was a huge agenda, and Keith's publishing career since 1961 has largely consisted in exploring its potential, and even in extending it to include attitudes to time, children's names, relations between the generations, and the history of manners and gesture. More than thirty years later the agenda is far from exhausted, least of all by historians of more recent periods.

His influential article of 1966, 'The Tools and the Job' in the *Times Literary Supplement*, reveals his reforming ardour undiminished. 'Keith Thomas raves in a muddle-headed doomsday way,' K. B. McFarlane grumbled to a graduate student; for G. R. Elton the article displayed 'an engaging arrogance'.[17] Keith pronounced A. J. P. Taylor's final volume in the Oxford History of England (published in the previous year) 'a brilliant swansong for the dying concept of real history as past politics, and social history as an unde-manding subsidiary'. Historians' 'dethronement of politics' would make social history 'not . . . a residual subject but a central one', reinforced by all the social sciences. 'The findings of social psychology . . . still await incorporation into the writing of history,' and sociology would sharpen up historians' use of such terms as 'feudalism', 'social class', and 'revolution'. Historians' many implicitly quantitative statements would become more self-conscious and rigorous; indeed, the 'genuine breakthrough' in historical demography was already lighting the way. The new econometric history was 'sweeping all before it' in the USA, promising 'a definitive solution' to such problems as slavery's economic efficiency or the railways' contribution to American eco-nomic growth. Historical research would henceforth advance, not through 'the individualist, prima donna tradition', but through 'cooperative scholar-ship and organized research, a world of seminars, workshops and graduate programmes'.[18]

---

[14] Thomas, 'Should Historians be Anthropologists?', 387.

[15] Thomas, 'History and Anthropology', 15–17.

[16] Ibid. 16; K. Thomas, 'The Social Origins of Hobbes's Political Thought', in K. C. Brown (ed.), *Hobbes Studies* (Oxford, 1965), 194 n. On drink and its place in social life, see K. Thomas, *Religion and the Decline of Magic: Studies in Popular Beliefs in Sixteenth and Seventeenth Century England* (1971), 17–19.

[17] McFarlane to Rees Davies, in K. B. McFarlane, *Letters to Friends, 1940–1966*, ed. G. Harriss (Oxford, 1997), 239; G. R. Elton, *The Practice of History* (1967; Fontana edn., 1969), 18 n. 5.

[18] K. Thomas, 'The Tools and the Job', *Times Literary Supplement*, 7 Apr. 1966, 275–6.

From this high point of Keith's historiographical radicalism, his one approach to polemic, there has been a gradual long-term retreat. It was already being sounded in the preface to the book that made his name, won the Wolfson Prize for History, and was included in 1994–5 by a distinguished panel of intellectuals among the hundred books to have been most influential since 1945 on Western public discourse:[19] *Religion and the Decline of Magic* (1971). 'I particularly regret not having been able to offer more of those exact statistical data upon which the precise analysis of historical change must so often depend,' he wrote. Given that 'the sources seldom permit such computation', he had been forced back upon 'the intellectual equivalent of the bow and arrow in a nuclear age': the historian's 'traditional method of presentation by example and counter-example';[20] Elton had already noted his failure to practise the quantification he preached.[21] There is a significant tension behind this discrepancy: on the one hand, Keith in his rationalism wanted historians to transcend the constraints of their raw material and settle large but disputed questions; but, on the other hand, he was acutely sensitive to diversity, nuances, and the intractability of the sources. His doubts about quantification are already implicit in his article of 1963, where, in highlighting the limitations of Marxism, he emphasized that 'economic wants are themselves culturally determined'.[22] For him, as also for many in the History Workshop movement (with whose aims he has shown a consistent, though discriminating, sympathy), statistics on closer inspection are not 'hard' at all, but are themselves cultural products. Nor would it be sensible for a historian's agenda to be determined by such few reliable statistics as survive. By 1983 Keith was amiably parodying quantitative history, noting in *Man and the Natural World* that there are thirty-five dogs in the David Loggan prints of Cambridge, but fifty-six in those of Oxford.[23]

Nor did his enthusiasm of 1966 stem from any major influence by sociology on his work. His article of 1963 made a bold early reference to Foucault, and in *Religion and the Decline of Magic* Max Weber and Malinowski are the theorists most cited. Norbert Elias has been important for him since his Neale Lecture on 'The Place of Laughter in Tudor and Stuart England' (1977).[24] Bryan Wilson and Shmuel Eisenstadt are sometimes cited, while Gramsci makes a cautious appearance in his Creighton Lecture of 1984.[25] But this does not amount to much; though Keith, like the sociologist, seeks pattern

---

[19] The list is in *Times Literary Supplement*, 6 Oct. 1995, 39.   [20] Thomas, *Religion*, p. x.
[21] Elton, *Practice of History*, 42 n. 15.
[22] Thomas, 'History and Anthropology', 7; cf. interview with Peer Vries, 102, and K. Thomas, 'Ways of Doing Cultural History', in R. Sanders *et al.* (eds.), *Balans en Perspectief van de Nederlandse Cultuurgeschiedenis* (Amsterdam and Atlanta, 1991), 68–9, 75.
[23] K. Thomas, *Man and the Natural World: Changing Attitudes in England 1500–1800* (1983).
[24] *Times Literary Supplement*, 21 Jan. 1977, 77–81.
[25] K. Thomas, *The Perception of the Past in Early Modern England* (Creighton Trust Lecture, University of London, 1984).

and explanation, he finds sociology's comparative and quantitative mood ultimately uncongenial, sometimes even clumsy. And, for all historical demography's substantial achievements, it could only ever constitute one ingredient of the 'total history' that he consistently sought. Psychology was somewhat more important for him. He was much influenced by Freud's *Civilization and its Discontents*, and in 1966 praised recent studies of the irrational and of crowd behaviour. He thought 'the greatest gap in the psychological field' was 'a historical study of methods of child-rearing at different periods',[26] and childhood recurs as a preoccupation in his writing, partly because family life is salient among his personal priorities, but mainly because it is during childhood that environment and culture most profoundly mould personality. *Religion and the Decline of Magic* invokes 'new methods of child-rearing' to explain the increasing appeal of 'an explanatory theory based on guilt'. *The Perception of the Past* notes that 'our most deeply-rooted images of the past are those acquired in childhood', and early modern children receive extended treatment in an essay of 1989.[27] As for theory, Freud is quoted most frequently, on topics ranging from dogs to demons,[28] and there are references to other psychoanalysts such as Ernest Jones and Otto Fenichel, psychologists such as Gustav Jahoda, and ethnopsychiatrists such as Margaret Field and Beatrice Whiting.[29]

The great incentive to intellectual collaboration is sophisticated equipment, but here again Elton in 1967 detected a discrepancy, for Keith was a stranger to the 'historical factories' that he saw as the historian's destiny: 'to the best of my knowledge, Mr Thomas . . . the author of some excellent articles, has never worked even within sight of one of these "factories".'[30] Yet his distance from technology (he has never driven a car, and bicycles round Oxford) has perhaps proved a long-term historical asset. Working alone; using typewriter, pen and paper; and coming to the word processor rather late—he could conserve his time, resources, style, and reputation in the 1970s and 1980s, while the high collaborative hopes of the 1960s ran into at least two problems. First, 'increasingly the structural, analytical, quantitative historians have found themselves talking to each other and no one else';[31] Keith has, by contrast, always prized the clarity of style that collaborative and quantitative

[26] Thomas, 'The Tools and the Job', 276.
[27] Thomas, *Religion*, 111; Thomas, *Perception of the Past*, 24; K. Thomas, 'Children in Early Modern England', in G. Avery and J. Briggs (eds.), *Children and their Books: A Celebration of the Work of Iona and Peter Opie* (Oxford, 1989), 45–77; cf. review of Lloyd de Mause (ed.), *The History of Childhood*, in *New Statesman*, 16 Apr. 1976, 511–12.
[28] Thomas, *Religion*, 481; Thomas, *Man and the Natural World*, 106, and the epigraph to ch. 6.
[29] Thomas, *Religion*, 111, 519, 647, 661.
[30] Elton, *Practice of History*, 42 n. 15.
[31] L. Stone, 'The Revival of Narrative: Reflections on a New Old History', *P&P* 85 (Nov. 1979), 15.

projects endanger. Behind this impulse lies no mere traditionalism but a conviction that history should help to mould public discussion. Professionalism, for him, should not entail mystification, nor can natural science offer history an appropriate model. Secondly, the big collaborative historical projects disappointed expectations. 'It cannot be denied that quantification has not fulfilled the high hopes of twenty years ago,' wrote Lawrence Stone in 1979; 'most of the great problems of history remain as insoluble as ever, if not more so,' and he cited 'huge piles of greenish print-out gathering dust in scholars' offices'.[32]

The 1960s were the decade of the 'national plan', a time when the two world wars still seemed lamentable but temporary interruptions to an ongoing secularized and rationalist late-Victorian liberal pursuit of peace, plenty, and progress. Open government, meritocratic social engineering, social science, and the application of intelligence by a cabinet of first-class brains would provide the means, assisted by an increasingly educated public. Yet already by the late 1960s these high hopes were fading, and Keith was not alone in his retreat from social science. With the travails of corporatism in the 1970s and the advent of Thatcher, the importance of politics (a subject that had not at first greatly interested Keith) became all too apparent. Partly for this reason, British political history—with the rise of early modern 'revisionists' and the growth of 'contemporary history'—possessed a vitality that Keith had not envisaged in 1963 when so dismissive about 'the endless analysis of the gymnastics of minor politicians'.[33]

For social anthropology, however, Keith's enthusiasm did not wane. It lies behind much of the impact made by *Religion and the Decline of Magic*, though critics sometimes exaggerate its influence on his work. Hugh Trevor-Roper claimed in 1963 that 'the history of the world, for the last five centuries, in so far as it has significance, has been European history'.[34] Elton complained that, 'when some writers can treat pre-industrial England, the economically most advanced society in the Europe of its day, as though it were like tribal Africa or nineteenth-century India, understanding is destroyed, not assisted'.[35] Influential Oxford gossips even surreptitiously dismissed Keith as 'Bonga Bonga Thomas'. Yet Keith, with Marc Bloch, has always been cautious in using such terms as 'primitive', 'totem', and 'taboo'. Never eager to reply to critics, he could none the less have repudiated such confident distancing of European from non-European experience even at the present day, let alone in earlier periods. He could also have pointed out that he did not allow social anthropology to impose crude parallels or rigid formulae upon his raw material. Social anthropology was no more and no less than 'an indispensable

---

[32] Ibid. 12.   [33] Thomas, 'History and Anthropology', 18.
[34] H. Trevor-Roper, 'The Rise of Christian Europe', *Listener*, 28 Nov. 1963, 871.
[35] Elton, *Practice of History*, 48.

stimulus to the historian. It stirs the imagination and suggests new ways of looking at a subject.[36] It was a preliminary to the historian's traditionally systematic and sensitive study of raw material: a prompt for that broad and sympathetic imagination that guides the historian when selecting and interpreting evidence. So Keith could pick and choose. Like most historians venturing into other disciplines, he is something of an intellectual bricoleur, drawing on functionalism, structuralism, and symbolic anthropology alike when a theory fits his data or preoccupations. Indeed, eclecticism about method pervades his work; as Hildred Geertz pointed out in 1975, he 'does not commit himself to the whole of any single approach'.[37]

In research procedure his methods were highly traditional, even old-fashioned, though this too proved a long-term advantage: his unflamboyant radicalism—all the more palatable given his conservatism in dress, manners, and family life—could gain a hearing in the most respectable circles. Though always coy about his research intentions, he is unusual among historians in describing his working methods openly. Like the social anthropologists, he approaches his material receptively: he keeps his reading broad, as was encouraged by the sheer range of the subjects that college tutors in Oxford's mid-century Modern History School were required to teach. But he also keeps his perspectives and sympathies broad. When reading and note-taking, he remains alert to a wide range of topics. In many ways severely rationalistic in his own thought processes and values, he aims when reading to attain 'a state of complete open-mindedness . . . to take nothing for granted': to recognize that 'the investigator has to begin by working out all the basic categories and silent assumptions implicit in the behaviour of the people he is studying'. A 'sense of otherness' is, he insists, 'essential for any historian approaching the past';[38] he is careful to cultivate the almost childlike naïvety that the imaginative historian requires when responding to the evidence, and to avoid imposing his own civility on recalcitrant subject matter. To quote the foreword to *Religion and the Decline of Magic*: 'astrology, witchcraft, magical healing, divination, ancient prophecies, ghosts and fairies, are now all rightly disdained by intelligent persons.' None the less, 'they were taken seriously by equally intelligent persons in the past, and it is the historian's business to explain why this was so'.[39]

Keith has spent time in archives opening up new manuscript sources (astrologers' and doctors' casebooks, for example) and on drawing new riches out of old sources such as church court records, especially when pursuing witches. But, as with Hill, most of his work draws on other sources, mainly

---

[36] Interview with Dr Francis Brooks, 29 July 1983, in the Australian Historical Association's *Bulletin*, 36 (Sept. 1983), 26.

[37] H. Geertz, 'An Anthropology of Religion and Magic, I', *Journal of Interdisciplinary History*, 6 (1975), 72.

[38] Thomas, 'Ways of Doing Cultural History', 74.   [39] Thomas, *Religion*, p. ix.

primary printed material, backed up by an impressively wide range of secondary literature: from journals of local history to histories of the Fire Service, from the *Annals of Eugenics* to the *Journal of the Society of Archivists*. He finds sorting his notes tedious, and to him the card indexes so widely used in the 1950s seemed 'too chilly'. Besides, they were difficult to reconcile with the Webbs' important principle (mediated to him through G. N. Clark) that there should be only one fact for each card. So in the late 1950s he pragmatically evolved the system of subject-sorted envelopes that he still uses. Into these he stuffs short summaries of points arising from his reading, cut up from larger sheets. A computer age would view this as a database both primitive and inflexible. It grew organically, with new categories added and old ones subdividing, and at any one moment neither possesses nor requires overall coherence. 'When the envelope starts to bulge, I tip it out and see what we have got. I then read more systematically so as to fill the gaps.'[40] There is, he disarmingly admits, 'a definite element of serendipity in it'.[41]

His most recent book, *The Oxford Book of Work* (1999), brings out the essentials of his approach. Covering a huge time-span and several cultures, it is no conventional anthology. By drawing upon a remarkable breadth of reading—from Aristotle and Aelfric to Michael Young and Zola—it brings out 'the human dimensions of a topic' that, if treated by historians at all, 'is usually discussed in a somewhat abstract way'. It transcends any narrowly economic or industrial-relations view of work by illuminating not just experience but also the attitudes and beliefs that experience generates. And by adopting an analytic structure with linking passages, it alerts readers to the 'huge variety of ways in which people have busied themselves' in the past.[42]

Here, as in all Keith's work, what matters are not the mechanics of the filing system but the imagination involved in choosing its categories, the resourcefulness that inspires the search for supplementary material on the selected topic, and the intelligence and care that go into building up a plausible and palatable synthesis. Keith brilliantly conjures up subjects out of very scattered, neglected, and unusual sources and from references often accumulated only incidentally while reading about something else. On almost all his topics there is no easily located cache of material, and much depends on 'incidental references picked up over a lifetime's reading', so these topics rarely attract graduate students or even seasoned scholars.[43] Having chosen his topic, he moves from 'reading in a rather random way' to reading 'rather exhaustively and systematically' in the selected area, soaking himself in relevant sources. He claims to have read 'every work anybody had ever written on the subject of witchcraft in seventeenth-century England when I wrote about it. I tried to

---

[40] Thomas, 'Ways of Doing Cultural History', 79.
[41] Interview with Caroline Moorehead, *The Times*, 2 Apr. 1983, 9.
[42] Thomas, *Work*, pp. vii, xvi.   [43] Thomas, 'Ways of Doing Cultural History', 79.

read every contemporary pamphlet on the subject and I went to all the church court records and to all the judicial records.'[44] Some reviewers of *Religion and the Decline of Magic*, as of *Man and the Natural World*, thought he cited too many examples to support generalizations: 'intellectual overkill', complained Stone, 'with a baroque display of examples for every point, supported by a barrage of recondite references'. Perhaps this reflects Keith's apology to himself for being unable to quantify his findings. *Religion and the Decline of Magic* was also criticized for giving examples 'without any indication of normality and abnormality'; there were complaints at the book's size and price, and even suggestions for an abridged edition.[45]

Innovators are often content to articulate a new idea without bothering to communicate it to others. To judge from his conversation, it is a danger of which Keith has himself been keenly aware, for he often mentions the failure of Lord Acton's great historical synthesis to emerge from the huge card index that Sir Charles Oman memorably observed gathering dust in his library after Acton's death, and quotes the passage at length in his *Work*.[46] Yet Keith has carefully steered between publishing nothing at all and publishing carelessly and hastily. He has if anything become increasingly aware of the need for careful presentation. He takes a long time over arranging his envelopes' contents into a coherent argument before beginning his first draft, and only then can he enjoy writing up. Perhaps philosophy at Balliol in the 1950s lies behind his almost moralistic commitment to writing lucidly and attractively. He repudiates the cant and pretension that since the 1960s have led some writers not just into occasional jargon but into an almost deliberate and pervasive obscurity in their writing and thinking. In 1989 he was equivocal about the new historicism, noting 'the tone of slightly precious over-ingenuity which seems to characterise this otherwise stimulating school of writers'. Style for him is not the icing on the cake, but is 'mixed up with the ingredients. For we cannot separate what we say from how we say it.'[47] Nor does he skimp the later stages; he knows that scholars' scrutiny will be specially alert when originality implicitly rebukes those who have gone before, so he gives no hostages to fortune with unverified references or inadequate documentation. His legendary skill at proof-reading, which can disconcert the most seasoned author, is fully applied to his own work. Nor does he rush into print. Between beginning research and the publication of his *Work* in 1999, he published only two books, and he has not been tempted by the recent rather lax academic practice of crowding occasional reviews unmodified between boards. He has even

[44] Interview with Peer Vries, 107.

[45] Stone, 'The Disenchantment of the World', *New York Review of Books*, 2 Dec. 1971, 17; cf. Noel Perrin on *Man and the Natural World*, in *New York Times Book Review*, 24 Apr. 1983, 8.

[46] Thomas, *Work*, 499–501.

[47] K. Thomas, *History and Literature* (Ernest Hughes Memorial Lecture, University College of Swansea, 1988; Swansea, 1989), 28 n. 18, 23.

refrained from collecting his many named lectures into the book that they would by now fully justify and amply fill.

III

Keith's two major books must now be analysed more closely for their originality and impact. His influence is so broad because he marries innovation with tradition in tone and subject matter as well as in method. 'The Tools and the Job' is an aberration from the less flamboyant image he was increasingly assuming after 1963; for a second self-reinvention, more gradual than the first, was now in train. He was becoming a quiet revolutionary, for whom exhortation and proselytism are not only bad form, but also ineffective, given that historians are professionally cautious. Better to assume a more respectable garb with unexceptionable lectures on main-line subjects in Oxford's History School and publications that can revitalize traditional subjects. His decision to lecture on a subject superficially so conservative as 'Aristotle, Hobbes and Rousseau' illustrates this well. In his first lecture he would repudiate assigning the ideas of these writers to the modern and relatively narrow category 'political'; his broader view of them enabled him to draw together his teaching and his research. Or take his 'The Social Origins of Hobbes's Political Thought'. In 1965 there were two approaches: on the one hand, the traditional, philosophical internal approach to Hobbes typified by (say) Warrender; and, on the other, the new Marxist approach of C. B. Macpherson. Keith neatly positioned himself between the two, criticizing Macpherson in order to substitute a social interpretation of his own that stressed the concept of honour.[48] He did not then refer to social anthropology, though that was the year when the famous volume on *Honour and Shame: The Values of Mediterranean Society* edited by J. G. Peristiany was published. Similarly his articles on the Diggers (1969) and 'The Levellers and the Franchise' (1972) discussed quite traditional topics, the latter effectively settling a much-debated issue. They sprang from the Hill tradition and from teaching part of Oxford's history syllabus.

Again, *Religion and the Decline of Magic*, though radical in its perspectives, illuminated the early modern British historian's more traditional concerns: the Reformation, puritanism, civil-war sects. 'One is impressed less with a sense of a new methodology', wrote E. P. Thompson, 'than with the evidence of the extension of a traditional historical discipline into new areas of research.'[49] The book emerged in a double sense from Oxford's conservative context.

[48] See J. H. Warrender, *The Political Philosophy of Hobbes* (Oxford, 1957); C. B. Macpherson, *The Political Theory of Possessive Individualism* (Oxford, 1962).

[49] E. P. Thompson, 'Anthropology and the Discipline of Historical Context', *Midland History*, 1/3 (Spring 1972), 47.

It owed something to an annual class Keith ran with John Cooper for third-year undergraduates on the 'Commonwealth and Protectorate' special subject; with some mutual rivalry, each in alternate weeks produced what was in effect a research paper on different dimensions of the subject. But the book also emerged from the depths of the Bodleian Library. There Keith's concern with the Levellers led him to Richard Overton, who referred to William Lilly's astrological casebook. From there he explored the many astrological items in the Ashmole manuscripts, moving on to witchcraft and religion. The book's witchcraft section was the most obviously original. Trevor-Roper's essay on the 'witch-craze' had appeared in book form two years earlier, and had ignored 'those elementary village credulities which anthropologists discover in all times and at all places', whereas Keith in the Hill tradition tried to show that such credulities also have a history.[50] But there is much else in the book, which continuously engages with popular culture, a subject that increasingly interested historians from the late 1960s. One of the book's major aims was to demonstrate the links between beliefs in different domains, and to delineate a 'mental climate'.[51] It also performs the remarkable feat of simultaneously accounting for change whilst acknowledging what Keith calls the 'self-confirming character' of 'systems of thought'.[52]

Religion and the Decline of Magic immediately began reshaping the historical agenda. The American Historical Association assigned it a session at their annual meeting in 1972. Hill saw it as 'perhaps the most important contribution to our understanding of English cultural history and indeed English history *tout court*, published in the past generation'.[53] It became a best-seller, bought by Penguin University Books (1973), transferred to Peregrine Books (1978) and Penguin Books (1991). It is displayed in occult bookshops, and no doubt witches as well as students consult it. Like Hill, Keith was relatively confident about the transition from magic to science,[54] but for John Bossy the terms religion and magic were 'none too clearly defined'. In approaching Christianity, which the book in no way privileged over non-Christian beliefs, Keith was as secular in outlook as E. P. Thompson in his influential *Making of the English Working Class* (1963), though less crudely so. Margaret Bowker criticized the chronology: one must go 'deep into the 18th century' to find the

---

[50] K. Thomas, 'The Relevance of Social Anthropology to the Historical Study of English Witchcraft', in M. Douglas (ed.), *Witchcraft: Confessions and Accusations* (1970), 47–79; H. R. Trevor-Roper, *The European Witch-Craze of the 16th and 17th Centuries* (Harmondsworth, 1969), 9; for Hill, see J. Bossy, 'Early Modern Magic', *History*, 57 (1972), 399–403.

[51] Thomas, *Religion*, 631 ff.

[52] Ibid. 432, 640; cf. E. Evans-Pritchard, *Witchcraft Oracles and Magic among the Azande* (Oxford, 1937).

[53] C. Hill, 'Partial Historians and Total History', *Times Literary Supplement*, 24 Nov. 1972, 1431–2.

[54] cf. C. Hill, *A Century of Revolution* (1961), 179–82; Hill, *Society and Puritanism in Pre-Revolutionary England* (1964), 486.

decline of magic; indeed, 'we may even wonder if it declined at all'.[55] Hildred Geertz thought it was 'not the "decline" of the practice of magic that cries out for explanation, but the emergence and rise of the label "magic"'.[56] Later commentators continue to scale down Keith's alleged eighteenth-century shift in attitudes not only to magic but also to medicine, astrology, and witchcraft. Capp could not accept 1700 as a turning point for astrology, and devoted thirty pages to its eighteenth-century decline.[57] For Roy Porter, the major eighteenth-century change in medicine was its commercialization, not its disenchantment: 'medical magic was to prove an unconscionable time a–dying.'[58] Patrick Curry later saw Keith as leaving 'unanswered questions': 'did astrology really die, or declining insofar as it did, why and how did that happen?'[59] As for Keith's view of witchcraft, it allegedly lacks a 'concern for the processes of cultural transmission' of ideas, as distinct from their plausibility or social functions.[60] Bostridge says that even élites took witches seriously until well into the eighteenth century; he brings politics back into explaining both the rise and decline of élite belief in witchcraft, an influence that he links to the rise and decline of what he calls the 'sacral state'.[61] Keith has himself admitted that he should 'have devoted more space to a proper semantic discussion of how the boundaries between "religion", "magic" and "science" shifted', and that 'more justice needs to be done to the symbolism of popular magic'.[62]

After this major work, he emptied envelopes of rich material into a sequence of articles and named lectures on unfamiliar topics. The 1970s were 'a fertile time . . . I had all sorts of subjects on the go, all at the same time.' Among the decade's most important pieces are *Age and Authority* and *Rule and Misrule in the Schools* (both 1976) and 'The Place of Laughter' (1977), drawing on classic functionalist anthropology. Two themes recur: a concern with authority, which links the pieces on women and on Hobbes with those on old age and schools; and a concern with attitudes or assumptions rather than with formal ideas. When asked after 1971 what he was working on, Keith's

---

[55] Bossy, 'Early Modern Magic', 399; M. Bowker, *Historical Journal*, 15 (1972), 363–6.

[56] Geertz, 'An Anthropology', 71–89. For Thomas's reply, see 91–109.

[57] B. Capp, *Astrology and the Popular Press* (1979), 141, 190, 279, 290–1.

[58] R. Porter, 'Medicine and the Decline of Magic', *Strawberry Fare* (Autumn 1986), 88–94, cf. N. C. Hultin, 'Medicine and Magic in the 18th Century', *Journal of the History of Medicine*, 30 (1975), 349–66; D. Harley, 'Mental Illness, Magical Medicine and the Devil in Northern England 1650–1700', in R. French and A. Wear (eds.), *The Medical Revolution of the Seventeenth Century* (Cambridge, 1989), 114–44.

[59] P. Curry, *Prophecy and Power: Astrology in Early Modern England* (Cambridge, 1989). See also M. MacDonald, 'The Career of Astrological Medicine in England', in O. P. Grell and A. Cunningham (eds.), *Religio Medici: Medicine and Religion in 17th Century England* (Aldershot, 1996), 62.

[60] J. Barry (ed.), *Witchcraft in Early Modern Europe* (Cambridge, 1996), esp. the introduction.

[61] I. Bostridge, *Witchcraft and its Transformations* c. *1650*–c. *1750* (Oxford, 1997), 204.

[62] Thomas, 'An Anthropology of Religion and Magic, II', *Journal of Interdisciplinary History*, 6 (1975), 97, 106.

characteristically laconic reply was 'animals'. Does his *Man and the Natural World* spring directly from his Welsh farming childhood? No, because this research interest emerged only slowly, and in childhood he had reacted against the farming life. He still vividly recalls his distaste at hearing the scream of pigs being slaughtered and at seeing his father's pitchfork belabouring a horse. As a child his rural skills did not extend beyond readily identifying flowers and grasses, nor have there been pets in his Oxford homes. His farming background did, however, lend him confidence in tackling a topic that interested him for purely intellectual reasons. His after-dinner talk in the mid-1970s on 'The Brute Creation: Changing Attitudes to Animals in Early Modern England' at London's Institute of Historical Research went down well. When invited to give the Trevelyan lectures at Cambridge, his recent special lectures had emptied so many envelopes that 'the only fat envelope at the time was one called "animals"'. The lectures delivered in 1979 grew into *Man and the Natural World*, published four years later.

Here, as earlier, Keith emphasizes 'the profound shift in sensibilities' in early modern England.[63] Once more his aim was 'to reconstruct an earlier mental world in its own right' and to 'expose the assumptions, some barely articulated, which underlay the perceptions, reasonings and feelings of inhabitants of early modern England towards the animals, birds, vegetation and physical landscape'.[64] Reviewers were again enthusiastic. Though the book's impact 'will perhaps not be quite so extraordinary as that of *Religion and the Decline of Magic*', Hill thought it would 'set historians and others thinking not only about early modern England but also about the nature of history itself—its methods, the evidence it uses'. Like other reviewers, Hill praised 'the elegance and wit' of Keith's writing, so the book was doubly appropriate for the occasion, in that it reflected both Trevelyan's preoccupation with the English landscape and his emphasis on history's affinity with literature.[65] E. P. Thompson, when reviewing *Religion and the Decline of Magic*, had regretted its failure to employ literary sources or refer to literary criticism; these Thompson thought as important as numeracy when dealing with literary texts—though, he added, 'it is not in fashion to mention this'.[66] By the 1980s Keith was pioneering Thompson's desired shift in historiographical fashion. *Man and the Natural World* was 'intended to do something to reunite the studies of history and of literature', and made 'heavy, though unrepentant, use of literary sources of a kind not currently fashionable among historians'.[67] Of Trevelyan Keith said that 'no one could be wholly immune to the poetic appeal of his writing', especially 'his moving evocation of the garden front

---

[63] Thomas, *Man and the Natural World*, 15.
[64] Ibid.
[65] *New Statesman*, 8 Apr. 1983, 22; cf. David Spring in *American Historical Review* (June 1984), 734, and David Holloway in *Daily Telegraph*, 21 Apr. 1983, 14.
[66] Thompson, 'Anthropology and the Discipline of Historical Context', 49.
[67] Thomas, *Man and the Natural World*, 16.

of St John's, witness of the last days of the courtiers of Charles I', which 'shaped my perception of my present college long before I ever set eyes upon it'.[68] The reviewers thought he had succeeded: he wore his scholarship lightly, and had an eye for the apt quotation, the curious illustration, and the apposite anecdote.[69] Indeed, he has always combined his strenuous pursuit of generalization and explanation with a taste for diversity and for the particular. His prose is often so seductive that it masks the originality of his apparently self-evident interpretation. Critics might question whether literary evidence is representative;[70] but for a period that lacks more systematic evidence, what is the alternative to a well-judged balancing of example against counter-example?

Keith returned to the theme in his lecture on *History and Literature* (1988), where he stressed their continuous interaction both in scholarship and in the world of action. Yet he saw such emphasis less as a novelty than as recovering an older theme, for as a child he had eagerly consumed historical novels by Harrison Ainsworth and Walter Scott as well as Dorothy Margaret Stuart's literary books for children about history. He now likened writing history to composing a painting, claiming in 1990 that successive historical interpretations do not cumulate or supersede one another, any more than 'a landscape of Cézanne supersedes a landscape of Constable. They are both perfectly valid landscapes'.[71] He had sometimes cited literary historians before: his essay on Hobbes discussed honour with reference to G. F. Jones, C. B. Watson, and C. L. Barber; his 'The Place of Laughter' appears to draw upon Mikhail Bakhtin's ideas of 'subversive laughter'; and a reference to the critic Erich Auerbach occurs in 1985. But he was becoming increasingly preoccupied with 'ways of doing cultural history', the title of his lecture in 1991; and he was applying them to a wide range of topics: 'The Perception of the Past' (1983), 'Literacy' (1986), 'Numeracy' (1987), 'Children' (1989), 'Conscience' (1993), 'Cleanliness' (1994), and 'Work' (1999). Bossy's comment on *Religion and the Decline of Magic*—that it does much 'to shift the centre of gravity of English 16th and 17th century historiography closer to . . . the daily experience of the ordinary Englishman or woman'[72]—applies to all Keith's writing. Yet his interest has never been confined to popular culture: the history of culture at any social level interests him;[73] cultural history includes all human experience and cannot be confined to activities commonly labelled 'cultural'. It should fertilize the whole of history, not be cramped within chairs reserved for the subject.[74]

[68] Ibid. 9 (preface).
[69] See e.g. Alan Ryan, *Listener*, 14 Apr. 1983, 29; Stuart Hampshire, *New York Review of Books*, 2 June 1983, 17; David Holloway, *Daily Telegraph*, 21 Apr. 1983, 14.
[70] As does E. L. Jones in *EcHR* 36 (1983), 630; cf. John Dixon Hunt, *Times Higher Education Supplement*, 6 May 1983, 14.
[71] Interview with Peer Vries, 106; cf. Thomas, *History and Literature*, 22.
[72] Bossy, 'Early Modern Magic', 403.   [73] Thomas, 'Ways of Doing Cultural History', 79.
[74] Interview with Peer Vries, 109.

Some criticize Keith's dependence on English sources. In *Religion and the Decline of Magic* he 'resisted the temptation to draw parallels with Scotland, Ireland or the Continent of Europe', preferring to postpone comparison 'until the data for each country have been properly assembled'.[75] For one historian his *Man and the Natural World* ignores 'the crucially pervasive and creative impact of the tropical and colonial experience', while a leading anthropologist sees his unwillingness to place Britain in comparative perspective as ethnocentric.[76] There are limits to what one scholar can achieve. Besides, in what is an increasingly international scholarly climate, Keith's Anglocentric approach is far less limiting than it would have been for a political historian. For in focusing on the broad trend of ideas and social change he was preoccupied with developments more likely to be replicated elsewhere, just as he was more likely to share preoccupations with historians writing about other societies. His ideas on witchcraft have been found relevant in work on America, on Luzern, on the Cambrésis, and on Lorraine.[77] *Religion and the Decline of Magic* has been translated into Italian and cited approvingly in studies from Bavaria, Hungary, Estonia, and Iceland.[78] *Man and the Natural World* has been translated into Swedish and French, while three of his essays, all concerned with senses of time, have been published as a book in German.[79] Both Keith's major books have been translated into Japanese, Portuguese, and Dutch. His reception has been especially warm in Holland, where students of witchcraft, animals, gesture, and laughter acknowledge his inspiration.[80]

IV

Our prime concern is with Keith the historian, but we must also recognize the teacher and the public figure who became prominent in the 1980s, if only because in him the past and the present interact in practical as well as

---

[75] Thomas, *Religion*, 197.

[76] R. Grove, *Green Imperialism* (Cambridge, 1995), 3; J. Goody, 'Man and the Natural World: Reflections on History and Anthropology', *Environment and History*, 2 (1996), 255–69, esp. 260–1.

[77] J. Demos, *Entertaining Satan* (New York, 1982), 298; R. Muchembled, *La Sorcière au village* (Paris, 1979), 35, 106, 159; R. Briggs, *Witches and Neighbours* (1996), 142, 209.

[78] W. Behringer, *Hexenverfolgung in Bayern* (Munich, 1988), 8, 72, 96, 128; B. Ankarloo and G. Henningsen (eds.), *Early Modern European Witchcraft: Centres and Peripheries* (Oxford, 1990), 243, 275, 397.

[79] i.e. K. Thomas, *Vergangenheit, Zukunft, Lebensalter: Zeitvorstellungen im England der frühen Neuzeit* (Berlin, 1988). An extract from *Religion* appeared in C. Honegger (ed.), *Die Hexen der Neuzeit* (Frankfurt am Main, 1978), 256–308.

[80] M. Gijswijt-Hofstra and W. Frijhoff (eds.), *Witchcraft in the Netherlands* (Rotterdam, 1991); H. de Waardt, *Toverij en Samenleving: Holland, 1500–1800* (The Hague, 1991), 29–33; C. Davids, *Dieren en Nederlanders: Zeven eeuwen lief en leed* (Utrecht, 1989), *passim*; J. Bremmer and H. Roodenburg (eds.), *A Cultural History of Gesture* (Cambridge, 1991); J. Bremmer and H. Roodenburg (eds.), *A Cultural History of Humour* (Cambridge, 1997), 7–8; R. Dekker, *Lachen in de Gouden Eeuw* (Amsterdam, 1997).

intellectual matters. Through understanding our past we broaden our tolerance and refine our perceptions; thereby we clarify the full range of options open to us, and by extending the scope of reason we enhance our control over the present. Not for nothing has Keith been on the editorial board of the journal *Past and Present* since 1968.

In St John's he held no major College office, yet he played the most important role of all, that of College Tutor, and his reputation as teacher and lecturer soon spread within Oxford. The approach to his Gothick room in the Holmes Building was increasingly encrusted by overflow from his library. The room was high-ceilinged and rather elegantly furnished, but it was not particularly tidy and was sometimes chilly. Tutorials were not relaxing occasions, though there was no parade of efficiency: reading lists were recalled from memory, papers littered the floor, and filing cabinets were slow to arrive. The young meritocrat from Barry Grammar School had no time for the dilettantism or sheer idleness of the few undergraduates who were still being admitted in the late 1950s on personal connection or sporting flair. Hard work and independent thought were expected. While essays were read out, he would sprawl rather untidily in his armchair, but his legs were restlessly crossed and recrossed. Did this speed up when the essay was good or when it was bad, we asked ourselves. He did not remain recumbent for long; books were often consulted, sometimes in the adjoining room, so offstage rummagings constituted another distraction. More frequently in the early years than later, he would also jump up to consult a book that he knew was being quoted extensively and without acknowledgement, alighting on the relevant passage and reading it out; pupils did not commit that sin twice. A contributor to this volume had not been sufficiently industrious one summer vacation, and on returning was told 'now I'm going to viva you for an hour on Aristotle'. There followed an hour of one-to-one grilling on extracts from the text, at the end of which, he recalls, 'I was like a floor-cloth.' Sweeping or vague generalizations were punctured, especially when sociological or social anthropological in nature. When Keith's characteristic 'yeees...' rose slightly in incredulity during an essay, trouble could be expected: it was a holding operation while he decided how precisely to disagree. Praise was not lavish; the best one could hope for was a 'lucid', or (very rarely) a 'commendably lucid'. Weaker pupils and entrance candidates sometimes understandably failed to recognize behind the interrogation a single-minded and unremitting search for and nourishing of talent, nor did they always perceive the distinction between inquisitiveness and inquisition. For inquisitive Keith certainly was and is, and the books on his shelves repeatedly suffered from the urgency of his desire to extract their contents. He could display an almost violent eagerness to 'gut' them, as he once put it. Underlying everything was ambition for his pupils and determination that they should make the most of what he saw as a precious opportunity.

Yet there was another side to Keith: a rumbustious conviviality that came as a revelation, even as a shock, to those who had seen him only in academic mode. One contributor was astonished, and even rather embarrassed, to see him after a schools dinner wildly hurtling croquet balls into the dim distance on the huge lawn of St John's. Then, as now, Keith was lively in gesture, youthful in appearance, quick in his movements, and receptive to new ideas. The young tutor dressed less formally than later, wearing a brown corduroy jacket or sometimes a rather faded grey suit. At his parties in the mid-1960s beer was poured from an enamel jug, but it soon gave way to sherry glasses and intellectual respectability, and a woman graduate was sometimes invited. A once-radical contributor still recalls Keith's 'wonderful politeness', on one such occasion, to the Vietnamese girlfriend he had acquired during the Vietnam war. Oxford's tutorial system, so repetitive for tutors, often encourages a routine processing of pupils; yet Keith treated the tutorial as a personal relationship, setting unorthodox essay topics, encouraging experiment, and making allowances for personal difficulties in the pace of the written work required. One contributor recalls him urging the merits of Carlo Ginzburg's *Il formaggio e i vermi* long before it was widely known outside Italy, and some years before it was translated into English. To be taught by him was a formidable and formative experience.

Still more was this so for his graduate students. He commented assiduously on the logic and presentation of scripts, and generously plundered his envelopes to help graduates even when they worked in areas close to his own. Possible social-anthropological approaches were mentioned but never pressed on his graduates. They found him a critical, stimulating supervisor, but intellectually permissive and never domineering or missionary. Books to review, people to meet, seminars to address, opportunities of every kind somehow came one's way. He was unusually conscientious and shrewd in giving advice about careers, important at a time when academic posts in history were scarce. 'If one approached Keith for a reference,' a contributor recalls, 'one could expect a pretty serious grilling as to whether this was the right thing to try for at this point in one's career. If he was convinced and agreed, he would support one with total commitment and the utmost generosity.' Graduates supervised by others experienced these benefits in diluted form through his influential graduate seminar on early modern British history, held from the 1970s in the magnificent Judges' Lodgings of St John's. In the early 1980s, one contributor recalls, 'it was *the* place to debate and hear debated issues at the cutting edge of early modern social and intellectual history'. Large audiences were attracted by Keith's astute eye for the essentials in an argument (usually, and sometimes disturbingly, raised in the often innocently phrased question with which he launched the discussion). There was also the *frisson* of the occasional eruption from John Cooper, who often attended. Keith's careful sociability rendered this graduate seminar—

unlike many in Oxford, which is not good at seminars—both intellectually demanding and fun.

By the early 1980s he was becoming so widely known that at least two of the contributors, precocious in their sixth forms, chose St John's as their undergraduate college because he was there. As a tutor he had become seasoned enough to devise tactics that would interest even the weaker among his pupils. In tutorials on Rousseau, for instance, he would ask the assembled company what was the first sentence in *The Social Contract*, usually getting a correct answer. He would then immediately ask what was the second sentence, only to encounter blank faces. 'Ah,' he would say, 'one day I shall find a student who has read as far as the second sentence of the work.' Word eventually percolated down the years, and a new device had to be invented. By the mid-1980s he was getting bored with some aspects of tutorial teaching, which had never closely matched his research interests, and it was time for the third of his four half-conscious self-reinventions. Fellows of St John's, if asked in the 1960s to predict his future, would have envisaged a lifetime's career as a successful College Tutor. But in 1980 he had been the Faculty's preferred candidate for the Regius Chair of Modern History and had not been appointed, though he held an *ad hominem* chair from January to September 1986. Not becoming Regius Professor was yet another of the accidents moulding a career that he sees as unplanned and as involving repeated responses to opportunity; his publications have often, for instance, originated as responses to invitations.

No invitation could have been more fortunate for Corpus Christi College than to attract him to succeed Sir Kenneth Dover as President in 1986. This humanist foundation of Bishop Fox—the smallest college in Oxford, but with a high academic reputation—gave him an appropriate setting. He immediately identified with the College, and revealed himself as an energetic 'hands-on' President, his competitive instincts harnessed to promote its interests. Social anthropology, like charity, should begin at home, and he was a shrewd observer of the Oxford college system. In contributing to the *History of the University of Oxford* (1994), he was uncompromising: the Oxford college could still, he said, 'provide its members with a living and working environment superior to that yet devised by any other academic institution'.[81] From two historian-presidents of St John's he had learned much of value for Corpus. With W. C. Costin he had often disagreed, and yet he shared Costin's conviction that an institution is ultimately more important than the individuals who pass through it. Immediately on arrival at Corpus, Keith highlighted Corpus traditions when addressing new members at their first dinner in Hall, dwelling light-heartedly yet seriously upon the College's symbols: the bees,

---

[81] K. Thomas, 'College Life, 1945–1970', in B. Harrison (ed.), *The History of the University of Oxford*, viii. *The Twentieth Century* (Oxford, 1994), 215.

the tortoise, the pelican, and the owl. He was equally at home when addressing the College's tenant farmers at their annual rent-audit dinner; indeed, as President his alertness to atmosphere elicited well-judged speeches attuned to the most varied types of occasion. His sense of the College's corporate identity made him especially popular with old members. He corresponded extensively with them and, learning from Sir Richard Southern's example at St John's, cultivated their loyalties with his thoroughly researched and witty after-dinner speeches at gaudies. These were repeatedly punctuated with shouts of laughter as he reminded old members what Corpus had been like in their day and explained how it had subsequently changed and yet how in many ways it had stayed the same.

At every point Keith's sense of history moulded his view of the presidency. Running an Oxford college is no easy task, but he soon found that he enjoyed it, and through his obvious dedication and sharpness of intellect he earned the respect he received. An alertness to the College's interests viewed over the very long term shaped a strategy on the major issues that was often courageous. He did not seek a cheap popularity by shirking the difficult decisions or taking the easy way out; when confronted by a challenge, his upper lip tightened and there would be no retreat. His concern for scholarship led him to assign much time to appointing new Fellows, and he readily seized opportunities for making the College better known and better funded. His incisive judgement, honed on thirty years' historical study, made him a brisk yet fair-minded chairman. With a close grasp of detail, he was also adept at giving a discreet lead and at defusing trouble with a well-timed joke. He gave much-needed encouragement and consolidated loyalties by dispatching timely and tactful notes to junior and senior members alike. Nor was the head of house's inevitably growing fund-raising role uncongenial to a President who had long relished exploring parts of English society that most Welshmen do not reach. On serious matters he was serious, and drove both the Fellows and the staff hard with his meticulousness on detail and his pursuit of high standards. Personal and institutional procedure and conduct must be correct, manners were important, and in term time he seldom wore anything other than a suit. His rapid response in argument, sharpened in three decades of tutorials, salutarily reminded the Fellows now and again what it was like once more to be a pupil. A quick intellect did not always grasp the strong feeling or real justification that inspired opinions unconvincingly articulated. It was a surprising fault in a President whose hallmark as historian was mapping the mental outlook of the uneducated, and offence was sometimes unintentionally given. His sense of the dignity and traditions of his office, his high intellectual standards, and his tall, fast-moving though unhurried presence sometimes made him seem more intimidating to the young than he intended. Yet he took trouble to get to know them, and on more light-hearted occasions had no difficulty in unbending. Those who knew only his elegant wit and ironic touch on public occasions soon came to relish the uninhibited and infectious humour that reflected his genuine zest for intellectual sociability. In his company, laughter is frequent, often at the wry anecdotes he adeptly recounts. He is, in short, good company.

Southern embodied Keith's ideal of the scholar-president. Keith did not allow his presidency to arrest the flow of scholarly publications; indeed, he gained stimulus in his writing from the daily challenge presented by a president's miscellany of simultaneous but diverse tasks. Nor did his duties preclude agreeing to give the Ford Lectures, the highest honour Oxford's history faculty has to bestow on historians of Britain, in the year 2000. Still, many other distractions from history now presented themselves, for he was moving towards the fourth of his self-reinventions: from respected Oxford historian to academic statesman and public figure. A head of house has many opportunities for serving the University. Keith has been a Pro-Vice-Chancellor and member of Hebdomadal Council since 1988 and has participated in several University committees, usually as Chairman. He has been closely involved with the Oxford University Press. He acted as Humanities Editor of its OPUS series from 1973 to 1989 and as General Editor of its Past Masters series from 1980 and of Oxford Studies in Social History from 1986. As a Delegate since 1980, and especially as Chairman of the Finance Committee since 1988, he has greatly influenced the growth and development of the Press, where his intellectual and academic integrity and breadth of interests make him widely consulted and widely respected.

Being head of house constitutes a good platform for venturing more widely afield. The young man who had sallied forth in the 1950s out of South Wales was not reluctant later in life to accept invitations to join major British institutions. Fellow of the British Academy from 1979, he was on the Economic and Social Research Council from 1985 to 1990 and a Trustee of the National Gallery from 1991 to 1998. In College committees making appointments he could often deploy relevant information acquired through being active in quite different spheres. Given all this, he was a 'natural' to chair the supervisory committee for the *New Dictionary of National Biography*. As a distinguished scholar, knighted for services to the study of history in 1988, with numerous connections and wide interests (reflecting what he once described as his 'grasshopper mind'[82]), he was the obvious person in the 1990s to mount a public defence of the humanities, which had been seriously on the defensive since the war. The most effective advocates of a cause are not always the most noisy, and he felt constrained in his public statements by his representative role as head of house and (from 1993 to 1997) President of the British Academy. Besides, such positions gave him many opportunities for lobbying government and wielding influence unobtrusively. In the mid-1990s he

[82] Interview with Peer Vries, 109.

promoted much-needed reforms within the Academy, found it a better site (in Carlton House Terrace near the Royal Society), and then obtained funds for it. So in 1996 he could point out, in his last presidential address to the Academy, that 'the symbolism of this juxtaposition of the two national academies in the centre of the capital is very potent. My hope is that it will serve as a reminder of the centrality to human life of the studies which we exist to foster.'[83] He seized the opportunities presented by his presidential addresses. 'We should do more to raise public awareness of the importance of the subjects we represent,' he told the Academy in 1994.[84] Referring two years later to inadequate government funding, he said that 'democracies have to be educated and . . . until both the social utility and the life-enhancing quality of our studies are more generally appreciated, the humanities and social sciences cannot hope for much better treatment'.[85]

G. M. Young says that 'a man's birth-year is only of importance because it directs us to look for what was happening in the world when he was twenty'.[86] In Britain in 1953 Keynes's predictions of 1930 on 'economic possibilities for our grandchildren' still seemed attainable: that early in the twenty-first century 'the *economic problem* may be solved'; that the competitiveness and greed entailed by wealth-getting might at last give way to more elevated impulses; and that we might 'once more value ends above means and prefer the good to the useful'.[87] In 1953 the afterglow of wartime triumph had not yet been dispelled; the collapse of empire did not yet seem imminent; the goodwill of liberated European countries towards Britain had not yet been squandered; German, French, and Japanese economic success had not yet exposed Britain's relative economic weakness; poverty had not yet revealed its capacity for perpetual self-renewal within the welfare state; and the limits to the social impact of secularized intelligence through political structures were as yet unclear. Keith shares many of the attitudes, and values many of the character traits, that in 1953 seemed peculiarly British. He has consistently advocated the highest standards of research and publication, and has resolutely defended meritocratic educational élitism. He was 'quite sure' in 1995 'that in the humanities it is infinitely more important that publications should be high in quality than that they should be numerous'.[88] And, while welcoming the 1960s for undermining class prejudice and creating a more open society, he did not relish that decade's informality and populism. Still less congenial was the robust commercialism that so unexpectedly gained ground after 1979. He had never taken a utilitarian or vocational view of university education, and

---

[83] British Academy, *Annual Report, 1995–6*, 11 (4 July 1996); cf. *Annual Report, 1993–5*, 10, 15.
[84] British Academy, *Annual Report, 1993–5*, 10; cf. *Annual Report, 1995–6*, 8.
[85] British Academy, *Annual Report, 1995–6*, 8.
[86] G. M. Young, 'Burke', *Proceedings of the British Academy*, 1943, 24.
[87] J. M. Keynes, *Essays in Persuasion* (1931), 372.
[88] British Academy, *Annual Report, 1993–5*, 12 (Presidential address, 6 July 1995).

deplored Thatcher's attack on the professions. 'The University should remain a critical and uncommitted observer of the economic process,' he had written in 1961, as the *Oxford Magazine*'s young editor, opposing the advent of business studies in Oxford, 'rather than become a tame accessory of the business world'.[89] In the 1990s he was disconcerted by the discredit that then at least temporarily engulfed so many once-respected British institutions.

Nowhere was there more cause for concern in the 1990s than at the heart of the cultural institutions within which he had spent his career. It was, he thought, a 'depressing generalisation' of Tocqueville's that love of truth for its own sake is the mark only of an aristocratic soceity.[90] Mass culture, pop music, mass tourism, mass spectator sport, demotic values, egalitarian fashions, and populist politics seemed to threaten the underfunded museums, art galleries, universities, libraries, high-class publishing ventures, and humane studies that he valued and to which he had given so much. He was nostalgic for the early twentieth-century tradition of working-class self-education that came out of the Welsh valleys, and deplored the waning cultural standards of a public-library system that had prompted such educational achievement in South Wales before the 1960s. If such things were in danger, were the benefits of mass affluence undiluted? If meritocratic recruitment, public funding, and harder work among Oxford's students were accompanied by narrow specialization, vocationalism, undue pressure to publish, populist lifestyles, and the indiscriminate application of the natural-science model, was there not more to be said for the *ancien régime* than he had once allowed?

Given these attitudes, there is at first sight something surprising about Keith's oft-repeated refusal to defend history as a distinct subject or department in universities. 'I do not think there is a unique historical method,' he said in 1990; historians are 'totally parasitic for their ideas upon other disciplines . . . Historians don't have any ideas of their own. They on the whole tend to employ what they think of as common sense, which is really a debased version of the economics, philosophy or sociology of a generation or two ago.'[91] Yet he takes up this position precisely because he sees history as a civilizing form of study. If the historical approach were confined within departments of history, the many other subjects that it should fertilize might lose their historical component, and historians might simultaneously be assigned mere leavings and lose contact with the important intellectual developments occurring elsewhere. 'It would be better', he thinks, 'to regard every subject as having its historical dimension.'[92] There is ample room for argument here. Historians may have no distinctive method, but their outlook is distinctive:

---

[89] *Oxford Magazine*, 18 May 1961, 347.
[90] British Academy, *Annual Report, 1995–6*, 7.
[91] Interview with Peer Vries, 101; cf. K. Thomas, 'The Past in Clearer Light, a Beacon on our future', *Times Higher Education Supplement*, 2 Dec. 1988, 16.
[92] Interview with Dr Brooks, 26.

they are professionally alert to change over time, just as the geographers are alert to contrasts across space. If fragmented into departments dominated by other disciplines, the historian's distinctive insights might gradually be lost. But there is no room for argument about the importance Keith attaches to the humanities and to history's place among them. The humanities 'enlarge our experience, enhance our self-consciousness, widen our sense of what is humanly possible and, most important of all, enable us to step outside the assumptions of our own day and to escape the tyranny of present-mindedness'.[93]

Keith cannot readily be pigeon-holed, still less can he be accused of sectarian alignment. Independent of fashion, though sometimes anticipating it, he has pioneered a distinctive view of historical study through practice more than through preachment, though he has often shown a practical concern about the health of the scholarly environment. There are limits to how far one scholar can hold out against the trends of his time, but his influence has been enhanced through his pupils. In later career he has seen them take over many of 'his' subjects, but this is a price he gladly pays for knowing that his agenda of the 1960s is still alive. His ideals are civilizing and humane, so it would be incongruous if he ever tried to impose them; they are best advanced through encouragement and setting an example. Besides, he wants for his pupils the intellectual freedom that he has himself enjoyed, so he has never sought to create a school of disciples. And, despite encouraging so many pupils and graduate students into areas where historical research is peculiarly difficult, and where he is a master, he has never inhibited them from publishing. So we, the contributors to this volume, take pleasure in acknowledging our debt to him and our admiration for what he has achieved.

[93] Thomas, 'The Past in Clearer Light', 16.

2

A Civil Tongue: Language and Politeness in Early Modern Europe

PETER BURKE

One of the domains in which the concept of civility was employed in early modern Europe was that of language. When a naval officer in Conrad's *Lord Jim* complains that 'it was as much as I could do to keep a civil tongue in my head', he was using a term with a long tradition, referring to the refusal to engage in the war of insults discussed elsewhere in this volume. However, this was not the only link between language and civility, as a recent study of the topic shows very clearly.[1] In the seventeenth century, George Wither referred to unseemly jests which 'every civil ear detests', while James Howell claimed that French had 'civiliz'd and smoothed' the English tongue.[2] In the sixteenth century, Sir Philip Sidney described the 'rude style' of traditional ballads as examples of an 'uncivil age', while George Puttenham discussed the language proper to 'men civill and graciously behavoured and bred'.[3]

Language, spoken or written, was viewed as one of the most obvious if not the most important ways of demonstrating status, manners, or breeding, a point made again and again in the treatises on good behaviour that proliferated in early modern Europe. To discuss the place of politeness in language and of language in politeness is the aim of this essay in what might be called 'historical pragmatics', a field to which Keith Thomas has contributed more than once.[4]

I

Two forms of linguistic behaviour will be studied here, 'altruistic' and 'egotistic' politeness. In the first place, consideration for others. In the second

---

[1] A. Bryson, *From Courtesy to Civility: Changing Codes of Conduct in Early Modern England* (Oxford, 1998), esp. 151–92.

[2] G. Wither, *Britain Remembered* (1628), 29; J. Howell, *New English Grammar* (1662), 'to the reader'.

[3] P. Sidney, *Miscellaneous Prose*, ed. K. Duncan-Jones and J. van Dorsten (Oxford, 1973), 97; G. Puttenham, *The Arte of English Poesie* (1589; repr. Menston, 1968).

[4] K. Thomas, 'Yours', in C. Ricks and L. Michaels (eds.), *The State of the Language* (1990), 451–6; his paper on accent unfortunately remains unpublished.

place, distinction from others, via 'higher' or 'purer' forms of language. The basic assumption in what follows is that polite language of both types changes over time, just as it varies from place to place, from one social group to another, and from individual to individual.

This assumption might appear to have been contradicted, if not completely demolished, by a major study of the subject published some twenty years ago by two British linguists. The central point of Brown and Levinson's lucid and elegant essay is that 'politeness phenomena' can be explained by 'universal strategies of verbal interaction'.[5] Inspired by the work of the sociologist Erving Goffman, the philosopher H. P. Grice, and the linguist John Gumperz, the authors analyse expressions of politeness in three unrelated languages (English, Tamil, and Tzeltal), centring on the concepts of 'face' and 'face-threatening acts' (FTAs). They distinguish between 'negative face' (the need not to be impeded) and 'positive face' (the need for one's wants to be desired by others).

Politeness, described as a way of minimizing these threats, is also divided into positive and negative forms. The authors list and discuss fifteen strategies of positive politeness ('seek agreement', 'joke', 'promise', and so on), and ten of negative politeness ('give deference', 'apologize', etc.). Their emphasis falls heavily on human rationality (sometimes analysed in terms of 'costs' and 'benefits'), and on universality. Criticizing what they call 'the once-fashionable doctrine of cultural relativity', the authors argue that 'superficial diversities can emerge from underlying universal principles and are satisfactorily accounted for only in relation to them'.[6]

What has happened to cultural differences? The authors note that what counts as an FTA varies from one culture to another, and they draw a contrast between 'positive politeness cultures' with low social distance (the USA, for example), and more hierarchical 'negative politeness cultures' (such as Britain and Japan).[7] However, they do not take their analysis of difference very far. In the revised version of their essay, they note the relevance of 'folk theories' of face, tact, and so on, but they do not develop this point either.[8] In similar fashion, in his classic essay on the subject, Erving Goffman glided from what he called 'the Chinese conception of face' to his own analysis of the USA without discussing differences between the two cultures.[9]

In this essay, on the other hand, the aim is to discuss variations and changes

[5] P. Brown and S. Levinson, 'Universals in Language Usage: Politeness Phenomena' (1978), revised as *Politeness: Some Universals in Language Usage* (Cambridge, 1987); cf. C. A. Ferguson, 'The Structure and Use of Politeness Formulas', *Language in Society*, 5 (1976), 137–51.
[6] Brown and Levinson, *Politeness*, 56.   [7] Ibid. 13–14, 48.
[8] For criticisms by linguists, see R. Watt *et al.* (eds.), *Politeness in Language* (Berlin, 1992), esp. 10, 107.
[9] E. Goffman, 'On Face-Work' (1955), repr. in his *Interaction Ritual* (Harmondsworth, 1972), 5–45.

in the rules of civility. I have no intention of denying the existence of universal human strategies, linguistic or otherwise. However, the importance of these strategies cannot be assessed without a study of what is not universal, of what varies between places or changes over time. Rather than assuming that what varies is necessarily 'superficial', as Brown and Levenson put it, the idea will be put to the test. In order to demonstrate the importance of universals, Brown and Levenson adopted the strategy of comparing polite language in three unrelated cultures. To show the importance of variation and change, it may be useful to adopt the opposite strategy to theirs and focus on three related cultures, England, France, and Italy.

A basic concept in this enterprise of historicization is that of different systems, codes, or 'regimes' of civility, which are embedded in larger regimes of everyday life.[10] By a 'regime' is meant a repertoire of practices, consisting of gestures and words (spoken and written), including modes of address such as 'Madam', or 'Your Majesty', formulaic phrases such as 'please' or 'yours sincerely', unspoken rules such as 'don't interrupt', and so on. Each element in the repertoire may have parallels elsewhere, but the regime is distinctive in its combination of items and also in its inflections or emphases, revealing cultural differences and contrasts at the level of tact (or tactics), if not at Brown and Levenson's deeper level of strategy. For these reasons a regime may be regarded as a system. Needless to say (among historians, at least), a linguistic regime is never static, any more than a political regime. In both cases, however, the structures usually have a longer life than individuals.

Regimes of civility are, of course, related to social structures, even if they are not simply translations of these structures into words. A working hypothesis might take the form of the proposition that, the more hierarchical (highly stratified or more sharply stratified) the society, the more formal or elaborate its civility will be. This hypothesis will be discussed, if not tested in the strict sense of that term, in the pages that follow. At this point in the argument what may need emphasis is the distinctiveness of different regimes. The evidence for the distinctiveness comes in particular from the history of encounters between people from different cultures, and the distance (not to mention misunderstandings) that these encounters reveal.

II

Take the case of 'oriental' politeness, for instance, as perceived by Westerners. What Brown and Levenson call the 'humiliative mode' of politeness, praising

[10] Cf. the notion of different 'politeness systems' employed in M. Sifaniou, *Politeness Phenomena in England and Greece: A Cross-Cultural Perspective* (Oxford, 1992), 41.

the other and depreciating the self and its possessions, has often been described as remarkable, exaggerated, and even servile.[11] These descriptions obviously have their place in the occidental construction of Orientalism, especially 'Oriental Despotism'. They also reveal perceptions of cultural distance that tell us something about the perceivers.

For example, the contemporary account of the embassy to the emperor of China sent by the Dutch East India Company in the mid-seventeenth century is full of references to the 'civility' of the Chinese. They treated the Dutch with civility, excused themselves with civility, refused with civility, and so on. The account notes 'the courtly and polite modish way of speaking' in China, in which the speaker refers to himself as 'He, or such a one'.[12] George Macartney, British ambassador to China in 1793–4, was more ambivalent. He commented on 'the most refined politeness and sly good breeding' of the mandarins he met, the slyness referring to 'an immediate acquiescence in words with everything we seemed to propose', combined with 'evasion' in practice. George Staunton, who accompanied the embassy and published a description of it soon afterwards, commented not only on the 'urbanity' of high-status Chinese but also on the 'excess' of Chinese manners, which 'require, in the mention of one's self, that the most abject terms should be employed, and the most exalted towards those who are addressed'. In other words, the British distanced themselves from the 'abject' language of the Chinese, the verbal equivalent of the kowtow to the emperor that the ambassador famously refused to perform.[13]

As for India, even in the seventeenth century, when Englishmen made a considerable use of compliments, they already perceived the polite forms of that country as distant from theirs. The English clergyman Edward Terry noted that 'this people of East India are civil in their speeches', while his successor John Ovington described 'the Orientals' as 'much more tender and insinuating in their language' than Europeans, so much so that whoever is accustomed to their style of speaking 'can hardly bear the roughness or be brought to digest the rudeness of the others'.[14] By the nineteenth century, attitudes had changed. Francis Day, an English medical officer stationed in Cochin, noted what he called the 'cringing servility' of the low-caste Permauls, while the missionary Samuel Mateer, who worked among the Pulayan of Travancore, described what he called the 'abject' language that the lower castes were compelled to use when speaking to their superiors, including the terms

[11] Brown and Levinson, *Politeness*, 179, 185.
[12] J. Nieuhoff, *Het Gezantschap der Neerlandsche Oost-Indisch Compagnie aan den Grooteen Tartarischen Cham* (Amsterdam, 1665); English trans. *An Embassy sent by the East India Company* (1699), 62, 83, 85, 173.
[13] G. Macartney, *An Embassy to China*, ed. J. Cranmer-Byng (1962), 87; G. Staunton, *An Authentic Account of an Embassy* (2 vols.; 1797), ii. 29, 35, 240.
[14] E. Terry, *A Voyage to East-India* (1655), 214; J. Ovington, *A Voyage to Surat* (1692), 276.

'your slave' (instead of 'I'), 'dirty gruel' (for 'rice'), 'hut' (for 'house'), and 'monkeys' (for children).[15]

The point is not to assert that Europeans never practise the humiliative mode (which some English people, for example, still do in a mild form), but simply to note that for centuries some of them perceived Chinese and Indian forms and formulas of civility to be different from their own. It is time to investigate whether these forms change over time as well as varying over space and whether they are related to social and political structures such as differences in degrees of liberty or equality.

III

The year 1789 might be considered an appropriate date at which to end an article on 'old regimes' of civility, partly because the best historical evidence for the importance and significance of the rules governing everyday life, including everyday language, comes from breaking them, or more exactly from investigating the moments at which, occasions on which, and contexts in which they are broken. Indeed, the traditional regime of French politeness broke down after 1789 precisely because it was associated with and taken to symbolize the *ancien régime* in general. Reciprocal *tu* replaced the asymmetrical system of *tu* and *vous*, the variety and hierarchy of modes of address were replaced by *citoyen* and *citoyenne*, and so on, in order to symbolize equality and fraternity.

In Europe before 1789 there was no such revolution in everyday language, apart from the practice of a few radical religious groups. The sixteenth-century Anabaptists addressed their fellow-believers as 'brother', 'sister', or 'thou'. The seventeenth-century Quakers shocked their contemporaries and anticipated the French revolutionaries by calling everyone 'thee' in what has been called a 'rhetoric of impoliteness' designed to show that 'Christ respects no man's person'—in other words, that worldly distinctions had no importance for true Christians.[16]

All the same, the European regime of civility was gradually modified in significant ways, especially in the later eighteenth century. Linguistic and other practices changed, and so did the 'folk categories' through which they were discussed in this period. Three at least of these categories may be regarded as central: 'honour', 'civility' itself, and finally 'politeness'. They require consideration here because they offer access to insiders' views of change.

---

[15] F. Day, *The Land of the Permauls* (Madras, 1863), 327, 391; S. Mateer, *The Land of Charity* (1871), 45.

[16] C.-P. Clasen, *Anabaptism: A Social History, 1525–1618* (Ithaca, NY, 1972), 146; R. Bauman, *Let Your Words be Few: Symbolism of Speaking and Silence among Seventeenth-Century Quakers* (Cambridge, 1983), 43–62.

Peter Burke

The term 'honour' (*onore, honneur*), as used in England, Italy, and France between 1500 and 1800, was a reasonably close equivalent of what Goffman preferred to call 'face'. The concept had a double meaning, but it may be argued that its very ambiguity or circularity was essential to its usefulness. It signified both the outer respect paid to men and women of a certain status, and the qualities that made this respect appropriate, especially courage in the case of men and modesty in that of women. People were honoured because they were honourable, and one knew that they were honourable because they were honoured.[17]

Equally ambiguous was the answer to the question, who possessed honour? According to the treatises on the subject, honour was a prerogative of the nobility. However, judicial records show that ordinary people, at least in towns, often claimed to have honour, and also that the courts took this claim seriously, at least on occasion.[18] The courts were involved because of attacks on the honour of the plaintiffs—in other words, insults. The concern they showed reveals the importance attributed to forms of language in the social life of the period.

The second keyword is 'civility' (*civiltà, civilité*). The concept developed first in Italy, where its associations with 'city' were taken very seriously. The countryside was for animals, the city for humans and the *vita civile* (a life that was at once civilized, civilian, and civic, and so appropriate for citizens of independent city-republics). Both the term and the idea of civility became increasingly important in western Europe in the sixteenth and seventeenth centuries, partly at the expense of the medieval term 'courtesy' (*cortesia, courtoisie*).

At the same time civility changed its meaning, referring less and less to political systems and more and more to elegant behaviour, including the practice of collecting statues and other objects. It is tempting to relate this change in the meaning of civility to the decline of city-republics in favour of absolute monarchies, small ones such as the Grand Duchy of Florence as well as large ones such as France.[19] The rise of civility in the new sense was both expressed and encouraged by Erasmus's treatise on good manners for small boys, *De civilitate morum puerilium* (1530), followed by Giovanni Della Casa's *Galateo* (1558), Stefano Guazzo's *La civil conversazione* (1578), Antoine de Courtin's *Nouveau traité de civilité* (1671), and many others. The translation of these texts reveals how far civility or politeness was becoming a European ideal. Della Casa was

---

[17] A. Jouanna, 'Recherches sur la notion de l'honneur au 16ᵉ siècle', *Revue d'histoire moderne et contemporaine*, 15 (1968), 597–623.

[18] Y. Castan, *Honnêteté et relations sociales en Languedoc* (Paris, 1974); cf. P. Burke, *Historical Anthropology of Early Modern Italy* (Cambridge, 1987), 109.

[19] J. Revel, 'Les Usages de la civilité', in P. Ariès (ed.), *History of Private Life*, iii (Cambridge, Mass., 1989), 167–205; R. Chartier, *Lectures et lecteurs dans la France d'ancien régime* (Paris, 1987), 45–86; A. Pons, 'Sur la notion de la civilité', in A. Montandon (ed.), *Etiquette et politesse* (Clermont-Ferrand, 1992).

translated into French, English, Latin, and Spanish, and Guazzo into French, English, and Latin, while Courtin was adapted into English and German.

A seventeenth-century English writer summed up the new ideal by declaring civility to consist in three things, two negative and one positive. In the first place, 'not expressing by actions or speeches any injury, disesteem, offence or undervaluing any other'. In the second place, 'in receiving no injuries or offences from others, i.e. in not resenting every word or action which may (perhaps rationally) be interpreted to be disesteem or undervaluing' (this fits the case of Conrad's sailor, quoted at the opening of this paper). On the positive side, 'in being ready to do all good offices and ordinary kindness for another'.[20] The rejection of an earlier honour-based system is particularly clear in this passage, in the recommendations both to refrain from honour-threatening acts and also to show less sensitivity to threats from others. The plural form 'civilities' came into use to refer to compliments and other polite expressions or gestures. As in the case of honours and honour, there was a revealing circularity here. The practice of civilities was a sign that the speaker was civilized.

An alternative term to civility was 'politeness'. La Rochefoucauld associated the two concepts in an epigram: 'La civilité est un désir d'en recevoir et d'être estimé poli.' In similar fashion, in his dictionary, Antoine Furetière defined *civilité* as 'une manière honnête, douce et polie d'agir, de converser ensemble'. *Politesse* became fashionable in seventeenth-century France, where Madame de Scudéry devoted one of her dialogues to the subject, defining it as 'savoir vivre'. According to the duc de Saint-Simon, Louis XIV was a paragon of politeness, 'Jamais homme si naturellement poli', drawing attention to the king's skill in 'measuring' his politeness to fit 'l'âge, le mérite, le rang'. The point made earlier about the influence of social structures on regimes of politeness could hardly be illustrated more clearly. In similar fashion, Bellegarde, the author of model conversations 'pour les personnes polies', distinguished different varieties of *politesse* as suitable for the *homme d'épée*, the *magistrat*, and so on.[21]

The terms *politezza* and *polite* had less success in Italian, but, in England, so common was the word 'polite' in the early eighteenth century that one scholar has coined the phrase 'the culture of politeness' to refer to this period, while another has entitled a history of England in 1727–83 *A Polite and Commercial People*, taking the phrase from the lawyer William Blackstone.[22] Eighteenth-century book titles include *The Polite Philosopher* (1734), *The Polite Student*

---

[20] O. Walker, *Of Education* (1673; Menston, 1970), 211.

[21] La Rochefoucauld, *Maximes* (1685; ed. F. C. Green, Cambridge, 1946), 67; Saint-Simon, *Mémoires*, i (Paris, 1983); J. B. de Bellegarde, *Réfléxions sur la politesse des mœurs* (Paris, 1703), 46. Cf. M. Lacroix, *De la politesse* (Paris, 1990); P. France, *Politeness and its Discontents* (Cambridge, 1992).

[22] L. E. Klein, *Shaftesbury and the Culture of Politeness* (Cambridge, 1994); P. Langford, *A Polite and Commercial People* (Oxford, 1989).

(1748), *The Polite Lady* (1760), *The Polite Academy* (1762), *The Polite Traveller* (1783), and so on.

Like 'civility', 'politeness' had a political origin—derived from the very terms 'polis' and 'political'—but in the seventeenth and eighteenth centuries it came to refer to elegant or 'polished' as opposed to 'rough' manners. As Lord Chesterfield, considered one of the authorities on manners in eighteenth-century England, wrote to his son, 'Good company, if you make the right use of it, will cut you into shape and give you the true brilliant polish' (6 July 1749). When Chesterfield's views were presented to a wider audience in the form of 'Principles of Politeness', the topics included cleanliness, dress, and spitting.[23]

Politeness often took the form of ritualized gestures, of 'making legs' (bowing), making genuflexions, or making curtseys (an expression of 'courtesy', from which the word is derived). However, the verbal genuflexion, what the English were coming to call a 'civil tongue', was considered one of the most important ways of expressing politeness. Thus Courtin devoted specific chapters of his treatise to conversation, compliments, and salutations, as well as to posture and gesture. These practices, ranging from competence in the current formulas of respect to the mastery of the art of conversation, showed family resemblances and, so far as language is concerned, might be defined by contrast to the ideal of plain speech, a frankness that in 'civil' circles was considered a breach of good manners.

The number of treatises published on the art of conversation at this time bear witness to the interest in the subject—'polite conversation', as it was often called.[24] In her *Conversations nouvelles*, for instance, Madame de Scudéry included 'savoir toujours parler à propos' in the definition of *politesse*, and advised her readers 'ne vouloir pas être le tyran de la conversation'.[25] Lord Shaftesbury argued that conversation was a means of 'polish'. Lord Chesterfield's frequently expressed opinions on the subject were soon summarized by his popularizers in the form of thirty-five 'rules for conversation'. It may be worth emphasizing that Chesterfield recommended politeness to inferiors. A master was advised to say to his servant that he would be 'much obliged' if the servant would carry out a certain task. In order to avoid misunderstanding, 'Indicate by your language, that the performance is a favour, and by your tone that it is a matter of course.'

How many people or even how many kinds of people followed the rules it is obviously impossible to say with precision. The rules were associated

---

[23] Chesterfield, *Letters* (1774); J. Trussler, *Principles of Politeness* (1775).
[24] D. A. Berger, *Die Konversationskunst in England 1660–1740* (Munich, 1978); C. Strosetzki, *Konversation: Ein Kapitel gesellschaftlicher und literarischer Pragmatik im Frankreich des 17. Jhts* (Frankfurt, 1978); E. C. Goldsmith, *Exclusive Conversations: The Art of Interaction in 17th-Century France* (Philadelphia, 1988); P. Burke, *The Art of Conversation* (Cambridge, 1993); M. Fumaroli, *Trois institutions littéraires* (Paris, 1994), 111–210.
[25] M. de Scudéry, *Conversations nouvelles* (Paris, 1685), 67.

with the upper classes, and they may be analysed in the manner of Pierre Bourdieu as a strategy for distinguishing themselves from those whom they perceived as their social inferiors. Complaining in the 1780s that 'all external evidence of rank' was disappearing, an English gentleman stressed the importance of 'politeness of expression; it is the only external distinction which remains between a gentleman and a valet, a lady and a mantua-maker'.[26]

The rules were codified at the time of the rise of absolute monarchy, so that they may also be analysed in the style of Norbert Elias as one of the means by which rulers tamed their nobilities. The role of aristocratic women, particularly the hostesses of the French salons, in the rise of politeness must not be underestimated. After all, as sociolinguists point out, women in many societies are more polite than men.[27] Italian and French models were consciously followed in England and elsewhere. As Thomas Sheridan, one of the specialists in the subject, remarked in 1780, 'The Italians, French and Spaniards, in proportion to their progress in civilisation and politeness, have for more than a century been employed, with the utmost industry, in cultivating and regulating their speech.'[28]

That many members of the 'middle classes' (the families of merchants, lawyers, and physicians, for example) were participating in this movement by 1700, if not before, is extremely likely. It would be difficult to explain the many editions of the treatises on conversation without such a hypothesis. Politeness in speech, as in other forms of behaviour, was a way for the middle classes to show that they were close to the upper classes. In England in particular, it has been argued that, in the eighteenth century, wealth and politeness were coming to replace (or at least to join) birth as a basis of social status. That certain forms of politeness were practised further down the social scale is likely, but the evidence is sparse. The generalizations about Italy, France, and England offered here should, therefore, be taken as applying to a minority of the population.

IV

It is time to be more concrete and to focus more sharply on some of the linguistic forms through which politeness was expressed in the period. Six of these forms will be discussed in turn—the avoidance of contradiction; accent; euphemisms; compliments; forms of address; and finally the humiliative mode of speech to social superiors.

[26] Quoted in K. Cmiel, *Democratic Eloquence: The Fight over Popular Speech in Nineteenth-Century America* (Berkeley and Los Angeles, 1990), 38.

[27] J. Holmes, *Women, Men and Politeness* (1995).

[28] Quoted in L. Mugglestone, *Talking Proper: The Rise of Accent as Social Symbol* (Oxford, 1995), 28.

1. *Negative civility*, sometimes described at the time as 'complaisance', the avoidance of what used to be called 'offence' (in other words, FTAs), is perhaps best illustrated by the advice not to contradict other people, especially one's superiors. Della Casa, for example, recommended his readers to avoid expressions such as 'it wasn't like that' (*Non fu così*) or 'you are wrong' (*Voi errate*). In France, Nicole Faret, whose adaptation of Castiglione became one of the most popular manuals of good behaviour in the seventeenth century, also warned his readers not to contradict.[29] Contradiction was considered an offence against 'complaisance', a seventeenth-century term for politeness in the sense of accommodating one's behaviour to the expectations of others. As the anonymous author of *The Art of Complaisance* (1673) put it, 'dissimulation is part of the essence of complaisance'. Similar points might be made about refusal. However, the rise of the ideal of sincerity or 'frankness', especially if not exclusively in England, led to the weakening if not the abandonment of this form of politeness. By the end of the eighteenth century, if not before, it could be perceived (as we have seen) as a peculiarly oriental form of evasiveness.

2. A second way of expressing politeness was by *accent*. In the sixteenth and seventeenth centuries, discussions of accent centred on the 'sweet and low'. In France, Nicole Faret, for example, remarked on the need to speak to superiors with what he called a 'sweet' tone of voice or 'un accent plein de soumission'. The critic Jean Chapelain argued that social intercourse between the sexes contributed 'à rendre les langues polies', because in talking to women, 'les hommes apprennent à adoucir la rudesse de la prununciation, que la mollesse naturelle des organes des femmes ammolit'. This sweetness, or something like it, appears to have been the target of Furetière's satirical *Roman bourgeois* (1666), in which a young abbé 'affectoit de parler un peu gras, pour avoir le langage plus mignard'.[30]

Accent was also a way to distinguish between élites and ordinary people. Chesterfield told his son 'to pronounce properly: that is, according to the usage of the best companies'. When, where, and among whom a regional accent came to be stigmatized in different cultures as a vulgar accent remains a problem for historians. An early example of such stigmatization comes from the rules drawn up for the seminary established in Milan in 1590. The teachers were instructed to correct 'the mispronunciations which the pupils brought with them from their places of origin' (*vitiosas quasdam inflexiones vocis . . . quas a patria secum extulerunt*).[31] As this rule suggests, the English were not unique in their preoccupation with accent. The duc de Saint-

[29] G. Della Casa, *Galateo* (1558; ed. D. Provenzal, Milan, 1950), ch. 18; N. Faret, *L'Honnête Homme* (1630; Paris, 1925), 54.

[30] Faret, *L'Honnête Homme*, 53; J. Chapelain, *Lettres*, ii (Paris, 1883), 169; A. Adam (ed.), *Romanciers du 17ᵉ siècle* (Paris, 1968), 906.

[31] A. Prosperi, *Tribunali di Coscienza* (Turin, 1996), 314 n.

Simon condemned the duchesse de Chaulnes because she had 'le ton, et la voix, et des mots du bas peuple'. By the eighteenth century, however, England had probably become the part of Europe in which these matters were taken most seriously. Sheridan, for example, emphasized the need to avoid 'rusticity of accent'. In the 1760s, an English clergyman, confiding to his diary the bad impression made on him by the bishop of Lincoln, declared that prelate's 'humble education and mean extraction' to have been revealed by his 'want of behaviour and manners', including his clumsy way of walking and his 'Yorkshire dialect'. The speech of some prominent people continued to reveal their place of origin—'Addington still spoke as a Hampshireman, Peel as a Lancastrian, even Gladstone employed a slightly northern brogue'— but these details are recorded precisely because they were breaches of the norm.[32]

3. *Vocabulary*, even more than accent, was the way in which high-status, civilized, or polite people were distinguished from others in this period. What is often called 'Victorian' language, in the sense of a series of euphemisms for sexual matters in the presence of ladies, is in fact much older than the nineteenth century and was far from a monopoly of the English. The word 'interesting', in the place of 'pregnant', for instance, was in use not only in England but also in nineteenth-century Spain. Or take the well-known example of euphemisms for 'leg'. On occasion, Charles Dickens even describes male trousers as 'unmentionables'. However, in seventeenth-century Portugal, a famous conduct book, modelled on Castiglione's *Courtier*, had already argued that the word *perna* could be used in the presence of ladies only if it referred to a man's leg. Ladies were not supposed to have legs.[33] In Italy, Della Casa devoted considerable space to the problem of linguistic 'indecency' (*disonestà*), noting in chapter 22 of the *Galateo* that 'our ladies' speak about 'chestnuts' when they mean 'figs', in order to avoid embarrassing double meanings, and advising female speakers or speakers to women to avoid the word *puttane*, a term that should be replaced by 'women of the world' (*femine del mondo*).

However, the practice of euphemism spread well beyond the 'private parts'. If we are to trust Pietro Aretino, who satirized the practice, ladies, or would-be ladies, in sixteenth-century Rome no longer called a window *finestra* but *balcone*, while a door, formerly *uscio*, became *porta*, presumably because the new terms sounded less vulgar.[34] When Magdelon, in *Les Précieuses Ridicules* (Act 1, Scene 5) called a servant *un nécessaire* and translated 'si vous êtes au

<hr/>

[32] Saint-Simon, *Mémoires*, i. 589; Sheridan quoted in Mugglestone, *Talking Proper*, 117; W. Cole, *The Bletchley Diary* (1931), 35; the reference to Addington etc. in R. J. W. Evans, *The Language of History and the History of Language* (Oxford, 1998), 15. Cf. Bryson, *Courtesy to Civility*, 189–91.

[33] Galdos, *Fortunato y Jacinta* (1886–7; Madrid, 1971), 935; F. Rodrigues Lobo, *Corte na Aldeia* (1619; Lisbon, 1972).

[34] P. Aretino, *Sei giornate* (*c*.1530; ed. G. Aquilecchia, Bari, 1975), 82.

logis' into 'si vous êtes en commodité d'étre visibles', she was not the first woman to distance herself from everyday language. In Spain, Francisco de Quevedo satirized the Spanish equivalent of the *précieuses*, the 'female latinist' (*hembrilatina*), who had coined pretentious new words for 'quarrel', 'fright', and 'stupidities'.[35]

The *précieuses* and their equivalents were mocked only because they went too far. Gentlemen were proceeding more slowly in the same direction. The preface to the first volume of the *Dictionnaire de l'Académie* (1694) declared that it was deliberately limited to 'la langue commune, telle qu'elle est dans le commerce ordinaire des honnêtes gens'. Excommunicated, therefore, were technical terms, 'les termes des arts et des sciences qui entrent rarement dans le discours', together with vulgarities, words that are 'bas et de style familier', associated with low-status people.

The concern with social class and its linguistic signs is sometimes thought to be a peculiarly English preoccupation, not to say malady. Hence it may be of interest to note a French nobleman of this period discussing what he calls 'espèces de classes différentes qu'on reconnait par leurs façons de parler'. Among the 'façons de parler bourgeoises' stigmatized in his dialogue is the use of the phrase 'mon époux', rather than 'mon mari, qui est la bonne manière de se nommer'.[36] Conversely, although no academy came into existence to control the English language, there was a movement to found one. Gentlemen were advised to avoid 'vulgarisms' (a word that is first recorded in English in 1644). 'Vulgar expressions are carefully avoided by those who want to write politely,' declared the anonymous *Art of Speaking* in 1676. It was on these grounds that Lord Chesterfield warned his son against using proverbs in his conversation.

4. The term 'compliments' was used first in Italian and then in French, while from the middle of the seventeenth century it is documented in English, suggesting that the custom, at least in its elaborated forms, followed a similar itinerary (in French, the word *galanteries* occupied some of the same conceptual space). In the narrow sense of the term, compliments were a kind of euphemism used to maintain the face of others by praising them and their possessions. In the wider sense, the term 'compliments' was used to describe formulas of respect, including the term 'respect' itself, as in the seventeenth-century English phrases 'my due respects' or 'my very kind respects'. The practice was known as 'paying' one's respects.

So important were compliments in the seventeenth century—to judge by the treatises on how to use them—that a German scholar has described the period as one of 'the culture of compliments' (*Komplimentierkultur*).[37] In

[35] F. de Quevedo, *Obras satíricas* (*c*.1650; Madrid 1924), 160.
[36] F. de Callières, *Des mots à la mode* (Paris, 1692), 43, 65.
[37] M. Beetz, 'Negative Kontinuität: Vorbehalte gegenüber barocker Komplimentierkultur', in K. Garber (ed.), *Europäische Barock-Rezeption* (Wiesbaden, 1991), 281–302.

England too treatises with titles such as *The Complete Academy of Compliments* (1705) were published at this time. There was a geography as well as a chronology and a sociology of compliments. The cultural distance between Italy and England in this respect is apparent from reactions of English travellers. In Siena, the English gentleman Fynes Moryson remarked that the term 'Palaces' was used in Italy to refer to houses of 'small magnificence' as a form of civility to their owners, while his visit to Verona prompted the observation that 'The Italian epitaphs are often more extravagant than those of other countries, as the nation is more given to compliment and hyperbole'.[38]

5. *Forms of address*, like other compliments, appear to have been more elaborate on the Continent than in Britain, as travellers sometimes noted. Thus Thomas Palmer noted what he called (like Brown and Levenson) the 'humilious phrases and kind compliments of kissing their hands' in both Italy and France, while Sir John Lauder commented with admiration on the manners of the French peasants. 'A man might have seen more civility in their expressions . . . than may be found in the first compliments on a rencontre between two Scots gentlemen tolerably well bred'.[39] Modes of address also made explicit the employment of different forms of language to different kinds of people, when speaking to one's superiors, equals, or inferiors.

There is apparently the least to say about England in this respect. However, even here a shift in modes of address between fathers and children among the English gentry has been noted by Lawrence Stone. 'In the first half of the seventeenth century a son, even when grown up, would commonly address his father in a letter as 'Sir', and sign himself "your humble obedient son", "your son in continuance of all obedience", or "your most obedient and loving son".' By the 1720s, however, a shift from what Stone calls 'deference' to what he calls 'respect' was already noticeable, and by the 1770s it was at its 'height'. 'Sir', for example, was replaced by 'Dear Papa'. Stone discusses this change as evidence for changing relationships within the family, but it should also be placed in the context of the history of forms of address.[40]

In France, Saint-Simon was, as might have been expected, much concerned with forms of address, especially among the nobility. Again and again he returns to the uses of *Monseigneur* and *Altesse*, with occasional observations on *Monsieur*, *Mademoiselle*, and *Madame*.[41] The impression he gives of an old 'formalist' who is shocked by the increasing informality of the younger

[38] F. Moryson, *An Itinerary* (4 vols.; Glasgow, 1907–8), i. 307, 378.
[39] T. Palmer, *An Essay of the Means how to Make our Travel into Foreign Countries more Profitable and Honourable* (1606), 68; J. Lauder, *Journals 1665–76*, ed. Donald Crawford (Edinburgh, 1900), 82.
[40] L. Stone, *The Family, Sex and Marriage in England 1500–1800* (1977), 171, 412–14.
[41] Saint-Simon, *Mémoires*, i. 64, 188, 597, 661, etc.

generation is consistent with the English evidence. However, the richest vein of evidence for changing forms of address comes from Italy.[42] It suggests two phases, an increase in formality in the sixteenth century countered by a movement towards informality in the eighteenth. Going still further than Stone's young noblemen, Cosimo de' Medici, future Grand Duke of Tuscany, wrote to his father as 'Illustrissimo signore mio padre', and to his mother as 'Magnifica et dilectissima madre'. From the middle of the sixteenth century onwards, honorific titles proliferated; *La Vostra Signoria*, *Excellenza*, *Magnificenza*, or even *Sublimità*, together with adjectives such as *illustrissimo*. The hyperbolic mode already discussed had spread to forms of address.

This inflation of titles did not take place without protest. Most complaints emphasized the debasement of the linguistic currency, but a few were more political in thrust. Andrea Spinola 'the philosopher', for example, a Genoese patrician who defended the tradition of civic equality when it was going into decline at the beginning of the seventeenth century, denounced the use of *illustrissimo*. His was a self-consciously republican civility.[43] All the same, the trend towards titles continued. Only in the mid-eighteenth century did it go into reverse, when men of letters such as Gasparo Gozzi and Pietro Verri argued for a more informal mode of address. Gozzi pleaded in the *Gazzetta Veneta* (2 April 1760) for a simplification of both language and ceremonies, while Verri denounced *le formalità* in the journal *Il Caffé* and praised the English Quakers for their simplicity of language.

6. The *humiliative mode* of politeness was quite common in early modern Europe. In the sixteenth and seventeenth centuries, in Spain and Italy in particular, expressions such as 'I kiss your hand' or even 'I kiss your foot' were in use in speech and writing, not to mention gesture. It was not unknown for nobles to describe themselves in a letter to their sovereign, the emperor Charles V, for instance, as 'your slave and servant' (*vostre esclave et serviteur*). In his famous conduct book Giovanni Della Casa cites the example of 'your slave in chains' (*vostro schiavo in catena*). Letters to the pope might be signed by 'quello che sta sotto i piedi di V. Beatudine'.[44]

The English did not normally go so far in this direction, and the Cambridge rhetorician Gabriel Harvey, writing to his friend the poet Edmund Spenser, associated Della Casa's *Galateo* with what he called 'cringing'. All the same, traces of this mode can be found, leading Keith Thomas to write, in a rare lapse from his normal detachment, of an Elizabethan 'tendency to undue obse-

[42] B. Croce, *La Spagna nella vita italiana durante la rinascenza* (Bari, 1917); J. Brunet, 'Un "langage colakeitiquement profane", ou l'influence de l'Espagne sur la troisième personne de politesse italienne', in *Presence et influence de l'Espagne dans la culture italienne de la Renaissance* (Paris, 1978), 251–315.

[43] A. Spinola, *Scritti scelti*, ed. C. Bitossi (Genoa, 1981), 247.

[44] Della Casa, *Galateo*, ch. 16; M. Pensa, *La Biblioteca Vaticana* (Rome, 1590), 42.

quiousness'.[45] It has been argued that it was the court environment in the period 1500–1800 that produced 'phrases of submission and devotion', such as offering 'humble thanks' for 'favours' and describing oneself as 'your humble (or obedient) servant'.[46] Even more important, in my opinion, was the prevalence of patron–client relationships in English society at this time. Formulas of a kind that would later be denounced as oriental can be found in the letters of noblemen in the Tudor and early Stuart period, as in the following three examples. In a letter to Lord Lisle in 1534 about the plans for a marriage alliance between the two families, Sir Francis Lovell contrasted 'your noble blood' with 'my poor stock', although a baron was only one degree above a knight in the social hierarchy. When Sir Christopher Hatton wrote to William Cecil about the house he was having built, magnificent even by Elizabethan noble standards, he called it his 'rude building'. When the Earl of Arundel wrote to Sir Dudley Carleton in 1619 about their common interest in collecting pictures, he thanked him for his care 'to satisfy my foolish curiosity in enquiring for the pieces of Holbein'.[47]

In the eighteenth century we see a strong reaction against this humiliative style. Already by 1673 the author of one English conduct book was associating compliments with 'duplicity and deceit'. 'They consist in praising immoderately and pretending greater love and friendship than either is deserved by or intended to him to whom they are offered'. They are examples of 'an abusing of language', for example offering 'imaginary services' or engaging in imaginary 'humiliations'.[48] A few years later, a sermon by Archbishop Tillotson denounced the conversation of his day as 'swelled with vanity and compliment' and 'surfeited' with 'expressions of kindness and respect'. The *Spectator* made similar points, and was praised by Samuel Johnson for its campaign against what he called 'the impertinence of civility'. In France, *Les Règles de la bienséance* (1781), discussing compliments, warned its readers against what it called 'hyperboles démesurées'.[49]

The positive aspect of this shift was the rise of sincerity. Montaigne was a pioneering critic of the inflation of what he described in his essays as the 'abjecte et servile prostitution de presentations; la vie, l'ame, devotion, adoration, serf, esclave, tous ces mots y courent si vulgairement que, quand ils veulent fair sentir une plus expresse volonté et plus respectueuse, ils n'ont plus de manière pour l'exprimer' (bk. 1, ch. 40). The cult of sincerity reached its apogee at the end of our period, when Rousseau and Herder, among others, attacked the culture of civility on these grounds. The permeation of

[45] Thomas, 'Yours', 453.

[46] C. McIntosh, *Common and Courtly Language* (Philadelphia, 1986), 69 ff., 82 ff., 137 ff.

[47] *The Lisle Letters*, ed. M. St Clare Byrne (1983), no. 61; Hatton quoted in C. Read, *Mr Secretary Cecil* (1925), 216; Arundel quoted in J. Brown, *Kings and Connoisseurs: Collecting Art in Seventeenth-Century Europe* (New Haven, 1995), 19.

[48] Walker, *Of Education*, 212–13; cf. Beetz, 'Negative Kontinuität'.

[49] Berger, *Konversationskunst*, 179, 225; *Règles*, 320.

everyday life by the new values was symbolized by such epistolary forms as 'yours sincerely' and 'yours truly'.[50] The reaction against hyperbole would eventually lead to such a deflation of the language of politeness that, by the nineteenth century, Englishmen in India would be astonished, as we have seen, by the 'servility' of the humiliative mode.

V

Cultural difference, notably the difference between the hyperbolic Italians and the less demonstrative English, has been the minor theme of this article, but the major emphasis has fallen on the direction and significance of linguistic change. In the case of Italy, some at least of the hyperbole developed in the course of the sixteenth century, rather than forming part of an unchanging 'national character'. The essential point, most clearly illustrated by the decline of elaborate forms of address and the humiliative mode of politeness, is the decline of formality in the eighteenth century. The old regime of politeness was undermined generations before the French Revolution.

Why did these changes take place? The 'folk theories' on the subject make an excellent point of departure for analysis, though they may be in need of development or qualification. Andrea Spinola, as we have seen, linked the rise of *Illustrissimo* to the decline of republican values. According to him, civic modesty and equality were giving way to display and hierarchy. In similar fashion Pietro Verri denounced the people who wanted to be addressed as *Vostra Signoria* as despotic 'sultans'. The rise of titles may be viewed as an outward sign of the process of social and political change in Italy that historians often describe as 'refeudalization'—in other words, a shift of wealth and power away from merchants and cities and back to aristocratic landowners.[51]

In the eighteenth century, what has to be explained is the shift from the 'honour system' (aggressive, masculine, and sharply hierarchical) to the 'politeness system' (gentler, oriented towards the opposite sex, and more egalitarian, at least in appearance). Shaftesbury gave a political explanation of the new politeness, which he defined by contrast to the flattery of courts, linking it to the rise of liberty and the Whig party. Some historians of eighteenth-century Britain have recently put forward a less partisan version of the same thesis, to the effect that the 'language of manners' was

[50] Thomas, 'Yours', 452. On the early modern period, L. Trilling, *Sincerity and Authenticity* (1972); J. Martin, 'Inventing Sincerity, Refashioning Prudence', *American Historical Review*, 102 (1997), 1309–42.

[51] R. Villari, *Ribelli e riformatori* (Rome, 1979), 95–6.

incorporated into political controversy and used as a means of moderating its violence.[52]

If the shift had been confined to Britain, the point would be persuasive. However, as we have seen, the Italians and the French were moving in the same direction without the aid of the Whigs or even of increasing liberty. Indeed, the same treatises on polite language were current in all three countries. Bellegarde, for instance, was translated into English and Italian. There must, therefore, have been other forces at work to civilize tongues besides the political one.

In the history of European rituals, a parallel shift towards informality has been noted more than once.[53] The painted portrait is another cultural domain where a shift towards the informal presentation of self has been dated to the eighteenth century. Famous examples include van Loo's Diderot, with dishevelled hair, and Reynolds's Baretti, peering short-sightedly at a book. These clues point in the direction of a major cultural shift that affected more than one region and more than one domain of behaviour. If we wish to explain the shift, we might reasonably invoke the parallel rise of commercial society, most obvious in eighteenth-century England, but also visible in France at this time and to a lesser extent in northern Italy, in the Venice of Gozzi or the Milan of Verri.

To explore the connection further, we might once again take a folk theory as a point of departure—for example, the idea of Philip Withers, quoted above, that the rise of polite language was a reaction to the decline of 'external evidence of rank'. It was a new way for upper-class people to distinguish themselves from others at a time when mass production was making it possible for the first time for ordinary people to imitate the dress of their social superiors. Polite language could, of course, be imitated in its turn and the proliferation of treatises on the subject suggests that this was precisely what happened. All the same, at least as an explanation of the rise of the English preoccupation with accent at this time, Withers's explanation has much to be said for it.

There is much more to be said on this subject than is possible in a short article. All the same, even a limited number of examples from early modern English, French, and Italian may be sufficient to suggest that, even if the same strategies of politeness can be found in many cultures, as Brown and Levinson argue, these strategies have not been used to an equal extent everywhere. Hence the surprised or even contemptuous reactions of

[52] Klein, *Shaftesbury*; N. Phillipson, 'Politics and Politeness in the Reigns of Anne and the Early Hanoverians', in J. G. A. Pocock (ed.), *The Varieties of British Political Thought 1500–1800* (Cambridge, 1993), 211–45.

[53] Burke, *Historical Anthropology of Early Modern Italy*, 223–38; E. Muir, *Ritual in Early Modern Europe* (Cambridge, 1997), 269–75.

Englishmen in Italy or Westerners in China to forms of politeness that they found excessive or even servile.

As in the case of clothes, so in that of language, the apparently 'superficial' deserves to be studied as a system of signs expressing what lies underneath. However, the language of 'surface', of 'expression', or 'reflection', or even 'refraction', may not do justice to the power of everyday actions, including linguistic actions. Trivial in themselves, a multitude of such acts—acts of deference, acts of identity, and so on—are capable of reinforcing or even reconstructing a political regime.

3

'Civilized Religion' from Renaissance to Reformation and Counter-Reformation

EUAN CAMERON

Many writers who advocated 'civilized' behaviour in the early modern period wrote in an overtly religious spirit. Erasmus, whose *On the Civility of the Manners of Children* inaugurated the early modern conduct book, treated refinement of manners as one of the minor branches of his broader project to create a sincere, rational Christian ethic.[1] In Giovanni della Casa's *Galateo*, written *c.*1551–5, it is a bishop who corrects the manners of a duke through his servant (the eponymous Galateo).[2] The followers and imitators of Friedrich Dedekind's *Grobianus* were largely written by German Protestant clerics.[3] The *Oráculo manual y arte de prudencia* written by the Jesuit Baltasar Gracián in 1647, and Jean-Baptiste de La Salle's *Règles de la bienséance et de la civilité chrétienne à l'usage des écoles chrétiennes*, first published in 1703, became key texts for 'civil' conduct.[4] The clerics who wrote conduct manuals undoubtedly believed that religion, and religious instruction in particular, could make people more 'civilized': that it could restrain their passions and moderate the excesses of their natures.[5] An important revision of Norbert Elias's thesis has proposed that the early modern conduct book derived ultimately from the rules of disciplined behaviour cultivated in medieval monasteries, rather than manuals of courtly etiquette.[6]

---

[1] N. Elias, *The Civilizing Process: The History of Manners and State Formation and Civilization*, trans. E. Jephcott (Oxford, 1994), 43 ff.; Erasmus's original text was entitled *De civilitate morum puerilium* (1st edn., ?1526; certainly 1530; 30 edns. by 1536).

[2] Elias, *The Civilizing Process*, 65; Giovanni Della Casa, *Galateo*, ed. Saverio Orlando (Milan, 1988); cf. M. P. Becker, *Civility and Society in Western Europe, 1300–1600* (Bloomington, Ind., 1988), 29.

[3] Elias, *The Civilizing Process*, 60; Friedrich Dedekind, *Grobianus, et Grobiana . . . Libri tres* (Leiden, 1642).

[4] Elias, *The Civilizing Process*, 538 n. 134; Baltasar Gracián, *Oráculo manual y arte de prudencia*, ed. M. Romera-Navarro (n.p., 1954). On this see H. Phillips, *Church and Culture in Seventeenth-Century France* (Cambridge, 1997), 81 ff.; on the religious background to instilling 'civility', see Phillips, *Church and Culture*, 77 ff. and refs.

[5] See e.g. the comment of Francis Hutchinson from 1716 quoted by I. Bostridge, *Witchcraft and its Transformations* (Oxford, 1997), 151.

[6] D. Knox, '*Disciplina*: The Monastic and Clerical Origins of European Civility', in

Yet 'civility' is not associated just with Christianity as such. Rather, it has been linked with a particular shift in the cultural styles and tastes of western Europe between the late Middle Ages and the Renaissance. It saw 'civil' and 'civility' displace 'courteous' and 'courtesy' as the fashionable terms to denote approved conduct.[7] It is associated with behavioural changes, crudely definable as a move from chivalric and feudal honour to courtly refinement or bourgeois respectability. Practically, this entailed a preference for privacy versus life in the public view; for restraint versus the exhibition of emotion; and for selective and discreet generosity rather than extravagant displays of munificence. It also intersected with a more rational, individualistic attitude to the place of man in society: merit was to be preferred over hierarchy or lineage, ethical standards over the liens of patron and client, and positive law over the force of tradition and convention.[8] How far did the influences run in the other direction? Was there such a thing as 'civilized religion'—that is, religion reshaped under the influence of the Renaissance cultural developments just described? Even to ask this question entails a particular attitude to religious belief and practice. It requires that religion be treated, not just as the expression of timeless absolute principles in daily life and thought, but as a cultural phenomenon, reflecting the values of the society that cultivates it.

I

The obvious point at which to start is the change in religious priorities associated with the Renaissance. Renaissance 'humanist' religion was overwhelmingly concerned with the ethical life of the individual (hence, *inter alia*, the conduct books). Erasmus laid himself open to the charge of turning Christ into nothing more than an ethical example.[9] Religious writers who shared this preoccupation tended to identify and oppose two particular evils in religion: dogma and 'superstition'.

Erasmus mercilessly traduced those intellectual clerics who elaborated a bewilderingly complex, linguistically barbarous dogmatic theology. He argued that they wasted their energies and failed to instil real (that is, ethical) piety.[10] The key to theology, for Erasmus, was, first, to keep it short and

J. Monfasani and R. G. Musto (eds.), *Renaissance Society and Culture: Essays in Honor of Eugene F. Rice Jr.* (Ithaca, NY, 1991), 107–35.

[7] Elias, *The Civilizing Process*, 83 ff.

[8] This is the broad interpretation of 'civility' favoured in Becker, *Civility and Society*, *passim*, though there are others in current use.

[9] A charge discussed implicitly by Luther in *Martin Luthers Werke: Kritische Gesamtausgabe* (Weimar, 1883–1948), viii. 53 ff.

[10] For Erasmus's attacks on theologians, see his *Praise of Folly*, in *Collected Works of Erasmus* (Toronto, 1974–), xxvii (1986), 127 ff.

simple; and, secondly, not to insist on absolute uniformity in details of belief. In a letter written to a Bohemian nobleman in 1519, Erasmus condensed the 'sum of Christian philosophy' into less than a dozen lines, then encapsulated the principle of doctrinal pluralism in words both astonishing and ironic in view of the date of the letter: 'If any man wishes to pursue more abstruse questions . . . he is welcome to do so with this restriction, that to believe what commends itself to this or that man should not at once become compulsory for everybody.'[11] In the adage *quot homines, tot sententiae* ('there are as many opinions as there are people'), Erasmus warned that 'the apostle Paul also seems to have alluded to this [proverb], when he advises that to prevent rivalry we ought to allow everyone to abound in his own opinion. If the mob of theologians were to listen to this advice, there would not nowadays be so much strife over trivial little issues.'[12]

Erasmus's indifference to uniformity of dogma had its parallels in the Renaissance papal curia, where (according to Pier Antonio Bandini) no one was considered a courtier or a gentleman unless he held, in addition to the approved doctrines, his own private heresy;[13] or in the eclectic, Neoplatonic theology of German humanists such as Mutian, Celtis, or Reuchlin.[14] Most undogmatic humanists (unlike Erasmus) kept their religious speculations private, the preserve of an inner circle of initiate friends.[15] Many were moderate and cautious, distrusting enthusiasm and fervour. They tended to express themselves ambivalently or ironically, and favoured discussion of alternatives over the rhetoric of absolutes.[16]

Secondly, the early Renaissance humanists reacted against a medieval practical theology where ritual observances and abstinences earned specific rewards, and where the Church formed a great collective forum for the exchange of grace between God, the priesthood, and the souls of the living and the dead. Fasting and penance, for example, came to be regarded as 'uncivilized' or 'barbarous' to the extent that they claimed to exchange fleshly

---

[11] L.-E. Halkin, *Erasmus: A Critical Biography*, trans. J. Tonkin (Oxford, 1993), 133, 177, based on P. S. and H. M. Allen (eds.), *Opus epistolarum Desiderii Erasmi*, iv (Oxford, 1922), 118. See also *Collected Works of Erasmus*, vii. 126–7.

[12] Erasmus [and others], *Adagia, id est: prouerbiorum, paroemiarum et parabolarum omnium, quae apud graecos, latinos, hebraeos, arabas, &c. in vsu fuerunt, collectio absolutissima*, ed. J. J. Grynaeus ([Frankfurt], 1643), 31; modern translation in *Collected Works of Erasmus*, xxi (Toronto, 1982), 240–1. The passage quoted was excised by Paolo Manuzio in his expurgated *Adagia* (Rome, 1575).

[13] For Pier Antonio Bandini's reminiscences, see P. McNair, *Peter Martyr in Italy: An Anatomy of Apostasy* (Oxford, 1967).

[14] See ch. iii, entitled 'The *Theologia Platonica* in the Religious Thought of the German Humanists', in L. W. Spitz, *Luther and German Humanism* (Aldershot, 1996), esp. ch. iii, pp. 124 ff. (chapters are separately paginated).

[15] Spitz, *Luther and German Humanism*, ii. 48; cf. with the seventeenth-century French *libertins*, as in Phillips, *Church and Culture*, 237.

[16] Becker, *Civility and Society*, p. xv; cf. ibid. 54–7.

mortifications for spiritual benefits.[17] Lives and legends of saints that promised rewards for the mechanical observance of their cults, or that celebrated holy men for reconciling people through mutual restitution and social reintegration, came likewise to be condemned as 'uncivilized'.[18] Saints were no longer expected to behave like the unscrupulous and partial patrons of unruly feudatories: ethics, and the individual's moral standards, became all-important.

Erasmus continued the critique of the fifteenth-century Italians in his own way. He ridiculed as 'superstition' at best, and cynical exploitation at worst, the popular piety that traded in special vows, bogus relics, or abstinences unfounded in scripture.[19] To criticize 'superstition' was not, of course, distinctive to humanists: scholastics, led by Thomas Aquinas, had done the same for generations.[20] However, humanists tended to ridicule as human folly what medieval clerics had denounced as the deception of demons.[21] Moreover, Renaissance humanists extended their critique beyond the obviously forbidden areas of the folk magic that lived parasitically on the official cult, into more areas of sanctioned and approved religiosity than anyone before them.

If the writers of the Renaissance represent 'civility' in the religious sphere, then it is reasonable to regard their *bêtes noires*, elaborate dogma and vulgar superstition, as the epitome of 'uncivilized', or, as they said themselves, 'barbarous' religion. Without the value judgements, one might still claim that both scholastic theology and traditional catholic piety, with its quantifiable grace and performative rituals, were the religious embodiments of medieval culture, of 'archaic' society with its organic structure and feudal, reciprocal values. The humanists' opposition to dogma and superstition may not exhaust the attributes of 'civilized religion', but it offers a starting point.

What became of this attitude after the Reformation? Before *c.*1520, there appeared no serious risk that the great edifice of sacerdotal authority and sacramental ministry could be shaken. It had been safe for a few choice intellectuals to raise learned doubts about doctrine, or quietly to mock the credulity of the piously uneducated. After the schism, that relaxed attitude

---

[17] Becker, *Civility and Society*, 160 n. 23, and refs.; L. W. Spitz, *The Religious Renaissance of the German Humanists* (Cambridge, Mass., 1963), 137–9.

[18] Becker, *Civility and Society*, 14, with refs. on p. 160 n. 23 to Francesco Novati (ed.), *Epistolario di Coluccio Salutati* (4 vols.; Rome, 1891–1911), ii. 303–4; Eugenio Garin, *Italian Humanism: Philosophy and Civic Life in the Renaissance*, trans. P. Munz (New York, 1965), 28; R. G. Witt, *Hercules at the Crossroads: The Life, Works, and Thought of Coluccio Salutati* (Durham, NC, 1983).

[19] See e.g. Erasmus's *Praise of Folly*, in *Collected Works of Erasmus*, xxvii. 114–15; *The Colloquies of Erasmus*, ed. and trans. C. R. Thompson (Chicago, 1965), esp. *Rash Vows* (4 ff.), *The Shipwreck* (138 ff.), *A Pilgrimage for Religion's Sake* (285 ff.).

[20] Defining the boundaries between superstition and religion forms the main issue in St Thomas Aquinas, *Summa theologica*, iia iiae, qq. 92–6, and in a large expository and occasional literature based on these questions.

[21] The whole rhetorical structure of Erasmus's *Praise of Folly* is based on the premiss that Folly earns the blame (or credit) for people's superstitions: see sects. 40–1, as in n. 10 above.

could no longer be sustained. Humanists chose a side to take, and defended it vigorously.[22] To argue, as Erasmus did, that issues like predestination simply did not need to be discussed, would no longer do. When Luther commented, criticizing Erasmus's religion, that 'the Holy Spirit is no sceptic', he was not accusing Erasmus unfairly of sheer unbelief. He was identifying a cultural gulf, a difference of principle over the legitimate scope of certainty in religion, which divided the early Renaissance from the early Reformation.[23]

The humanist aversion to dogma appears largely dormant until the mid-seventeenth century. A handful of freethinkers and spiritualists refused to submit to any rigid form of Protestantism, such as Sebastian Franck or Caspar Schwenckfeld, or critical individualists like Sebastian Castellio.[24] Hendrik Niclaes and the Familists practised an urbane, secretive dissent apparently attractive to some of Elizabeth I of England's courtiers.[25] Spiritual *libertins* and religious sceptics of seventeenth-century France like Gabriel Naudé would, from different standpoints, oppose both superstition (especially that of vulgar Catholicism) and fanatical dogmatism (especially that of militant Protestantism), in the name of a rational, non-credal faith.[26] However, these individualist freethinkers were an infinitesimal minority among the religiously minded of early modern Europe.

The task here is to analyse what became of 'civilized religion' in the confessional age: specifically, what became of the Renaissance humanists' aversion to rigid doctrinal definitions, and their mockery of a traditional religion that 'bargained' with the deity and with the dead for protection and favour. In the mainstream churches, one finds a highly complex and paradoxical state of affairs. The cultural and religious legacy of the Renaissance could not be ignored, but it was certainly transformed.

II

The humanists opposed any attempt to pin down the faith to detailed dogmas. In contrast, as Wilhelm Dilthey put it in the nineteenth century, Luther's faith 'is not the exit of dogma . . . on the contrary, it has this dogma in all respects

---

[22] See Spitz, *Luther and German Humanism*, ch. iv, p. 109; ch. v, p. 209.

[23] See Luther's *De servo arbitrio*, as trans. in E. G. Rupp (ed.), *Luther and Erasmus: Free Will and Salvation* (1969), 105–9; on humanist scepticism, see Becker, *Civility and Society*, 58.

[24] See P. M. Hayden-Roy, *The Inner World and the Outer World: A Biography of Sebastian Franck* (Renaissance and Baroque Studies and Texts, 7; New York, 1994); R. E. McLaughlin, *Caspar Schwenckfeld, Reluctant Radical: His Life to 1540* (New Haven, 1986); S. Zweig, *Ein Gewissen gegen die Gewalt, Castellio gegen Calvin* (Frankfurt am Main, 1979).

[25] See C. W. Marsh, *The Family of Love in English Society, 1550–1630* (Cambridge, 1994); but cf. K. Thomas, *Religion and the Decline of Magic: Studies in Popular Beliefs in Sixteenth and Seventeenth Century England* (1971), 322.

[26] Phillips, *Church and Culture*, 230 and refs.

as its necessary presupposition. It stands and falls with the dogma.'[27] Paradoxically, the Renaissance humanists' *skills* of persuasive rhetoric, a fluent and attractive written style, and progressive and systematic schooling were used in the era of confessional orthodoxy to inculcate precisely the sort of dogma that Erasmus so decried.[28] More bewilderingly still, one can see a plausible connection between the credalism of the post-Reformation era and the humanists' desire for a *personal* commitment to faith. This shift towards the individual's religious commitment marked a distinct change from the 'archaic' modes of social organization identified by historians like Marvin Becker.[29] Whereas medieval popular religion, with its priestly and saintly intercessions, embodied the contemporary social principles of reciprocity, patron–client relationships, and vicarious atonement,[30] none of the early modern churches officially encouraged the idea that one person could be godly on behalf of another, or that one godly action was interchangeable with another.[31] This ideal of conscious, educated commitment required a trained clergy, and a trained laity. Both Protestant and Catholic churches set about this task with similar aims and similar techniques. However, the frameworks within which they worked led, ultimately, to very different outcomes.

In Protestant countries, clergy education was reformed either by recasting the existing universities to provide for the new style of clergy training; or by setting up new colleges and academies specifically to train pastors. Generally speaking, the first route was followed in kingdoms and principalities where old universities were already available to be adapted, as in most Lutheran states, and also in England and Scotland. The second route was chosen either where the existing universities were beyond the control of the reformed church (as in France) or where the state was too small to have supported a full university (as in Strasbourg, Geneva, Herborn, or Neustadt).

Where possible, Protestant clergy were trained within the mainstream of academic life. The medieval philosophies that had supported traditional theology were stripped out of the curriculum—for instance, by Philipp Melanchthon for Lutheran Germany. One might have expected Melanchthon to have imposed theological standards on everything. In fact, the reverse seems to be true. Melanchthon resisted becoming a member of a theological

[27] W. Dilthey, 'The Interpretation and Analysis of Man', in L. W. Spitz (ed.), *The Reformation: Basic Interpretations* (2nd edn., Lexington, Mass., 1972), 18.

[28] See e.g. Spitz, *Luther and German Humanism*, ch. ix.

[29] Becker, *Civility and Society*, passim but esp. 140–2.

[30] Note the phrase 'the debt of interchanging neighbourhood', which was used in the *Golden Legend* to describe one of the reasons for reverencing the saints: E. Duffy, *The Stripping of the Altars: Traditional Religion in England 1400–1580* (New Haven, 1992), 160–70.

[31] See Becker, *Civility and Society*, 62, for decline of the idea of vicarious holiness; see also ibid. 71, 182.

Name: GRUNWALD-HOPE, Kerstin Newton Park

Number: | 0 | 3 | 3 | 6 | 8 | 3 | | | | |

Expiry date: 15|2|21

Thank you for using our Click and Collect service

Your books are already issued to your account, but they may be recalled if someone reserves one of them. Please check your university email for updates.

Do you need the whole book? If not we can scan a selected chapter and email you a copy.

Email **Library@bathspa.ac.uk** for details.

Need help writing your assignment, referencing, or with other study skills? The Writing and Learning centre are here to help you. Email **WLC@bathspa.ac.uk** for details.

Can't find the books you need, or are you struggling to navigate through all our online resources? Our Subject Librarians are happy to help.

Email **Library@bathspa.ac.uk** for details.

BATH SPA UNIVERSITY Library

faculty, and regarded his true home as in the Arts.[32] His humanistic natural philosophy was certainly made *consistent* with his Protestantism; but the attempt recently made to tie his philosophy in with rigid Lutheranism does not seem fully persuasive.[33]

On the whole, Protestant centres of education were not like seminaries. Most did not just teach clergy; seldom were they hermetically sealed from the ideas current in the world outside. Even rare exceptions, like the 'cloister schools' of Württemberg, fed their products into the (quite cosmopolitan) University of Tübingen for final training.[34] The Genevan academy's primary *raison d'être* was to train ministers: yet soon after Calvin's death the Genevan bourgeoisie gave it the substance, if not the name, of a university by introducing other disciplines besides theology.[35] Cultural and intellectual diversity was guaranteed by the refugee or transient communities of foreign students and pastors-to-be.[36] Zurich sent its students abroad to both Calvinist and Lutheran (especially Philippist) universities to complete their education.[37] The theoretically 'Calvinist' university of Heidelberg continued to use Melanchthon's textbook of theology.[38] Scotland, with four universities by 1600, still sent students not only to Calvinist centres, but also to Baltic Lutheran universities such as Rostock or Helmstedt.[39] Exposure to diversity of opinions was not sought for its own sake. In some countries, especially strict Lutheran states, foreign education was seen as positively dangerous and to be discouraged.[40] It took place, first because there was often no alternative; and, secondly, because many Protestants, especially Calvinists, were inclusive rather than exclusive in their attitudes to the orthodoxy of brother churches.

The same plurality of voices was heard in the instruction of the Protestant laity. Laypeople were introduced to dogma through catechesis. While the ideal

[32] See H. Scheible (ed.), *Melanchthons Briefwechsel: Kritische und kommentierte Gesamtausgabe* (1977–), vol. T2 [Texte 255–520] (Stuttgart-Bad Cannstatt, 1995), nos. 268 (T2, 57–8), 342 (T2, 178); see also H. Scheible, 'Melanchthon, Philipp (1497–1560)', in *Theologische Realenzyklopaedie*, xxii. 373.23–6; and cf. *Briefwechsel* 432, T2, 365.1–9.

[33] See S. Kusukawa, *The Transformation of Natural Philosophy: The Case of Philip Melanchthon* (Cambridge, 1995), 188–9; cf. E. Cameron, 'Philipp Melanchthon: Image and Substance', *Journal of Ecclesiastical History*, 48/4 (1997), 705–22, esp. 712.

[34] B. Tolley, *Pastors and Parishioners in Württemberg during the Late Reformation 1581–1621* (Stanford, Calif., 1995), 10–11, 24 ff.

[35] K. Maag, *Seminary or University? The Genevan Academy and Reformed Higher Education, 1560–1620* (Aldershot, 1995), 24 ff., 186 ff.

[36] On the Genevan academy, see G. Lewis, 'The Genevan Academy', in A. Pettegree, A. Duke, and G. Lewis (eds.), *Calvinism in Europe 1540–1620* (Cambridge, 1994). On refugee religious culture, see H. A. Oberman, *The Reformation: Roots and Ramifications*, trans. A. C. Gow (Edinburgh, 1994), 218 ff.

[37] Maag, *Seminary or University?*, 129–40; see also O. P. Grell and B. Scribner (eds.), *Tolerance and Intolerance in the European Reformation* (Cambridge, 1996), 115.

[38] Maag, *Seminary or University?*, 168.

[39] *Letters of John Johnston c.1565–1611 and Robert Howie c.1565–c.1645*, ed. J. K. Cameron (Edinburgh, 1963), pp. xviii ff.; Grell and Scribner (eds.), *Tolerance and Intolerance*, 116.

[40] See e.g. Tolley, *Pastors and Parishioners*, 10–11.

of Protestant education may have been to inculcate absolute verbal uniformity on teaching, among the young especially,[41] no reformed catechism actually achieved total ascendancy even within the major denominations. When Luther's two catechisms appeared in 1529, many rivals were in print in Germany, often with Luther's encouragement.[42] In the reformed tradition, Calvin's catechism came too late on the scene to influence Zurich or Strasbourg, for example. The widely used Heidelberg catechism of 1563 followed a slightly different line of development from Genevan thought.[43] Moreover, as the Protestant confessions suffered internal fissures and schisms, rival factions produced competing credal documents; attempts to mediate and reconcile often simply increased the number of documents in circulation, like the Zurich consensus of 1549, the Second Helvetic Confession of 1566, or the Lutheran Formula of Concord.[44] The catechism in the English Book of Common Prayer was so short and summary (as John Knox complained very early on) that it encouraged the formation of new, unofficial catechisms for the ready market in religious instruction.[45]

Of course, many of these catechisms and confessions expressed the same essential ideas, but at different levels of sophistication and with different emphases. Credal diversity was not embraced deliberately. Nevertheless, because the reformed doctrine of the Church did not require any supranational unity of churches, it was inevitable that the church in each region or nation would acquire its own style and formulas. Minor differences in creeds or worship did not prevent churches from regarding each other as fellow members in the invisible Christian communion.[46] As confessions of faith and catechisms multiplied, it would become harder to believe that one form of words, and only one, was eternally correct. This semantic diversity must, in the fullness of time, have made easier the acceptance that *all* verbal expressions of the faith were provisional and relative.

The process reached a peak in mid-seventeenth-century England. The claims of so many rival religious leaders to exclusive truth—quite contrary to their intentions, one need hardly add—cancelled each other out. As Thomas

---

[41] G. Strauss, *Luther's House of Learning: Indoctrination of the Young in the German Reformation* (Baltimore, 1978), *passim*.

[42] For the diversity of early German catechisms, see F. Cohrs, *Die evangelischen Katechismusversuche vor Luthers Enchiridion* (2 vols.; Berlin, 1900–2), *passim*; Strauss, *Luther's House of Learning*, 164–5.

[43] A. Cochrane, *Reformed Confessions of the Sixteenth Century* (1966), 305–31; K. Barth, *The Heidelberg Catechism for Today*, trans. S. C. Guthrie (Richmond, Va., 1964), 12, 22 ff.

[44] R. Kolb, *Confessing the Faith: Reformers define the Church, 1530–1580* (St Louis, Mo., 1991); G. Strauss, 'The Mental World of a Saxon Pastor', in P. N. Brooks (ed.), *Reformation Principle and Practice: Essays in Honour of A. G. Dickens* (1980), 164–7.

[45] For Knox, see *The Works of John Knox*, ed. D. Laing (6 vols.; Edinburgh, 1854–64), iv. 26. For English catechisms see I. Green, *The Christian's ABC* (Oxford, 1996), *passim*, but esp. 45–92, and 51 for an estimate of numbers.

[46] Calvin, *Institutes*, IV. i. 10–16.

Hobbes put it, 'it is unreasonable in them, who teach there is such danger in every little errour, to require of a man endued with reason of his own, to follow the reason of any other man, or of the most voices of many other men; which is little better, than to venture his salvation at crosse and pile'.[47]

The wave of humanist-inspired education that followed in the wake of the Counter-Reformation presents some interesting contrasts to its Protestant equivalent. It became axiomatic that priests should receive a formal academic training, even if the seminaries envisaged by the Council of Trent in many instances took a long time to appear. The Society of Jesus, which led the first wave of educational reforms,[48] adopted Renaissance educational techniques enthusiastically. Like the French secular colleges and Johann Sturm's Strasbourg *Gymnasium*, Jesuit colleges structured their teaching around graded classes, where examinations had to be passed before students could move from one grade to another.[49] Antique texts, carefully expurgated and selected, formed the core of the Arts curriculum. Jesuits like Nadal tried to retrieve some works of Erasmus from their blanket condemnation in the *Index*, and continued to use his grammatical writings.[50] The florid 'copious' rhetoric of the early Renaissance came back into vogue, after it had fallen from favour elsewhere in Europe, as a means to an emotive, alluring pulpit style.[51] Ciceronian Latin survived longer than nearly anywhere else, save perhaps some English public schools.[52]

Catholic educators, Jesuits above all, gathered the harvest of the literary Renaissance. However, Jesuits then and later pointed out that scholarship was cultivated not for itself, but as a means to Godliness.[53] Educators presumed that religious truth was unique and indivisible, and reflected that unity through strict uniformity. The Jesuit *Ratio studiorum*, approved in 1599, was one of the most prescriptive documents ever produced, as to the content, form, and method of what was taught. Sympathetic commentators, let alone critics, speak of its 'pedagogic totalitarianism' and its 'authoritarian humanism'.[54] Even Catholics engaged in internal controversy over the content of orthodox tradition insisted that truth was indivisible.[55]

---

[47] Thomas Hobbes, *Leviathan*, ed. C. B. Macpherson (Harmondsworth, 1968), 711.
[48] A. Scaglione, *The Liberal Arts and the Jesuit College System* (Amsterdam, 1986), 58–9.
[49] Scaglione, *Liberal Arts*, 71–2; cf. A. Schindling, *Humanistische Hochschule und freie Reichsstadt* (Wiesbaden, 1977); L. Junod and H. Meylan, *L'Académie de Lausanne au xvi⁰ siècle* (Lausanne, 1947), 11–17.
[50] Scaglione, *Liberal Arts*, 78–9.   [51] Ibid. 98–109.   [52] Ibid. 86.
[53] Ibid. 84; cf. F. Cesareo, 'Quest for Identity: The Ideals of Jesuit Education in the Sixteenth Century', in C. Chapple, *The Jesuit Tradition in Education and Missions: A 450-year Perspective* (1993), 17–29.
[54] Scaglione, *Liberal Arts*, 84, 95. See the claim from a Jesuit lecturer in the Philippines quoted by J. O'Hare, 'Jesuit Education in America', in Chapple, *The Jesuit Tradition*, 147–8, that 'not only is Jesuit education the finest system of education ever devised by the mind of man, it is the finest that ever could be devised by the mind of man'.
[55] See the Simon–Bossuet debate in Phillips, *Church and Culture*, 126 ff.

Counter-Reformation educators took steps to protect their students from any exposure to heterodox ideas. To discuss opinions from sources not officially approved was forbidden in the *Ratio studiorum*. In-house textbooks were written by such Jesuits as Orazio Torsellini, author of manuals on grammar and history.[56] In the universities of Spain and Portugal, the *cursus philosophicus* detached Aristotelianism from many of the contentious debates that had troubled early Renaissance Italy.[57] Pupils could be secluded from the wider intellectual world, principally future clergy but also members of the lay élite. Such seclusion could be achieved by the seminary system (often run by Jesuits) but also became current in seventeenth-century France.[58] This conviction of the absolute unity and permanence of their teaching materials could not fail to have a paralysing effect. In Jesuit hands, humanist literary techniques went hand in hand with an entirely unhumanistic dependence on Aristotle and Thomas Aquinas, prescribed by Loyola at the start. Late scholasticism itself had been anything but static, and the adoption of Thomas's *Summa*, rather than Peter Lombard's *Sentences*, as a set text carried on the most forward-looking trends in fifteenth-century theology.[59] Jesuit Aristotelianism in the sixteenth century exploited the new scholarly work on the text of the philosopher.[60] However, and despite the claim that neo-Aristotelianism offered some autonomy to the natural sciences, the doctrine of substances and accidents was held sacrosanct when challenged by Descartes, precisely because to deny it would cast the official dogma of transubstantiation into doubt.[61] Nothing could be less humanist than to enthral natural philosophy to a religious dogma, expressed in scholastic categories.

The same conviction about the absolute unity of truth is seen in the production of an official catechism for the Church, the *Roman Catechism*, authorized after Trent and published in 1566. After its appearance other individuals' catechisms, very numerous in the period *c.*1530–60, became much rarer, in complete contrast to the position in Protestant countries.[62] Even the three scrupulously orthodox catechisms of the Jesuit Peter Canisius were controversial in some quarters.[63] There were obvious dangers inherent in adopting a particular written formula of over 500 pages, as 'a book in which to find

[56] Scaglione, *Liberal Arts*, 90–1.

[57] See C. B. Schmitt, Q. Skinner, and E. Kessler (eds.), *The Cambridge History of Renaissance Philosophy* (Cambridge, 1988), 512 ff., 606 ff.

[58] Phillips, *Church and Culture*, 89.   [59] Scaglione, *Liberal Arts*, 97–8.

[60] See C. H. Lohr, 'Les Jésuites et l'aristotélisme du xvie siècle', in L. Giard (ed.), *Les Jésuites à la Renaissance* (Paris, 1995), 79–91, esp. his comment that metaphysics in the Jesuit college resembled a body of systematic doctrine rather than an exposé of Aristotle as such.

[61] Phillips, *Church and Culture*, 163 ff.

[62] Originally entitled *Catechismus ad parochos* (Rome, 1566); later *Catechismus Romanus*. On pre-1566 Catholic catechisms, see *Theologische Realenzyklopaedie*, xvii/5, article 'Katechismus' (Berlin, 1988), 729 ff.

[63] Petrus Canisius, *Summa doctrinae christianae* (Vienna, 1555), *Catechismus minimus* (Ingolstadt, 1556), and *Catechismus minor* (Cologne, 1558); Scaglione, *Liberal Arts*, 84.

catholic truth in all certainty'.[64] One of the lessons of the early Renaissance
was, allegedly, that the relationship between words and the things that they
describe is not fixed, but can entail ambiguities and uncertainties.[65] If that is
so of language in general, it must be infinitely more so of religious language.
Yet a recent analyst of the Roman Catechism describes it as a 'timeless exposition of a timeless faith'.[66] The new redaction of the *Catechism of the Catholic
Church* in 1994[67] provoked criticism from some Roman Catholic theologians
over whether a single catechism could be produced and imposed by authority to be appropriate to all peoples across the world.[68] If a single catechism is
not appropriate to all countries, *a fortiori* it is not appropriate to all times. Yet
this insight, a cliché in Protestantism since late-nineteenth-century liberalism,
presents Catholicism with some difficulty, such is the influence of its Counter-
Reformation heritage.

   The different outcomes of the Protestant and Catholic handling of dogma
reflect, to a large measure, their different doctrines of the Church, and, behind
that, different ideas about the relationship of the divine to the human. An
admirer of the Catholic system might argue that Protestantism succumbed to
credal pluralism—and thereby equipped itself to face the modern era—
through failure, while Catholicism became petrified because of its very
success.

III

The second aspect of this problem, the outcome of the Renaissance critique
of 'superstitious' worship, sheds further light on the question. Both confessions, by inculcating a more reasoned and conscious obedience to their
principles, sought to 'civilize' early modern belief. The churches educated
their priests or ministers before sending them into the parishes. When they
returned to rural life in a perhaps unfamiliar parish, they at once stood at a
cultural and intellectual distance from most or even all of their parishioners.[69]
The new style of priest or minister was aware of himself as a professional individual, rather than as one of an organic community; parish religion in the
early modern period lost some of its communal, traditional quality.[70] Priests

---

[64] From the preface to *Catéchisme du Concile de Trente* (Paris, 1969), 3.
[65] Becker, *Civility and Society*, 83.
[66] R. I. Bradley, *The Roman Catechism in the Catechetical Tradition of the Church* (Lanham, Md.,
1990), 3.
[67] *Catechism of the Catholic Church* (1994).
[68] See M. J. Walsh (ed.), *Commentary on the Catechism of the Catholic Church* (1994), esp. 2–3;
J.-B. Metz and E. Schillebeeckx (eds.), *World Catechism or Inculturation?* (Edinburgh, 1989).
[69] Tolley, *Pastors and Parishioners*, 5 ff.; cf. Phillips, *Church and Culture*, 298.
[70] For communal versus individual religion in the Counter-Reformation, see M. R. Forster,
The Counter-Reformation in the Villages (Ithaca, NY, 1992).

and ministers were, in theory, predisposed to question traditional attitudes to folk religion. Their own educators attacked the belief that words, gestures, shapes drawn on parchment, or anything else could secure spiritual or material graces. The custom of divining the weather, or good or evil fortune, from chance occurrences of various kinds was denounced. This campaign to remould the popular mind clearly forms part of a move towards a more rational outlook on the causes of things in the universe.[71]

Protestant theologians did not immediately take up the Renaissance critique of 'popular religion' in so far as it was *popular*, rather than *Catholic*. They struck first and foremost at medieval Catholicism itself, its ideals as well as its debasements and corruptions. However, in the mid-sixteenth century several lines of argument enabled Protestant theologians to move the critique of 'superstitions' on from the stage reached in the later Middle Ages. Preachers and writers such as Johannes Spreter, Augustin Lercheimer, or Jakob Heerbrand insisted that no ritual or form of words had power to change the properties of matter, or to instil into objects any qualities that were not there in all species of the same kind at their creation.[72] Therefore the charms of folk magicians, or the spiritual or magical significance ascribed to particular objects at particular times, were futile and meaningless. Words were just words: shapes or letters written on parchment had no power other than to contain a message. Protestants, of course, had no need so to cover their condemnations of magical charms as to protect the consecration of the Eucharist or the blessing of 'sacramentals', holy water, bread, herbs, palms, and so forth. On the contrary, they went out of their way to exploit the obvious parallels between Catholic rites and magical spells: they noted the resemblances and condemned both equally.[73]

A second characteristic of Protestant thought was Providentialism. Given that late medieval pastoral theologians had taught that misfortune or sudden illness might often arise from the malice of sorcerers or witches,[74] Protestants risked encouraging more, not less, recourse to folk magicians by stripping

---

[71] On the early modern critique of superstition, see e.g. S. Clark, *Thinking with Demons: The Idea of Witchcraft in Early Modern Europe* (Oxford, 1997), 472–88; cf. E. Cameron, 'For Reasoned Faith or Embattled Creed? Religion for the People in Early Modern Europe', *TRHS*, 6th ser., vol. viii (1998), 165–87.

[72] Johannes Spreter, *Ein Kurtzer Bericht, was von den Abgoetterischen Saegen und Beschweren zuehalten* (Basel, 1543), sigs. A ii^{r–v}, A iii^{r–v}; Augustin Lercheimer, *Ein Christlich Bedencken und Erinnerung von Zauberey*, in *Theatrum de veneficis* (Frankfurt-am-Main, 1586), 289; Jacobus Heerbrandus, *De magia disputatio* (Tübingen, 1570), 12.

[73] Spreter, *Kurtzer Bericht*, sig. Aiii^v; Lercheimer, *Christlich Bedencken*, 289–90; Heerbrandus, *De magia disputatio*, 13–15; Johann Georg Godelmann, *Tractatus de magis, veneficis et lamiis* (Frankfurt, 1601), 55–8; Antonius Praetorius, *Gründlicher Bericht von Zauberey* (Frankfurt, 1629), 63–5.

[74] Johannes Nider, *Formicarius*, republished as *De visionibus ac revelationibus* (Helmstedt, 1692), bk. 5, ch. 3; Silvestro Mazzolini Prierias, *De strigimagarum demonumque mirandis libri iii* (Rome, 1521), bk. 2, ch. 7, sigs. bb ii^v ff. Cf. E. E. Evans-Pritchard, *Witchcraft, Oracles and Magic among the Azande* (Oxford, 1976), 18.

away ecclesiastical protective magic. They responded that spiritual defences against evil or misfortune were beside the point. Everything that happened proceeded from the judgement and wisdom of a loving God; one should use natural means of protection, and trust to prayer.[75] This message, though anticipated by a late medieval nominalist like Martin Plantsch of Tübingen,[76] laid a far more one-sided stress on God's sovereignty than had been customary in the past.

Such extreme providentialism led, eventually, to the decline of the devil as a serious factor in religious thought. It was a small step from dissuading defence against demons, to play down the role of personified evil until it disappeared altogether. Mainstream Protestant theologians wished no such thing. Luther wrote about the presence and power of the devil frequently—too frequently for some humanists.[77] Even Melanchthon, who lacked Luther's gothic near-Manichaean imagination, lectured conventionally on the nature and power of demons.[78] Later in the century, Protestants allowed themselves, to their disadvantage, to be drawn into exorcism contests with their more impressive Catholic brethren.[79] Yet the logic of providentialism tended to set aside, if not demons as such, at least their power to shape events. Reginald Scot's *Discoverie of Witchcraft* reads in many respects like a classic Protestant work: it denounces the ignorance of the old clergy and appeals to religious knowledge and trust in the divine dispensation. However, so rigorously does it exclude the devil from serious consideration that it strays closer to unorthodoxy than most of its counterparts. Some collusive evidence has appeared to link Scot with the Familists.[80] More orthodox in his beliefs, Sir Thomas Browne nevertheless thought the chief harm done by the devil was not physical damage, but the sowing of error—including the error, which Browne thought widespread enough to mention, that the devil did not exist.[81]

Some parts of Thomas Hobbes's *Leviathan* seemed impeccably Protestant in their reasoning. In book IV, 'Of the Kingdome of Darknesse', Hobbes reinterpreted the Protestant demonological tradition to suit his own unorthodox ideas. He attacked, in terms close to (for example) Heinrich Bullinger's *Decades*, the idea that consecrations, whether of the Eucharist or any other

[75] Thomas, *Religion*, 90–103.

[76] Martin Plantsch, *Opusculum de sagis maleficis* (Phorce, 1507), sigs. a iv^r–b iv^r.

[77] H. A. Oberman, *Luther: Mensch zwischen Gott und Teufel* (Berlin, 1982); see also Oberman, 'Martin Luther: Forerunner of the Reformation', in Oberman, *The Reformation: Roots and Ramifications*, 56–70.

[78] A story told by Melanchthon in his lectures about the illusory resuscitation of a dead musician by demonic magic is reported by Caspar Peucer, *Commentarius, de praecipuis divinationum generibus* (Frankfurt, 1607), 14.

[79] See the instances described below, nn. 97–8.

[80] Reginald Scot, *The Discoverie of Witchcraft* (1584); on Scot's possible links with the Familists, see Clark, *Thinking with Demons*, 543–5.

[81] Sir Thomas Browne, *Pseudodoxia epidemica*, in *The Works of Sir Thomas Browne*, ed. C. Sayle (3 vols.; Edinburgh, 1927), i. 182–93.

cult object, could change the nature of the thing consecrated. He objected that the word 'consecrate' in the Bible meant nothing of the sort.[82] He departed from the traditional view in his doctrine of souls and spirits. As a materialist and a mortalist, Hobbes despised the Aristotelian and Thomist idea of 'separated essences' or 'incorporeal spirits', and not only because belief in such spirits, and especially in souls in purgatory, reinforced the politically divisive authority of the pope.[83] The whole science of 'demonology' he dismissed as derived from wrong-headed ancient philosophy. Possession and lunacy were one and the same thing; most scriptural language concerning possession was figurative. If scripture spoke of 'spirits corporeall (though subtle and invisible)', they played no part in his scheme of things.[84] Hobbes represents an extreme example: yet he shows what could happen when Aristotelian philosophy (largely protected in the Protestant universities of the sixteenth century) was discarded, and the Protestant critique of the traditional religious world view was taken to its logical conclusion. By the late seventeenth century, the fear of intellectual 'atheism', the fear that intellectuals who took the new philosophies to their logical conclusion would undermine *all* supernatural beliefs, largely replaced the fear of superstition and magic.[85] Many bold thinkers were themselves Protestant clergy. Besides the numerous English sceptics, the Cartesian Balthasar Bekker in his *The Enchanted World* blew open the whole question of spirits and apparitions from within the heart of the Dutch Reformed Church.[86]

Protestant critiques of popular superstitions began from identical standpoints to their Catholic counterparts. Yet the logic of Protestant beliefs about the transcendence of God led inexorably to a different view of the devil, and therefore of superstition itself. Without demonology, wrong religion became less the result of demonic seductions than a product of human folly and ignorance. This attitude to wrong religion both looked backwards to the Renaissance humanists, and foreshadowed the more sweeping critiques of 'superstition' (meaning most traditional religions) made in the Enlightenment.

Roman Catholicism inherited from its late medieval past a campaign against 'vulgar errors' expressed through penitentials, confessional manuals, sermons,

[82] Hobbes, *Leviathan*, 633–5.

[83] Ibid. 638, 691–2. Cf. H. Bullinger, *The Decades of Henry Bullinger*, trans. 'H. I.' and ed. T. Harding (4 vols.; Parker Society; Cambridge, 1849–52), iv. 254–60.

[84] Hobbes, *Leviathan*, 657–64. See R. Tuck, 'The "Christian Atheism" of Thomas Hobbes', in M. Hunter and D. Wootton (eds.), *Atheism from the Reformation to the Enlightenment* (Oxford, 1992), 111–30.

[85] Thomas, *Religion*, 309; see N. Smith, 'The Charge of Atheism and the Language of Radical Speculation, 1640–1660', in Hunter and Wootton, *Atheism*, 159–81; J. Redwood, *Reason, Ridicule and Religion: The Age of Enlightenment in England, 1660–1750* (1976), 29 ff.

[86] Balthasar Bekker, *De betoverde weereld* (Amsterdam, 1691–3); editions appeared in German, French, and English; A. Jelsma, 'The Devil and Protestantism', in A. Jelsma, *Frontiers of the Reformation* (Aldershot, 1998), 25–39.

and treatises such as *Dives and Pauper*.[87] It brought new weapons to the task, notably the inquisitions (in Spain and Italy) and diocesan pastoral visitations (nearly everywhere).[88] However, even to scrape the surface of this issue reveals new complexities. In the first place, the Roman Catholic Church of the Counter-Reformation had to preserve continuity with its heritage, while purging that heritage of un-Catholic or corrupt elements. The frontier between popular and magisterial Catholicism was marked by a string of hard cases. In the later Middle Ages, many cults grew up that claimed to ensure certain spiritual benefits, in this world or in the next, for their devotees. Lady Fasts gave protection against sudden death, offerings in honour of St Onofrius protected against demons, the *Bulla Sabbathina* shortened the time Carmelite friars spent in purgatory, and so on.[89] In the early modern period— and indeed before—individual theologians tried to dissuade people from trusting to rites of this sort. However, short of an absolute papal condemnation, or indeed renunciation of the whole idea of the intercession of saints, others could continue to uphold such practices.[90]

Secondly, some Catholic writers used the argument that special divine favours had been 'delegated' to particular cults, to justify, or at least bring into a disputable grey area, various quasi-magical charms and curative spells. If God had endowed particular saints, or particular sacraments, with special holiness for human benefit, might he not also have given particular places, or particular people, or other forms of words, other spiritual properties? This sort of reasoning was found in highly reputable and otherwise orthodox Catholic sources such as Hieronymus Llamas and the Jesuit Leonardus Lessius. Rigorous rationalists, who denied *any* automatic benefits to acts of worship of any kind, may have been in a minority in the late sixteenth and early seventeenth centuries.[91]

[87] *Dives and Pauper*, ed. P. H. Barnum (Early English Text Society os 275, 280; 2 vols.; Oxford, 1976–80), exposition of the First Commandment, chs. 31–50; Nikolaus von Dinkelsbühl, 'Ain Tractat von den zehen Poten', in K. Baumann (ed.), *Aberglaube für Laien* (Quellen und Forschungen zur europaeischen Ethnologie, 6; 2 vols.; Würzburg, 1991), ii. 503–50.

[88] M. R. O'Neil, 'Magical Healing, Love Magic and the Inquisition in Late Sixteenth-Century Modena', in S. Haliczer (ed.), *Inquisition and Society in Early Modern Europe* (1987), 88–114; M. R. O'Neil, '*Sacerdote ovvero strione*: Ecclesiastical and Superstitious Remedies in 16th Century Italy', in S. Kaplan (ed.), *Understanding Popular Culture* (Berlin, 1984), 53–83; U. Mazzone and A. Turchini, *I visiti pastorali: Analisi di una fonte* (Bologna, 1985).

[89] *Dives and Pauper*, bk. i, ch. 42, i. 172–3; Nider, *De visionibus ac revelationibus*, 420ff.; Emanuele do Valle de Moura, *De incantationibus seu ensalmis opusculum Primum . . .* (Evora, 1620), fo. 9ᵛ–p. 13.

[90] Valle de Moura reports different views on the *Bulla Sabbathina*: *De incantationibus*, 12ff., citing Fr Thomas de Jesus, *De antiquitate et sanctitatis ordinis carmilitani*, bk. 2 ch. 1.

[91] Valle de Moura, *De incantationibus*, 29ff., with refs. to Nicolaus Serarius, *Commentarii in sacros Bibliorum libros, Josuae, Judicum, Ruth, Tobiae . . .* (Paris, 1611), on Tobit, ch. 8; and to Francisco Valles, *De iis quae scripta sunt physice in libris sacris, sive de sacra philosophia liber singularis* ([Geneva], 1595), ch. 28; see de Moura's discussion of Llamas and Lessius, in *De incantationibus*, 65ff.; also Martinus Delrio SJ, *Disquisitionum Magicarum Libri Sex, in tres tomos partiti* (Lyon, 1599–1600), i. 37–42, on *saludadores*.

Two circumstances encouraged Catholic defenders of the 'magical' power of ritual to press the point further than their late medieval predecessors. First, there was the mission field. Missionaries in Asia and the New World, especially those in central and southern America, struggled with indigenous religions (which they regarded as demonic) like dark-age missionaries in northern Europe.[92] Ultimately, Roman Catholicism would arrive at an accommodating syncretism at variance with its official outlook.[93] In the short term, the pressures of mission provoked eager reporting of miracles, special providences, and dramatic demonstrations of spiritual power. Missionary friars, for instance, reputedly forced devils to carry water or stones for them during the building of monasteries or mission stations.[94] Such stories found their way, via the published reports of the missions,[95] into the works of Martín Delrio or Friedrich Forner as proofs of the spiritual power inherent in Catholicism. Indigenous Americans had been exorcized, or converted to Catholicism, or both, through the power inherent in the sacraments, holy water, or the sign of the cross.[96]

The confessional struggle within Europe provided another reason for Catholic writers and preachers temporarily to suspend their rationalism. Propagandists could not resist demonstrating the superiority of their faith by its power to work special miracles, above all miracles of exorcism. Tales were told of possessed people, or even haunted houses, whom Protestant prayer had failed to help, but whose demons had quailed and vanished in the presence of priests or holy objects.[97] On occasions clerics from both creeds were drawn into contests of exorcizing power, leading in turn to pamphlet controversies over what had actually happened.[98]

These Roman Catholic responses to popular religion may ultimately prove to have been marginal examples: certainly there was little scope for future development. Nevertheless, if Protestantism's logic tended towards providentialism, Catholicism's belief that divine power was delegated downwards into holy rituals and consecrated objects tended to confirm rather than

---

[92] V. I. J. Flint, *The Rise of Magic in Early Medieval Europe* (Oxford, 1991); A. Murray, 'Missionaries and Magic in Dark-Age Europe', *P&P* 136 (1992), 186–205.

[93] Jacques Lafaye, *Quetzalcoatl and Guadalupe*, trans. B. Keen (Chicago, 1976); N. S. Davidson, *The Counter-Reformation* (Oxford, 1987), 70 ff.

[94] Valle de Moura, *De incantationibus*, fo. 5ʳ, with refs. to Joannes dos Santos, *Ethiopia Oriental* (Evora, 1609), and [Diego] Ortiz, *Compendium summarum*.

[95] Accounts used to this effect include: Luis Frois, *Brevis Iapaniae insulae descriptio* (Cologne, 1582); Pedro de Cieza de Leon, *Cronica del Peru* (Seville, 1553, and subsequently), pt. 1, ch. 118.

[96] Delrio, *Disquisitionum*, iii. 237 ff., 247 ff., 263 ff., 284 ff.; Friedrich Forner, *Panoplia armaturae Dei* (Ingolstadt, 1626), 141, 148–9, 255, 262 ff.

[97] Delrio, *Disquisitionum*, ii. 75 ff., iii. 285; Forner, *Panoplia*, 98–9, 268–9.

[98] e.g. the 'Miracle at Laon' of 1566, in D. P. Walker, *Unclean Spirits* (1981), 19–28; or Peter Canisius's exorcism of Anna von Bernhausen at Altötting, in Martin Eisengrein, *Unser liebe Fraw zu Alten Oetting* (Ingolstadt, 1571), and Johannes Marbach, *Von Mirackeln und Wunderzeichen* (Strasbourg, 1571), as analysed by Philip Soergel.

discourage an immanentist, even a 'magical' view of spiritual power. The consequences of this approach were seen in Rome's uneasy relationship with emergent science, and remain today in the official papal recognition of miracles. This outlook would have required preserving elements in late medieval religion that the humanists would certainly have regarded as 'uncivilized'.

IV

The differences between Protestant and Catholic attitudes to dogma and superstition arose not from mere coincidence or circumstances, but from fundamental differences in assumptions. Protestantism believed in an absolutely sovereign transcendent God. The churches on earth carried out his revealed will, but neither institutions nor their teaching had any prerogative access to spiritual power. In any case, the reformed churches right from the start were several, not one. Multiplicity forced Protestants to come to terms with the provisional character of much of what they wrote. Initially, this was only possible because they set Scripture apart from every other form of religious writing. They uncoupled it from the continuous hermeneutic tradition within the Church, in which medieval theologians had believed. In the short term this made religious pluralism easier to live with. These basic assumptions predisposed the Protestant theologians, ultimately, to adopt an attitude towards religious language and the power of ritual that had obvious affinities with the rationalism of the Renaissance humanists.

Roman Catholicism entered the early modern world with a renewed emphasis on the absolute unity of the church on earth and its teachings, and a conviction—expressed in controversy and confrontation—that it, and it alone, represented the divine dispensation on earth. This outlook tended to dampen down any doubts about the power of human language to express the faith absolutely, and to look for supernatural confirmation of its powers and authority. Yes, Roman Catholicism adopted many of the trappings of the Renaissance: its rhetoric, its educational methods, some of its textual criticism. In some respects the Jesuit tradition followed the Renaissance more enthusiastically than the Protestant. This humanist 'civility', however, took shape under the mantle of idealized uniformity, and of studied continuity with many of the traditions of the past. Continuity and uniformity made it difficult for the Catholic Church to respond with any suppleness to the rapidly changing cultural environment of the Counter-Reformation centuries.

One has come a long way from books on manners and courtesy. However, what the humanists approved in religion, and contrasted to 'uncivilized' or 'barbarous' religion, was in fact Christianity on the threshold of modernity:

religious thought awakening to a sense of the provisional, as opposed to the absolute, character of all human creeds and rituals. Both the Protestant and Catholic traditions laid claim to the mantle of the Renaissance; yet it was ultimately easier for the former to embrace its effects on religion than for the latter, with consequences that can be seen in the development of religious thought up to the present.

4

Civility and Civil Observances in the Early Modern English Funeral

RALPH HOULBROOKE

In 1645 the *Directory for the Publique Worship of God* forbade the performance at burials of any religious ceremonies, including praying, reading, and singing on the way to, or at, the grave, because (it claimed) they had been grossly abused, did not benefit the dead in any way, and had proved 'many wayes hurtfull to the living'. But any 'civill respects or differences at the Buriall, suitable to the ranke and condition of the party deceased whiles he was living', were specifically exempted from these proscriptions.[1] The significance of the word 'civill' in this place is somewhat ambiguous. Besides its root meanings (of or pertaining to citizens or the body of citizens) the word had by 1645 acquired an enormous range of other connotations and shades of meaning. 'Polite' and 'decent' may well have been intended here. It seems likely that the authors of the *Directory* also wished to make a broader distinction between religious observances and secular ones. 'Pertaining especially to the *ordinary* life and affairs of a citizen, as distinguished from *military*, *ecclesiastical*, etc.', is the relevant definition in the *Oxford English Dictionary*.

The words 'civil' and 'civility' were sometimes used in English discourse about funeral practices several decades before the publication of the *Directory*. Anthony Anderson, preaching in 1581 at the funeral of the famous lawyer Robert Keylwey at Exton in Rutland, speculated that his audience had not come for what he considered the right reasons: 'But you of the greater sort, take you care, that ye come not to heare what the lord saith, only for civility or neiborly courtesie, in respect of these funerals . . .'. Halfway through his long sermon, he offered to defer the second part of it, because the 'ciuill solemnities'—that is, the heraldic ceremonies—might otherwise run on too long. Anderson implicitly distinguished between 'ciuill' and religious observances and used the word 'civility' to refer to politeness or courtesy.[2]

[1] *A Directory for the Publique Worship of God, Throughout the Three Kingdoms* (1645), 73–4.
[2] A. Anderson, *A Sermon of sure Comfort, preached at the Funerall of Master Robert Keylwey Esquire, at Exton in Rutland, the 18. of Marche 1580* (1581), 43, 47.

This essay explores the idea of civility with particular reference to aspects of funerals that were not in the strictest sense religious or liturgical. It illustrates the nature of civility in three main ways: by contrast with practices that English commentators found uncivil or barbaric; by discussion of some observances that served as touchstones of courtesy and decorum, and by identification of certain important changes in those observances. In early modern England there were various aspects of funerals that were considered to be both 'civil' as opposed to religious and also marks of 'civility' in the sense of the politeness appropriate to a civilized society. They included mourning dress, hospitality, alms, heraldic ceremonies, and funeral processions, all of which will be discussed here. In practice it was impossible to separate religion from civility. In all civilized societies concepts of civility have been largely shaped by religious beliefs. Protestant Christianity was an essential element of post-Reformation England's conception of the truest civility. Fully civil behaviour had to be compatible with true religion. Early modern commentators knew of many ancient and modern societies that, though distinguished by both advanced material culture and some formality or even politeness of manners, were also disfigured by 'superstition' in various forms, including not only pagan, Muslim, and Hindu, but also Roman Catholic and Greek Orthodox.

I

Several writers of the late sixteenth and seventeenth centuries considered and compared the variety of ancient and modern funeral rites. Comparative observations of this sort flowed both from the Renaissance study of classical antiquity and from the increasing number of published European travellers' reports about Asian, African, and American customs. Among the earlier books devoted to the subject published on the Continent were Lilio Gregorio Giraldi's *De sepulchris, et vario sepeliendi ritu* (Basle, 1539) and Thomaso Porcacchi's *Funerali antichi di diversi popoli, et nationi* (Venice, 1574). In England, learned interest in the history of funeral ceremonies was signalled in 1600 by the delivery of a series of discourses to the Society of Antiquaries by Sir William Dethick, Garter King of Arms, and other scholars.[3]

Some peoples were considered to have disposed of their dead in utterly inhuman and barbaric ways. Sir William Segar, Dethick's successor, discussing funerals in his *Honor Military, and Ciuill* (1602), implicitly condemned as

---

[3] *A Collection of Curious Discourses written by Eminent Antiquaries upon Several Heads in Our English Antiquities*, ed. T. Hearne (expanded edn., 2 vols.; 1771), i. 199–221.

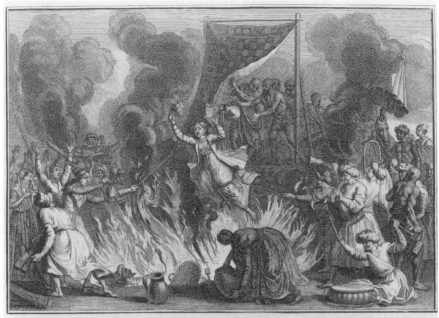

Maniere dont les FEMMES se BRULENT aux INDES apres la Mort de leurs EPOUX.

1. Performance of sati, from B. Picart, *Cérémonies et coutumes religieuses de tous les peuples du monde* (Amsterdam, 1728–43)

'vnciuill or sauage' the Lotophagi, who cast dead bodies into the sea, the Scythians, who ate the flesh of the dead at their feasts, and the Hircani and Massagetae, who had corpses eaten by dogs.[4] The funeral customs described with the deepest abhorrence by European observers of the contemporary world were, however, those that involved the sacrifice of the living to act as servants or companions of the dead, such as had been found in Guinea, Mexico, and Peru. The Chinese, by contrast (Sir Thomas Browne noted), burned great numbers of printed pictures of slaves and horses over the grave, 'civilly content with their companies in effigie which barbarous Nations exact unto reality'.[5]

The Hindu custom of sati, the burning of the widow with her husband's body, was described by several European travellers. English observers such as Edward Terry and Ralph Fitch noted that it was theoretically voluntary, but

[4] Sir W. Segar, *Honor Military, and Ciuill, contained in foure Bookes* (1602), 252.
[5] Sir T. Browne, *Hydriotaphia: Urne Buriall; or, a Discourse of the Sepulchrall Urnes lately found in Norfolk* in *The Religio Medici & Other Writings of Sir Thomas Browne*, with an introduction by C. H. Herford (1906), 99.

essential for the preservation of the widow's honour.[6] The belief underlying
sati was the antithesis of the Christian doctrine that there was no marriage or
any other exclusive partnership in heaven, which facilitated the acceptance of
remarriage in England. This spirit of acceptance was well expressed in Henry
King's poem *The Legacy*, addressed by a husband to his wife:

> Those were barbarian wives, that did invent
> Weeping to death at th'husbands monument;
> But in more civil rites she doth approve
> Her first, who ventures on a second love;

where the word 'civil' neatly encapsulates two meanings: civilized as opposed
to barbarous, and courteous in showing respect to the dead.[7]

The best-known comparative discourse of funerals by an English author is
Sir Thomas Browne's *Hydriotaphia: Urne Buriall* (1658). Disposal of mortal
remains was almost universal in human societies, he asserted, and could even
be discerned among some animal and insect species. The 'civill society' of the
bees 'carrieth out their dead, and hath exequies, if not interrments'. The cautious and sceptical Browne tended to judge favourably those rites that
appeared to be grounded on reasonable if speculative conceptions of the
natural world, and those that seemed to be informed by some glimmering of
Christian revelation, but he condemned those that were based on superstition. He pointed out that inhumation and burning had been the methods of
disposing of the body maintained by the 'sobrest Nations'. Inhumation was
the method of disposal most conformable to the Word of God and scriptural
example. But different scientific doctrines had provided grounds for cremation 'according to severall apprehensions of the most rationall dissolution'.
Thus some had believed that it was most natural to end in fire, the master
principle, or element, that would in the end consume all the rest; others had
relied on this purifying element to free the ethereal particles in their composition. He distinguished between these 'rationall' conceptions and the superstitions of those who 'too much affected, or strictly declined' cremation on
mistaken religious grounds.[8]

Of all pagan funeral customs, those of classical antiquity were the most
widely familiar among early modern authors. Browne commended some of
them because they conveyed an intimation of immortality: opening the eyes
of the corpse towards heaven before lighting the funeral pyre, using wood
from evergreen trees as fuel, and making music symbolizing the soul's participation in the harmony of heaven. But he also disparaged various aspects

---

[6] S. Purchas, *Hakluytus Posthumus or Purchas His Pilgrimes. Contayning a History of the World in Sea Voyages and Lande Travells by Englishmen and others* (20 vols.; Glasgow, 1905–7), ix. 44–5, x. 178.

[7] *Minor Poets of the Caroline Period*, ed. G. Saintsbury (Oxford, 1905–21), iii. 182.

[8] Browne, *Hydriotaphia*, 96–8, 101.

of ancient rites. To see a good omen in a quick burning pyre, or to offer sacrifice to the winds to achieve this result, 'was a low form of superstition'; to bury money with the dead to pay Charon's fee 'was a practise full of folly'.[9] Other commentators found in Roman rituals such as the carrying of the deceased's trophies in his funeral procession and the delivery of a laudatory oration antecedents of modern funeral practices. Joshua Stopford in his *Pagano-Papismus* (1675) condemned much of Roman Catholic funeral ritual precisely because of its pagan Roman ancestry.[10]

Sir Thomas Browne appraised the funeral customs of antiquity in the light of shared conceptions of civility, as well as reason and Christian revelation. The solicitude for the body widely shown among the ancients was not to be condemned: Christians had 'handsomely glossed the deformity of death, by careful consideration of the body, and civil rites which take off brutall terminations'. Their belief in a resurrection had not caused them to neglect the interment of bodies acknowledged to be 'the lodging of Christ, and temples of the holy Ghost'. Of all the ancient peoples, it was the children of Israel whose customs most closely prefigured Christian practices. Jewish observances recorded in Scripture were conventionally accorded greater respect than the rites of any other non-Christian nation. The fact that many funeral ceremonies, such as feasts, lamentations at the grave, music, weeping mourners, the washing, anointing, and kissing of the dead, and the closing of their eyes, were practised not only by the Greeks and Romans, but by the Jews as well, showed that 'these were not meere Pagan-Civilities', in Browne's opinion.[11]

Several English observers who described the funerals of other peoples nevertheless emphatically deprecated the ostentatious displays of grief customary among several Christian nations as well as Jews and pagans. They contravened Saint Paul's injunction that Christians should not mourn as others did who had no hope. A show of unrestrained grief at funerals in either spontaneous or ritual form was taken as one of the surest signs that true Christian belief was absent. Among the ostensibly Christian, it signalled hypocrisy or superficiality of faith. It was also widely practised by the savage or 'ethnic', the heathen unenlightened by religion. The American Indians furnished several good examples of such behaviour described by English travellers. The inhabitants of Guinea, a people 'altogether wild, rough, and uncivill', also displayed a grievous sorrow for their dead, howling and crying.[12]

Excessive lamentations were also a frequently noted element of obsequies in lands under the sway of the Greek Orthodox church. When a Russian died,

---

[9] Ibid. 124–7.

[10] *Curious Discourses*, ed. Hearne, i. 206–7, 209–11; J. Stopford, *Pagano-Papismus: Or, An Exact Parallel betweene Rome-Pagan and Rome-Christian, in their Doctrines and Ceremonies* (1675), 278–87.

[11] Browne, *Hydriotaphia*, 101, 123.

[12] Purchas, *Hakluytus Posthumus*, vi. 289, 344, xvi. 348, xviii. 449–50, xix. 388.

according to Giles Fletcher, women mourners would 'stand howling over the body after a prophane and heathenish manner . . . asking him what he wanted, and what he meant to die'. In their funerals, noted George Sandys, the Greeks living under Turkish rule retained several of their ancient and heathen ceremonies. 'Their lamentations are the same that they were, and beyond all civilitie.' William Forde, preacher to the English ambassador at Constantinople, vividly evoked in a funeral sermon the hideous noises and self-inflicted disfigurements that manifested the sorrow of female mourners at Greek funerals. St Paul condemned 'this excessive, vnmeasurable, immoderate lamentation'.[13]

Their laments were one of the distinctive features by which the Irish, so close to England, and avowedly Christian in religion, showed themselves in English eyes to be primitive and savage. In *A View of the Present State of Ireland*, Edmund Spenser expressed through the mouth of 'Irenius' the opinion that their 'disparefull outcryes, and ymoderate waylinges' at burials pointed to the possibility that the Irish were related to the Scythians, perhaps the fiercest barbarians of the ancient world. Even though this 'evill custome' might be a religious abuse rather than a matter for 'civill reformacion', it was nevertheless 'vncyvill'.[14]

II

Ostentatious grief formed no part of the decent, orderly solemnity of an English funeral. The Italian humanist Polydore Vergil commended before the Reformation the English avoidance of lamentation on such occasions.[15] Sadness was, however, signalled by the dark and dreary colours of mourning, especially black. Between the fifteenth and early seventeenth centuries the funeral processions of important or wealthy people customarily included scores or even hundreds of individuals dressed in mourning apparel, such as the servants, kinsfolk, and colleagues of the defunct, and a contingent of poor folk near the head of the procession. The house where the corpse lay prior to the funeral was usually hung with black cloth, as was the church where the services took place. The cost of 'blacks' often amounted to three-quarters of the funeral account.[16]

[13] Purchas, *Hakluytus Posthumus*, viii. 169, xii. 620–1; W. Forde, *A Sermon preached at Constantinople . . . at the Funerall of the vertuous and admired Lady Anne Glover, sometime Wife to the Honourable Knight Sir Thomas Glover* (1616), 50–1.

[14] E. Spenser, *A View of the Present State of Ireland*, ed. W. L. Renwick (1934), 72–3. John Aubrey described singing at Yorkshire funerals as 'Irish Howlings' in his *Remaines of Gentilisme and Judaisme*; see *Three Prose Works*, ed. J. Buchanan-Brown (Fontwell, 1972), 176.

[15] Quoted by G. W. Pigman III, *Grief and English Renaissance Elegy* (Cambridge, 1985), 138 n. 8. For Italian humanist denunciations of excessive mourning, see M. B. Becker, *Civility and Society in Western Europe, 1300–1600* (Bloomington, Ind., 1988), 99.

[16] L. Stone, *The Crisis of the Aristocracy 1558–1641* (Oxford, 1965), 576, 784–5.

Before the Reformation, costly gifts of mourning garb had been intended not merely to represent or encourage sorrow, but to help mobilize prayers for the soul of the deceased in its greatest need. Some religious conservatives may have hoped even after 1559 that they still would have this effect. Rejection of intercessory prayer was implicit in the Protestant criticism that this 'outrageous mourning' showed doubt about the fate of the dead.[17] Christians should rather rejoice in the deaths of their friends. The 1572 *Admonition to the Parliament* alleged that mourning, even when it was not hypocritical, was 'superstitious and heathnish, bicause it is used onely of custome'.[18] Thomas Cartwright added that mourning blacks provoked sorrow beyond the moderation appointed by St Paul. In controversy with Cartwright, John Whitgift asserted that the wearing of mourning was 'no matter of religion, but of civility and order'. To 'put religion in it' was superstitious; to use it to provoke sorrow was not to be excused, but it might usefully serve to remind the wearer of his own mortality.[19] Richard Hooker defended the wearing of mourning as a fitting sign of grief and love for departed friends. It seldom happened, he ironically remarked, that men were 'fain to have their mourning gowns pulled off their backs for fear of killing themselves with sorrow that way nourished'. To show sorrow was natural, and, even if it was absent, 'yet the signs are meet to shew what should be'. Hooker may be said to have regarded mourning as a mark of civility towards the dead.[20]

The clothing of scores of participants in black at the expense of the deceased's family nevertheless went beyond the demands of civility. Religious arguments may have prepared the way for a change in practice, but its heavy cost was perhaps the decisive consideration. When around 1600 many of the nobility and gentry sought to limit the amount spent on their funerals, the cost of mourning blacks was the item most often specifically mentioned. Sir Francis Knollys, treasurer of Queen Elizabeth's household (d. 1596), claimed that his goods were insufficient to meet his children's needs. He firmly prohibited any 'costly pomp of ceremonies or great gifts of blacks for mourning' at his burial, whereby his children might 'anyways be hindered'. Apostrophizing Knollys in a funeral elegy, the poet Thomas Churchyard assured him that

> Thy friends shall mourne, not with long clokes of black
> But with sad looks, of doell behind thy back.

[17] Will of Thomas Brudenell, d. 1549, quoted by J. Wake, *The Brudenells of Deene* (1953), 48.
[18] *An Admonition to the Parliament* in *Puritan Manifestoes*, ed. W. H. Frere and C. E. Douglas (1954), 28.
[19] J. Whitgift, *The Defence of the Answer to the Admonition, against the Reply of Thomas Cartwright*, in *Works*, ed. J. Ayre (Parker Society; 3 vols.; 1851–3), iii. 368–70.
[20] R. Hooker, *Of the Laws of Ecclesiastical Polity*, in Hooker, *Works* (2 vols.; Oxford, 1841), ii. 153.

Requiring a Christian burial without extraordinary show or spectacle, the earl of Salisbury, the foremost statesman of James I's reign (d. 1612) requested blacks only for his own servants and some few friends.[21]

The ostentatious display of cumbersome mourning dress did not always impress observers. John Chamberlain found Queen Anne's immensely lavish funeral in 1619 'but a drawling tedious sight'. The great number of lords and ladies made but a poor show 'which perhaps was because they were appar-elled all alike, or that they came laggering all along even tired with the length of the way and waight of theyre clothes, every Lady having twelve yardes of broade cloth about her and the countesses sixteen'.[22] Here was another reason for a lightening of processional mourning dress and a reduction in the number of participants for whom it was provided. Fynes Moryson, travelling in Lutheran northern Germany towards the end of the sixteenth century, noticed that, apart from the chief mourners at funerals, the other men who followed the hearse had no mourning cloaks nor gowns, such as were used in England, 'but only hattbandes of black Sipres hanging downe behynde, Called Trawerbandes that is mourning bandes'. The fashion for funeral hatbands, clearly imported from the Continent, became established in England during the following century. In France too, Moryson noticed, mourning apparel was worn at funerals only by close relatives, who bought it for themselves.[23]

During the seventeenth and early eighteenth centuries the mourning clothes once provided for large numbers of individuals at funerals were largely replaced by gifts, which ranged from memorial rings for special friends to the gloves presented to all guests, including silk hatbands and scarves for inter-mediate categories of participant. All these items might be provided in dif-ferent qualities, according to the standing of the individual concerned. At the higher levels of society this change in practice may have represented a financial saving. Further down the social scale, among new aspirants to gentility, esp-ecially in the towns, many families may have faced an increase in expenditure to provide such gifts.

The distribution of funeral gifts required nice judgement and a good deal of care. It was notoriously easy to cause offence by neglecting neighbours

---

[21] J. Edmondson, *A Complete Body of Heraldry* (2 vols.; 1780), i, 'Funerals' (unpaginated), had already noticed in late Elizabethan wills provisions curtailing funeral expenditure. See also Stone, *Crisis*, 577; *The History of Parliament: The House of Commons, 1558–1603*, ed. P. W. Hasler (3 vols.; 1981), ii. 414; T. Churchyard, *A sad and solemne Fvnerall, of the right Honorable sir Francis Knowles, knight* (1596); E. M. Tenison, *Elizabethan England: Being the History of this Country 'In Relation to all Foreign Princes'* (14 vols.; Leamington Spa, 1933–61), xii. 487.

[22] J. Chamberlain, *The Letters of John Chamberlain*, ed. N. E. McClure (2 vols.; Philadelphia, 1939), ii. 237.

[23] Fynes Moryson, *Shakespeare's Europe: Unpublished Chapters of Fynes Moryson's Itinerary, Being a Survey of the Condition of Europe at the end of the 16th Century*, ed. C. Hughes (1903), 333–4; Corpus Christi College, Oxford, MS 94, fo. 644. I am grateful to Dr Alastair Duke for referring me to *Shakespeare's Europe*, and to Christine Butler, Archivist of Corpus Christi College, for enabling me to read passages in Moryson's MS omitted by Hughes.

or kinsfolk, or by giving them presents that did not match their own estimate of the closeness of their connection with the deceased. In 1718, when Christopher Little of Whitton (Northumberland) buried his young wife, he gave nothing to a neighbour, Mr Hall. The curate urged Little to make good the unintended yet resented slight. Mrs Hall at first 'said her husband should not take any thing if they offered', but her pride was sufficiently gratified by the gift of a scarf and 18d. to buy gloves.[24]

In course of time the convention became established that mourning for kinsfolk, friends, and benefactors was to be donned at one's own expense. Mourning etiquette grew ever more elaborate, but the responsibility for observing social rules and making fine judgements concerning degrees of recognition was largely transferred from the closest kinsfolk or executors of recently deceased persons to the members of their larger circle of friends and relatives. True civility now appeared to lie in making life as easy as possible for the recently bereaved and in offering them support without waiting for an initiative on their part. After the death of Lady Bunbury in 1744, the earl of Bristol assured Sir Thomas Hanmer that he would take the first opportunity of showing the honour that he had in being related to them both as soon as Hanmer let him know when he intended to go into mourning for her. The distribution of memorial rings, the costliest of mourning presents, also lost favour. Horace Walpole sneered at the ill-advised gift of a ring from his nephew Lord Orford after Orford's mother's death in 1781 as 'too vulgar. . . . Mourning rings are as much out of fashion amongst people of rank as plum porridge.'[25]

Funeral feasts were placed by Sir Thomas Browne in that class of civilities that were not 'meere Pagan', in view of their prevalence among the Jews.[26] Richard Hooker saw the chief purpose of these Jewish banquets as 'the comfort of them whose minds are through natural affection pensive', and a good precedent for their modern counterparts.[27] Funeral eating and drinking had, however, also been intended to encourage prayer for the deceased before the Reformation, and a paternoster for the dead often accompanied funeral banquets in Lancashire around 1590.[28] The notion that those who partook of the hospitality of the dead took upon themselves a share of the burden of their sins survived in some parts of England till the late nineteenth century.[29]

[24] *The Diary of the Rev. John Thomlinson*, in *Six North Country Diaries*, ed. J. C. Hodgson (Surtees Society, 118; 1910), 141.

[25] R. Trumbach, *The Rise of the Egalitarian Family: Aristocratic Kinship and Domestic Relations in Eighteenth-Century England* (1978), 34–41; *Letter Books of John Hervey, First Earl of Bristol, with Sir Thomas Hervey's Letters during Courtship and Poems during Widowhood, 1651–1750* (3 vols.; 1894), iii. 298–9; *The Yale Edition of Horace Walpole's Correspondence, 1717–1797*, ed. W. S. Lewis (48 vols.; Oxford, 1937–83), xxv. 124.

[26] Browne, *Hydriotaphia*, 101.   [27] Hooker, *Laws*, ii. 154.

[28] *A Description of the State, Civil and Ecclesiastical, of the County of Lancaster, about the year 1590*, in *Chetham Miscellanies*, v, ed. F. R. Raines (Chetham Society, os 96; 1875), 6.

[29] R. Richardson, *Death, Dissection and the Destitute* (Harmondsworth, 1989), 8–9.

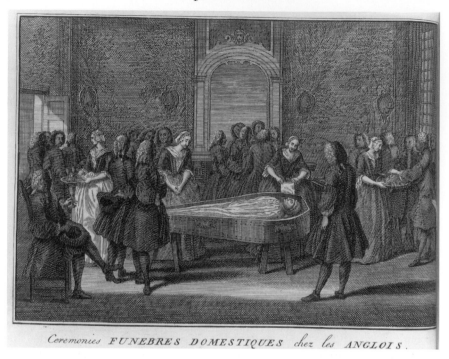

Ceremonies FUNEBRES DOMESTIQUES chez les ANGLOIS.

2. Moderate refreshment, distribution of rosemary, and viewing of the dead, before an English funeral, from Picart, *Cérémonies et coutumes religieuses*

Hospitality was seen by many good Protestants as essential to preserve the reputation of the dead and those who represented them. The most lavish feasts were doubtless staged at the upper end of the social scale, but the meal or 'drinking' (as it was very often described) took a larger proportion of the funeral expenditure of families of middling and small means. To withhold such hospitality was an incivility likely to cause resentment and unfavourable comment. A 'dry' funeral disappointed guests.[30]

Respect for the memory of the dead nevertheless precluded excessive 'mirth in funeral'. Various observers remarked upon the deep incongruity or indecency in this context of merriment or laughter. Here was an area of potentially serious tension between the different functions of the last rite of passage. The widespread practice of dispensing refreshments before as well as after the burial itself sometimes resulted in undue levity during the procession. Moderation, in convivial refreshment as well as in the manifestation of grief, was seen as the ideal way of lessening the tension between the different

[30] *Letters of Chamberlain*, ii. 483.

demands of the funeral occasion. Contemporary descriptions of feasts give the impression that their scale gradually declined in the course of time. The Londoner Henry Machyn often mentioned in the journal that he kept during the middle years of the sixteenth century the great plenty of meat and drink at a funeral.[31] By the eighteenth century, refreshments at genteel funerals in London and much of southern England consisted of wine, often burnt or spiced, together with cakes or biscuits. The names of some of these delicacies, such as macaroons and Naples or Savoy biscuit, betrayed their continental origins. A historian of London social life could assert in 1811 that funeral feasts were by then almost forgotten in the capital. The custom had degenerated, through the intrusion of sensuality where grief and solemnity ought to have presided. 'In the country, it was perfectly excusable to furnish persons who had assembled from a considerable distance with a substantial meal; but the Londoners became sensible in process of time, that indulgence on such occasions was almost impious; hence, cakes and wine now supply the place of the "funeral baked meats".'[32]

One means of maintaining good order at funeral dinners was the segregation of social ranks or groups and sexes. The fare given might also vary according to the status of the recipients. The concern for regulation and control in the interest of decorum appears strongest in some instructions for the conduct of eighteenth-century funerals. When Mrs Anne Phelips of Montacute (Somerset) was buried in 1707, the servants were enjoined to hinder all indecent mirth and noise. Planning his own funeral in 1708, Sir Richard Newdigate envisaged that four parish officers would be on hand to put disorderly people in the stocks.[33]

In the course of his late-sixteenth-century travels, Fynes Moryson noted the absence of funeral banquets in France, Italy, and Poland. In Denmark only friends coming from afar were privately entertained at home.[34] Other travellers reported that immoderate feasting and drinking were common among the American Indians. 'Whether they use any superstition in this custome I know not,' wrote Robert Harcourt in his account of a voyage to Guiana; 'time will reveale, and also reforme it'.[35] The gradually changing character of refreshments at English burials during the early modern period may have been one aspect of a larger process of adoption of standards of civility and decorum already widely accepted in various European countries. The old belief that

---

[31] *The Diary of Henry Machyn, Citizen and Merchant-Taylor of London, from A.D. 1550 to A.D. 1563*, ed. J. G. Nichols (Camden, os 42; 1848), 68, 112, 113, 160, 161, 166, 167, 188, 307.

[32] Quoted in review of J. P. Malcolm, *Anecdotes of the Manners and Customs of London from the Roman Invasion to the Year 1700*, in *Gentleman's Magazine*, 81 (1811), 463.

[33] Somerset RO, Taunton, Phelips MS DD/PH 239; Lady Newdigate-Newdegate (A. E. Newdegate), *Cavalier and Puritan in the Days of the Stuarts* (1902), 355.

[34] Corpus Christi College, Oxford, MS 94, fos. 537, 644; Moryson, *Shakespeare's Europe*, 395, 456–7.

[35] Purchas, *Hakluytus Posthumus*, xvi. 376–7, 429, xviii. 76.

the credit of the dead and their surviving representatives depended upon dispensing generous hospitality nevertheless died out only slowly in remoter parts of the country.

Alms-giving was an important element of many funerals for a long time after the Reformation. Until the seventeenth century, carefully chosen poor people in mourning dress very often occupied a prominent place near the front of genteel funeral processions. Enormous doles had already been major elements of the funerals of the wealthy before the Reformation, but it was only afterwards, in the later sixteenth century, that alms of this type reached the height of their popularity among folk of moderate means.[36] In the course of time, the poor were to be gradually excluded both from a share in funeral conviviality and from their place in funeral processions. Charitable doles were either greatly reduced in scale, discreetly distributed to deserving poor away from the funeral site, or replaced by contributions to the support of the poor of the parish.

There were probably three main reasons for the declining participation of the indigent. First, some Protestants were wary of funeral alms because of their long-standing association with intercessory prayers. It is hardly surprising that the separatist Henry Barrow should have claimed that the poor recipients of gowns and doles were expected to say a paternoster for their benefactors' souls. More unexpected is the open plea of Anthony Anderson, preaching at Robert Keylwey's burial in 1581, that the organizers of the funeral should prevent its being abused by the wicked 'to father their popish prayer for the deade' on charitable devotion to the poor.[37] (He somewhat uncivilly asserted that the majority of his 'huge' audience had come in hope of a dole.) Secondly, the inception and gradual improvement of a national system of poor relief, together with a growing preference for carefully targeted lifetime or testamentary benefactions on the part of the wealthy, made such doles seem wasteful and superfluous. Finally, the confluence of large numbers of poor sometimes created confusion, and even fatal accidents. Such scenes were incompatible with civility and order.[38]

Funeral doles nevertheless died out only very slowly, especially in the north. When Alice Wandesford was buried in 1659, over 1,500 poor had a dole at the door of the house, and others in Catterick church. In 1705 Sir Walter Calverley attended another Yorkshire funeral where over 600 poor people received a dole. They greatly outnumbered the other people who attended the funeral,

[36] I. W. Archer, *The Pursuit of Stability: Social Relations in Elizabethan London* (Cambridge, 1991), 167, 169; D. Levine and K. Wrightson, *The Making of an Industrial Society: Whickham 1560–1765* (Oxford, 1991), 341.

[37] H. Barrow, *A Brief Discoverie of the False Church* (1590), in *The Writings of Henry Barrow 1587–1590*, ed. L. H. Carlson (Elizabethan Nonconformist Texts, 3; 1962), 461–2; Anderson, *Sermon of sure Comfort*, 43–4.

[38] See e.g. *Letters of Chamberlain*, i. 135.

and were so much more numerous than had been expected that the organizers increased the amount set aside for distribution by nearly ten shillings. The conviction that a generous dole helped to maintain the reputation of deceased gentlefolk and their families was by no means dead in the eighteenth century.[39]

The 'civill respects or differences' appropriate to the status of the deceased and sanctioned by the *Directory* of 1645 were most clearly expressed by means of the heraldic funeral. Controlled and developed by the Tudor monarchy through the agency of the heralds, such funerals differentiated each of the upper ranks of society by means of rules concerning such matters as the ensigns and achievements to be borne in procession, the number of supporters and assistants to accompany the chief mourner, and the size and design of the hearse in which the corpse would be placed within the church. The royal coat of arms worn by the heralds who organized such obsequies reinforced the authority requisite for this task. It also made clear to all that the defunct had 'died honourably in the Kings allegeance, without spot of infamie, or other disworship to his Name, Blood, & Family', and served to ratify the public transfer of his achievements of honour to his heir. Proper maintenance of the hierarchy of rank, in which the heralds theoretically played so important a part, was a mark of the truly civil society.[40]

The formalities of heraldic obsequies survived the Reformation with relatively little adaptation because they were for the most part civil as opposed to religious ceremonies.[41] The intrusive way in which heraldic rituals brought the elaborate pomp and brilliant colour of secular ceremonial into the very heart of places of worship nevertheless caused some unease among Protestants. The religious radical Henry Barrow was exceptional in his outright mockery of the inappropriateness of militaristic rites redolent of the obsequies of mythical heroes to the funerals of men who were 'but stept into the gentrie'.[42] James Pilkington, bishop of Durham, dared not utterly condemn this solemnity added by 'civil policy', yet wished it 'more moderately used' than it often was.[43] Lord Burghley claimed in 1589, not entirely convincingly, that the display of the arms of his wife's noble relatives on her hearse, which showed God's favour towards her stock, was not inspired by 'any vain pomp of the world, but for civil duty towards her body; that is to

---

[39] *The Autobiography of Mrs Alice Thornton of East Newton, Co. York*, ed. C. Jackson (Surtees Society, 62; 1875), 117; *Memorandum Book of Sir Walter Calverley, Bart.*, ed. S. Margerison, in *Yorkshire Diaries and Autobiographies in the Seventeenth and Eighteenth Centuries*, ii (Surtees Society, 77; 1886), 105.

[40] C. Gittings, *Death, Burial and the Individual in Early Modern England* (1984), 166–87; Segar, *Honor*, 238 (*recte* 254).

[41] J. Woodward, *The Theatre of Death: The Ritual Management of Royal Funerals in Renaissance England, 1570–1625* (Woodbridge, 1997), 37–60, 204.

[42] Barrow, *Brief Discoverie*, 459.

[43] J. Pilkington, *A Godlie Exposition vpon Certeine Chapters of Nehemiah* (1585), in Pilkington, *Works*, ed. J. Scholefield (Parker Society; 1842), 317.

be with honour regarded, for the assured hope of the resurrection thereof at the last day'.[44]

The demand for heraldic funerals may have been most widespread during Elizabeth's reign, which witnessed a remarkable increase in the number of claims to bear arms conceded by heralds in their county visitations. At the same time, however, the supply of honours bestowed more directly by the Crown, knighthoods and peerages, was tightly controlled. John Vernon of Sudbury (Derbyshire), grandson and son-in-law of knights, but only an esquire himself, was perhaps just the sort of man whose family most prized the distinction of a heraldic funeral. The rhyming chronicle of Vernon's life tells how, after his death in 1600, his widow's 'cheefest care of all / Was to provyde a comlie Funerall', which was worthily performed by the heralds.[45]

To fail to give a man the honourable funeral due to his rank was a gross incivility. In *Hamlet*, Shakespeare has Laertes claim that the 'obscure burial' of his father Polonius—

> No trophy, sword nor hatchment o'er his bones,
> No noble rite nor formal ostentation—

cried to be heard 'as 'twere from heaven to earth'.[46] It is none the less clear that many members of the nobility and gentry were choosing to dispense with the full formalities of the heraldic funeral from the later years of Elizabeth's reign onwards. This was largely due to the cost of blacks. But, in addition, the heralds' own charges and perquisites, their quarrels over the sharing of profits, and their appointment of ill-supervised deputies of comparatively humble birth were all resented.[47] During the 1620s it proved increasingly difficult to levy funeral fees from the Lancashire gentry, many of whom preferred to display escutcheons and hatchments produced cheaply by unlicensed 'hedge paynters' rather than pay the full costs of heraldic obsequies. Such people resented what they saw as the uncivil importunities of the deputy heralds.[48] In the 1590s Fynes Moryson had noticed that in the United Provinces, where funerals were usually conducted with little or no pomp, the arms of some 'gentlemen and others of the best sorte' were set up on their doors for a year following the burial. Later, as many paintings of Dutch church

[44] J. Strype, *Annals of the Reformation and Establishment of Religion . . . during Queen Elizabeth's Happy Reign* (4 vols.; Oxford, 1824), iii (2). 129.

[45] Stone, *Crisis*, 67, 72, 98; J. C. Cox, 'The Rhymed Chronicle of John Harestaffe. Sudbury and the Vernons', *Journal of the Derbyshire Archaeological and Natural History Society*, 10 (1888), 107.

[46] *Hamlet*, IV. v. 212–14.

[47] Sir A. Wagner, *Heralds of England: A History of the Office and College of Arms* (1967), 200–5, 209, 215, 235–6, 237–8, 240.

[48] *Letters on the Claims of the College of Arms in Lancashire, in the time of James the First: by Leonard Smethley and Randle Holme, Deputy Heralds*, in *Chetham Miscellanies*, v, pp. vi–viii, xi–xii, xviii–xix, 1–10, 19–21, 28–31, 34–7.

interiors show, they were hung up in the church.[49] In England, hatchments came to be widely used by armigerous families in a similar fashion.

Heralds would long be seen, however, as indispensable participants in the obsequies of men who had performed exceptional public service. Philip Sidney was an outstanding early example of a national war hero who received an especially lavish funeral. It was, however, very largely paid for, not by the Crown, but by Sidney's father-in-law Francis Walsingham, whose debts led him to stipulate a simple funeral for himself.[50] The costs of a number of later funerals, including those of the earl of Essex (1646), the duke of Albemarle (1670), and the earl of Sandwich (1672), were mainly met by the state.

Those who arranged funerals that manifested pretensions beyond their proper station were always vulnerable to ridicule or contempt. In the later seventeenth and eighteenth centuries, the 'middling sort of people' adopted many of the trappings of the genteel funeral. Undertakers enabled them to ape their betters more cheaply than would otherwise have been possible, while also encouraging them to spend more than was desirable or necessary. It is difficult to say whether civility to the dead or self-aggrandisement was the more important motive. 'This absurd notion of being *handsomely buried* has given rise to the most contradictory customs, that could possibly be contrived for the advantage of death-hunters,' observed 'The Connoisseur' in 1754. It was particularly ridiculous, he thought, that an urban tradesman should be carried scarcely a hundred yards from his own house 'with the equipage and retinue of a lord', or have an achievement fixed over his door. An increasing proportion of the funeral disbursements of the urban 'middling sort' went to the undertaker for such things as coaches, the coffin, mutes, pages, and coach-men, and mourning either hired or bought for servants, family members, and attendants.[51]

The procession to the church was the most public part of the funeral spec-tacle. A heraldic procession demonstrated particularly effectively the ability or willingness of the head of a family to do his predecessor or relative due honour, and his success in attracting support. The majority of the participants were in some sense his dependants: his immediate relatives, household and estate officers, and tenants. Poor bedesfolk came near the head of the proces-sion. Paid professionals included the officers of arms and, before the Refor-mation, several clergy. But the most sensitive indicator of the success of the occasion for an experienced observer would have been the presence of persons

---

[49] Moryson, *Shakespeare's Europe*, 380; J. Farrington, *An Account of a Journey through Holland, Frizeland, etc. in severall Letters to a Friend* (Leiden, 1994), 56.

[50] J. F. R. Day, 'Death Be Very Proud: Sidney, Subversion, and Elizabethan Heraldic Funerals', in D. Hoak (ed.), *Tudor Political Culture* (Cambridge, 1995), 179–203; *Wills from Doctors' Commons. A Selection from the Wills of Eminent Persons proved in the Prerogative Court of Canterbury, 1495–1695*, ed. J. G. Nichols and J. Bruce (Camden, os 83; 1863), 69.

[51] *Gentleman's Magazine*, 24 (1754), 466–9; Richardson, *Death, Dissection and the Destitute*, 272–3; P. Jalland, *Death in the Victorian Family* (Oxford, 1996), 195–6.

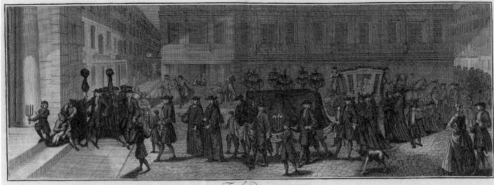

CONVOI Funebre des ANGLOIS.

3. A decorous and fashionable English funeral procession approaches the church at dusk, from Picart, *Cérémonies et coutumes religieuses*

whose incentive to attend was less directly material in character: kinship, friendship, or neighbourly courtesy. Some of these individuals played a crucial role at the heart of the procession as pall-bearers and supporters or assistants of the chief mourner. The number of gentlefolk was an indicator of the regard in which the deceased and his or her family were held. Marshalling a procession called for tact and judgement. Failure to give participants the places that they considered appropriate could cause great resentment.[52]

Attendance at the funerals of middle-ranking folk was an important obligation of fellow members of their craft guilds or religious confraternities. Members of corporations could expect to be followed to the grave by their colleagues in office. Such attendance was not only a matter of personal regard or courtesy, but also an important means of displaying fraternal or institutional solidarity. Invitations or instructions had to be sent by letter or word of mouth to all those who were to play a leading part in the procession. Within the immediate neighbourhood, a death would already have been signalled by the passing bell and the knell that followed the departure of the soul. A bell might toll for an hour or forty-five minutes immediately before the burial itself. In towns, funeral arrangements were often announced beforehand by a bellman or town crier. As late as 1855 it was allegedly still quite common around Carlisle to send out messengers to invite all and sundry. In the seventeenth century, the more discreet method of invitation by tickets (often elaborately decorated) was adopted by Londoners with aspirations to gentility.[53]

Various developments tended to reduce attendance at funerals between the

---

[52] Segar, *Honor*, 253; R. C[roshawe], *Visions, or Hels Kingdome, and the Worlds Follies and Abuses, strangely displaied* (1640), 135.

[53] Machyn, *Diary*, 68, 71, 106, 112, 166; *The Diary of Samuel Newton, Alderman of Cambridge*

Reformation and the Industrial Revolution. Religious confraternities were dissolved in 1547–8, the numbers of priests participating fell sharply after the Reformation, full-blown heraldic funerals rapidly lost their popularity after the later years of Elizabeth's reign, guilds became weaker, and the poor were very gradually excluded from both processions and refreshments. The upper classes increasingly preferred 'private' funerals. The growth of privacy in the celebration of English rites of passage, emphasized by their most recent historian, served many different purposes. In funerals, however, decorum was the overriding concern.[54]

The survival throughout this period of the custom of asking friends or kinsfolk to bear the pall or coffin nevertheless ensured that most funerals included a solid core of participants from outside the immediate family. Funerals often drew many more people than had been invited. There were several instances during the seventeenth and eighteenth centuries of seemingly spontaneous gatherings of large numbers of gentlemen to give a civil farewell to valued members of a county community. The funeral of the eminent London Huguenot merchant and 'country' politician Thomas Papillon in 1702 was designed to be a 'private' occasion, but the last journey from London to his burial at Acrise in Kent developed into a public demonstration of respect by men of the county on horseback and in their coaches. Welcome though such a friendly manifestation might otherwise have been, the unavoidable confusion that ensued made Papillon's son order in his own will that he should be buried 'in the *most* private manner'.[55]

Interest in a funeral was not always so benign. It was allegedly the risk of a popular tumult that persuaded Charles I's government to have the duke of Buckingham buried privately at night. The funeral cavalcade of Gilbert Burnet, the celebrated Whig bishop, was subjected to the outrageous incivility of stoning by a Tory–Jacobite mob in 1715. Even worse was the interruption of the funeral of a London undertaker and pawnbroker in October 1758. During the funeral a mob gathered 'and committed such enormous outrages out of resentment to the deceased, that the clergyman who officiated had great difficulty to perform his office'.[56]

One form of tribute to the newly dead enjoyed its greatest popularity

---

(1662–1717), ed. J. E. Foster (Cambridge Antiquarian Society, 23; 1890), 24–6; *Notes and Queries*, 1st ser., 11 (1855), 414, 455; J. Litten, *The English Way of Death: The Common Funeral since 1450* (1991), 21, 77, 131, 162, 164. Invitation to funerals by means of 'billetts' was already widespread in France before 1600: see Corpus Christi College, Oxford, MS 94, fo. 644.

[54] D. Cressy, *Birth, Marriage and Death: Ritual, Religion, and the Life-Cycle in Tudor and Stuart England* (Oxford, 1997), esp. 446–9.

[55] A. F. W. Papillon, *Memoirs of Thomas Papillon, of London, Merchant (1623–1702)* (Reading, 1887), 381–2 (emphasis added).

[56] *Calendar of State Papers, Venetian*, xxi. 1628–9, ed. A. B. Hinds (1916), 337; T. E. S. Clarke and H. C. Foxcroft, *A Life of Gilbert Burnet, Bishop of Salisbury* (Cambridge, 1907), 474; *Gentleman's Magazine*, 28 (1758), 500.

during this period: the biographical account included in the funeral sermon. In the Reformed churches there was a widespread suspicion of such sermons. In Scotland, the Book of Discipline of 1560 explicitly forbade them. In debate with John Whitgift, Thomas Cartwright, the leading Elizabethan Presbyterian, argued that they nourished an opinion that the dead were the better for them, and introduced into the church an invidious distinction between the rich and the poor. In ancient times funeral orations had been better used at Athens than among the Christians. 'For there it was merely civil, and the oration at the death of some notable personage made not by a minister, but by an orator appointed therefore; which I think may well be done.'[57] This was the heart of the matter: only by keeping praise for the dead firmly within the civil sphere could such rhetorical civility be prevented from adulterating the preaching of the Word with false comforts begotten of mercenary incentives. English clergy of all shades of churchmanship had nevertheless become so firmly attached to the funeral sermon by the 1640s that the issue proved an irreconcilable difference between Scots and English representatives at the Westminster Assembly. The *Directory* of 1645 accorded such sermons only a rather oblique approval when it permitted the minister to remind the Christian friends of the deceased of their duty at a burial. But this passage was soon cited as sufficient authorization.[58]

Although funeral sermons were largely devoted to the exposition of a scriptural text, it was the testimony concerning the character of the deceased that most interested the audience. Many preachers declared their determination not to flatter, yet these discourses were not without their own special civilities. The faults of the departed were usually mentioned in the vaguest terms, or quietly concealed, while distinguished ancestry and public achievements were often described at some length. It was notoriously difficult to achieve the right balance, and to avoid either giving offence or causing derision by saying too little or too much. In the eighteenth century, funeral sermons lost much of their acceptance among the genteel. Yet during the period of their greatest popularity, between *c*.1610 and *c*.1720, no other comparable medium came anywhere near achieving their success. Funeral orations were delivered in some milieux, especially the universities. Verses were pinned to the coffins of celebrated individuals, and broadside elegies on public heroes were distributed through the streets. But no form of secular memorial speech appears to have become established as one of the normal civilities at funerals of the gentry and the middling sort. In England words spoken in tribute to the dead have never entirely freed

[57] F. B. Tromly, '"According to Sounde Religion": The Elizabethan Controversy over the Funeral Sermon', *Journal of Medieval and Renaissance Studies*, 13 (1982), 293–312; *Defence of the Answer*, 375.

[58] Robert Baillie to William Spong, 6 Dec. 1644, in *The Letters and Journals of Robert Baillie A. M. Principal of the University of Glasgow* (3 vols.; Edinburgh, 1841–2), ii. 245; *Directory*, 74; B. Spencer, Ἀφωνόλογος, *A Dumb Speech: or, A Sermon made, but no Sermon preached, at the Funerall of the Right Vertuous, Mrs Mary Overman* (1646), sig. A4ᵛ.

themselves from a religious context. Even today they are more often delivered at funerals or memorial services than in any other setting.[59]

III

'The presumed superior wisdom of most modern nations', a contributor to the *Gentleman's Magazine* remarked in 1795, 'has induced them to omit much of the pomp and ceremony which formerly attended funerals. Interest being the prevailing object of the present day, it is thought in general absurd to expend in decorating the dead what might be applied to the advantage of the living.'[60] This writer's reference to the 'decoration' of the dead is somewhat misleading, if only because the previous century had probably seen a considerable increase in the amount spent on coffins and grave clothes by the middling sort of people.[61] Yet the scale and cost of the most expensive funerals had diminished. 'Obsequium' or dutiful service, root of the word 'obsequies', was a major purpose of the magnate funerals of the later Middle Ages. The recently departed stood in greatest need of the prayers of the living. Magnificent largesse nurtured their reputations and encouraged recipients to pray for them. The Protestant repudiation of intercessory prayer opened the way to a gradual reappraisal of funeral expenditure. The distinction between 'civil' and 'religious' funeral observances was drawn as a result of a continuing desire on the part of many Protestants to purge burial rites of everything that savoured of superstition. But the distinction could never be watertight.

The advance of 'civility' in various related senses is evident in the development of the English funeral between the Reformation and the Industrial Revolution. The simplification or abandonment of ritual, ceremony, and mourning apparel enhanced the importance of individual comportment and self-control. Changes in the scale and nature of hospitality gradually closed an important social and psychological safety valve and helped to enforce a greater uniformity and sobriety of demeanour. The end of alms-giving removed the sight, sound, and smell of poverty, making decorum easier to maintain. As tangible incentives to attend became less important, participation came to depend increasingly on respect for the dead and desire to comfort the bereaved, and on civility in the sense of a flexible code of good manners designed to cope with every social situation.[62]

[59] R. A. Houlbrooke, *Death, Religion, and the Family in England, 1480–1750* (Oxford, 1998), 295–330.

[60] *Gentleman's Magazine*, 65 (1795), 389.

[61] Litten, *English Way of Death*, 76–81, 99–109.

[62] The formulation of this conclusion was assisted by A. Bryson, *From Courtesy to Civility: Changing Codes of Conduct in Early Modern England* (Oxford, 1998), esp. 281–2. The meanings of 'civil' and 'civility' explored in this essay overlap, but do not correspond exactly, with those emphasized by Dr Bryson.

5

Sexual Manners: The Other Face of Civility in Early Modern England

MARTIN INGRAM

Sex is a slippery subject for the historian; but then so is civility. That the two themes have not been much explored in tandem, at least in an English context,[1] is none the less surprising. Since the 1960s there has been an explosion of research into sexuality in early modern society. On the other side, Norbert Elias's *Civilizing Process*, which has been so important in setting the agenda for studies of civility, included changing attitudes to sex within its compass of cultural change: he envisaged in this sphere, as in so many other areas of social life, a rising threshold of shame and embarrassment.[2] It is true that issues of 'sex' in the sense of 'gender' are of recognized importance for anyone who approaches the theme of civility via the most obvious route—that of contemporary courtesy literature.[3] But even this avenue has been only partially explored, and until very recently studies focusing primarily on gender and the role of women in the early modern period have engaged surprisingly little with concepts of civility.[4] There are thus large gaps; and, while this essay goes some way towards filling them, its limits should be recognized.[5] It cannot address directly the sexual component of Elias's grand theory, which, though only a segment of the larger whole, itself poses so many large questions that he himself baulked at

---

[1] Cf. R. Muchembled, *Popular Culture and Elite Culture in France, 1400–1750*, trans. L. Cochrane (Baton Rouge, La., 1985), 74–5, 100, 189–96.

[2] Norbert Elias, *The Civilizing Process: The History of Manners and State Formation and Civilization*, trans. E. Jephcott (Oxford, 1994), 148.

[3] F. A. Childs, 'Prescriptions for Manners in English Courtesy Literature, 1690–1760, and their Social Implications', D.Phil. thesis (Oxford, 1984), ch. 5; J. Bremmer and H. Roodenburg (eds.), *A Cultural History of Gesture: From Antiquity to the Present Day* (Cambridge, 1991), 8 and *passim*; A. Bryson, *From Courtesy to Civility: Changing Codes of Conduct in Early Modern England* (Oxford, 1998), 38–9, 127–8, 161–2, and chs. 6–7 *passim*.

[4] But see G. J. Barker-Benfield, *The Culture of Sensibility: Sex and Society in Eighteenth-Century Britain* (Chicago, 1992), *passim*; A. Vickery, *The Gentleman's Daughter: Women's Lives in Georgian England* (New Haven, 1998), ch. 6.

[5] A much fuller discussion of some aspects is provided by D. M. Turner, 'Representations of Adultery, c.1660–c.1740: A Study of Changing Perceptions of Marital Infidelity from Conduct Literature, Drama, Trial Publications and Records of the Court of Arches', D.Phil. thesis (Oxford, 1998).

treating them.[6] Its more modest aims relate to what has been the main focus of my research since I began it under the supervision of Keith Thomas: to explore how notions of civility and incivility impinged on the public regulation of sexuality in early modern England, investigating how contemporaries 'on the ground' rather than writers of conduct books thought of and used these ideas. The survey reveals that, far from civility's being an exclusively élite commodity concerned with polite behaviour, versions of the concept had resonance much further down the social scale and had a hard moral edge.

The context was very different from modern Western society. Nowadays we assume that religion and personal morality are, within limits, essentially matters for the private conscience. In the early modern period the morals of everyone were very much a public concern and subject to official censure. Adultery and fornication were not only sins but also crimes, and Tudor England had inherited from the Middle Ages an elaborate set of institutions, procedures, and laws designed to curb the passions. At least into the sixteenth century, some sexual misdemeanours were dealt with by manorial courts. Moreover, London, Westminster, and many provincial cities and towns claimed jurisdiction over sexual offenders by special custom; while the principal target was prostitution, individual fornicators and adulterers were not immune from prosecution. Around 1500 the royal courts not only exercised jurisdiction over rape and brothel-keeping, but also claimed the right for constables and other local officers to invade suspect houses and take sexual offenders before a justice to be bound over to the good behaviour. Later, secular jurisdiction was to be extended to buggery and to the discretionary punishment of the parents of bastard children; and for ten years after 1650 adultery was made subject to the death penalty, while fornication became punishable by imprisonment.[7] However, the main agent of moral regulation was the Church and its elaborate, omnipresent system of courts, where suspects were reported by means of 'presentments' made by the churchwardens, sidesmen, and other representatives of parishes in town or country. Operating at a high level of activity in the late sixteenth and early seventeenth centuries, the courts were swept away amid the collapse of Charles I's personal rule and the subsequent civil wars and Interregnum. But they were restored with the monarchy after 1660, and the eventual decay of their jurisdiction over religion and

---

[6] Cf. Elias, *Civilizing Process*, 494 n.

[7] K. Thomas, 'The Puritans and Adultery: The Act of 1650 Reconsidered', in D. Pennington and K. Thomas (eds.), *Puritans and Revolutionaries: Essays in Seventeenth-Century History Presented to Christopher Hill* (Oxford, 1978), 257–82; R. M. Karras, *Common Women: Prostitution and Sexuality in Medieval England* (New York, 1996); M. Ingram, 'Reformation of Manners in Early Modern England', in P. Griffiths, S. Hindle, and A. Fox (eds.), *The Experience of Authority in Early Modern England* (1996), 47–88; M. K. McIntosh, *Controlling Misbehavior in England, 1370–1600* (Cambridge, 1998).

morals, though accelerated by the Toleration Act of 1689, was a protracted and patchy process.[8]

The view of human nature in general, and sexuality in particular, that underlay and justified secular and more particularly ecclesiastical jurisdiction over sin was a commonplace of contemporary Christian thinking, deriving from an amalgam of Judaeo-Christian elements and Stoic and other late classical ideas with a strong ascetic component. Fallen man was corrupt, his higher faculties or reason constantly under threat from the lusts of the flesh. Those who allowed themselves to be swept away easily on these torrents of passion were guilty of 'luxury' or 'intemperance', and by definition far gone in sin; those who were betrayed by mere frailty, yet remained aware of the need for restraint and of the sinfulness of their actions, were said to have incurred the somewhat more pardonable sin of 'incontinence'.[9] These ideas lent themselves to metaphors deriving from the handling of horses or other beasts: to guard against sin by maintaining a balance between reason and 'affection' required the application of spurs to goodness and bridles to curb lust. Humoral theory provided further levels of explanation—for example, accounting for the proclivities of particular individuals towards certain sins, and postulating broader differences between the sexes. Until the seventeenth century, women, in whose constitution cold and moist humours were supposed to predominate, were conventionally regarded as more lustful than men.[10]

Some of these ideas are implicit in the language of the period, such as the use of the word 'folly' by churchmen, moralists, and the people to mean sexual immorality.[11] Fuller expressions of the underlying philosophy by ordinary layfolk are only rarely found, and it is, of course, doubtful how far the more restrictive aspects of this system of thought ever recommended themselves to the majority.[12] But, with variations, such ideas were the common coin of contemporary moral, political, and theological writings. 'The most part of men follow vice', lamented Thomas Starkey around 1530, 'and in their hearts do as it were conspire against the dignity of virtue and nature of man, they consider

[8] R. Houlbrooke, *Church Courts and the People during the English Reformation, 1520–1570* (Oxford, 1979); M. Ingram, *Church Courts, Sex and Marriage in England, 1570–1640* (Cambridge, 1987); R. A. Marchant, *The Church under the Law: Justice, Administration and Discipline in the Diocese of York, 1560–1640* (Cambridge, 1969).

[9] J. A. Brundage, *Law, Sex and Christian Society in Medieval Europe* (Chicago, 1987), 420–30. For a contemporary account, see William Vaughan, *The golden-grove, moralized in three bookes* (2nd edn., 1608), sigs. H5–H6ᵛ.

[10] I. Maclean, *The Renaissance Notion of Woman: A Study in the Fortunes of Scholasticism and Medical Science in European Intellectual Life* (Cambridge, 1980), ch. 3; A. Fletcher, *Gender, Sex and Subordination in England, 1500–1800* (New Haven, 1995), 74.

[11] e.g. Matthew Griffith, *Bethel: or, a forme for families* (1633), 301; Thomas Tuke, *A treatise against painting and tincturing of men and women* (1616), 38; Wilts. RO, D1/39/2/8, fo. 106ʳ.

[12] For an example—a drunkard's account of his own nature—see Wilts. RO, D5/19/33, fo. 134ᵛ; cf. McIntosh, *Controlling Misbehavior*, 204–5.

not the frailty of man, which seeing the best followeth the worst, overcome by sensual pleasure'. 'How then', demanded John Turner in 1698, 'shall we vindicate the dignity of our diviner nature, but by keeping up the dominion and superiority of our reason over the vile affections and inclinations of the body? Or in what can we more dishonour or debase ourselves, than in subjecting the noble faculties of the soul, to the tyrannic, usurped power of our depraved appetites and lusts?'[13]

I

Control of the body and of the passions is the connection between sex and civility, but, of course, the overlap is only partial, as a semantic survey will show. 'Courtesy', down to the seventeenth century a more common term to describe polite behaviour than 'civility', had little to do with sex or even with gender. 'Politeness', current by the eighteenth century, had in itself even less of a sexual resonance; but 'rudeness', with which it was often contrasted, did have a place in sexual discourse, and at least as a nursery word does so to the present day. 'Decency' is another important term. Nowadays its usage is perhaps narrowing towards the exclusively sexual, as is certainly the case for 'indecent' and 'indecency'. In the sixteenth and seventeenth centuries these words were of broader significance; yet, unlike such bland modern near-synonyms as 'acceptable' or 'appropriate', they did have a moral edge and could certainly carry a strong sexual meaning. 'Manners' as a term was deeply ambiguous. It often meant the rules of polite behaviour, a usage dating from the fourteenth century at least. But well into the eighteenth century, and in certain contexts beyond, it was frequently used in a sense much closer to our notion of 'morals', albeit with the emphasis on the externals of behaviour and relations with other people. Historians have long been familiar with the term in the phrase 'reformation of manners', which they have tended to associate exclusively with the anti-vice campaigns of the Societies for Reformation of Manners in the 1690s and 1700s, and with the so-called puritan attempts at moral reform in the century after 1560. However, these were merely variants on a persistent theme of 'reformation of manners' that long pre-dated the Reformation. Sexual offences were always prominent among the 'ill manners' that were targeted. The association with moral activism must always have coloured usages of the term 'manners', even when the forms of polite behaviour were meant.[14]

---

[13] Thomas Starkey, *A Dialogue between Pole and Lupset*, ed. T. F. Mayer (Camden Society, 4th ser., 37; 1989), 13 (spelling modernized); John Turner, *A discourse on fornication: shewing the greatness of that sin* (1698), 42.

[14] Ingram, 'Reformation of Manners', *passim*.

What of 'civility', together with the adjective 'civil' and the inverse forms 'uncivil' and 'incivility'? This terminology, which provides the focus for much of what follows, was burgeoning rapidly in the late sixteenth century: the dialogue *Of cyvile and uncyvile life* (1579) is a showcase of usages. References to 'civil wars', 'civil dissension', 'martial and civil', and 'laws civil and common' remind us that concepts of civility originated in ideas about political and legal relations. More interesting is the antithesis between 'the savage nations' and 'a most civil country' such as England. This association of 'civil' with what would later be termed 'civilized' was a keynote of the propaganda associated with the Elizabethan conquest of Ireland; it could also be used of remote areas of England, such as Durham; and it was to be increasingly in demand in the seventeenth century as authors engaged with the experiences of transoceanic trade and colonization.[15] On a different scale of social interaction, the author of *Cyvile and uncyvile life* also equated civility with the 'ceremonies' of visiting, dining, and so forth; yet there is a conceptual link with the broader notion, since the absence of such civilities is seen as 'barbarous'. At the heart of this tract is a vision that associates towns and cities with a more ordered, sophisticated, and refined mode of behaviour. Characterized as 'civil' and 'civility', it is contrasted with 'country conditions', 'bluntness and rusticity', and 'manners' that are 'rude', 'clownish', 'uncomely'.

This author had a particular purpose in insisting so firmly on the linkage between cities and civility, concerned as he was to argue that an educated, urban-based gentry was advantageous to the commonwealth.[16] In contrast, Stefano Guazzo's *The civile conversation* (1574; English translation, 1581–6), a central text in the tradition of courtesy literature, played down the connection. 'Conversation', in this context, denoted not just verbal utterance but conduct of all kinds; and hence Guazzo argued that 'we would have understood, that to live civilly, is not said in respect of the city, but of the qualities of the mind: so I understand civil conversation, not having relation to the city, but consideration to the manners and conditions which make it civil . . . [and] so I will that civil conversation appertain . . . to all sorts of persons of

---

[15] *Of cyvile and uncyvile life. The English courtier, and the cu[n]trey-gentleman* (1586 edn.), repr. in *Inedited Tracts: Illustrating the Manners, Opinions, and Occupations of Englishmen during the Sixteenth and Seventeenth Centuries*, ed. W. C. Hazlitt (Roxburghe Library, n.p., 1868), 1–93, here p. [5]; cf. Edmund Spenser, *A View of the Present State of Ireland*, ed. W. L. Renwick (1934), p. [3] and *passim*; C. Maxwell, *Irish History from Contemporary Sources (1509–1610)* (1923), 105–6, 107, 112–13, 117, 164, 173, 174, 181; D. Marcombe, 'A Rude and Heady People: The Local Community and the Rebellion of the Northern Earls', in Marcombe (ed.), *The Last Principality: Politics, Religion and Society in the Bishopric of Durham, 1494–1660* (Nottingham, 1987), 121; K. O. Kupperman, *Settling with the Indians: The Meeting of English and Indian Cultures in America, 1580–1640* (1980), 46–54, 58–63, 81–2, 105–6, 186–7; K. O. Kupperman (ed.), *America in European Consciousness, 1493–1750* (Chapel Hill, NC, 1995), 8–10.

[16] For a similar view with a different political purpose, see Spenser, *View of the Present State of Ireland*, ed. Renwick, 213.

what place or of what calling so ever they are'.[17] In English usage, the idea of
'civility' gradually sloughed off its specific association with civic society and
government, while retaining the more general connotations of urbanity and
without, therefore, the contrasts with 'ignorance' and 'rusticity' ever losing
any of their force. None the less the idea of people living in close proximity
and having to get along—neighbours or fellow citizens—remained with the
idea of civility and informed the usages that will be explored in the later parts
of this essay.

    The relationship with sexual regulation is complicated by the fact that 'civil-
ity' was a multi-stranded phenomenon of which certain elements were much
more closely related to Christian morality than others—an issue of no small
relevance to the much-debated question of the social circles in which notions
of 'civility' were generated.[18] Most obviously congruent with the prescriptions
of Christian sexual morality are texts that dealt with the basics of the subject,
tellingly directed at *children*. Pre-eminent among these was Erasmus's *De civilitate morum puerilium* (1530; English translation, 1532). Though some of its
theme and content had been anticipated in earlier works, the eminence of its
author, the elegance and pedagogic utility of its language (Renaissance Latin
adapted to the level of a well-schooled boy of 10), and its systematic treatment and firm basis in Ciceronian and other classical ideas ensured that the
work had immense influence not only of itself but also as the model for many
later texts. Dealing with many matters of polite behaviour that were outside
the sphere of morality ordinarily defined, Erasmus was at pains to emphasize
that 'these things be not here spoken for that intent, as though no man may
be honest without them'. But a very close link with Christian morality was
everywhere apparent. In view of the intended readership, there was naturally
no explicit reference to the adult sins of fornication and adultery. But apparel
that failed to cover the privy members while stooping was declared 'ever
dishonesty'; while

to disclose or show the members that nature hath given to be covered, without necessity, ought to be utterly avoided from gentle nature. Also when need compelleth to
do it, yet it must be done with convenient honesty, yea though no person be present,
for angels be ever present, to whom in children bashfulness is a tutor and follower of
chastity. The sight of the which to withdraw from the eyes of men is honest. Much
more we ought not suffer other to touch them.

---

    [17] Stefano Guazzo, *The civile conversation*, trans. George Pettie and Bartholomew Young (1586),
fo. 22.
    [18] C. S. Jaeger, *The Origins of Courtliness: Civilizing Trends and the Formation of Courtly Ideals,
939–1210* (Philadelphia, 1985); J. W. Nicholls, *The Matter of Courtesy: Medieval Courtesy Books and
the Gawain-Poet* (Woodbridge, Suffolk, 1985), ch. 2; D. Knox, 'Erasmus' *De Civilitate* and the Religious Origins of Civility in Protestant Europe', *Archiv für Reformationsgeschichte*, 86 (1995), 7–55;
D. Knox, '*Disciplina*: The Monastic and Clerical Origins of European Civility', in J. Monfasani
and R. G. Musto (eds.), *Renaissance Society and Culture: Essays in Honor of Eugene F. Rice Jr.* (New
York, 1991), 107–35.

Underlying these prescriptions was the conviction, well established in Christian thought long before Erasmus wrote, that the body was the outward reflection of the soul; though 'grace of honest behaviour' might be nurtured by education, fundamentally 'this outward honesty of the body cometh of the soul well composed and ordered'.[19] This core element of civility—aptly conveyed in the phrase 'decency in conversation'[20]—was obviously not the preserve of the Court (though Erasmus ostensibly wrote for a prince), nor of aristocratic society more generally, nor of the city. Indeed, it is in some ways more plausible, as Dilwyn Knox has argued, to identify the main impetus towards self-restraint with monastic and clerical *disciplina*—and hence, one may add, with the church courts' work of moralizing lay society.[21]

De civilitate and other basic works stand in contrast to many of the more sophisticated treatments of civility and related issues, which were directed at adults or, at least, those on the threshold of adult life. The key texts of the sixteenth century, mostly penned in Italy, generally originated in courtly circles, as did the French treatises of Antoine de Courtin and others that superseded them in the seventeenth. Imbued as they were with aristocratic ideals of honour, they inevitably had a more ambiguous relationship to Christian morality. It is true that the *Galateo* of Giovanni Della Casa, archbishop of Benevento (1556; English translation, 1576), deliberately veered towards a universal morality, asserting that the matter in discussion was 'either a virtue, or the thing that comes very near to virtue', and offering a set of prescriptions that were not the monopoly of courtiers but 'very necessary and profitable for all gentlemen, or other'; the text even embodies, like a plum in a pudding, a miniature diatribe against sexual sin and other 'foul and filthy' vices.[22] More generally, it may be said that all these adult texts at least paid lip service to the ideal of Christian chastity—especially with regard to women, for whom the ideals of civility and sexual modesty were virtually conflated. But Baldesar Castiglione's *Book of the Courtier* (1528; English translation, 1561), breathing the refined air of Renaissance Urbino, depended in part on an elusive ideal of *sprezzatura*—inadequately translated as 'recklessness' or 'nonchalance'—that had precious little to do with the Ten Commandments or the Epistles of St Paul.[23]

More generally, the ideal of 'civility' as it had developed by the seventeenth century embodied the powerful notion of accommodating oneself to others. In the words of Della Casa refracted through his Elizabethan translator, 'every act that offendeth any the common senses, or overthwarteth a man's will and

[19] Desiderius Erasmus, *De civilitate morum puerilium: a lytell boke of good maners for children*, trans. Robert Whytyngton (1540), sigs. A2ᵛ, B1ʳ, B3ʳ, D3ʳ.

[20] Cf. the English subtitle of a later work on civility designed for children: *Youths behaviour, or decencie in conversation amongst men*, trans. Francis Hawkins([c.1640]; 7th edn., 1661).

[21] Knox, 'Erasmus' *De Civilitate*'; Knox, '*Disciplina*'.

[22] *Galateo of Maister Iohn Della Casa*, trans. Robert Peterson (1576), title page, 2, 106–7.

[23] *The courtyer of Count Baldessar Castilio*, trans. Thomas Hoby (1561).

desire, or else presenteth to the imagination and conceit, matters unpleasant, and that likewise, which the mind doth abhor, such things, I say, be naught, and must not be used'. This duty of complaisance was likely, in the long run, to blunt the edge of moral condemnation, and indeed might create an alternative morality that radically parted company with traditional Christian teaching. One indication of unease emerged in the use of language. Della Casa prescribed the use of euphemisms to avoid direct mention of unsavoury or scandalous subjects: for example, 'it better becomes a man's and woman's mouth to call harlots, women of the world'. His purpose was moral, deriving from the biblical precept that 'evil communications corrupt good manners'.[24] But it was a commonplace of moralist criticism that 'every vice hath a cloak of virtue to cover it: as, for example . . . they that violate women and ravish virgins, we call that bearing of love'; 'if he be a whoremaster, they say he is an amorous lover and Venus bird'; 'our ancestors were but bunglers at vice . . . they could but call a spade a spade . . . we are become far more exquisite'.[25] Over time the suspicion grew that the soft words of civility—'mistress', 'miss', 'gallant', 'intrigue', 'gallantry'—were a cloak for sin.[26] The broader social context of civility—the places of resort of polite society, such as the Spring Gardens at Vauxhall in London or the growing spa town of Bath; occasions of sociability, such as play-going and assemblies; fashion and its excesses in dress and demeanour—also stimulated moral condemnation, which grew louder, shriller, and more insistent in response to the growth of London, the development of the 'season', and changes in aristocratic and genteel behaviour as the Stuart century progressed. 'In this sad age', lamented Clement Ellis as early as 1660, a gentleman was 'one who has studied to bring sin so much into fashion . . . that he is now accounted a clown that is not proud to be thought a sinner'; 'no better than an uncivil fellow, and no companion for gentlemen'.[27]

But this was only one current of moralists' thinking; and their works—which of course encompassed a very wide range of genres, written in a variety of registers by laypeople as well as clergy—were not always so critical of civil-

[24] Della Casa, *Galateo*, trans. Peterson, 5, 82; cf. 1 Cor. 15: 33.

[25] Anon., *The pilgrimage of man, wandering in a wilderness of woe* (1612), sig. D2ᵛ; John Northbrooke, *A treatise wherein dicing, dau[n]cing, vaine plaies or enterludes with other idle pastimes, &c. commonly used on the sabboth day, are reprooved* (1579), sig. A4ʳ; Barnaby Rich, *My ladies looking glasse* (1616), 17; see also Lewes Bayly, *The practise of pietie* (11th edn., 1619), 199–200.

[26] Jeremy Collier, *Essays upon several moral subjects. Part III* (3rd edn., 1720), 113–14; C. Lasch, 'The Suppression of Clandestine Marriage in England: The Marriage Act of 1753', *Salmagundi*, 26 (Spring 1974), 95–6 (quoting Edward Ravenscroft, *The London Cuckolds*, III.1). These issues are developed in Turner, 'Representations of Adultery', ch. 3.

[27] Clement Ellis, *The gentile sinner, or England's brave gentleman* (Oxford, 1660), 11, 189 (while this particular quotation refers in context partly to drunkenness, the argument applied equally to sexual sins and the 'lip-adultery' of filthy talk: ibid. 12–13, 36–7, 142). See also Jeremy Taylor, *'Holy Living' and 'Holy Dying'*, ed. P. G. Stanwood (2 vols.; Oxford, 1989), i. 70–1. On the changing social context, see Bryson, *From Courtesy to Civility*, 128–50.

ity. Indeed, as many modern commentators have pointed out, the boundary
between courtesy literature and conduct literature with a strong moral component was very blurred. Differences of intent, reflected in differences of
emphasis and vocabulary, are none the less evident, as some contemporaries
made clear: thus Jeremy Taylor, in discussing behaviour, distinguished
between the strictures of his own devotional tract and what '*in civil account*
are called undecencies, and incivilities'.[28] The sins that were centrally the
concern of Christian moralists were mostly crying ones that invited condemnation in no uncertain terms. Echoing the Bible, adultery and fornication were
characteristically presented as 'filthy', polluting acts, or as bestial and animal-
like behaviour; but in this context these metaphors evoked, not lack of
manners, but the dire iniquity of sexual transgression.

Yet, increasingly in the seventeenth century, moralists did appeal to the idea
of civility, or notions dependent on it, to buttress their arguments in certain
situations. Allestree repeatedly prodded his readers' conscience by enquiring
why duties towards God were not observed with the same rigour as the everyday code of civility. From a different perspective, some writers stressed the
difference between the deep, heartfelt morality of dedicated Christians and
that of 'civil men'—that is, individuals who were not 'open blasphemers,
drunkards, whore-masters, and the like' but 'yet remain mere worldlings, and
. . . lukewarm professors'. A more appreciative attitude to the animal world
could turn bestial metaphors on their head. Man had much to learn, mused
Matthew Griffith, from the habits of the elephant: not only was he strictly
monogamous, but he copulated for only five days every three years, 'and so
secretly, that he is never seen in the act'; afterwards 'the first thing he doth is
to go directly to some clear river, and to wash his body, not willing to return
to his companions till he be cleansed'. By a parallel logic, the laxness of the
contemporary treatment of adultery and incest was castigated by reference to
the uncompromising punishments meted out by heathen societies past and
present: incestuous marriages, according to Thomas Beard, were 'inhibited
not only by the law of God, but also by civil and politic constitutions, where-
unto all nations have ever by the sole instinct of nature agreed and accorded,
except the Ægyptians and Persians'.[29]

Moralists also used the language of civility and incivility to set limits on
actions that were not of themselves obviously sinful, or to persuade readers
of the sinfulness of behaviour that some regarded as lawful or neutral. Not all
the targets of attack related to sexual immorality as such. For example, the
stern mid-century Presbyterian Thomas Hall insisted that long hair in males
was condemned by 'every civil, grave and gracious man'; while the same

---

[28] Taylor, '*Holy Living*' and '*Holy Dying*', ed. Stanwood, i. 104 (emphasis added).
[29] Richard Allestree, *The ladies calling* (2 pts.; Oxford, 1673), i. 45, 138; ii. 10, 57; Henry Scudder,
The Christians daily walke in holy securitie and peace (6th edn., 1635), 228–9; Griffith, *Bethel*, 316;
Thomas Beard, *The theatre of Gods iudgements* (1597), 327.

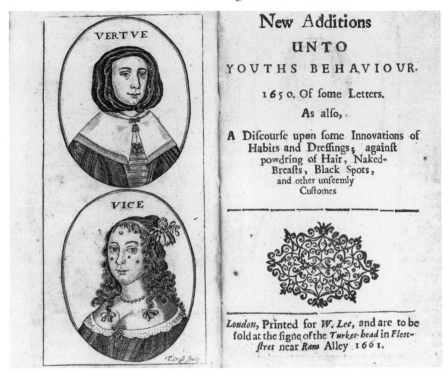

New Additions

UNTO

YOUTHS BEHAVIOUR.

1650. Of fome Letters.

As alfo,

A Difcourfe upon fome Innovations of
Habits and Dreſſings; againſt
powdring of Hair, Naked-
Breaſts, Black Spots,
and other unfeemly
Cuſtomes

London, Printed for *W. Lee,* and are to be
fold at the figne of the *Turkes-head* in *Fleet-
ſtret* near *Ram* Alley 1661.

4. 'Vertue' and 'Vice', from *Youths behaviour, or decencie in conversation amongst men*, trans. Francis Hawkins (7th edn., 1661), [40–1]

author repeatedly inveighed against the 'rudeness' of Maygames and similar pastimes.[30] However, part of Hall's case was that such sports were the means to debauchery and whoredom, and civility was often brought into play in discussions of relations between the sexes and related matters. Thus Thomas Beard condemned sexual intercourse between couples who had been secretly contracted but not publicly married, 'warning how unlawful all such conversation is, and how contrary to good manners, and to the laudable customs of all civil and well governed people'. John Downame distinguished between kissing and embracing 'used after a civil and honest manner to express our love one to another' or 'civil courtesy'—kissing was in fact a common means of salutation in this period—and similar gestures used 'in wanton dalliance between those who are light and lascivious'. And the additions to Hawkins's

---

[30] Thomas Hall, *Comarum ακοσμια: the loathsomnesse of long haire . . . with an appendix against painting, spots, naked breasts, &c* (1654), 23; Thomas Hall, *Funebria florae: the downfall of may-games* (2nd edn., 1661), title page, 5.

Youths behaviour in 1650 engaged with the 'baring of the breasts and shoulders' of women: 'I know their excuse is at hand, 'tis the fashion, and fashion is a custom, and custom is a law, or a nature, or both. But admit it a custom, and a fashion, yet it is so far from civil, that the civil heathens would from all ages downward have abhorred it, even to jealousy.'[31] Behind all such cases may be inferred a growing apprehension—stimulated by the greater knowledge of the classics, of ancient and modern history, and of contemporary geography and anthropology that all educated people were beginning to enjoy by the seventeenth century—that Christian revelation was not the only basis for morality.

II

Works concerning civility are for the most part texts without contexts, and students of the genre have had little success in positively identifying their readers or demonstrating their influence in concrete terms. The same may be said for much moralist literature.[32] And so we must turn to sources relating to specific, real-life individuals. There are some indications that we should not expect explicit notions of civility to be very prominent in the everyday discourse of most members of society, even by the late seventeenth century. Richard Gough's *History of Myddle* (1701) contains numerous miniature biographies of the inhabitants of this and neighbouring parishes in Shropshire within the author's lifetime, and is an unusually rich source for evaluative discourse. Some individuals are praised for being 'courteous', 'obliging', 'comely', 'modest', 'orderly'; others are castigated as 'rude', 'untowardly', and so forth—all terms that find their echo in the conduct literature. Yet the words 'civil' and 'civility' were apparently not part of Gough's active vocabulary. Myddle was, of course, remote from the metropolis, but it was adjacent to the fashionable town of Shrewsbury and at no great distance from the provincial centres of Chester and Ludlow, while Gough was a man of considerable education. The omission is, therefore, telling.[33] Even more so is the fact that Samuel Pepys, moving in and out of the highest circles of Restoration London, used 'civility' and related terminology quite sparingly in his diary:

[31] Beard, *Theatre of Gods iudgements*, 321; John Downame, *Foure treatises, tending to disswade all Christians from foure no lesse hainous then common sinnes* (1609), 201; *Youths behaviour*, trans. Hawkins, 57–8.

[32] Bryson, *From Courtesy to Civility*, 5–6; Childs, 'Prescriptions for Manners', 3–6, 34–40. The fact that most works of civility current in England were translations or based on foreign models compounds the problems.

[33] Richard Gough, *Antiquities and Memoirs of the Parish of Myddle* (Shrewsbury, 1875), 55, 57, 61, 65, 94, 122, 124, 146, 147; cf. A. McInnes, 'The Emergence of a Leisure Town: Shrewsbury, 1660–1760', *P&P* 120 (1988), 53–87.

about once a month on average in 1664, for example, only slightly more often in 1668, the last full year of journal entries.[34]

Court records, the main focus of attention here, are not inconsistent with these observations; but when batches of them are read *in extenso* they do provide some more positive indications. Taking the terms 'civil', 'civility', and their opposites as the index, they suggest that usages were rare down to the end of the sixteenth century, but were widely current by the 1620s and had become fairly common by 1700. The adjectival forms were more common than the nouns. They may have been more current in urban circles, particularly London, but occurred in rural locations too. Of course they cannot be taken as a simple index of people's ordinary use of language. Usages tended to be either *reflexive*, echoing the terminology of official articles of inquiry or interrogatories (predetermined sets of questions directed at witnesses, presumably drawn up by professional lawyers); *conventional* or formulaic, occurring in set phrases that were or became commonplaces of legal discourse; *rhetorical*, reflecting a careful choice of words to make a case or otherwise persuade judges, justices, or the like; or a combination of these modes. But this does not mean that the terms were meaningless or alien to the individuals who used them. Moreover, official formularies and the promptings of lawyers were not the only means whereby ordinary people were exposed to this language: similar usages to those found in the court records occurred in literature designed for a popular audience, especially materials such as murder pamphlets or 'last dying speeches' that themselves had some affinity to legal records.[35] The overall impression is of a concept being encountered, slowly added to existing linguistic repertoires, gradually appropriated, and turned to advantage as occasion offered.

A reference point is offered by the transcription of the records of the Essex village of Earls Colne for the period 1400–1750, carried out by a team headed by Alan Macfarlane. The computer-generated index yields only a small clutch of references to 'civil', 'civility', and related terms, used at various points in time between 1620 and 1723.[36] Yet, though employed rarely, the words could certainly be used to powerful effect, as will appear later when some of this material is examined. My other examples are drawn mainly from an extensive trawl though church court, quarter sessions, city and borough court, and some central court records relating mainly to Dorset, Wiltshire, Berkshire, Oxfordshire, and the cities of London and Westminster and adjacent metro-

[34] *The Diary of Samuel Pepys*, ed. R. Latham and W. Matthews (11 vols.; 1970–83), v. 30, 61, 66, 90, 111, 144, 176, 255, 270, 336, 341, ix. 12, 92, 112, 114, 118, 169, 176, 189, 220, 228, 264, 274, 317, 380.
[35] e.g. K. U. Henderson and B. F. McManus (eds.), *Half Humankind: Contexts and Texts of the Controversy about Women in England, 1540–1640* (Urbana, Ill., 1985), 281, 308, 355, 362.
[36] *Records of an English Village: Earls Colne, 1400–1750*, ed. A. Macfarlane *et al.* (Cambridge, 1980–1), [microfiche] nos. 7.00042–7.02063 *passim*, 177.00005–177.02064 *passim*, 323.00741, 323.00795.

politan areas in the sixteenth, seventeenth, and early eighteenth centuries. The situation in other parts of England, including the north, would repay further investigation.[37]

While sex and civility provide the main focus of this discussion, the discourse was never confined to sexual matters and some other usages must be explored to establish context. First it should be noted that the Church, through the rubrics of the Prayer Book and visitation articles and injunctions, demanded that the fabric and furnishings of churches, the state of graveyards, the dress and conduct of the clergy, and the behaviour of laypeople in church should be 'orderly', 'decent', and 'comely', and sought information on 'rude and immodest behaviour' and other circumstances that contravened these orders.[38] No doubt these prescriptions were often flouted.[39] However, they did mean that the Church was setting standards of religious behaviour based on concepts very close to those of civility. Such concepts were apparently absorbed by local officers, or at least reflected back in the terminology of presentments and parochial reports; and, as the language of civility became established in common usage, specific references to 'civil', 'uncivil', and so on were grafted on. As early as 1599 Alexander Goozey of Salisbury was prosecuted 'for unreverently, uncivilly, rudely and barbarously behaving himself, especially for violently pulling off his wife's hat from her head in the church in time of divine service'; in 1619 John Francklin of Everleigh (Wiltshire) was prosecuted on the grounds that 'being distempered and overcome with immoderate drinking he behaved himself very unreverently and uncivilly in the church to the disturbance and offence of the whole congregation'; while in Lyme Regis in 1635 there were complaints of young and old behaving themselves in church 'very unreverently and uncivilly' by keeping their hats on and neglecting to kneel.[40]

Such material offers some support for Knox's argument that church and clergy were standard-bearers of civility; in the post-Reformation English context the concept was especially useful, since decorum and decency were the main arguments for retaining ceremonies that otherwise might be

---

[37] For examples of some northern usages, see *Depositions from the Castle of York, relating to Offences Committed in the Northern Counties in the Seventeenth Century*, ed. J. Raine (Surtees Society, 40; 1841), 57, 63, 91, 100, 118; *Yorkshire Diaries and Autobiographies in the Seventeenth and Eighteenth Centuries*, ed. H. J. Morehouse (Surtees Society, 65; 1877), 91.

[38] *Visitation Articles and Injunctions of the Period of the Reformation*, ed. W. H. Frere and W. M. Kennedy (Alcuin Club Collections, 14–16; Oxford, 1910), iii. 20, 113, 175, 266, and *passim*; *Elizabethan Episcopal Administration*, ed. W. P. M. Kennedy (Alcuin Club Collections, 25–7; Oxford, 1924), ii. 58, 72, and *passim*, iii. 188, 194, 230, and *passim*; *Visitation Articles and Injunctions of the Early Stuart Church*, ed. K. Fincham (Church of England Record Society, 1, 5; 2 vols.; Woodbridge, Suffolk, 1994–8), i. 7, 10, and *passim*, ii. 1, 2, and *passim*.

[39] K. Thomas, *Religion and the Decline of Magic: Studies in Popular Beliefs in Sixteenth and Seventeenth Century England* (1971), 161–2; A. Macfarlane, S. Harrison, and C. Jardine, *Reconstructing Historical Communities* (Cambridge, 1977), 197–8; but cf. Ingram, *Church Courts*, 108–9.

[40] Wilts. RO, D1/39/1/27, fo. 65ᵛ; D1/39/2/9, fo. 21ᵛ; D5/28/35, no. 73.

condemned as superstitious, and neatly fitted the proposition that such usages might legitimately be left to the magistrate to order.[41] However, there were also contexts where the secular no less than the church authorities insisted on personal restraint, and where ideas of civility likewise had an important purchase. This was especially so in relation to encounters, particularly in public, between individuals of unequal status or authority—above all in formal settings such as a court of law, or where office was actually being exercised. While behaviour was to an extent duly shaped by expectations in these situations, there were weak points in the web of deference that could lead to abrasive exchanges: for example, lesser officers such as constables might well fail to command the respect of their neighbours; the same was true of clergymen, especially if they were perceived to be proud, grasping, incompetent, or immoral, as also of upstart or self-styled gentlemen (or gentlewomen); even individuals of apparently secure status could find themselves affronted. Frequently on such occasions the abusive speech or disrespectful behaviour was characterized in terms invoking standards of civility. John Dod, a barber of St Margaret's Westminster, was bound over in 1630 'for giving uncivil speeches' to a Justice of the Peace. To take a provincial example, in 1654 Walter Woodman of Malmesbury, commanded by an overseer of the poor to perform an order to maintain his bastard child, 'did then uncivilly and unmannerly clap his hand upon his breech and bade him . . . kiss his arse'. In 1671, in a case that illustrates both status challenge and religious profanation, John Hawkins, Esquire, was affronted by Thomas Carter in the church of Ashton Keynes (Wiltshire) with 'incivility' in 'many scurrilous and opprobrious speeches . . . in a brawling and brutish manner', in 'breach of good manners and in dishonour of the church'.[42]

All these cases involved males. What of women who uttered invective? Traditionally females were regarded as particularly prone to sins of the tongue (though some moralists insisted that men were just as bad),[43] while, on the other hand, it was a contemporary commonplace that, among women's main duties, along with chastity and obedience, was silence—not literal soundlessness, as writers such as William Gouge in the early seventeenth century and Robert Codrington a generation or two later hastened to add, but at least a 'reverend and meek' restraint and avoidance of 'over-much tattling'.[44] Ignoring such qualifications, some historians have assumed that women's speech

[41] Knox, 'Erasmus' *De Civilitate*'; Knox, '*Disciplina*', *passim*.

[42] London Metropolitan Archives, WJ/SR (NS) 27, no. 20, cf. Guildhall Library, MS 9064/20, fos. 10ᵛ, 19ᵛ; Wilts. RO, A1/110/1654E, no. 50; D1/42/61, fos. 29ʳ, 30ᵛ; see also Oxon. RO, MS Oxford Dioc. Papers c. 4, fos. 102ᵛ, 107ʳ.

[43] Edward Reyner, *Rules for the government of the tongue* (1656), 30–1, 52; William Gearing, *A bridle for the tongue* (1663), 417 and *passim*; Richard Allestree, *The government of the tongue* (Oxford, 1674), 73; but cf. Stephen Ford, *The evil tongue tryed and found guilty* (1672), 123, 284.

[44] William Gouge, *Of domesticall duties* (1622), 281–2; Robert Codrington, *The second part of youths behaviour, or decency in conversation among women* (1664), 31–2.

was subject to rigorous restraint, and that loquacity could incur such severe physical punishment as the cucking-stool and scold's bridle. Elsewhere I have argued for a more conservative interpretation: 'scolding' as a crime generally involved not mere talkativeness but serious verbal and sometimes physical harassment.[45] This is not to deny that women were more prone than men to be condemned for insulting, ribald, or merely assertive speech, and the language of incivility—sometimes explicitly coupled with that of unwomanliness—was used to censure them. In 1631 Jane Winter of Weldon (Northamptonshire) was said to be a 'reviler of her honest neighbours in most uncivil and unwomanly term[s]'. Margaret Davis of Nettleton (Wiltshire), ultimately ducked as a scold, was in a Star Chamber case of 1614 said to have been accused of brawling, reviling, and chiding 'in most barbarous and uncivil manner . . . far unfit for any sober woman' (the actual presentment in the local manor court did not explicitly refer to civility, but stated that Margaret and another inhabitant had been 'unruly women of their tongues' who, though admonished to reform, 'have not amended their manners').[46] The vulnerability of women (particularly poor women) in this respect may be further illustrated by a case of a different kind from Abingdon (then in Berkshire) in 1671. Joan Broughton went into a victualling house, not for the first time, to induce John North to pay 'above forty' shillings that he owed her husband. 'What the pox! What would you do with John North?', exclaimed his friend Charles Sherwood, described as a 'farmer or yeoman' of some substance; and he went on to abuse her in a torrent of coarse invective that called her sexual honesty in question and 'forced . . . [her] to go out of the house crying'. The telling circumstance in this case was that a woman, guilty of no more than pertinacity in collecting a debt, and the victim of gross verbal abuse, had to defend herself against the imputation that she had provoked it by her own incivility. Witnesses on her behalf insisted that she did not 'give any the least provoking or uncivil words to the said Charles Sherwood, but that . . . [they] heard her call him after a seemly and civil manner, "Mr Sherwood" at every word'.[47]

In the language of abuse, of the kind to which Joan Broughton was subjected, sexual matters were often prominent. This was especially (though not exclusively) so when it referred to women, since the stock means of abusing or slandering a female was to call her a whore, or words to similar effect.[48] In

[45] M. Ingram, '"Scolding Women Cucked or Washed": A Crisis in Gender Relations in Early Modern England?', in J. Kermode and G. Walker (eds.), *Women, Crime and the Courts in Early Modern England* (1994), 48–80, esp. 67–9; cf. D. Underdown, 'The Taming of the Scold: The Enforcement of Patriarchal Authority in Early Modern England', in A. Fletcher and J. Stevenson (eds.), *Order and Disorder in Early Modern England* (Cambridge, 1985), 116–36.

[46] *Quarter Sessions Records of the County of Northampton*, ed. J. Wake and S. A. Peyton (Northants Record Society, 1; Hereford, 1924), 99; PRO STAC 8/123/16, m. 3; cf. BL Add. MS 23, 151, fo. 52. For another example, see PRO STAC 8/266/29, m. 1.

[47] Wilts. RO, D1/42/61, fos. 236ᵛ–31ʳ [from reverse of volume].

[48] L. Gowing, *Domestic Dangers: Women, Words and Sex in Early Modern London* (Oxford, 1996), ch. 3.

discussion of such cases in the records, the emphasis was, as one might expect in a legal context, usually on the actual *defamatory* nature of such accusations and the specific kinds of legal, economic, and social jeopardy that they entailed. However, slanders imputing sexual immorality, whether adultery, fornication, or 'whoredom' more vaguely defined, were sometimes described as 'undecent' or 'unmannerly', with the emphasis on the lack of decorum that their use entailed; they were frequently condemned as 'base' or 'vile'; slanderers, whether men or women, were castigated as 'foul mouthed'; and the actual words were sometimes expurgated by witnesses as 'not seemly to be related'.[49] Sometimes lack of civility was explicitly invoked. In the London Consistory Court in 1635, for example, it was reported that Mary Delaney 'fell into discourse of Margaret Delaney her mother-in-law and used base and uncivil language of her . . . and called her whore and bawd in an angry and malicious manner'. The abuse uttered by an Oxford man in 1621 was similarly characterized; William Kelsall, in an altercation over a debt, declared that Joan Sympson was a whore and her husband a cuckold, 'and that her man[servant] had carnally known her, expressing that in a more uncivil and obscene term'.[50]

Was the language of civility used to refer not merely to talk about sex but to actual sexual behaviour? In these court records (as in the pages of moralists), out-and-out adultery, fornication, and other forms of sexual trangression were condemned in explicit terms; and, like the moralists, ordinary people often chose to characterize such behaviour as 'filthy' or 'bestial'. Again in line with moralists' usages, specific reference to civility and incivility was usually made only in *marginal* situations: to refer to (often to condemn) sexual behaviour that fell short of full intercourse, or to defend an individual against charges of sexual misdoing by claiming a reputation for unimpeachable conduct. The commonest usage is found in witnesses' statements on behalf of female plaintiffs in sexual slander suits of the kind that have already been introduced. The utility of suits for defamation was precisely that they turned the tables, transforming the accused person, the victim of slander, into the accuser. To buttress their actions plaintiffs often brought evidence of character. In the sixteenth century, it was commonly said that women were 'virtuous', 'chaste', 'honest', 'modest', 'of good credit and reputation'. Increasingly, in the seventeenth century, such formulas were augmented by the language of civility. In a typical case in London in 1635, Margaret Bloise was said to have 'been accounted a woman of honest life and conversation and of good name and fame till this report [of immorality] was raised . . . and a woman of civil behaviour and carriage'. Provincial cases were similar: in 1618 it was

[49] London Metropolitan Archives, WJ/SR (NS) 2A, no. 2; WJ/SR (NS) 17, no. 7; WJ/SR (NS) 2B, no. 40.

[50] London Metropolitan Archives, DL/C/234, fo. 116ʳ; cf. Guildhall Library, MS 9064/17, fo. 25ᵛ; Oxon. RO, MS Oxford Archd. Papers Oxon c. 10, fos. 27–9.

alleged that Jane Seymour of Ramsbury (Wiltshire) was always 'reputed and taken to be a modest, civil and honest young woman' till Anthony Ryder claimed to have 'had the breaking of her . . . up', whereupon she was 'like to be put by of a good match which otherwise had proceeded'.[51]

Similar usages occurred in the secular courts. In 1610 seven of the inhabitants of Broad Chalke (Wiltshire) complained to the JPs in Quarter Sessions of a certain Robert Cane, 'being wholly given to contention and to raise strife and enmity between neighbour and neighbour'; among other abuses, it was said, he had brought a false and damaging accusation of whoredom against Elizabeth Line, 'known to be of an honest and civil life'. In the Westminster sessions in 1620, Elizabeth Sandes petitioned the justices for redress against Charles Chambers, gentleman, who (she claimed) had seduced her under colour of 'his many and deep vows and protestations of marriage' and then abandoned her 'contrary to all humane honesty'. Before his appearance, she protested, she had been an apprentice for six years and a servant for a further seven in the households of substantial citizens, 'in both which places she behaved herself in very civil and honest manner'. The equivocal circumstances of this and other cases are a reminder, if any is needed, of the rhetorical or deliberately persuasive nature of these usages, and hence the fact that the claims should not necessarily be taken at face value.[52]

The term 'civil', used in this fashion, occurs mostly in relation to women, but could also be applied to men; it might also refer to a household. A petition to the Westminster justices in 1629, subscribed by the minister, churchwardens, and about thirty of the inhabitants of St Martin in the Fields, stated that Priscilla Knuckle, widow, was 'of honest life and conversation, approved with us, and doth keep a civil and well governed house free from all scandalous imputations', while her son was 'a man of honest and civil life and well demeaned'.[53] Yet again, 'civil' could be applied to a whole category of inhabitants, usually in contrast to the alleged demerits of a named person. Thus in 1623 a man of Grays Thurrock (Essex) was said to be 'a very poor and indigent fellow of no credit or esteem with any man that liveth a civil and honest course of life';[54] while in 1619 Cecily Springbat, wife of John Springbat, miller, of Wilsford (Wiltshire), was presented to the bishop's court for behaviour that raised persistent suspicions of adultery, 'to the great offence of all honest and civil people and will not reform herself'.[55]

---

[51] London Metropolitan Archives, DL/C/234, fo. 49ᵛ; Wilts. RO, D1/42/32, fos. 119–20ᵛ; for other examples, see Guildhall Library, MS 9057/1, fo. 11; Wilts. RO, D1/42/61, fo. 57.

[52] Wilts. RO, A1/110/1610H, no. 142; London Metropolitan Archives, WJ/SR (NS) 2, no. 145; cf. WJ/SR (NS) 15, no. 130.

[53] London Metropolitan Archives, WJ/SR (NS) 26, no. 88; cf. P. M. Humfrey, '"I saw, through a large chink in the partition . . .": What the Servants Knew', in V. Frith (ed.), *Women and History: Voices of Early Modern England* (Toronto, 1995), 63.

[54] Guildhall Library, MS 9189/1, fos. 22ᵛ–3ʳ.

[55] Wilts. RO, D1/39/2/9, fo. 21ᵛ.

The counterpart to these claims of 'civil' demeanour were allegations of 'incivility' in the sense of improper behaviour. These might be brought by presenting officers or other accusers against men, women, errant couples, or even groups of, for example, young people. A participant at a dancing match at a mill in Broad Chalke (Wiltshire) on St John's (midsummer) night 1639 claimed that she 'saw no abuse offered or incivility committed by any'. What was at issue emerged from the statements of other witnesses: one admitted that in the darkness of the night when the candles had burnt out she 'heard some of the maids cry out', while another young woman reported that one of the young men present 'termed himself to be the bishop', and that a certain Catherine Sangar of Knoyle 'was set upon her head and was bishopped'.[56] Occasionally charges of uncivil behaviour were brought by women against men, and are of particular interest. Women had to tread warily, since in making a complaint they ran the risk of having their own chastity brought in question.[57] In such a situation the language of incivility was particularly useful: it implied the woman's own claim to respectable status and forestalled some stock male defences, as that the gestures complained of had been designed to test the woman's honesty (to make coarse advances was hardly the way to go about it) or were merely 'in merriment' (all the writers of conduct books and courtesy manuals concurred in condemning indecent jokes). To take an example, in 1634 Julian Daves, an Oxford man's wife, appeared voluntarily before the archdeacon's court, and complained that John Hunt, a married mercer, had 'several times attempted her chastity, soliciting her sometimes by earnest entreaty and persuasion, and other times laying violent hands upon her . . . and in uncivil manner thrusting his hands under her coats [i.e. skirts] and striving to handle her privities'. She claimed that 'besides his evil talk he would often pull out his privities and labour to show them to this allegant and to put them in her hand'. 'These things being come to the knowledge of her husband [had] bred much discontent betwixt them', and she begged the court to take action to restore both 'her credit and . . . her husband's good opinion of her'.[58]

Yet another usage of the language of civility in these court records remains to be discussed. Although fornication and adultery were subject to legal penalty, they were, as 'acts of darkness and great secrecy',[59] notoriously difficult to prove; the exception was the case of unmarried women who became pregnant, and even then the fact of paternity could be hard to substantiate.

[56] *Records of the County of Wilts, being Extracts from the Quarter Sessions Great Rolls of the Seventeenth Century*, ed. B. H. Cunnington (Devizes, 1932), 131–2. Sexual horseplay was the main issue but there may have been a satirical reference to the Bishops' War.

[57] S. Hindle, 'The Shaming of Margaret Knowsley: Gossip, Gender and the Experience of Authority in Early Modern England', *Continuity and Change*, 9 (1994), 391–419.

[58] Oxon. RO, MS Oxford Archd. Papers Oxon. c. 12, fos. 264ᵛ–5; cf. ibid., fo. 167ᵛ; Wilts. RO, A1/110/1724M (unnumbered bundle), information of Mrs Mary Hauckins.

[59] John Ayliffe, *Parergon juris canonici anglicani* (1726), 44.

'Though one should see a man upon the very body of a woman, with her coats up above her middle,' warned the early eighteenth-century commentator John Ayliffe, 'yet it does not necessarily follow from thence, that carnal copulation did intervene or ensue between them'. Moreover, it was really only the full sexual act that was of interest to the law: kissing, cuddling, 'tumbling', and the like were very rarely, in themselves, the subject of prosecution. In practice, evidence of sexual immorality was usually circumstantial and cumulative in nature. Private meetings, too-frequent 'companying', undue familiarity, untoward pregnancies, suspicious removals, the intuition of fellow servants and neighbours, or the rash speeches of the parties, gradually led to the build-up of 'vehement suspicion' or 'common fame' of incontinence sufficient to justify legal action.[60] However, it was sometimes necessary to prove a 'fame', if it was challenged or not authenticated by the presentment of the churchwardens; and occasionally, as a prelude to separation proceedings or a common-law prosecution for 'criminal conversation',[61] it was necessary to undertake formal proof of adultery. Two devices came into play here. The first, which has already attracted historical attention, was a deliberate breach of privacy more determined and more invasive than the general context of neighbourly surveillance on which the system of sexual regulation always depended. Exploiting their legal powers, constables or other local officers, with the aid of neighbours on duty as members of the watch, sometimes made sure that their search was fruitful by 'staking out' dwellings where immorality was suspected of taking place, seizing the best opportunity to invade the house to catch the couple in the act. More commonly, neighbours or fellow servants followed up suspicious signs (which might include, for example, the locking of doors against intrusion) by spying on couples through windows or through chinks in floors, doors, or walls—actions that were both facilitated by the flimsiness and disrepair of many contemporary houses and outbuildings and recognized and sanctioned in canon law.[62] The second device was to provide, as a complement to or substitute for direct evidence of carnal knowledge, testimony of unseemly behaviour that might constitute a presumption of guilt; the language of 'incivility', 'rudeness', and so forth was frequently invoked to this end. On occasion both strategies were employed to enmesh the accused couples as securely as possible in a web of circumstantial evidence.

A case from Halstead (Essex) in 1620, evidently relating to a wealthy yeoman household, vividly evokes both the moral and material context. A maidservant called Alice March deposed that one afternoon she found her

[60] Ibid. 44–5; Ingram, *Church Courts*, 239–45, 253–5.
[61] On the action of 'criminal conversation', whereby a deceived husband could obtain cash damages from his wife's lover, see L. Stone, *Road to Divorce: England, 1530–1987* (Oxford, 1990), ch. 9.
[62] Thomas, *Religion*, 527; Ingram, *Church Courts*, 244–5; cf. Ayliffe, *Parergon*, 51.

mistress, Isabel Collins, alone by the fireside with a certain Robert Carter. Her suspicions were aroused when she noticed that they had gone into the 'old parlour', and, alerting a fellow servant, the two went to investigate. The 'latch of the . . . door' being 'pulled out', they had perforce to open it with a 'fire fork'. But not finding the couple, they concluded that they must be in the cheese house, and went outside to look in through the window. This proved to be too high for them to see through, but on their meeting another servant, Thomas Jones, he took them 'into his chamber which was directly over the cheese house', where they were able to take turns to look down into the room through a crack in the floorboards. What they saw, they all claimed, was Carter and Collins in what appeared from their position and disordered clothes to be the act of adultery. Their accounts were embellished with vivid detail, including, in the words of one of the witnesses, the fact that she had a bird's-eye view of 'Robert Carter's bald head, his hat lying by him, and she perceived that he was very hot for his head did reek'.

This literally steamy account was, despite its apparent plausibility, under-mined by other witnesses who claimed that it was physically impossible to get an adequate view into the cheese house through the crack. So the next phase of testimony broadened into an evaluation of Isabel Collins's character, the defence claiming that she 'did always carry and demean herself soberly, civilly and modestly' and was 'a very honest and civil woman'. The prosecution coun-tered by trying to prove, amongst other things, that she habitually 'gadded abroad' haunting alehouses, was commonly drunk, used unseemly talk, and was suspected of immorality with other men besides Carter. John Prentice, a 60-year-old Halstead husbandman, testified 'that he hath once seen her so dis-tempered with drink that she pissed as she sat in . . . [his] presence in the hall of her own house, and at other times he hath often seen her idle and he think-eth the occasion thereof to be through over much drinking'. Rose Chapman, wife of a linendraper, deposed that 'knowing . . . Isabel to nurse her child and give suck she asked her . . . whether her breasts did not prick and she made answer that her breasts did not prick but she had one part about her would have a prick'. Finally, Agnes Leonard reported that seven years before she had seen Isabel Collins with a certain John Freeman in 'the chamber over the kitchen . . . being there alone together . . . very suspiciously, he having one hand in her placket and the other about her neck and was kissing her in a very lascivious manner'. A little later she had 'found the said Freeman almost out of breath and the said Isabel had her ruff beaten down behind and bruised flat, whereby this deponent did suspect that there had been some ill act passed between them'. It went without saying that incontinence (in both the con-temporary and modern senses), inebriety, saucy talk, and a crushed collar were incompatible with 'civility'.[63]

---

[63] *Records of an English Village*, ed. Macfarlane *et al.*, [microfiche] nos. 7.00042–7.02798 *passim*; for quotations see nos. 7.00084, 7.00165, 7.00717, 7.02318, 7.02370, 7.03370.

Cases like this embody a certain paradox. The detailed testimony about intimate activities, however contrived it might be, implies an acceptance of the
propriety of neighbourly surveillance. Court records reveal that proof of adultery based on deliberate spying, particularly by servants, continued to be commonplace into the eighteenth century.[64] Yet there were contrary currents in
contemporary culture. 'Never listen at the doors or windows,' warned Jeremy
Taylor in 1650, 'for besides that it contains in it danger and a snare, it is also
an invading my neighbour's privacy'.[65] The complaisance stressed by
seventeenth-century writers on civility might likewise be thought to have discouraged snooping. Moreover, as time went on, changes in the physical layout
of houses and the growing availability of bedcurtains and other aids to seclusion may have made privacy less easily violable. The impact of such changes,
gradual though they were, are hinted at in a case from James II's reign. An
innkeeper and his wife from Alderbury (Wiltshire) testified that John Venice
and Joan Lawrence, wife of Matthew Lawrence, had come to their inn and
stayed the night in a room with only one bed. Venice asked for another to be
brought in, but did not demur when told that this was impossible; 'Cousin,'
he was alleged to have asked his companion, 'you will not be afraid to lie down
upon the bed by me?' The innkeeper's wife left them 'in private about
bedtime', but 'passing in the next room, did by the help of their candle, and
the conveniency of a great hole in the door of that room wherein they were,
see and observe the said Joan Lawrence leaping up into the bed in her shift,
but the curtains being drawn about the bed she did not see the said Venice,
and the candle was soon put out'. The couple came to the inn again shortly
afterwards and stayed in the same room. On this occasion, the landlady 'being
unwilling of their company did not much attend them, nor particularly
observe any incivilities between them'. However, the next morning a tragi-
comedy was acted out. Joan's husband arrived and took up position in the
room onto which the adulterous couple's bedchamber opened. Having
looked through the door and satisfied himself that his wife was there with
Venice, he sat down and made himself at home. The couple within soon
became uncomfortably aware of his presence by the sound of his voice, and
consulted with the landlady how to extricate themselves from their predica-
ment. To Venice's suggestion that Joan should make her escape through the
window, the innkeeper's wife indignantly replied that 'she should not go out
at any window there'. With some spirit, Joan declared that she would 'pack
up my things and go out by him'. She did so, but there were no immediate
recriminations, her husband merely doffing his hat to her as she went by.
Venice came out next, and there was a further show of courtesies: 'as he passed
one of the company drank to him; and he staying to pledge drank to Matthew
Lawrence'. But these attempts at politeness soon broke down, and Lawrence

---

[64] Stone, *Road to Divorce*, 211–15; for some examples, see Humfrey, '"I saw, through a large
chink in the partition . . . "', 63–6.
[65] Taylor, *'Holy Living' and 'Holy Dying'*, ed. Stanwood, i. 100.

and Venice came to blows in which the landlady, caught in the middle, sustained cuts and bruises. 'Civility', in the sense of polite accommodation, could not contain the raw emotions aroused by sexual bad 'manners'.[66]

III

Approaching the topic of civility through court records is of considerable historical interest. It shows that, far from being the preserve of élites of gentle or aristocratic status, versions of the concept did have resonance, indeed utility, for people from a much wider social spectrum. The particular face of civility that is exposed here is less to do with the niceties of polite behaviour than with conduct and qualities that a later age would term respectability, propriety, and decency. While they were not exclusively concerned with sexual behaviour, this was undoubtedly a strong component. Terms such as 'civil' and 'incivility' could apply to either sex, but they were gendered in the sense that usage reflected some much broader cultural assumptions, notably that sexual reputation was of much more central importance to women than to men. The ideas associated with this face of civility made sense to the individuals who peopled the courts because they were closely related to the long-established notions of reputation and moral status that underpinned defamation suits and other procedures in the church and secular courts, and to the habits of household and neighbourhood regulation that were so deeply engrained in contemporary society.

Some historians, probing the workings of the church courts, have questioned whether the religiously based notions of sin that ostensibly underlay them can possibly have had real purchase on the popular mind. A degree of scepticism is certainly in order, and it has always been recognized that popular attitudes to illicit sexuality were at most *broadly congruent* with the strictures of Christian morality, not in total conformity at every point.[67] But the absorption of the language of civility adds a further dimension to this discussion: the concept provided a complementary basis for moral conduct, an ethic consistent with Christian morality but based in social rather than religious bonds. Such an ethic, it may be suggested, had a particular utility in seventeenth-century society, both for the ordinary people who resorted to the courts and for the secular and ecclesiastical authorities that ran them. By the close of Elizabeth's reign, both the Catholic/Protestant split and Puritan zeal had rendered traditional Christian ethics problematic. The first divided the religious basis for morality, while the second made moral and religious demands that

---

[66] Wilts. RO, D1/42/60, fos. 110ᵛ–108ᵛ [reverse foliation].
[67] L. Gowing, 'Language, Power and the Law: Women's Slander Litigation in Early Modern London', in Kermode and Walker (eds.), *Women, Crime and the Courts*, 27–8; cf. Ingram, *Church Courts*, 164–5.

even the respectable often found excessive, and hence threatened if it did not actually disrupt social harmony. The idea of 'civility' helped to re-establish some common ground. The need for such an ethic was, moreover, underscored by the incivility of the civil wars and their contentious aftermath: even a cursory glance at the sources and secondary literature shows that there was frequent recourse to the concept in the 1640s and 1650s, as diverse individuals and groups (including, paradoxically, soldiers) claimed 'civil' status and either condemned the 'incivility' of their opponents or exhorted them to 'be civil'.[68] Religious differences were to prove persistent in the post-Restoration world, undermining the integrity of the national church and leading before 1700 to the permanent and recognized existence of dissenting groups both Catholic and Protestant. This divided situation was among the most important forces that led eventually to the collapse of moral regulation exercised by the church courts. Ideas of civility and incivility, it may be suggested, were to prove of increasing utility in a moral regime less dependent on courts of law. But, even while those institutions remained in operation—and they did so, albeit with declining levels of activity, throughout the eighteenth century— their pursuit of adulterers, bastard-bearers, and the like was itself partly sustained by their appeal to the broadly non-divisive standards of common decency that the term 'civil' implied. In reforming manners they could claim to punish both sins and incivility.

[68] R. Bauman, *Let Your Words Be Few: Symbolism of Speaking and Silence among Seventeenth-Century Quakers* (Cambridge, 1983), 54–6, cf. B. Reay, *The Quakers and the English Revolution* (1985), 71–2; A. Woolrych, *Soldiers and Statesmen: The General Council of the Army and its Debates, 1647–1648* (Oxford, 1987), 123; I. Gentles, *The New Model Army in England, Ireland and Scotland, 1645–1653* (Oxford, 1992), 156, 177–8; R. Ashton, *Counter-Revolution: The Second Civil War and its Origins, 1646–8* (New Haven, 1994), 200, 202, 387; A. M. McEntee, '"The [Un]Civill-Sisterhood of Oranges and Lemons": Female Petitioners and Demonstrators, 1642–53', in J. Holstun (ed.), *Pamphlet Wars: Prose in the English Revolution* (1992), 101.

6

The Civility of Women in Seventeenth-Century England

SARA MENDELSON

A superficial glance at the early modern literature of civility would yield a predominantly male model for this important social attribute. Most sixteenth- and seventeenth-century treatises and handbooks on the art of civility were composed by male authors, and were intended to instruct male readers in its basic elements. These included civil behaviour or *civilité*, the technique of 'self-fashioning' to promote success in the competitive game of court politics; civil letters, a style of prose whose foundations in the Greek and Latin classics were inaccessible to most women; and civil government, a civic duty from which all females other than queens were barred, because women were 'founden unapt' in 'wisedome and civile policy'.[1]

Yet if we examine a wider range of early modern sources, we find that the terms 'civil' and 'civility' and their synonyms crop up in a diversity of female contexts. At the Caroline court, a series of masques was staged in which Queen Henrietta Maria and other ladies of her circle were represented as imposing perfect harmony and civility on the entire cosmos through their feminine beauty and charm.[2] The earl of Cork noted his desire to educate his daughters in the 'foundations of religion and civility', and his son Robert Boyle

Many thanks to Sylvia Bowerbank, Patricia Crawford, Alan Mendelson, and Mary O'Connor for their comments on drafts of this chapter.

[1] N. Elias, *Power and Civility* (Oxford, 1982); S. Greenblatt, *Renaissance Self-Fashioning* (Chicago, 1980); M. Becker, *Civility and Society in Western Europe 1300–1600* (Bloomington, Ind., 1988); A. D. Hall, *Ceremony and Civility in English Renaissance Prose* (University Park, Pa., 1991); Thomas Elyot, *The Defence of Good Women* (1545), sig. B7ᵛ, cited in S. Mendelson and P. Crawford, *Women in Early Modern England 1550–1720* (Oxford, 1998), 349. Although Castiglione's influential *Book of the Courtier* includes female as well as male characters in its dialogues, neither Castiglione nor his successors wrote a companion piece for *The Courtier* entitled *The Courtesan*. In any case, by the early seventeenth century the term 'courtesan' no longer denoted a noblewoman attached to the court, but a high-class prostitute: 'Your whore is for every rascall, but your curtizan is for your courtier' (*Oxford English Dictionary*; usage cited is for 1607). For the significance of misogyny as a central theme in Castiglione's *Book of the Courtier*, see W. Rebhorn, *Courtly Performances: Masking and Festivity in Castiglione's Book of the Courtier* (Detroit, 1978), 123–31.

[2] S. Bowerbank and S. Mendelson, *Paper Bodies: A Margaret Cavendish Reader* (Peterborough, Ont., 1999), 'Introduction', 17–18 and nn. 1–3.

later expounded in his *Occasional Reflections* on the concept of civility as it applied to women, describing it as 'what the French call *Bien seance* . . . that Civility, and suppleness of Humour, which is requisite to endear Conversation, and is so proper to the softer Sex'. Civility as refined sociability, Boyle declared, was 'almost as Essential to a compleat Lady, as her Sex'.[3]

Women themselves were well aware of the vital importance of civility as a female attribute. In a diary entry written in 1702, Dame Sarah Cowper reminded herself of the need to practise the art of civility in her own day-to-day life. 'Civility', she asserted, 'is a chief part of the knowledge how to live. It is a kind of charm that attracts the love of all.'[4] Even in the mundane context of seventeenth-century court records, female witnesses frequently commended or reproved women of the middling and plebeian classes for their 'civil' or 'uncivil' speech and deportment.

What did the terms 'civil' and 'civility' mean for early modern women? Was the feminine ideal of civility simply a modified version of its masculine counterpart? To what extent did women create their own paradigms of civil behaviour? Within the female domain itself, how far down the class spectrum can we trace concepts of civility? Just as we might ask whether women had a culture of their own, distinct and perhaps different from that of men,[5] we can explore the possibility that both élite and ordinary women may have sustained their own cultural traditions of sociability and decorum, traditions that may have varied from one social setting or geographical locale to another.

Among the élite, women's civility was most often associated with generalized rules of manners and deportment rather than with specifically feminine attributes.[6] Aside from conferring a kind of irresistible charm on those who practised it, civility for Dame Sarah Cowper was understood as a system of paternalistic justice: 'Too much does better in civility than too little, but it ought not to be alike to all, for then it would degenerate into injustice. It is even a duty and in use among enemies, which shows the power of it.'[7] For élite women as well as their male counterparts, civility dictated the rules for

---

[3] Quoted in S. Mendelson, *The Mental World of Stuart Women* (Amherst, Mass., 1987), 65 and n. 12; Robert Boyle, *Occasional Reflections* (1665), sect. IV, 131.

[4] Herts. RO, Panshanger MSS, D/EP/F29, Dame Sarah Cowper, Diary, vol. i (1700–2), 291 (21 Oct. 1702). Dame Sarah was the wife of Sir William Cowper, 2nd baronet, and mother of William, first earl Cowper (d. 1723). Many thanks to Anne Kugler for sharing her scholarly expertise on the Cowper diaries.

[5] Mendelson and Crawford, *Women in Early Modern England*, ch. 4.

[6] For examples of general forms and rules of civility for élite women during the latter half of the seventeenth century, see the entry on 'Manners' in *The Ladies Dictionary* (1694), 314–19. Early modern manuals of female conduct were not quite analogous to male handbooks of civility; in fact, such works tended to highlight the dangers of courtly civility in undermining the all-important female virtues, chastity, piety, and silence; see e.g. Richard Brathwait, *The English Gentlewoman* (1631), 'Complement', 59–79.

[7] Cowper, Diary, i. 291.

appropriate modes of social interaction. The rules were not the same for all, however, but varied according to the relative status of the parties concerned. True civility for Dame Sarah could be defined as the art of giving to individuals their due according to their rank or place in society. Because anyone in the civic community could lay claim to a place in the social order, everyone merited some measure of civility, even enemies.

Notions of civility for Dame Sarah were thus intimately connected with the perception and outward expression of authority and hierarchy in a communal framework. Civility required a kind of self-referential mapping of the social system, a precise negotiation of competing (and sometimes contradictory) claims of authority. Conversely, the lack of civility implied the forfeiture of membership in the ranks of the élite. As Dame Sarah commented, 'clownishness makes one hated and despised. For if incivility proceeds from pride it deserves to be hated, if from brutishness it is contemptible.'[8] 'Clownishness', the opposite of 'civility', denoted not only rural origins but peasant or plebeian status. Indeed, most of the early modern antonyms for 'civil' were also used to refer to the plebeian or illiterate masses, such as the 'vulgar' or the 'rude multitude'.

For the duchess of Newcastle, the practice of civility was even more clearly associated with the duties and prerogatives of rank. In her brief autobiographical memoir (in which she used the terms 'civil' and 'civility' eleven times), the duchess explained why she and her siblings had not been 'sufferd to have any familiaritie with the vulgar servants, or conversation'. Instead, the Lucas children were taught to keep their social distance by demeaning themselves to the servants 'with an humble civillity towards them, as they with a dutifull respect to us'. As the duchess explained, 'not because they were servants were we so reserv'd . . . but by reason the vulgar sort of servants, are as ill bred as meanly born, giving children ill examples, and worse counsel'.[9]

For both sexes, the refinements of civil behaviour represented a crucial component in reinforcing the dichotomy between rich and poor, educated and illiterate, civilized gentility and brutish vulgarity. Élite commentators might interpret what they perceived as plebeian incivility in a negative sense, as the near-bestial condition of mankind in a Hobbesian state of nature. According to this scenario, the poor of both sexes were lumped together with other 'uncivilized' groups such as the Irish or Native Americans.[10] Alternatively,

---

[8] Ibid.

[9] Margaret Cavendish, duchess of Newcastle, 'A True Relation of my Birth, Breeding, and Life', in *Natures Pictures drawn by Fancies Pencil to the Life* (1656), 370–1.

[10] J. Leerssen, 'Wildness, Wilderness, and Ireland: Medieval and Early-Modern Patterns in the Demarcation of Civility', *Journal of the History of Ideas*, 56 (1995), 25–39; P. Mason, *Deconstructing America: Representations of the Other* (1990); B. W. Sheehan, *Savagism and Civility: Indians and Englishmen in Colonial Virginia* (Cambridge, 1980). See also M. Hendricks and P. Parker (eds.), *Women, 'Race', and Writing in the Early Modern Period* (1994).

some writers invoked the positive stereotype of the 'merry peasant' as a free and happy contrast to the repressive precepts of aristocratic self-restraint. In one of the duchess of Newcastle's imaginary sociable letters, she made an unfavourable comparison between the artificial decorum of the nobility, 'Constrain'd and bound with Forms and Rules', with what she supposed was the freer and more 'natural' behaviour of the lower orders:

whereas the Countrey Peasants meet with such Kind Hearts and Unconcerned Freedom as they Unite in Friendly Jollity, and Depart with Neighbourly Love, the Greater sort of Persons meet with Constrain'd Ceremony, Converse with Formality, and for the most part Depart with Enmity . . . for there is amongst the Better sort a greater Strife for Bravery than for Courtesie, for Place than Friendship, and in their Societies there is more Vain-glory than Pleasure, more Pride than Mirth, and more Vanity than true Content . . .[11]

Yet whether plebeian lack of manners was interpreted in a positive or negative sense, either stereotype of plebeian behaviour was based ultimately on the same aristocratic credo, the presumption that a refined and formalized code of civility was the prerogative of the upper ranks.

Although literate sources can tell us a good deal about the way notions of civility facilitated the 'self-fashioning' of élite women as civilized exemplars of their own class, we cannot assume that these sources supply us with direct knowledge of the manners and mores of the plebeian majority. The very importance of élite ideals of civility as a class marker led parents to try to shield their children of both sexes from the social contamination of their uncivil inferiors, as exemplified by the duchess of Newcastle's own childhood experiences. Indeed the duchess acknowledged her own ignorance of plebeian manners, implying that her depiction of peasant women as happy and free was a fantasy of her own creation. The minds of men are too various to be known, she concluded her sociable letter, 'and since we cannot Know our Selves how shall we know Others?'[12] If plebeian women sustained their own traditions of civil behaviour, we are unlikely to obtain an accurate account of their rites and ceremonies from élite commentators of either sex.

In enquiring about the civility of ordinary women, we encounter all the manifold obstacles that confront historians who try to investigate virtually any aspect of the beliefs and behaviour of the illiterate majority. Because early modern women were about 90 per cent illiterate with respect to writing ability, we do not have access to personal memoirs that we might compare with those of authors such as Dame Sarah Cowper or the duchess of Newcastle. Moreover, the rules of polite behaviour were more often than not expressed and perpetuated by example and other non-verbal means that

---

[11] Margaret Cavendish, *CCXI Sociable Letters* (1664), letter LV.
[12] Ibid., letter LV.

rarely evoked descriptive comment.[13] As Keith Thomas has pointed out, although the body is itself as much a historical document as a charter or diary or parish register, it is 'unfortunately one which is a good deal harder to preserve'.[14]

Even for aristocratic women, our evidence about the civility of gesture and bodily comportment in relation to the parameters of class and gender is relatively sparse. One of few such descriptive comments for early modern England is Mandeville's observation that children assimilated gender differences in deportment at an early age: whereas a girl of 3 had already learned by example to cover her legs modestly, a boy of the same age was urged to 'take up his Coats, and piss like a Man'.[15] More infrequent still was the depiction of plebeian women's bodily expressions of civility. Occasionally we can catch a glimpse of such formal gestures, as in Robert Boyle's account of the deferential bow of a pretty milkmaid: 'judging by our Cloaths, and more by *Lindamors* meen, that we were of a Quality differing from theirs she was wont to converse with, she gave us a Salute low enough to let us see that she forgot not her Condition, but attended with so much Gracefulness, as made *Lindamor* conclude she merited a better . . .'.[16]

Yet at least one early modern source offers us a wealth of explicit and implicit commentary on the civility of plebeian women, the records of the church courts. As far as gender is concerned, some types of litigation (for example, defamation suits, where civility was often a central issue) feature women in equal or greater numbers than men as litigants.[17] In the testimony of witnesses, we can observe ordinary men and women disputing over what was or was not considered civil behaviour. Frequently, deponents used the term 'civil' and its synonyms and antonyms to characterize, defend, or condemn the speech and behaviour of the parties in dispute. By examining the language and usage of the courts, and by analysing the implications of complex social interactions that were later shaped into detailed narratives in court depositions, we can reconstruct some of the elements of a code of civility for women in village society, which we can then compare with more familiar patterns typical of élite women.

---

[13] Bourdieu remarked that societies set such store on seemingly insignificant details of physical and verbal manners because 'treating the body as a memory, they entrust to it . . . the fundamental principles of the arbitrary content of the culture' (P. Bourdieu, *Outline of a Theory of Practice*, trans. R. Nice (Cambridge, 1977), 94, quoted in J. Tribby, 'Body/Building: Living the Museum Life in Early Modern Europe', *Rhetorica*, 10/2 (Spring 1992), 141).

[14] K. Thomas, 'Introduction', to J. Bremmer and H. Roodenburg (eds.), *A Cultural History of Gesture from Antiquity to the Present Day* (Cambridge, 1991), 2.

[15] B. Mandeville, *The Fable of the Bees: Or, Private Vices, Public Benefits*, ed. F. B. Kaye (2 vols.; Oxford, 1924), i. 71–2.

[16] Boyle, *Occasional Reflections*, sect. IV, 18.

[17] For women's role in defamation suits, see L. Gowing, 'Gender and the Language of Insult in Early Modern London', *History Workshop*, 35 (Spring 1993), 1–21, and, more generally, L. Gowing, *Domestic Dangers: Women, Words, and Sex in Early Modern London* (Oxford, 1996).

From the range of commentary in court records that refers to civil or uncivil conduct, we can distinguish two connotations of the term 'civil' in relation to female speech and behaviour. The first sense, already noted in the writings of élite women, is that of polite or appropriate modes of social interaction, whether with friends, relations, neighbours, strangers, or even enemies, for the rules of civility covered not only the ceremonies of friendship and neighbourliness, but the mediation of conflict and strife as well. Typically, accusations of incivility in this sense were likely to arise on occasions when questions of relative status in the local community were at issue. A common context for allegations of uncivil behaviour was in the course of disputes about church seating, the archetypal setting for plebeian women's contests over social status.[18] In a Devon suit in 1635, for example, witnesses alleged that Susan Richardson not only sat in the church pew where Mary Blight was accustomed to sit, but refused to allow Mary to sit in her usual place. When rebuked for doing so, Susan used 'many ill words and railing speeches' to Mary, and 'in railing uncivil manner' called her 'giglet[19] and young thing', 'proud minx', and the like. Susan concluded by telling Mary that 'thy husband hath better fed thee then taught thee, go home and learn more manners'.[20]

The words 'young' and 'proud' reiterated in Susan Richardson's 'railing speeches' point to the crux of the problem on this occasion, the question of which parameter of social ascendency, age or rank, should have taken precedence in public interactions between the two women. Mary Blight had acted on the assumption that her rank (defined by her husband's status) entitled her to the seat in question. But Susan Richardson employed a mode of 'uncivil' behaviour to call attention to her conviction that Mary Blight had violated the tenets of civility in the first instance, for she had failed to concede to her neighbour the extra deference due to age. The fact that two witnesses who had been sitting in the same pew were 'ancient' women aged 60 and 54 respectively would have added weight to Susan Richardson's claim.[21]

The arrangement of church seating always entailed the negotiation of diverse (and often conflicting) forms of authority in the local community, including the hierarchies of social or economic class, gender, age, marital status, civic office, and more nebulous factors such as personal repute. The number of disputes over church seating presented to the church courts during the early modern period suggests that neither churchwardens nor parishioners found it easy to resolve these competing claims to social ascendency. Age was in practice one of the more difficult parameters to accommodate to other

---

[18] K. Dillow, 'The Social and Ecclesiastical Significance of Church Seating Arrangements and Pew Disputes, 1500–1740', D. Phil. diss. (Oxford, 1990), 129–42.

[19] Giglet: a giddy, romping girl.

[20] Devon RO, Chanter 866, Diocesan Court Depositions 1634–40 [not foliated or paginated], *Blight* v. *Richardson*, 13 Mar. 1635, testimony of Mary Bawler and Elizabeth Caseley.

[21] Ibid.

forms of authority, because the idealized status of the elderly in a patriarchal society was so often at odds with their actual power and prestige in everyday life.[22] It may have been partly for this reason that the code of village civility demanded an extra margin of courtesy from more prosperous women towards their elderly friends and neighbours, just as women of the upper ranks were supposed to be scrupulously polite and attentive to their aged relations, including those of inferior social status.[23]

The second connotation of civil behaviour in church court records refers to civility as modesty or sexual propriety, especially in relation to female conduct. The word 'civil' frequently appears in depositions as a synonym for 'modest', 'sober', or 'chaste' as a description of a woman's speech and deportment. Defamation causes in particular were apt to focus on female civility in the sense of modesty or sexual decorum. This usage of the word was constrained at least in part by the legal framework of defamation suits: if it could be proved that the plaintiff was uncivil in the sense of being immodest or unchaste, then the alleged insult was no defamation. Thus, for example, a witness in a 1616 Oxfordshire suit affirmed that Joan Rose had never been suspected of any kind of 'lewdness', but 'did always behave her self civilly and honestly'. In a Devon suit, Ellen Searle was described as a 'modest civil woman' who could not have been the wife of a cuckold, as her defamer had insisted. In London in 1632, a witness defended Margaret Eddise (who had been called a whore) by assuring the court that Margaret had 'behaved herself very civilly and well'.[24]

On the other hand, lack of civility in the sense of immodesty or sexual impropriety was also well documented in the records of the church courts. In 1627 in the London parish of St Botolph Aldgate, Elizabeth Hobridge claimed she saw some 'uncivil behaviour' of Mary Peters in the company of Michael Drayton: to wit, Mary Peters 'did show her tail unto and before the said Mr Drayton'. Men too could be characterized as uncivil in the sense of sexual impropriety, if their behaviour was sufficiently aggressive. James Vesey was described as 'rude and uncivil' to a maidservant whom he tried to rape; in contrast, Vesey's wife was depicted by a dozen witnesses as 'modest, chaste and civil in her life and conversation'.[25]

[22] K. Thomas, *Age and Authority in Early Modern England* (1977).

[23] For more on the topic of women and ageing, see Mendelson and Crawford, *Women in Early Modern England*, 184–94. The principle that age trumps class in the female code of civility was not limited to the early modern period. Susan Richardson's admonition to Mary Blight that her husband should teach her better manners reminds us of the scene in Jane Austen's *Emma* in which Mr Knightly delivers a stern lecture to Emma on the duties of civility and *noblesse oblige*, after Emma's uncivil treatment of her poor old neighbour Miss Bates.

[24] Oxon. RO, MS Archd. Papers Oxon. c. 118, 1616–20, fo. 36; Devon RO, Chanter 878, Consistory Court Depositions 1679–81, fo. 16; Guildhall Library, London, MS 9057, vol. i, fo. 11 (*Eddise* v. *Sadd*, 1 Dec. 1632).

[25] Guildhall Library, London, MS 9189, vol. ii, fo. 21 (*Welch* v. *Peters*, 29 May 1627); Greater London RO, DL/C/241, fos. 1–14 (*Vesey* v. *Vesey*, 7 Apr. 1684).

Witnesses' depositions attached to an Oxfordshire suit and counter-suit for defamation presented in 1616 and 1617 reveal some of the ambiguities and contradictions inherent in notions of plebeian female civility as modesty.[26] Both the suit and counter-suit were part of the fallout from a prior incident in which James Bonham had assaulted Margaret Woodbridge when she was alone in her house in Halton:

> one Bonham did come to [Margaret], and by force [did] pluck off some part of the hair of her privy parts, and . . . her husband William Woodbridge coming in and finding her and the said Bonham to be there alone together she . . . [complained] unto him of the said Bonhams force and abuse towards her and [did] take up her clothes and show her privities unto one Bledlowe happening into the said house a very little while before the coming in of her said husband . . .[27]

The story quickly spread and Margaret became the butt of masculine village humour. When a man was pestering a young woman at Thomas Wyse's mill, Wyse told him to let her alone, for she was 'not as Goodwife Woodbridge is . . . Bonham did fetch off a handful of hair of the one side of her, using the bawdy name of her privy parts, and the other side is bald'.[28] Margaret sued Thomas Wyse for defamation, claiming her good name had been 'much impaired' by his scandalous words. But Wyse quickly retaliated with a counter-suit, presenting several male witnesses who portrayed Margaret as a drunken and disorderly woman who had brought scandal on herself through her immodest and uncivil deportment. Defending Wyse, Richard Bledlowe described how Margaret Woodbridge did 'uncivilly and beastly . . . take up her clothes above her navel to show her wrong or hurt unto her husband' in Bledlowe's presence.[29] Although on this occasion Margaret Woodbridge was herself the injured party, whose exposure of her injury was not intended as a sexual act, she was nevertheless cast in the role of offender because of her immodest display of that which should have been concealed from all men except her husband.

As we sift through the various usages of the words 'civil' and 'civility' in church court records, we begin to see a gender dimension in concepts of civility among the plebeian classes. There were important implications for women's status *qua* women in the notion that ideals of female civility had a sexual component. Just as the lack of civility in the social sense was liable to lead to the forfeiture of social rank, a defect in civility in the sexual sense implied the loss of gender status for women, since 'uncivil' was taken to be a synonym for 'immodest' or 'unchaste'. It was for this reason that the early modern judiciary allowed prostitutes to be stripped to the waist when

---

[26] Oxon. RO, MS Archd. Papers Oxon. c. 118, 1616–20, fos. 34–34ᵛ (*Woodbridge* v. *Wyse*, 9 Dec. 1616); ibid., fos. 60ᵛ–62ᵛ (*Wyse* v. *Woodbridge*, 22 Mar. 1617).

[27] Oxon. RO, MS Archd. Papers Oxon. c. 118, 1616–20, fo. 60ᵛ.

[28] Ibid., fo. 34.   [29] Ibid., fo. 62ᵛ.

subjected to a public whipping as a punishment for sexual misconduct: a convicted prostitute had forfeited her place in the civil order, and with it she had lost the prerogatives of female modesty, including the right to be shielded from men's predatory gaze.[30]

But civility for ordinary women was not a simple dichotomy or 'double standard', whereby social courtesy was required for both sexes and all classes, and sexual modesty or propriety was imposed upon women. The practice of plebeian civility was far more complicated, for, while the social and sexual connotations of the word 'civil' can be differentiated in theory, in practice they were apt to blur into each other, especially in the context of female behaviour and gender relations in village society. Moreover, the existence of hierarchical gender domains in early modern England itself generated a series of overlapping codes of civility which sometimes reinforced and sometimes conflicted with each other.

First, ordinary women were taught to practise the civility of deference, which related both to the class hierarchy and the gender order. The courtesy of deference was always a double burden for plebeian women, who were obliged to show dutiful subservience to the rich of both sexes, their social superiors, as well as to men, their 'natural' superiors. Secondly, women *qua* women cultivated the civility of female friendship and neighbourliness, a more-or-less egalitarian code that dictated polite modes of sociable interaction within the female domain. It is particularly difficult to reconstruct the rites and ceremonies of female-to-female civility at the plebeian level, since women valued their privacy within their own sphere, and were generally reluctant to reveal in mixed company what they had been doing or talking about while men were not around. Thus we have few details about plebeian social rites and customs that accompanied the archetypal setting for the exchange of female civilities, the ceremony of lying-in or childbed.[31] Yet on occasion the courts, for purposes of their own, asked female witnesses to bring private matters to the public view. If we pay close attention to witnesses's reports of conversations and their narrative reconstructions of events, we can catch a glimpse of complex social interactions in which women dexterously negotiated the different codes of plebeian civility that helped give structure and meaning to the sociable interactions of daily life.

In the 1631 Oxfordshire suit *Office* v. *Godman et Scoulter alias Godman* we can observe women from different sectors of village society attempting to

---

[30] Men were well aware of the ironies inherent in this situation: 'Why dost thou lash that whore? Strip thine own back, | Thou hotly lusts to use her in that kind | For which thou whipp'st her' (*King Lear*, Act IV, Sc. vi).

[31] See P. Crawford, 'The Construction and Experience of Maternity', and A. Wilson, 'The Ceremony of Childbirth and its Interpretation', both in V. Fildes (ed.), *Women as Mothers in Pre-Industrial England* (1990).

impose plebeian norms of civil behaviour in a situation fraught with conflict, where the civil authorities had themselves failed to stem the tide of disorder. The suit was a promoted office (or disciplinary) cause brought to the attention of the Oxford Diocesan court by a third party.[32] In 1631 the court heard a number of depositions concerning allegations against a young unmarried woman named Elizabeth Scoulter living in the village of Kencot. During the summer of 1630, Elizabeth's aunt, Katherine Hulot, had gone to the rector of Kencot with complaints about Elizabeth, who was living at the time with her grandmother, the widow Hulot. Widow Hulot had told her daughter Katherine Hulot that James Godman was in the habit of visiting her granddaughter Elizabeth at 'unseasonable times' of the night, that she 'much misliked' James Godman's frequenting of her house, and feared there might be 'mischief done and a child begotten between him and Besse [Elizabeth]'.[33] Widow Hulot had appealed to Katherine to deal with Elizabeth, since she herself was too 'old and blind' to be able to 'see to it'.

Katherine later reported that she had tried to admonish Elizabeth, but got only 'churlish and froward speeches' from her. Katherine Hulot then brought her story to the local rector, Mr James Fretherne, telling him it concerned him to see such matters reformed, 'for you are our minister and teacher'. Fretherne's response was to 'advise and persuade . . . James Godman to marry the said Elizabeth Scoulter or else not to frequent her company any more'.[34] Nevertheless, Godman continued to visit Elizabeth at 'unseasonable times' but gave no indication he intended to marry her.[35]

Some months later, rumours circulated in the village that Elizabeth Scoulter, while very weak and ill, had been escorted by James Godman from her grandmother's house to her mother's house during the night in order to bear an illegitimate child in secret with her mother's help. Local suspicions were aggravated by the fact that she returned to her grandmother's house within a day. No material evidence of the birth came to light, but rumour and scandal had reached such a pitch that a 'search' or examination of Elizabeth Scoulter's body by 'ancient women' of the village was organized by Mr and Mrs Fretherne, to determine whether Elizabeth 'had had a child and concealed the same',[36] presumably disposing of it afterward with her mother's aid or connivance.[37]

The search or inspection of a woman's body by a duly constituted 'jury of matrons' to determine physical signs of pregnancy or recent childbirth was

[32] For the depositions associated with this cause and with a related suit for defamation, see Oxon. RO, MS Oxford Dioc. Papers c. 26, Consistory Court Depositions 1629–34, fos. 141ᵛ–148, 153ᵛ–159 (*Giles Swet* v. *James Godman et Elizabeth Scoulter alias Godman*), and fos. 167–71 (*Scoulter* v. *Fretherne*).

[33] Ibid., fo. 155ᵛ.   [34] Ibid., fo. 156.   [35] Ibid., fo. 141ᵛ.   [36] Ibid., fo. 167ᵛ.

[37] For the general topic of single women's maternity and concealed births, see L. Gowing, 'Secret Births and Infanticide in Seventeenth-Century England', *P&P* 156 (1997), 87–115; see also Mendelson and Crawford, *Women in Early Modern England*, 148–51.

a common feature of early modern criminal trials involving plebeian female suspects who appeared before the secular courts.[38] In the case of Elizabeth Scoulter, however, the search was not the result of a court order, but a much more informal and impromptu affair. The coercive powers of this unofficial 'jury of matrons' were debatable, since the search itself had been prompted by nothing more substantial than village gossip and rumour. Yet the enquiry into Elizabeth Scoulter's alleged crime was ultimately unsuccessful in its aim of putting an end to village suspicions, not only because the search lacked the seal of official judiciary approval, but also because the ambiguities inherent in the situation were heightened by contradictions between conflicting models of civility that patterned the ceremonial of the investigation and its aftermath.

The enquiry into the activities of James Godman and Elizabeth Scoulter had its inception in the civility of deference, as female members of the Hulot–Scoulter family appealed to the authority of James Fretherne in his acknowledged civic role, the 'political responsibilities of the Priest-Magistrate', as it was expressed in the discourse of civil letters.[39] It is difficult to imagine where else the Hulot women might have turned for paternalistic aid. Not only were they a poor and powerless female-headed household trying unsuccessfully to control a young girl who showed herself defiantly uncivil towards family authority.[40] The village constable, the representative of secular civil order in the local community, was none other than James Godman, who was cited together with Elizabeth Scoulter in the promoted ecclesiastical suit. According to witnesses' testimony, Godman appears to have adopted a schizophrenic attitude towards his dual role as village constable and seducer of young women. He remarked to his friend the village tithingman that he thought Elizabeth Scoulter ought to clear herself of suspicion, because he was worried about his 'oath' as constable; meanwhile he told the rector that he would not marry Elizabeth if the rumours about her proved true, 'for he said he would not marry a whore'.[41]

Just as the Hulot women brought their complaints of civil disorder to their minister in his role as 'Priest–Magistrate', they showed an analogous form of the civility of deference by simultaneously appealing for help to his wife, Mrs Anne Fretherne. As Mrs Fretherne later reminded the widow Hulot, 'you told me that I was the chiefest woman in the town and that it behoved me to look to this'.[42] In so doing, the widow Hulot acknowledged the existence of a parallel female hierarchy, whereby women of élite status might serve informally

[38] J. C. Oldham, 'On Pleading the Belly: A History of the Jury of Matrons', *Criminal Justice History*, 6 (1985), 1–64.

[39] Hall, *Ceremony and Civility*, 139–47.

[40] There is no mention of a male Hulot or Scoulter in the depositions for this cause.

[41] Oxon. RO, MS Oxford Dioc. Papers c. 26, Consistory Court Depositions 1629–34, fo. 143[v].

[42] Ibid., fo. 146[v].

in a magisterial capacity in the local community, especially as mediators or advocates, even if they held no formal office. While discourses of civil government warned that a woman was forbidden to exercise judicial power over men in a general sense, she might be permitted to do so in a compassionate context—for example, in securing the pardon of a wrongly convicted prisoner.[43]

Aside from the civility of deference owed to Anne Fretherne as the highest female representative of her class in village society, she was also called to take a leading role in subsequent events because Elizabeth Scoulter's alleged misdeeds fell into the realm of 'female matters' from which men were normally excluded. Once the enquiry into Godman and Scoulter's activities was brought into the female sphere, however, social interactions became subsumed into ideals of female friendship and neighbourliness, whose essential spirit was at odds with the disciplinary aims of male institutional authorities.

The ceremonies of female friendship were designed to allow women to display the appropriate degree of concern for each others' welfare, comfort, and self-esteem. We can observe the women of Kencot exchanging such tokens of courtesy and mutual concern, even as they plunged more deeply into their investigation of the Godman–Scoulter affair. Indeed, all the female-to-female conversations between members of the Hulot–Scoulter ménage and their neighbours (later recounted by female witnesses in court testimony) had been prefaced with the universal formula of plebeian civility, of asking a friend or neighbour 'how she did', and then enquiring how other members of the extended family 'did' as well. Even Mrs Fretherne was constrained by *noblesse oblige* to use the same formula when, seated astride her horse, she encountered the widow Hulot standing in her daughter's doorway: 'did not I call to you and asked you how your kinswoman did and you made answer that she was very ill.'[44]

Nor were these enquiries about the health and welfare of the Hulot–Scoulter family mere empty formalities. When the Widow Hulot replied to neighbours that her granddaughter Besse was 'very ill', several village women immediately responded by paying a visit to the ailing Elizabeth at her mother's house, to learn 'how she did' and to ask 'what she ailed'. After Elizabeth's mother gave the visiting female delegation 'frivolous' answers to their enquiries, refusing to supply details about what precisely was wrong with

---

[43] For women's right to take part in civil government solely in a compassionate context, see Sir Thomas Elyot, *The Boke named the Gouernour* (1531), bk II, vii, 'Mercyfuless'. As an example from real life, the countess of Warwick served as neighbourhood peacemaker to all and sundry during the 1670s, arbitrating quarrels between family members, neighbours, and even three ministers on one occasion. In this informal role her social ascendancy and her reputation for unbiased rectitude outweighed any disadvantages represented by her sex. See Mendelson, *Mental World*, 110–15.

[44] Oxon. RO, MS Oxford Dioc. Papers c. 26, fo. 145.

Elizabeth, village matrons put together rumour and scandal with their own suspicions about the true nature of Elizabeth's malady.[45]

Even the search itself had the atmosphere of a sick visit or childbed gathering almost as much as of a judicial enquiry. Although it began like a parish procession with James Fretherne at its head, as the Frethernes collected various 'ancient matrons' of the village from their homes and marched them in a body to the Widow Hulot's house, the search was immediately transformed into an all-female occasion. As soon as James Fretherne had explained matters to the Scoulters, he left the house, delegating the examination of Elizabeth Scoulter's body to his wife and the other respectable matrons who had accompanied the Frethernes. This strict separation of male and female spheres was dictated by early modern notions about the civility of dress and nakedness as they related to gender domains. Just as Native Americans were categorized by Europeans as beyond the pale of civilization because they did not wear clothes, a woman who allowed her unclothed body to be seen by a man other than her husband was judged to be outside the bounds of civilized society.[46]

Within the private realm of female relationships, in contrast, the civility of friendship not only allowed but encouraged women to reveal intimate details of their bodily condition to each other, especially during the travails of pregnancy and childbirth.[47] Yet this form of bodily intimacy was permitted between female friends and neighbours for a specific purpose, to enable them to show attentive concern and to give appropriate aid and advice. Because of the fragile physical and emotional state of the childbearing woman, those who were invited into the ritual space of lying-in or childbed were scrupulous in observing the ceremonies of courtesy towards her. For example, any form of quarrelsome or contentious behaviour was strongly discouraged in this setting.[48]

Once they had been commandeered by the Frethernes into conducting a search of Elizabeth Scoulter's body, the matrons of Kencot thus found themselves torn between two conflicting ideals of plebeian female civility. Had they come in the spirit of female friendship, to show neighbourly concern for a dangerously ill young woman who may or may not have been suffering from the trauma of recent childbirth? Or were they, in their compliance with the civility of deference, being manœuvred into exploiting the special intimacy of female-to-female relations to serve the disciplinary objectives of external authority? If the latter, then the searchers' confirmation of recent childbirth

---

[45] Ibid., fo. 143.

[46] Mason, *Deconstructing America*, 170–2; note the extreme repugnance with which witnesses described Margaret Woodbridge's 'beastly' behaviour (above, n. 29).

[47] Mendelson and Crawford, *Women in Early Modern England*, 151, 239.

[48] See e.g. Folger Shakespeare Library, Washington, DC, Rich MSS, X. d. 453, no. 46, cited in Mendelson and Crawford, *Women in Early Modern England*, 214.

might have rendered Elizabeth Scoulter vulnerable to possible capital punishment, under the 1624 Statute 'to Prevent the Murthering of Bastard
Children'.[49]

When Elizabeth Scoulter showed herself unwilling to be searched, weeping
and 'affirming earnestly that she had had no child', the ancient matrons of
Kencot appear to have been reluctant to press her, as they vacillated between
duty and compassion. Alice Goodenough testified that 'Mrs Fretherne wished
. . . that they might see [Elizabeth's] breasts whereupon . . . Elizabeth opened
her breast a little and this deponent put her hand into . . . Elizabeths bosom
and felt her breast and her nipple and drew her nipple a little but finding
her so poor and weak this deponent was loath to tamper further with her'.[50]
At this point, witnesses reported, Mrs Fretherne pulled out her own breast
and said 'look you here huswife[51] your breast is not as mine is'. Although
intended to coerce Elizabeth Scoulter into confessing her guilt, Anne Fretherne's action had the opposite effect of calling attention to her own alien status
in this quasi-childbed gathering, for she herself at age 40 had never borne a
child. Indeed, she conceded her own lack of matronly expertise, assuring the
Scoulters that 'if you dislike me because I have had no child . . . then take
whom you will'.[52]

Nevertheless, her officious intervention was singled out by the Hulot–
Scoulter ménage as a manifestation of malice and bad faith, of punitive
authority rather than neighbourly concern. When Mrs Fretherne asked
Goodwife Scoulter why she would not allow her daughter to be searched, she
replied, 'because you come to disgrace my daughter'.[53] Countering Mrs
Fretherne's threat that the matrons of Kencot would support her contention that Elizabeth had been 'newly delivered of a child' ('here be two neighbours that bear witness what I say'), Goodwife Scoulter adroitly turned the
remark around, representing it as a slander uttered by Mrs Fretherne: 'they
shall witness that Mrs Fretherne says thee hast a child.'[54] Meanwhile, the Scoulters launched a suit for defamation against Anne Fretherne in the church
courts.[55]

Detailed analysis of conversations reported in depositions attached to the
Scoulter case would reveal more subtle features of the plebeian art of civility,
such as women's skilful use of wit and circumlocution to obfuscate and deflect
the inquisitorial efforts of their social superiors.[56] But even the brief account

[49] 21 Jac. I, c. 7; for the context of this statute, see Mendelson and Crawford, *Women in Early Modern England*, 44–5; see also Gowing, 'Secret Births'.
[50] Oxon. RO, MS Oxford Dioc. Papers c. 26, fo. 144[v].
[51] i.e. 'hussy', an ill-behaved or mischievous girl.
[52] Oxon. RO, MS Oxford Dioc. Papers c. 26, fos. 146–146[v].
[53] Ibid., fo. 158[v].   [54] Ibid., fo. 147[v].   [55] Ibid., fos. 167–70.
[56] Many of these plebeian conversational strategies found their echoes in élite prescriptive rules for civil behaviour. For example, *The Ladies Dictionary* advised its readers, 'when you answer *no* in contradiction to some person of quality, you must not say bluntly or positively, *no*, but by way of Circumlocution' (*The Ladies Dictionary*, 314).

of the case presented here has shown that patterns of civility formed an essential part of the structure of women's everyday life in village society. The case also illustrates the complexity of plebeian norms of polite behaviour, for the civility of ordinary women was governed not by one but by multiple codes of sociability and deportment. In a society where both the maintenance of social hierarchy and the perpetuation of self-contained gender domains were fundamental concerns, the coexistence of different codes of civility entailed the continual mediation of conflict—in this case between class and gender, the civility of deference and the tenets of female friendship.

It is clear from our examination of the various usages of the terms 'civil' and 'civility' in different female contexts that ideals of civility were highly significant for women of every social class. Indeed, the records of the church courts suggest that concepts of civility among the illiterate female populace were at least as complex, and certainly as important to their practitioners, as those of the upper ranks. Much like their aristocratic sisters, plebeian women understood the practice of civility as a process of negotiating the boundaries of authority, of conferring on each person the courtesy and concern due to his or her place in the civil order. And for both élite and ordinary women, gender introduced further complications into their sociable lives, as they navigated the shifting contours of divergent codes of propriety and decorum generated by the separate domains in which they had their social being.

Yet we might argue that the practice of civility called for even more creative skill and finesse on the part of ordinary women, as compared with those situated at the apex of the social order. Participating in an oral rather than a literate culture, plebeian women had no access to handbooks of courtesy and civility, to written rules of precedence, to the numerous literary and material artefacts of civilized gentility produced by and for the educated élite. Because they were not 'constrain'd and bound with Forms and Rules' codified in written records, plebeian women confronted a much more fluid and ambiguous situation. Without a village Garter King of Arms to pronounce on matters of precedence and decorum, they were obliged to settle conflicting claims of status and authority for themselves *in medias res*, in the very act of behaving civilly or uncivilly to each other.

7

Civilization and Deodorization?
Smell in Early Modern English Culture

MARK S. R. JENNER

> An eminent professor of mathematicks affirmed to me, that, chanc-
> ing one day in the heat of summer, with another mathematician
> . . . to pass by a large dunghil . . . in *Lincoln's-Inn Fields*, when they
> came to a certain distance from it, they were both . . . surprised to
> meet with a . . . strong smell of musk, (occasioned, probably, by a
> . . . kind of putrefaction,) which each was for a while shy of taking
> notice of, for fear his companion should have laughed at him for
> it; but, when they came much nearer . . . that pleasing smell was
> succeeded by a stink proper to such a heap of excrements.
>
> (Robert Boyle (1772))[1]

If natural philosopher acquaintances of Robert Boyle were reluctant to discourse about smells for fear of ridicule, university-based historians, seeking
to establish the civil and cerebral nature of their discipline, were even warier
of discussing such grossly corporeal themes.[2] Only a few social historians
remarked upon the importance of smell in the cultures that they were studying. Keith Thomas, for instance, remarked how in witchcraft cases 'stinking
. . . living-quarters were . . . taken as evidence' of animal familiars, noted the
importance of odours in herbalists' classification of plants, and drew attention
to the opinion of the eighteenth-century physician George Cheyne that God
made horses' excrement sweet-smelling because humans would spend so
much time near it.[3]

I am grateful to the audiences in Cambridge, Leicester, and London who commented on
my papers on smell in early modern England, and to Fay Bound, Justin Champion, James
Robertson, Jenny Smith, and Adrian Wilson. Above all my profound thanks to Patricia Greene
for her encouragement and her perceptive comments.

[1] R. Boyle, 'Experiments and Observations about the Mechanical Production of Odours', in
R. Boyle, *Works*, ed. T. Birch (6 vols., 1772), iv. 271.

[2] On how the professionalization of history denigrated research into 'manners' and other
bodily themes, see M. S. R. Jenner and B. O. Taithe, 'The Historiographical Body', in R. Cooter
and J. V. Pickstone (eds.), *Medicine in the Twentieth Century* (forthcoming).

[3] K. Thomas, *Religion and the Decline of Magic: Studies in Popular Beliefs in Sixteenth and Sev-*

With the recent somatic turn in the humanities, historians have begun to pay increasing attention to the history of sensibilities and the senses, including the olfactory. Alain Corbin's *The Foul and the Fragrant* (1982; English translation, 1986) was indubitably *the* pioneer in this cultural history of smell. As Frank Kermode noted, it 'created . . . a stir . . . partly . . . because no respected historian had ever before written . . . so explicitly, about shit'.[4] Despite the unsystematic nature of its arguments and chronology, Corbin's work has been widely influential. But he was neither the sole progenitor of this new historiography, nor simply a historical byway in the denigration of sight in twentieth-century French thought.[5] Historians' interest in the olfactory coincided with an increased use of odours in representations of the past.

In 1984 the York Archaeological Trust opened Jorvik, one of the first museum experiences in which you could 'smell the past'. Despite the Adornoesque ruminations of some sniffy commentators, Jorvik essayed a pioneering new historical and museological poetics of the sensorium, which sought to communicate directly with the public.[6] No matter how much historians grub around in archives and no matter how colourful and evocative the vocabulary we employ, we are not going to produce work that is as pungent as the scratch and sniff cards of the Viking privy that you can buy at the end of your trip under Coppergate.[7] As Barthes concluded in his study of De Sade, 'Written down, shit does not smell; Sade can drench his partners in it, we receive no effluvia from it, only the abstract sign of something disagreeable.'[8] In history and anthropology the real and the written are inevitably severed.

Although Jorvik transgressively foregrounds behaviour normally confined to what Erving Goffman termed 'back space',[9] its smellscapes contain some highly conventional stories about history, hygiene, and olfaction. First, it reinscribes what the celebrated Chaucer scholar Terry Jones has dubbed the toilet-training theory of history—the notion that the remote past was marked by

enteenth Century England (1971), 731; *Man and the Natural World: Changing Attitudes in England 1500–1800* (1983), 53, 82, 19.

  [4] F. Kermode, 'With the Aid of a Lorgnette', *London Review of Books*, 16/8 (28 Apr. 1994), 14.

  [5] M. Jay, *Downcast Eyes: The Denigration of Vision in Twentieth-Century French Thought* (Berkeley and Los Angeles, 1993).

  [6] On its search for directness, see P. V. Addyman, 'Reconstruction as Interpretation: The Example of the Jorvik Viking Centre, York', in P. Gathercole and D. Lowenthal (eds.), *The Politics of the Past* (1990), 259–63.

  [7] Recent claims by some anthropologists that abandoning the social-scientific conventions of ethnographic writing 'would take us beyond the mind's eye and into the domain of the senses of smell and taste' miss the fundamental distinction between the *textual* invocation of a sense and its lived reality: P. Stoller, *The Taste of Ethnographic Things* (Philadelphia, 1989), 27 and *passim*. Cf. D. Howes, 'Controlling Textuality: A Call for a Return to the Senses', *Anthropologica*, 32 (1990), 55–73; C. Classen, 'Sweet Colors, Fragrant Songs: Sensory Models of the Andes and the Amazon', *American Ethnologist*, 17 (1990), 732.

  [8] R. Barthes, *Sade, Fourier, Loyola* (Paris, 1971), 140 (my translation).

  [9] E. Goffman, *The Presentation of Self in Everyday Life* (1959).

squalor and stench, and modernity by a *nostalgie de la merde*. The past, the visitor learns, *smelt*. These excremental odours construct a narrative of progress and deodorization. They reinforce the way in which dirt signifies otherness and the past in popular and not-so-popular historiography, and ignore how dirt is a culturally relative concept, being what offends 'the eye of the beholder', the nose of the inhaler, and the cultural rules of a particular society.[10] Secondly, the Jorvik experience (consciously or not) suggests that smell was more central to earlier societies than our own. Simpler peoples and less literate cultures, it is often argued, were more attuned to sounds, tactile experiences, and above all to variations in smell. Drawing on studies that stress how far perceptions are culturally mediated,[11] this paper will explore the meanings of certain smells in early modern England and challenge these two grand narratives of smell and civilization.

I

Freud's *Civilization and its Discontents* is perhaps the most elegant and influential account of the devaluing of smell over the centuries. Significantly he related the repression of the olfactory and increasing recourse to 'modern' hygienic practices. 'The diminution of the olfactory stimuli' in human beings, he suggested, was a necessary part of 'the fateful process of civilization'. It was concomitant with the adoption of an upright gait. 'A social factor', he added, 'is also unmistakeably present in the cultural trend towards cleanliness. . . . The incitement to cleanliness originates in an urge to get rid of . . . excreta, which have become disagreeable to sense perceptions.' But this revulsion towards faeces 'would scarcely be possible if the substances that are expelled from the body were not doomed by their strong smells to share the fate which overtook olfactory stimuli after man adopted the erect posture'.[12]

Freud's speculations traversed a grandly Darwinian timescale; more historically minded thinkers have located similar shifts in the more recent past. Corbin suggested that between the mid-eighteenth and late nineteenth centuries urban space was deodorized. Other authors have claimed that the early modern period saw a significant shift from olfaction and from hearing to the cultural primacy of sight and that the sixteenth century placed particular emphasis upon the sense of smell. 'Observation, from the seventeenth century

[10] Cf. M. Douglas, *Purity and Danger* (1966), 2.

[11] On the cultural conditioning of olfactory perception, see E. Cohen, 'The Broken Cycle: Smell in a Bangkok Soi (Lane)', *Ethnos*, 53 (1988), 37–49; W. E. A. van Beek, 'The Dirty Smith: Smell as a Social Frontier among the Kapsiki/Higi of North Cameroon and North-Eastern Nigeria', *Africa*, 62 (1992), 38; P. Rodaway, *Sensuous Geographies* (1994), ch. 4.

[12] S. Freud, *Civilization and its Discontents*, in *Civilization, Society and Religion* (Penguin Freud Library, 12; 1985), 288–9 n.

onwards,' declared Foucault, 'is a perceptible knowledge furnished with a
series of systematically negative conditions. Hearsay is excluded . . . so too are
taste and smell.' 'The eye', declared Norbert Elias, 'takes on a very specific
significance in civilized society,' becoming the principal 'mediator of pleasure'.
Like touch, 'the sense of smell, the tendency to sniff at food or other things,
comes to be restricted as . . . animal-like'.[13] 'Whereas today smell and taste
are relatively unimportant by comparison with the other three senses,' wrote
Robert Mandrou, 'the men of the sixteenth century were extremely suscep-
tible to scents and perfumes.' Mandrou was developing Lucien Febvre's claim
that the 'sixteenth century did not see first: it heard and smelled'. Its inhabitants, Febvre continued, 'were open-air men, seeing nature but also feeling,
sniffing . . . breathing her'.[14] Like Freud, Mandrou and Febvre represent olfaction as a more 'natural' sense and as one that has atrophied with the development of culture.

Such ideas have a long pedigree. In 1667 Henry Oldenburg reported John
Beale's suggestion that humans 'by . . . drink of water only, bread, and food
of litle odor, clean lodgings &c. may have . . . a more universall extent in
smelling, than Dogs or Vulturs'.[15] Meanwhile, in a narrative that anticipated
the Enlightenment fascination with the sensory skills of the wild boy of
Aveyron,[16] Kenelm Digby wrote of a boy who had grown up living alone in
a forest in the Ardennes on a diet of roots and who consequently 'could att a
great distance wind by his nose, where wholesome fruites or rootes did grow'.
However, 'a litle while after he came to good keeping and full feeding, [he]
quite lost that acutenesse of smelling'.[17]

Febvre's and Mandrou's portrayals of Ronsard and Rabelais as unalienated
organic intellectuals sniffing the air is massively overdrawn. It is not as if
sixteenth- and seventeenth-century people possessed a highly elaborated
vocabulary for smells that has been lost over the last three hundred years.
Tudor and Stuart people did not subtly distinguish between many different
types of odour in the ways that the Inuit were once alleged to be capable
of differentiating between a myriad qualities of snow.[18] Comenius's mid-

---

[13] Corbin, *Foul and Fragrant*, pt. II; M. Foucault, *The Order of Things*, Eng. trans. (1970), 132;
N. Elias, *The Civilizing Process*, trans. E. Jephcott (Oxford, 1978), 203.

[14] R. Mandrou, *Introduction to Modern France 1500–1640*, trans. R. E. Hallmark (New York,
1976), 54; L. Febvre, *The Problem of Unbelief in the Sixteenth Century*, trans. B. Gottlieb
(Cambridge, Mass., 1982), 432, 424.

[15] *The Correspondence of Henry Oldenburg*, ed. A. R. Hall and M. B. Hall (13 vols.; Madison
and London, 1965–86), iii. 509.

[16] C. Classen, 'The Sensory Orders of "Wild Children"', in D. Howes (ed.), *The Varieties of
Sensory Experience* (Toronto, 1991).

[17] K. Digby, *Two Treatises. In the one of which, the Nature of Bodies; in the Other, the Nature of
Mans Soule; is Looked into* (Paris, 1644), 247–8. A garbled version of this story was retold in C. N.
Le Cat, *A Physical Essay on the Senses* (1750), 31–2.

[18] L. Martin, '"Eskimo Words for Snow": A Case Study in the Genesis and Decay of an
Anthropological Example', *American Anthropologist*, 88 (1986), 418–23.

seventeenth-century educational text *Orbis pictus* noted that the nose scented 'smels and stinks'—that was it.[19] Other early modern dictionaries reveal a similarly impoverished vocabulary with which to treat the sensations of the nose. Both the widely diffused iconography of the five senses,[20] and dominant strands of Aristotelian philosophy, concurred on the primacy of sight.[21]

Nevertheless, odours did arouse more explicit concerns in areas of early modern English culture than today. As Mary Dobson has recently shown, the olfactory quality of airs was a standard feature of topographical description.[22] Smells that we might consider simply unpleasant could be as fatal as mustard gas. During the late 1640s two London apprentices who had participated in Royalist demonstrations fled to Paris. There one of them fell ill. His companion's diary records that he came downstairs and met their landlord who 'made great complaints yt [he, the sick man] going to stoole in ye Chamber did anoy his howse & would bring the plague in his house . . .'. 'I made them answer', the diarist continues, 'yt what came from him [i.e. the sick apprentice] was only Jelly and water & had no sent', but nevertheless resolved that they should seek fresh accommodation.[23]

The landlord's fear of the disease-bringing power of smell would have made perfect sense on the other side of the Channel. Throughout the sixteenth and early seventeenth centuries the olfactory drove social policy with regard to the regulation of London's public space. An examination of the orders about street cleaning and environmental regulation throughout this period indicates that the City's mayors and aldermen were preoccupied with the extirpation of stench and noisome air. In June 1580, for instance, the Lord Mayor, Nicholas Woodroffe, ordered that the streets be cleansed and the kennels run for 'the Avoydinge of the infection of the plague and the lothesome Stinckes and savours that are in the severall streetes of this Cyttie'.[24] In May 1634 a precept complained that the streets were 'much annoyed with soyle, dunge and other noysome . . . things and by noysome smells therefrom arrisinge'; just over thirty years later another command explained that its purpose was 'to pr[e]vent those unsavory and noysome smells and stenches . . . wch hath a pestiferous Influence on Mans Body'.[25] Up till the final third of the

[19] J. A. Comenius, *Orbis pictus* (1659; facs. edn., 1968), 87.

[20] On the iconography of the five senses, see L. Vinge, *The Five Senses: Studies in a Literary Tradition* (Lund, 1975); F. Kermode, 'The Banquet of Sense', repr. in his *Shakespeare, Spenser, Donne* (1971); C. Nordenfalk, 'The Five Senses in Late Medieval and Renaissance Art', *Journal of the Warburg and Courtauld Institutes*, 48 (1985), 1–22; *Immagini del sentire*, ed. S. Ferino-Pagden (Cremona, 1996).

[21] I. Maclean, 'Foucault's Renaissance Episteme Reassessed: An Aristotelian Counterblast', *Journal of the History of Ideas*, 59 (1998), 149–66.

[22] M. Dobson, *Contours of Death and Disease in Early Modern England* (Cambridge, 1997), ch. 1.

[23] Centre for Kentish Studies, Maidstone, U1015 F4, fo. 13ᵛ.

[24] Corporation of London RO, Journal of the Common Council 21, fo. 41.

[25] Ibid., Journal 36, fo. 265; Journal 46, fo. 60.

seventeenth century their concern above all was to ensure that the streets and thoroughfares were kept clean and sweet.[26]

Preservatives against epidemic disease were similarly olfactory. In 1631 the mayor and aldermen of York recommended the use of sponges soaked with camphor and white wine vinegar to ward off the infection of the plague and ordered that all infected houses be perfumed with juniper, rosemary, bay leaves, vinegar, 'Tarr, pitch, or Rosin'.[27] In every plague epidemic in sixteenth- and seventeenth-century London churchwardens invested in frankincense and other fumigants to burn in vestry rooms and churches. The College of Physi- cians' official recommendations suggested a battery of pomanders, perfumes, and ferocious fumigants.[28] Among the alternatives listed in advice books were sniffing tarred rope or herbal nosegays. Thomas Dekker noted sardonically how during the London plague of 1603 'rosemary, which had wont to be sold for twelvepence an armful, went . . . for six shillings a handful'.[29]

Such smells were understood to have a direct effect upon the body. Aro- matics consequently featured more prominently within early modern learned discourse than they do today. During the 1650s and 1660s, for instance, John Evelyn and John Beale entertained ambitious schemes for social, religious, and metaphysical transformation through the odours of flowers and blos- soms, while the Royal Society discussed the effects of tobacco smoke and rank smells on silkworms.[30] Johanne St John's late-seventeenth-century collection of cures included the recommendation that you should sniff hot hog's dung to cure nosebleed and inhale the smoke of burning rosemary as a remedy for headache.[31] One remedy for the palsy was 'the strong scent . . . of a fox'. Com- bined with energetic rubbing of the head, it would disperse the humours to the outer parts of the body.[32]

Women, particularly their wombs, were held to be particularly sensitive to odours. The early seventeenth-century French surgeon Jean Guillemeau recommended that, if a woman retained the placenta after delivery, you should cause her 'to smell unto bad, and stinking odors, as old shoes, and Partridge feathers burnt, *Assafoetida, Rue*'. Applied to the nose, such vapours would cause the uterus to expel the afterbirth. Women with a post-partum hernia or prolapsed womb, by contrast, were to be treated with '*Pessaries, Parfumes*', and '*Suffumigations*'. 'Let the woman', he wrote, 'receive this fume beneath, sitting

[26] M. S. R. Jenner, 'Early Modern English Conceptions of "Cleanliness" and "Dirt" as Reflected in the Environmental Regulation of London *c*.1530–*c*.1700', D.Phil. thesis (Oxford, 1991), ch. 3.

[27] York City Archives, House Book 35, fo. 120.

[28] Jenner, '"Cleanliness" and "Dirt"', 146–75.

[29] G. Markham, *The English Housewife*, ed. M. R. Best (Montreal, 1986), 12; T. Dekker, *The Wonderful Year*, in E. D. Pendry (ed.), *The Stratford-upon-Avon Library*, iv. *Thomas Dekker* (1967), 48.

[30] M. Jenner, 'The Politics of London Air: John Evelyn's *Fumifugium* and the Restoration', *Historical Journal*, 38 (1995), 535–51; *Philosophical Transactions*, 1 (1665–8), 26.

[31] Wellcome Institute MS 4338, fos. 15, 80.   [32] Markham, *English Housewife*, 14.

in a chaire, with a hole in it,' and let the perfumes include assafoetida 'because the Matrice flyeth from any thing . . . of a bad savour'.[33] John Sadler, the Norwich physician, made similar recommendations for women suffering from suffocation of the mother. 'Hold under her nose *Partridge* feathers haire and old shoes burnt', he wrote, 'and . . . other stinking things: for evill odours are an enemie to nature, hence the Animall spirits doe so . . . strive against them, that the naturall heate is thereby restored'.[34]

II

Many classical authors stated that pestilence originated in bad airs, but one can perhaps better grasp how smell could be interpreted as a direct threat to bodily health and integrity if one examines contemporary understandings of olfaction. As Richard Palmer has outlined, within Galenic physiology 'to smell' was to take a substance into the brain.[35] According to Galen, two projections reached from the front ventricle of the brain down to the cribriform plate that separates the nasal cavity from the brain. These 'horn-like processes' were not nerves, Galen's anatomy explained, but in 'substance . . . exactly like . . . the brain'.[36] Furthermore, Galenic physiology reckoned that the bony area at the back of the nasal fossae was permeable. It allowed catarrh—the waste product produced by the cooling of hot vapours rising to the brain—to escape and it allowed part of the air that you inhaled to enter the cerebellum. There airborne odours were received directly by these two projections and thence the sensation communicated to the sensus communis.[37]

This account was endorsed by Avicenna,[38] and remained dominant during the first century of the anatomical renaissance. Part of the 'breath that we draw' in, wrote John Banister in 1578, 'ascendyng up by the nostrels into these . . . litle holes . . . part of the breath . . . passeth this way into the brayne'.[39] Helkiah

[33] J. Guillemeau, *Child-birth or, the Happy Deliverie of Women* (1612; facs. edn., Amsterdam, 1972), 181, 243–4.

[34] J. Sadler, *The Sick Womans Private Looking-glasse* (1636; facs. edn., Amsterdam, 1977), 72, also 71, 83.

[35] R. Palmer, 'In Bad Odour: Smell and its Significance in Medicine from Antiquity to the Seventeenth Century', in W. F. Bynum and R. Porter (eds.), *Medicine and the Five Senses* (Cambridge, 1993).

[36] Galen, *On Anatomical Procedures: The Later Books*, trans. W. L. H. Duckworth, ed. M. C. Lyons and B. Towers (Cambridge, 1962), 186, 195, also 4; B. S. Eastwood, 'Galen on the Elements of Olfactory Sensation', *Rheinisches Museum für Philologie*, 124 (1981), 268–90.

[37] R. E. Siegel, *Galen on Sense Perception* (Basle, 1970), ch. 3. In general Galen rejected the idea that particular parts of the brain received information from particular senses. His understanding of the olfactory bulb is a notable exception: R. E. Siegel, *Galen on Psychology, Psychopathology, and Function and Diseases of the Nervous System* (Basle, 1973), 94, 236.

[38] Palmer, 'In Bad Odour', 62.

[39] J. Banister, *The Historie of Man* (1578; facs. edn., Amsterdam, 1969), fo. 101ᵛ. Banister here cites Galen and Fernel. Cf. J. Berengario da Carpi, *A Short Introduction to Anatomy*, trans. L. R. Lind (Chicago, 1959), 148, also 145.

Crooke's *Microcosmographia* (published some forty years later) concurred. The nose, he wrote, 'leadeth the ayre, informed, as it were, with the formes of odours through the hole of the Spongie bone to the Mammillary processes as unto the principall organs of smelling'. He made the process clearer a few pages later: 'The Aire altred with Odors or by an aierie exhalation of odorifferous thinges is received by the Nose . . .'. At the top of the nostrils were two holes. The greater part of the air inhaled went to the lungs 'without any sense of odours; the rest ascendeth . . . to the instrume[n]ts of Smelling, but . . . is altred in the spongie bones' at the top of the nasal cavity. 'This aire thus altred in the Labyrinths of the spongie bones,' he continued, 'together with the species or forme of the odour passeth thorough the holes of the *Sive* [as he characterized these bones] into the *Mammillary processes*, or by them . . . is received and so conveyed to the common Sense . . . in the Braine.'[40] To, that is, the area of the brain that brought together the information provided by the five senses.

The boundaries of the human frame were thus permeable; what we might now term the olfactory environment penetrated the body and was absorbed by the brain. Consequently there were physiological reasons for Montaigne's declaration that odours altered his spirits 'according unto their strength and qualitie'.[41] Furthermore, some commentators argued that you were what you smelt as well as what you ate. There was a learned tradition deriving from the Pythagoreans that it was possible to be nourished from the smell of food and that Democrites sustained himself on the smell of honey or hot bread. Anatomists debated whether it was true that 'Cooks, who . . . are busie boyling and roasting viands for other men, doe receive so many odours from them that they scarse ever are hungry'.[42] By contrast, to ingest fetid smells was to introduce poison, 'a certaine venemous facultie', such as James VI and I detected in tobacco, 'to the braines'.[43] '*The best thing against the Plague*', there- fore, was that 'In the morning before you go far from your habitation', you should 'wash your mouth with water and vineger . . . then drink a quarter of a spoonfull of the . . . liqour, and so press your nose, that your brain being freed from all externall ayre infected, may . . . by the vapour and steem held in your mouth, be moistned'.[44]

Over the seventeenth century the notion that air reached the brain was dis- credited as physicians reconceptualized the process of respiration after Harvey. Van Helmont argued forcefully that catarrh was nasal mucus, not phlegm pro- duced by the cooling of animal spirits in the brain and excreted through the

---

[40] H. Crooke, *Microcosmographia: A Description of the Body of Man* (1616), 616, 620.

[41] M. de Montaigne, *The Essays*, trans. J. Florio (1603; facs. edn., Menston, 1969), 171.

[42] Crooke, *Microcosmographia*, 705.

[43] *Minor Works of King James VI and I*, ed. J. Craigie (Scottish Text Society, 4th ser., 14; 1982), 91.

[44] J. Wecker (rev. R. Read), *Eighteen Books of the Secrets of Art & Nature* (1660), 43.

cribriform plate.[45] In the 1650s and 1660s Conrad Schneider, professor of medicine at Wittenburg, argued at great length and after much anatomical work that, although nerves ran through it, the forehead bone was not permeable.[46] Thomas Willis's and Robert Lower's research into cerebral anatomy reached similar conclusions. As Lower wrote in 1672,

That nothing passes through the cribriform plate into the nostrils, is . . . proved by the conformation of this part of the body. For although in dry skulls the openings of this bone appear permeable and let light through, yet in a living creature they are wholly stuffed with the nerves and membranes coming from the olfactory bulbs . . .[47]

Doctors and other natural philosophers increasingly saw the *nerves* lining the upper part of the nose as the immediate organ of smell. Thomas Willis's anatomy of the brain explained,

although many Nerves belong to the Organ of Smelling, yet that sense is properly performed by the Fibres interwoven in the inward Coat of the Nostrils: for those Fibres being struck by the sensible object, move and contract themselves . . . according to the Idea of the impression; which Affection of them being carried by the passage of the Nerves to the Head . . . [and] there staid by the common Sensory, causes the perception of the sense.[48]

It is tempting to link Galenic physiology in which the mammillary processes directly encountered the air to Bakhtin's arguments, developed recently by Barbara Duden and Ulinka Rublack, about the openness of the early modern body, which continually 'swallows the world and is itself swallowed by the world'.[49] The shift towards nervous perception could then be seen as part of the emergence of the 'more tightly sealed, more leakproof' *homo clausus* of modernity.[50] Although by *c.*1700 both olfaction and hearing had come to be

[45] W. Pagel, 'Medieval and Renaissance Contributions to Knowledge of the Brain and its Function', in *The History and Philosophy of Knowledge of the Brain and its Functions* (Oxford, 1958), 109; W. Pagel, *Joan Baptista Van Helmont* (Cambridge, 1982), 162–71.

[46] A. M. Luyendijk-Elshout, 'The Cavity of the Nose in Dutch Baroque Medicine', *Clio Medica*, 8 (1973), 296; K. Dewhurst, 'Thomas Willis and the Foundations of British Neurology', in F. Clifford Rose and W. F. Bynum (eds.), *Historical Aspects of the Neurosciences* (New York, 1982), 334; C. V. Schneider, *De catarrhis* (5 books; 1660–64), II, sect. i, ch. 20, and sect. ii, ch. 1.

[47] R. Lower, *De catarrhis 1672*, trans. and intro., R. Hunter and I. Macalpine (1963), 6. Willis's position was less clear. Although when he explored skulls and brains with a probe he found that the mammillary processes did not enter the nose, his Oxford lectures of the 1660s talked of the nostrils as part of the brain's excretory system: K. Dewhurst (ed.), *Thomas Willis's Oxford Lectures* (Oxford, 1980), 80, 84 n.

[48] T. Willis, *Five treatises* (1681), 139. Cf. J. Keill, *The Anatomy of the Humane Body Abridg'd* (5th edn., 1714), 216.

[49] M. Bakhtin, *Rabelais and his World*, trans. H. Iswolsky (Bloomington, Ind., 1984), 317; B. Duden, *The Woman beneath the Skin*, trans. T. Dunlap (Cambridge, Mass., 1991), ch. 4; U. Rublack, 'Pregnancy, Childbirth and the Female Body in Early Modern Germany', *P&P* 150 (1996), 84–110.

[50] J. Barrell, *The Birth of Pandora and the Division of Knowledge* (Basingstoke, 1992), 150. More generally, see Elias, *Civilizing Process*.

understood in terms of nerves rather than internal air or *pneuma*,[51] we should resist such lines of interpretation. First, as many authors on eighteenth-century sensibility have demonstrated, the sensitive nerves of the man of feeling intensified the physical bond between the individual and the world around him: he was anything but sealed off from his surroundings.[52]

Secondly, claims that there was a shift from an open to a closed body hugely oversimplify the variety of physiological models in the pro-modern world. Just as not every account of the early modern body placed biological sex upon a continuum,[53] so not every sixteenth-century understanding of olfactory perception considered the brain to be as permeable as did the Galenic model. The Pythagorean belief that you could survive on the odour of food was widely discussed, but it was generally rejected for many of the same reasons that Aristotle advanced in *De sensu*. Moreover, the Aristotelian account of olfaction drew an ontological distinction between smells and vapours that is blurred in many cultural histories of perception. For Aristotle, and after him Averroes, odour was a dry exhalation that was transmitted through pneuma—air. It was a *species*—an immaterial quality possessed by and diffused from an object—not itself a form of vapour.[54] Throughout the Middle Ages and thereafter there was a debate over whether smell was a physical entity that was taken into the body, or an immaterial sign, transmitted through the air that you breathed in, and that the human mind could detect.[55]

This uncertainty permeates many early modern accounts of olfaction. Crooke, for instance, entangles the two, writing that odours could affect the body, sustain life, and so on, if the effect 'be understoode [to be] of that vaporous or aerie exhalation . . . wherein the odour is transported'. But, 'if we understand by odours the simple obiect of the smell, naked and separated from exhalations', then such claims were utterly false. For 'of an odour considered by it selfe and separately there is no knowledge, for so considered it is nothing, neither doth it fall under Sense, but as it is ioyned with the exhalation it mooveth the Sense and . . . falleth under Science or knowledge'.[56]

More importantly, learned physiology may have closed off the human brain from direct contamination by the odours of life, but doctors and laypeople

[51] On hearing, see P. Gouk, 'Some English Theories of Hearing in the Seventeenth Century: Before and After Descartes', in C. Burnett, M. Fend, and P. Gouk (eds.), *The Second Sense: Studies in Hearing and Musical Judgement from Antiquity to the Seventeenth Century* (1991).

[52] G. J. Barker-Benfield, *The Culture of Sensibility* (Chicago, 1992); A. J. van Sant, *Eighteenth-Century Sensibility and the Novel* (Cambridge, 1993).

[53] T. Laqueur, *Making Sex* (Cambridge, Mass., 1990); K. Park and R. A. Nye, 'Destiny is Anatomy', *New Republic* (18 Feb. 1991), 53–7.

[54] K. Park, 'The Organic Soul', in C. B. Schmitt and Q. Skinner (eds.), *The Cambridge History of Renaissance Philosophy* (Cambridge, 1988), 470–2, 474–5.

[55] S. Kemp, 'A Medieval Controversy about Odor', *Journal of the History of the Behavioral Sciences*, 33 (1997), 211–19.

[56] Crooke, *Microcosmographia*, 706, 708.

continued to be acutely conscious of the physical effects of particular smells upon the body—whether that impact was understood in terms of the chemical composition of these odours, the size and shape of the particles that comprised them, or their putrefying qualities. They thus attached great significance to the airs that one inhaled. Sir Richard Blackmore's 1725 *Treatise on the Vapours and the Spleen* was couched in iatromechanical terms, focusing on the tone of the nervous fibres. But he acknowledged that 'sweet and disagreeable Odours', 'by their Impulses and Impressions on the Spirits in the Brain, continued . . . by the Mediation of the Nerves to the inferior . . . Parts' of the body, could produce fainting, fits, convulsions, and palpitations of the heart. Like Sadler, a hundred years before, he reckoned that 'outward Remedies of a . . . foetid Scent' were of benefit to hysterical patients, though he cautioned readers about the dangers of traditional and (in his opinion) overstrong scents like burning feathers.[57]

Moreover, the neo-Hippocratic strands within Restoration and Augustan medicine probably increased the attention paid to the environmental origins of disease. Smell was often treated as indicating bad air *and* as being bad air. More importantly, throughout the early modern period and long into the nineteenth century airs were held materially to affect those who experienced them and who took them into their bodies. In the eighteenth century fears about the link between bad air and disease inspired innovations such as the erection of windmills to ventilate Newgate prison.[58] As William Buchan's *Domestic Medicine* (1772) warned, 'unwholesome air is a very common cause of diseases'; 'what goes into the lungs', he continued, was more dangerous than food or drink.[59]

Furthermore, throughout this period airs were the object of intense natural philosophical analysis, involving air pumps, retorts full of nitrous oxide, or diverse experiments *en plein air*; no matter what Foucault may have said in *The Order of Things*, smell continued to provide experimenters with valued information. Robert Boyle, for instance, recorded how he

inquired of my Lord of *Sandwich* . . . whether it be true which is reported of the Purity of the Air at *Madrid*, that though they have no Houses of Office, but every Night throw out their Excrements into the Streets, yet by the Morning there remains no more Smell of them. To which I was answered, That 'twas true the Excrements were so disposed of, but that *Madrid* is the stinkingst Town they ever came into.[60]

Claims for a fundamental shift in the cultural significance of olfaction during the early modern period thus seem to be at best overdrawn and at

---

[57] Sir Richard Blackmore, *Treatise on the Vapours and the Spleen* (1725), 54, and 122–3.
[58] J. C. Riley, *The Eighteenth-Century Campaign to Avoid Disease* (Basingstoke, 1987), 106–8 and *passim*.
[59] W. Buchan, *Domestic Medicine* (1772), 92.
[60] R. Boyle, *General History of the Air* (1692), 212.

worst misguided. Indeed, framing research in terms of whether there was a fundamental sensory tranformation, a shift from an odoriphile to an odoriphobe culture,[61] seems an unhelpfully crude way of approaching the cultural history of the senses and of scents. Not only is experience fundamentally synesthetic,[62] but people exploited (and exploit) their senses in different ways in different contexts, whether in cooking, dairying, carving, practising medicine, studying, or whatever. The practices of everyday life do not observe a fixed hierarchy of the senses; Corbin's call for historians to examine 'the hierarchy of the representations and uses of the senses at the heart of a culture' is thus utterly impossible, because such a research project would require us to be able to determine the heart of a society.[63] Nor, furthermore, are odours banished together. One odour can be decried while another is celebrated and cherished. It is surely more productive to begin to trace a history of smells, exploring the cultural meanings of particular odours in specific locations or within particular discourses, rather than a history of smell. I conclude, therefore, with a brief exploration of such a case study—the history of the smell of garlic (with occasional digressions into the olfactory history of onions and leeks).

III

The English aversion to the smell of garlic is stereotypically one aspect of the Victorian repression of sensuality swept away in the 1960s in a process initiated a decade earlier by Elizabeth David's *Mediterranean Food*, the preface of which evoked the interwar Mediterranean through the southern smells of garlic and rosemary.[64] I began research expecting to trace how first polite and then popular culture gradually rejected the herb as distasteful and foreign. However, early modern recipe collections, herbals, and household manuals do not suggest that Mrs Beeton's neglect of the root (garlic appears only in a faintly alarming Anglo-Indian curry recipe) was simply the result of nineteenth-century sensory deprivation. Rather, there is considerable evidence of English aversion to the pungent herb in previous centuries. By the mid-eighteenth century such discourse had permeated the political language of the urban middling sort. Rioters in Bristol in the 1750s apparently shouted out 'No Jews! No French . . . No Lowering Wages . . . to 4d. a Day and Garlick!' In Hogarth's painting *Calais Gate* (1749), the indigent

---

[61] For this dichotomy, see D. Howes, 'Le Sens sans parole: Vers une anthropologie de l'odorat', *Anthropologie et sociétés*, 10/2 (1986), 32.

[62] J. Leavitt and L. M. Hart, 'Critique de la "Raison" Sensorielle: L'Élaboration esthétique des sens dans une société himalayenne', ibid. 14/2 (1990), 77–98.

[63] A. Corbin, 'Histoire et anthropologie sensorielle', ibid. 13 (my translation).

[64] E. David, *Mediterranean Food* (1950), introduction.

Scottish exile in the foreground has, some scholars suggest, been reduced to eating garlic.[65]

While this construction of garlic-hating and xenophobic (particularly anti-French) Englishness probably intensified during the eighteenth century, there were many hostile or comic representations of the root throughout the early modern period. Garlic was included in the culinary anti-masque of Ben Jonson's *Neptune's Triumph*. As Culpeper wrote in 1653, the 'offensiveness of the breath of him that hath eaten Garlick will lead you by the Nose to the knowledg hereof'.[66] Describing roughly contemporaneous experiments into odours, Robert Boyle wrote how he had placed a 'fragrant liquor in stopped glasses . . . in a warm place'. After a while he found it 'so to degenerate in . . . scent, that one would have thought it to have been strongly infected with garlick'.[67] Whereas by the 1590s leek-eating was presented as particularly Welsh,[68] other national groups were denigrated by portraying them as raising and eating garlic. Samuel Colvil's late-seventeenth-century satire depicted louse-ridden Scottish Presbyterians and their Whig allies dining enthusiastically on pigs' tails and garlic, while another Hudibrastic satire of Scotland published a couple of years before the Union wrote dismissively of how north of the border

> The pregnant Roots that in the Garden settles
> Are Garlick, Poppies, Artichoks and Nettles.[69]

In the 1690s John Evelyn declared that, though garlic was 'both by *Spaniards* and *Italians*, and the more Southern People, familiarly eaten', he reckoned it 'more proper for our Northern Rustics . . . living in *Uliginous* and moist places, or such as use the *Sea*'.[70]

Importantly all these groups were poor. The reek of garlic was a marker of social (and not just national) distinction throughout the early modern period, as it had been in the classical world.[71] Many authors wrote of the stinking breath of the common people; garlic regularly functioned as a sign of poverty and of rusticity, contrasted with the costly scents of spices and perfumes. In *Measure for Measure*, for instance, Lucio declares that the Duke was so lecherous that he 'would mouth with a beggar though she smelt brown bread and garlic'.[72]

[65] L. Colley, *In Defiance of Oligarchy* (Cambridge, 1982), 155; L. Colley, *Britons* (New Haven, 1992), 33.

[66] *Ben Jonson*, ed. C. H. Herford, P. and E. Simpson (11 vols.; Oxford, 1925–52), vii. 690; N. Culpeper, *The English Physitian Enlarged* (1653), 111.

[67] 'Experiments . . . about the Mechanical Production of Odours', 269.

[68] e.g. *Henry V*, v. i. 21–79; J. Parkinson, *Paradisi in sole paradisus terrestris* (1629), 513.

[69] S. Colvil, *Mock Poem, or, Whiggs Supplication* (1681), pt. ii. 8; *A Trip Lately To Scotland With a True Character Of The Country and People* (1705), 12.

[70] J. Evelyn, *Acetaria. A Discourse of Sallets* (1699), 27.

[71] S. Lilja, *The Treatment of Odors in the Poetry of Antiquity* (Helsinki, 1972), 127–9.

[72] *Measure for Measure*, iii. ii. 177–8.

However, even when it was serving as an olfactory marker of alterity, garlic was a complex image. In the Roman world garlic was generally associated with the rustic and the barbarian, but was often represented as preferable to the perfumed and effeminate breath of the flatterer.[73] Similarly, on occasions in the sixteenth and early seventeenth centuries garlic and onions symbolized simple and authentic society or pious retreat. Arthur Warren's early seventeenth-century *Poverties Patience*, for instance, contrasted the terror of the rich man expecting to be poisoned at every feast with the carefree diet of the poor.

> Rootes, Onions, garlick, and the Hermits meale,
> Proves better feasting then this dangerous fare.[74]

Nor was a distaste for garlic an uncontentious expression of English national public opinion. The power of Hogarth's images, for instance, stemmed from their role in debates about the nature of Englishness in artistic style and in cultural forms. As with language and manners, garlic's French associations were enormously attractive to sections of eighteenth-century polite society.[75] Indeed, garlic featured in the 'overheated' sauces and cullis fashionable in the late seventeenth and eighteenth centuries and condemned by many moralistic and patriotic commentators.[76]

Garlic, like onion, was seen as heating—it was hot in the third or fourth degree, most herbals reckoned.[77] While thus good for asthmatics and those with cold, watery stomachs, this natural heat gave both roots, from the Middle Ages onwards, an association with lust. William Turner, for instance, noted in the 1550s that garlic stirred men to venery; Chaucer's Summoner, afflicted with a loathsome skin condition, was exceedingly partial to onions, garlic, and strong red wine and kept a concubine.[78] Such moral connotations were strengthened by garlic's walk-on part in the Bible. When the Israelites were crossing the desert, they complained that in Egypt they had dined on fish, onions, and garlic, not to mention melons and cucumbers; now they had to subsist on boring old manna.[79] Pious authors thus regularly used garlic to symbolize sensuality and its loathsomeness. The Puritan minister William Attersoll commented, 'In these words we see how carnall men conceive carnal things. They prefer their trash before Manna,' reminding his readers that 'all ye wealth of the world . . . is no better then onyons and garlike in comparison of spirituall things'.[80] As the poet, John Collop, asked in 1656,

[73] E. Gowers, *The Loaded Table* (Oxford, 1993), 289–310.
[74] A. Warren, *The Poore Mans Passions. And Poverties Patience* (1605), unpaginated.
[75] See M. Cohen, *Fashioning Masculinity: National Identity and Language in the Eighteenth Century* (1996).
[76] On cullis, see C. A. Wilson, *Food and Drink in Britain* (1973), 221–3.
[77] e.g. *The Grete Herball* (1526), sig. Bii; Gerard, *Herbal* (1597), 140; *An English Herbal* (1690?), 32; W. Salmon, *Botanologia. The English Herbal* (1710), 408.
[78] W. Turner, *A New Herball* (1551), sig. Bᵛ; R. E. Kaske, 'The Summoner's Garleek, Onyons, and eek Lekes', *Modern Language Notes*, 54 (1959), 481–4.
[79] Num. xi: 5.
[80] W. Attersoll, *A Commentarie upon the Fourth Booke of Moses, Called Numbers* (1618), 529, 531.

Can *Egypts* garlick, we or onyons need?
On th'milk of th'word can't our youth better feed?[81]

Furthermore, if, as such authors reiterated, carnality was a false god, what better demonstration could there be of this than Pliny's account of 'the foolish superstition of the Ægyptians, who use to sweare by Garlicke and Onions, calling them to witnesse in taking their othes, as if they were no lesse than . . . gods'?[82] This story was energetically reworked by Juvenal in his fifteenth satire, and many early modern versifiers exploited the topos for all it was worth. In *The Overthrow of the Gout*, for instance, Barnaby Googe, reminded the sore-toed

> Bothe Garlick, Rue and Onions soure
> expel them far from thee:
> Although the fond Egiptians doo:
> suppose them Gods to be.[83]

By the late seventeenth century the image had not only been incorporated into Hobbes's catalogue of possible gods,[84] but was finding its way into the language of philosophical denigration and even political ephemera. William Petty, for instance, dismissed the 'Vaporous garlick & onions of phantasmaticall seeming philosophy',[85] while one satirical poem on Titus Oates declared,

> Th'Egptians once (tho' it seems odd)
> Did worship *Onyons* for a *God*;
> And poor peel'd *Garlick* was with them
> Esteem'd beyond the greatest *Gemm* . . . [86]

Before we conclude that garlic-hating was a timeless peculiarity of the English, however, we need to look at other strands of discourse about the root. Commenting on the lines in Shakespeare's *Coriolanus* in which Menenius dismisses the commoners' opinions as the 'breath of garlic-eaters', E. K. Chambers rather literal-mindedly wrote in 1898 that 'Apparently the lower class Londoner ate more garlic than he does today.' In fact, the evidence for the practice is somewhat contradictory. Garlic seems to have been used quite extensively in the Middle Ages, suggesting that the City parish of St James Garlickhithe was, in the words of the Elizabethan chronicler John Stow, an area where 'of old time . . . Garlicke was usually solde'.[87] In 1333–4 the garden of Glastonbury Abbey supplied the monks with 8,000 heads of garlic;

---

[81] 'On Homer', in *Poesis Rediviva: or, Poesie Revived* (1656; facs. edn., Menston, 1972), 64.
[82] *The Historie of the World: Commonly called the Naturall Historie of C. Plinius Secundus*, trans. P. Holland (2 vols; 1635), ii. 20.
[83] B. Googe (trans.), *The Overthrow of the Gout* (1577), sig. Ciiv.
[84] T. Hobbes, *Leviathan*, ed. R. Tuck (Cambridge, 1991), 79.
[85] Quoted in S. Shapin and S. Schaffer, *Leviathan and the Air Pump* (Princeton, 1985), 304.
[86] R. Duke, *A Panegyrick upon Oates* (1679?).
[87] Quoted in *Coriolanus*, ed. J. D. Wilson (Cambridge, 1964), 222; J. Stow, *A Survey of London* ed. C. L. Kingsford (2 vols.; Oxford, 1971), i. 249.

medieval household and garden accounts make fairly regular reference to the herb.[88] In the 1550s William Turner described common or garden garlic as 'good meat', and other subsequent herbals noted that country people ate wild garlic.[89] However, other early modern writers declared that most of their contemporaries did not use the root for culinary purposes. The herbalist John Parkinson observed in 1629 that

The old World, as wee finde in Scripture . . . and no doubt long before, fed much upon Leekes, Onions, and Garlicke boyled with flesh; and the antiquity of the Gentiles relate the same manner of feeding on them, to be in all Countries the like, which howsoever our dainty age now refuseth wholly, in all sorts except the poorest . . .'[90]

Yet garlic *was* being cultivated and used. It appears occasionally in seventeenth-century household accounts; Gervase Markham's *English Housewife* (1615) advised that in February the good wife should sow garlic alongside other herbs. A century later Hannah Glasse's cookbook listed garlic among the products of the kitchen garden, while its 1796 edition listed garlic among the vegetables in season in February and March and from July to December.[91]

Not the least of its uses would have been medicinal. Culpeper may have decried its stench, but he also recognized it as a powerful and efficacious herb. As commentator after commentator from the early sixteenth to the early nineteenth centuries observed, Galen designated it the poor man's mithridate (or cure all).[92] As Sir John Harington's translation of the School of Salernum noted, garlic did not just make you wink and stink, it protected you against all kinds of diseases.[93] Taken internally, it killed worms; it was recommended for animal bites and as a protection against stagnant water.[94] By the 1790s

[88] C. Dyer, 'Gardens and Orchards in Medieval England', in Dyer, *Everyday Life in Medieval England* (1994), 127–8; C. M. Woolgar (ed.), *Household Accounts from Medieval England* (Records of Social and Economic History, 17, 18; Oxford, 1992–3), *passim*; C. Noble, C. Moreton, and P. Rutledge (eds.), *Farming and Gardening in Late Medieval Norfolk* (Norfolk Record Society, 61; 1997), 49–52.

[89] Turner, *A New Herball*, i. 224; R. Lovell, ΠΑΜΒΟΤΑΝΟΛΟΓΙΑ, *Sive Enchiridion Botanicum, Or A Compleat Herball* (1659), 182.

[90] Parkinson, *Paradisi in sole paradisus terrestris*, 513.

[91] T. Gray (ed.), *Devon Household Accounts, 1627–59 Part I* (Devon and Cornwall Record Society, 38; 1995), 20, 116, 150; Markham, *English Housewife*, 62; H. Glasse, '*First Catch Your Hare . . .*' [a facsimile of *The Art of Cookery Made Plain and Easy* (1747)] (Totnes, 1995), 165; H. Glasse, *The Art of Cookery made Plain and Easy* (1796; facs. edn., Wakefield, 1976), 2–6.

[92] W. Turner, *Libellus de Re Herbaria 1538. The Names of Herbes 1548* (Ray Society, 145, 1965), 85; J. Gerard, *The Herball or Generall Historie of Plantes* (1597), 140; Parkinson, *Paradisi in sole paradisus terrestris*, 514; J. K'Eogh, *Botanalogia Universalis Hibernica, Or, a General Irish Herbal* (Cork, 1735), 51.

[93] J. Harington, *The School of Salernum*, ed. F. R. Packard and F. H. Garrison (New York, 1920), 86.

[94] e.g. *Ane Herbal 1525* (facs. edn., New York, 1978), sig. B1–1ᵛ; Gerard, *Herball* (1597), 140–1; J. Archer, *A Compendious Herbal* (1673), 65; W. Salmon, *Botanologia* (1710), 408–9.

some doctors regarded garlic as, in Dr William Lewis's words, 'not only an offensive, but . . . a noxious drug', but other health advice books continued to recommend its therapeutic possibilities. Indeed its efficacy as a cure for tuberculosis found professional medical advocates during the early twentieth century.[95]

IV

This brief survey has delineated some of the multifaceted meanings of one smell and its representations. It has deliberately resisted the tendency in many histories of the senses to generalize about the sensory regime of an entire culture or to discourse about modernity. The sense of smell has a rich and various history, but we need to get away from grand evolutionary narratives such as Donald Lowe's *History of Bourgeois Perception*. In such histories of the sensorium, sight is always triumphing just as the middle class is always rising. In Georg Simmel's words, 'modern social life increases in ever growing degree the rôle of mere visual impression'.[96]

Most authors discussing the cultural history of the senses seem to assume that their interrelations constitute a zero-sum game—that any increase in the cultural significance of one sense automatically means an equal devaluing of another. Even though clinical psychologists working with blind and partially sighted people report that their sense of hearing may become more developed, there is no logical reason why the enhancing of one faculty should lead to a decline in another.[97] Moreover, it is not, I think, at the moment productive to ask whether olfaction played a greater or lesser role in modern and pre-modern cultures, or to ponder whether printing, Albertian perspective, or the telescope marked the decisive victory of ocularcentrism and the traumatic mirror phase of Western history.

We need to distinguish more clearly between the two narratives of deodorization that I outlined in my introduction and that Freud wove so artfully together. Cultures may banish faecal or other odours from public space without devaluing odours or olfaction in general.[98] Pronouncements like Zygmunt Bauman's that 'Scents had no room in the shiny temple of perfect order modernity set out to erect' sound very grand, but a cursory examination of nineteenth- or twentieth-century culture reveals the complete vacuity

---

[95] R. Hawting, 'The Use and Neglect of Garlic in the Treatment of Consumption', B.Sc. dissertation (Manchester, 1994), 5 and *passim*.

[96] D. Lowe, *History of Bourgeois Perception* (1982); G. Simmel, 'Sociology of the Senses: Visual Interaction', in R. E. Park and E. W. Burgess, *Introduction to the Science of Sociology* (3rd edn., 1960), 360.

[97] Jay, *Downcast Eyes*, is particularly sensitive to the complexities of even the most ocularcentrist discourses.

[98] Cf. Leavitt and Hart, 'Critique de la "Raison" Sensorielle'.

of such claims—after all, the deodorized house smelt *fresh*.[99] Every deodorizing is another olfactory encoding.

My ideas are partly inspired by recent lines of writing within the history and anthropology of literacy. Anthropologists and historians once linked the acquisition of writing with a fundamental mental transformation and a major realignment of the senses—the domestication of the savage mind. Increasingly, however, they are unwilling to categorize the peoples that they study as literate or illiterate in the style of UN education programmes. Many prefer to talk about *literacies*, recognizing that reading and writing constitute a range of practices just as, as Keith Thomas showed, they did in early modern society.[100] Perhaps the history of the senses should develop this kind of multiple ethnography and abandon its attempts to sniff out the origins of the modern sensorium.

---

[99] Z. Bauman, 'The Sweet Scent of Decomposition', in C. Rojek and B. S. Turner (eds.), *Forget Baudrillard?* (1993), 24.

[100] B. V. Street, *Literacy in Theory and Practice* (Cambridge, 1984); K. Thomas, 'The Meaning of Literacy in Early Modern England', in G. Baumann (ed.), *The Written Word: Literacy in Transition* (Oxford, 1986).

8

Civility and the Decline of Magic

ALAN MACFARLANE

One of the most puzzling aspects of the emergence of a new kind of world in the last few centuries in the West is the development of what we now call 'science'. The shift from a magical and religious-dominated cosmology to a mechanistic and secular one, though far from complete and far from confined to the period roughly between 1550 and 1850, is in general indisputable. Until that time it had not happened in other civilizations such as China, Japan, or the Islamic world, which had much earlier reached a higher level of craft knowledge than anything then current in Europe.[1] So why did it happen where it did, when it did, and why did it happen at all? A number of historians—for example, Thomas Kuhn and Michel Foucault—have drawn attention to the 'paradigmatic' or 'epistemic' shift manifested in the work of Galileo, Descartes, and others. Yet, while providing examples of the shift, neither has been able to put forward any plausible explanation of why the shift occurred. Indeed they both specifically state that they leave it to others to explain why.[2] More recently we have been given an excellent, revised, picture of the earlier magic cosmology and its continuity with the later 'scientific' one by Stuart Clark. Yet, once again, the author explicitly states that he is not attempting to provide any explanation of why the cosmologies changed over time.[3] Some of the most stimulating suggestions concerning the reasons for the change have, in fact, come from anthropologists, who draw attention to the importance of literacy, the 'trade-travel' complex, Protestantism, the clash of cultures and other factors in the movement to the 'Open society' of modern science and technology.[4] Yet they are unable to provide the detailed historical evidence and the assertions remain general.

[1] See e.g. T. E. Huff, *The Rise of Early Modern Science: Islam, China, and the West* (Cambridge, 1993).

[2] T. Kuhn, *The Structure of Scientific Revolutions* (2nd edn., Chicago, 1975), esp. the preface; M. Foucault, *The Archaeology of Knowledge* (1978), esp. 162–3, 175; M. Foucault, *The Order of Things: An Archaeology of the Human Sciences* (1977), esp. p. xiii.

[3] S. Clark, *Thinking with Demons: The Idea of Witchcraft in Early Modern Europe* (Oxford, 1997), esp. the postscript.

[4] See e.g. R. Horton, 'African Traditional Thought and Western Science', pt. ii, *Africa*, 37/2 (Apr. 1967), and E. Gellner, *Plough, Sword and Book: The Structure of Human History* (1988).

The most ambitious attempt to solve the problem is that given in the two major works by Keith Thomas, *Religion and the Decline of Magic* (1971) and *Man and the Natural World* (1983). It is worth reflecting on the ways in which these two books, so influential in both their content and their approach, have advanced our understanding of why a great cosmological shift occurred in western Europe in the early modern period. The argument in *Religion and the Decline of Magic*, somewhat simplified, can be summarized as follows. The central initial premiss is based on Malinowski's thesis that magic is 'to be expected and generally to be found whenever man comes to an unbridgeable gap, a hiatus in his knowledge or in his powers of practical control, and yet has to continue in his pursuit'. As Thomas notes, these theories 'constitute one of the few direct assaults on the difficult question of why it is that magical beliefs decline' and hence, inversely, why science emerges. He further quotes Malinowski to the effect that 'Magic is dominant when control of the environment is weak', and Evans-Pritchard to the effect that 'the advances of science and technology have rendered magic redundant'. Thomas's reaction is that, 'when applied to the facts of sixteenth- and seventeenth-century society, it makes a good deal of initial sense'.[5] What then, in Thomas's account, was this 'environment' and how did its change help to explain the decline of magic?

I

In the first chapter of *Religion and the Decline of Magic* Thomas provides an overview of the insecure world of the sixteenth and seventeenth centuries in England, which was 'still a pre-industrial society, and many of its essential features closely resembled those of the "underdeveloped areas" of today'. The preoccupations with 'the explanation and relief of human misfortune', we are told, 'reflected the hazards of an intensely insecure environment'.[6] The first insecurity is connected to 'the expectation of life'. Thomas cites evidence to show that 'Tudor and Stuart Englishmen were, by our standards, exceedingly liable to pain, sickness and premature death'. In relation to the latter, for example, he cites the low life expectancy of the aristocracy and, though noting expectations of life at birth as high as 40–45 in some country villages, concludes that contemporaries knew that 'life was short, and that the odds were against any individual living out his full span'.[7] The second insecurity was the food supply, which 'was always precarious'. 'About one harvest in six seems to have been a total failure, and mortality could soar when times of dearth coincided with (or perhaps occasioned) large-scale epidemics'. People died of

---

[5] K. Thomas, *Religion and the Decline of Magic: Studies in Popular Beliefs in Sixteenth and Seventeenth Century England* (1971), 647, 648 and n 2.
[6] Ibid. 3, 5.   [7] Ibid. 5, 6.

starvation and exposure in the streets, and most people suffered from vitamin deficiencies. People were 'chronically under-nourished and vulnerable to tuberculosis and gastric upsets'.[8]

The third insecurity was disease. 'There were periodic waves of influenza, typhus, dysentery . . . smallpox', but the most feared of all was bubonic plague, which 'terrified by its suddenness, its virulence and its social effects'. In this pain-filled environment, 'medical science was helpless before most contemporary hazards to health'. Doctors were unable to diagnose and hence to cure most diseases, and, in any case, physicians were too expensive for the majority of the population. The fourth insecurity was fire: 'Unable to prevent the outbreak of fire, and virtually helpless during the actual conflagration, contemporaries showed little more resource when it came to bearing the loss.'[9] Thomas finds that 'Poverty, sickness and sudden disaster were thus familiar features of the social environment of this period.' Given this background, he is not surprised to find that people were driven to alcohol, tobacco, and gambling on a large scale.[10] In a long review of Thomas's book, Lawrence Stone echoes and endorses this view in even more trenchant terms. 'Premodern man' lived in a world where

both groups and individuals were under constant threat, at the mercy of the hazards of weather, fire, and disease, a prey to famines, pandemics, wars and other wholly unpredictable calamities. This insecurity produced a condition of acute anxiety, bordering at times on hysteria, and a desperate yearning for relief and reassurance.[11]

The major part of Thomas's *Religion and the Decline of Magic*, some 600 pages of detailed historical evidence, is then devoted to showing the gradual erosion of the magical world view and the birth of modern science. What happened was the 'scientific and philosophical revolution of the seventeenth century'—that is, 'the triumph of the mechanical philosophy'. There was 'a rejection both of scholastic Aristotelianism and of the Neoplatonic theory', which killed off magic. 'The notion that the universe was subject to immutable natural laws killed the concept of miracles, weakened the belief in the physical efficiency of prayer, and diminished faith in the possibility of direct divine inspiration.'[12] This was Weber's great 'disenchantment of the world', without which 'modernity' could not have occurred. Yet why did it happen? The theory that the new mechanistic philosophy can be the explanation is clearly inadequate. Not only is it tautologous—one is trying to explain the growth of a new world view by the growth of that same world view, but the timing is wrong. This latter point is made, for example, by Lawrence Stone. 'The trouble with this explanation is that skepticism about magic and witchcraft was growing among clergy, lawyers, doctors and lay magistrates in the

---

[8] Ibid. 6, 7.   [9] Ibid. 7–8, 8–12, 16.   [10] Ibid. 17–21.
[11] L. Stone, *The Past and the Present* (1981), 155–6.   [12] Thomas, *Religion*, 643.

early seventeenth century, before the new natural science had made any real impact.'[13]

As Thomas admits, 'The most difficult problem in the study of magical beliefs is thus to explain how it was that men were able to break out of them.'[14] In relation to the early Malinowski thesis and the various types of insecurity that he has suggested were 'reflected' in early religious and magical beliefs, the obvious place for Thomas to search is for changes in those insecurities. At first he seems to find some evidence for a major change in the later seventeenth century. He notes that population pressure decreased and that this, with improvements in agriculture, began to overcome the danger of harvest fluctuations. He notices the absence of bubonic plague after 1665 and the fact that, by the end of the century, the English, alongside the Dutch, were the wealthiest nation in Europe. He notes improved communications, with the growth of newspapers, for example, which helped people to find lost property. The growth of deposit banking and fire and life insurance towards the end of the century, as well as improved fire-fighting equipment, mitigated some of the risks. Several of these developments were built on embryonic sociology, economics, and the statistical calculation of probabilities.[15] Yet, when all is considered, Thomas comes to the conclusion that the Malinowskian theory does not work: 'the more closely Malinowski's picture of magic giving away before technology is examined, the less convincing does it appear.'[16] He then proceeds to show the weakness in the argument.

Basically the problem is that, given the nature of the insecurities outlined in his first chapter, the developments of the later seventeenth century were far too little and far too late. As Thomas points out, many of the sceptical and anti-magical attitudes were already present in the Lollard works of the fifteenth century. As he notes, for example, 'Many later medieval theologians were strongly "rationalist" in temperament, and preferred to stress the importance of human self-help . . . They regarded the sacraments as symbolic representations rather than as instruments of physical efficacy.' Much of the most important development of 'science', whether that of Bacon, Galileo, Harvey, or others, had occurred well before the supposed improvements in insurance, fire-fighting, and so on. As for the treatment of disease, Thomas elaborates in detail how, despite increasing knowledge, 'so far as actual therapy was concerned, progress was negligible.'[17] Indeed, we now know that the later seventeenth century was unhealthier than the later sixteenth century in England, which again undermines the views of growing security.[18] Stone summarizes

---

[13] Stone, *Past and Present*, 168.   [14] Thomas, *Religion*, 643.   [15] Ibid. 643, 650, 651–4.
[16] Ibid. 656.   [17] Ibid. 47, 658.
[18] See e.g. E. A. Wrigley and R. S. Schofield, *The Population History of England 1541–1871* (Cambridge, 1981), 414, fig. 10.5.

this central weakness: 'during the critical period when magic was in decline and the magical properties of religion also in retreat in the fact of natural theology, there was really no great technological breakthrough.'[19]

Thomas is thus puzzled. He suggests that the change must have been mental, rather than technological. 'For the paradox is that in England magic lost its appeal before the appropriate technical solutions had been devised to take its place.' Indeed it was the reverse of Malinowski. 'It was the abandonment of magic which made possible the upsurge of technology, not the other way round', and this was one of the preconditions, as Weber had seen, for the 'rationalisation of economic life'.[20] If the change that occurred in the seventeenth century was 'not so much technological as mental', what caused that change? Here Thomas admits defeat. He is 'forced to the conclusion that men emancipated themselves from these magical beliefs without necessarily having devised any effective technology with which to replace them'. Yet, 'the ultimate origins of this faith in unaided human capacity remains mysterious'. Despite toying with the idea that 'the decline of the old magical beliefs' are connected to 'the growth of urban living, the rise of science, and the spread of an ideology of self-help', Thomas admits that 'the connection is only approximate and a more precise sociological genealogy cannot at present be constructed'.[21] He might have added that the 'rise of science' and 'spread of an ideology of self-help' are merely parts of the problem to be explained, as we noted in relation to mechanistic philosophy. Thus in terms of explanation of the decline of magic, the central theme of this work, Thomas has been unable to find a solution. The 'mystery' remains, just as it did after my own much more modest attempt at about the same period to 'explain' the decline of witchcraft.[22] We appear to be stuck.

The difficulty of solving the problem of the decline in witchcraft beliefs and accusations is illustrated in a recent collection which is specifically devoted to examining Keith Thomas's major work on *Religion and the Decline of Magic*.[23] In a helpful overview of developments in this field since Thomas's work was published, Jonathan Barry draws attention to a few possible contributing causes for the decline—for instance, the association of witchcraft beliefs with certain religious sects in the Civil War, both witchcraft and these groups being later discredited, and the decline of the interest in magic in the church courts after 1660.[24] Peter Elmer suggests tentatively that Quaker-witch stereotypes took over from pure witches as scapegoats in the 1650s, but admits that 'all

---

[19] Stone, *Past and Present*, 169.   [20] Thomas, *Religion*, 656–7.

[21] Ibid. 661, 663, 665, 666.

[22] A. Macfarlane, *Witchcraft in Tudor and Stuart England* (1970), ch. 16, and esp. pp. 202–3.

[23] J. Barry, M. Hester, and G. Roberts (eds.), *Witchcraft in Early Modern Europe: Studies in Culture and Belief* (Cambridge, 1998).

[24] In ibid. 31, 35.

mono-causal explanations for the decline of educated belief in witchcraft has proved highly elusive'.[25] All that we can be certain of is that, as Ian Bostridge writes, 'by the 1720s the ideological foundations of witchcraft had slipped'.[26] We are still left puzzled.

In his second book, *Man and the Natural World*, Keith Thomas studied a related problem—that is, the growing mastery over and estrangement from the natural world that occurred most markedly in England. His argument may be summarized as follows.[27] If we compare the start and end of the period he reviews, 1500 and 1800, a series of deep changes in perception and feeling had occurred; we have moved from a pre-modern, pre-capitalist, magical cosmology, into a modern, capitalistic, scientific one. Weber's 'disenchantment of the world' has occurred, Marx's alienation of man from the natural world is complete. In 1500 we are in an anthropocentric world of the Bible. All creatures are ordained for man's use; 'nature' is made for man alone and has no rights apart from man. 'Man stood to animal as did heaven to earth, soul to body, culture to nature.' This assumption of a man-ordained world was gradually eroded during this period. This 'revolution in perception—for it was no less' at the upper intellectual and social levels had a 'traumatic effect upon the outlook of ordinary people'. Basically what happened was the separation of man from nature. 'Crucial' to the older beliefs was the interblending of man and nature, 'the ancient assumption that man and nature were locked into one interacting world'. There then occurred the split between man and nature, between thought and emotion, which is part of the famed 'dissociation of sensibility'. The natural world was no longer full of human significance. No longer was every natural event studied for its meaning for human beings, 'for the seventeenth and eighteenth centuries had seen a fundamental departure from the assumptions of the past'.[28]

Why did this happen? Here Thomas falls back on roughly the same set of causes as those advanced in *Religion and the Decline of Magic*. There were scientific and intellectual discoveries: the telescope expanded the heavens and diminished man in space, geological discoveries diminished man in time, the microscope brought out the complexity of nature, exploration and empire brought unimagined species to light. There were economic and social causes.

The triumph of the new attitude was closely linked to the growth of towns and the emergence of an industrial order in which animals became increasingly marginal to the process of production. This industrial order first emerged in England; as a result, it was there that concern for animals was most widely expressed.

---

[25] In Barry *et al.*, *Witchcraft*, 171; cf. 157, 176.   [26] In ibid. 316.

[27] This summary is taken directly from A. Macfarlane, *The Culture of Capitalism* (Oxford, 1987), 79–82.

[28] K. Thomas, *Man and the Natural World: Changing Attitudes in England 1500–1800* (1983), 35, 70, 75, 90.

Kindness to animals, for example, depended on the newly created wealth; it was 'a luxury which not everyone had learnt to afford'.[29] Through the study of the attitude to trees, flowers, and animals he argues that it was rapid urbanization, the replacement of animal by artificial power, growing affluence and security, and a widening intellectual horizon that led to the revolution in ideas about the natural world.

The problem is, however, that Thomas himself gives a great deal of evidence to show that the separation of man and the natural world was not a new phenomenon, invented as mankind for the first time gained mastery over nature in the eighteenth century. For instance, concerning the 'disenchantment of the world', it is not clear that this occurred after the Reformation, for Thomas tells us that 'Since Anglo-Saxon times the Christian Church in England had stood out against the worship of wells and rivers. The pagan divinities of grove, stream and mountain had been expelled, leaving behind them a disenchanted world to be shaped, moulded and dominated'.[30] Although Thomas is right to point out that it is too simple to see this disenchantment as simply equated with Christianity, there is certainly an ascetic stress in Christianity, and particularly in the northern variety, that was hostile to the interfusion of man and nature, to 'magic' and 'symbolic thinking'. Closely related was the supposed shift from the anthropocentric classification of the world, a growing tendency to recognize the separateness and autonomy of the natural world. Having argued that this change was a central feature of the revolution in perception, Thomas continues that 'there was, of course, nothing new about the realization that the natural world had a life of its own'.[31] The view was fully propounded in Aristotle. Turning to specific instances, he shows that pet-keeping, far from being a new invention, was widely present in medieval England, and that the debate over animal cruelty was likewise an old one—for instance, being rehearsed in a poem of 1410. He concludes that the 'truth is that one single, coherent and remarkably constant attitude underlay the great bulk of the preaching and pamphleteering against animal cruelty between the fifteenth and nineteenth centuries', noting that 'so far as their main arguments were concerned there was a notable lack of historical development'.[32] Likewise the enthusiasm for gardening goes back to the Middle Ages, as does the love of wild nature. The anti-urbanism and the desire for country life were widely present well before the sixteenth century.[33]

Where then does this leave Thomas's thesis? It would be difficult to argue that 'urbanism' and 'industrialism' could have had serious effects in England before the second half of the eighteenth century. As in his earlier book on *Religion and the Decline of Magic*, the causes of the change came at least a

---

[29] Ibid. 181, 186. [30] Ibid. 22. [31] Ibid. 82. [32] Ibid. 153, 154.
[33] Macfarlane, *Culture*, 86–91.

couple of centuries too late to explain the phenomenon. As for 'science', this is a complex matter, for the growth of 'science' is one of the very things we are trying to explain and it can become tautological to explain the rise of 'science' by 'science'. Thomas's two attempts to chart the greatest intellectual change in modern history thus, ultimately, leave us with a 'mystery'.

II

In probing Keith Thomas's first book, Hildred Geertz draws attention to an epigraph used by Thomas, taken from Selden. 'The Reason of a Thing is not to be enquired after, til you are sure the Thing itself be so. We commonly are at *What's the Reason of it?* before we are sure of the Thing.' She continues with Selden's anecdote about Sir Robert Cotton, who 'was exclaiming over the strange shape of a shoe which was said to have been worn by Moses, or at least by Noah, when his wife, apparently a much more simple soul, asked: "But Mr Cotton, are you sure it is a Shoe?"'[34] Geertz uses this warning to lead into an attack on Thomas's use of the word 'magic', but it is equally worth looking at another part of the shoe that Thomas is investigating—namely, the links in his argument concerning the environment that led to the decline of magic and the utilitarian and 'scientific' attitude to nature.

Let us experiment by changing some of the parameters. First, as we have seen in relation both to nature and to the decline of magic, the process was already well advanced before the sixteenth century. As compared to most magical worlds, that of the Pastons, of Chaucer, of Bartholomaeus Anglicus or Bracton was already very secularized. In his effort to redress the previous balance, Keith Thomas has exaggerated somewhat the magical elements of the earlier period. Witchcraft and popular magic were already somewhat peripheral. Most explanation was this-worldly, even if people also invoked God, Hell, fairies, etc. This he admits on several occasions, as we have seen. If we reformulate the problem thus, we have less to explain. It was a slight tilting of a balance rather than a vast and revolutionary change from one world view to another. Hence much less of a causal revolution is needed. Secondly, it is worth examining briefly the central opposition between 'magic' and 'science'. As in the standard anthropological tradition since Frazer, these are treated as antithetical and opposed systems. But, given the questioning of the epistemological purity of science,[35] the more sympathetic accounts of the intellectual framework of magic,[36] and the critique of anthropologists on this very

[34] Quoted in H. Geertz, 'An Anthropology of Religion and Magic, I', *Journal of Interdisciplinary History*, 6 (1975), 71.

[35] See e.g. B. Latour and S. Woolgar, *Laboratory Life: The Social Construction of Scientific Facts* (1979).

[36] See e.g. F. Yates, *Giordano Bruno and the Hermetic Tradition* (1964); Clark, *Thinking with Demons*.

point,[37] it now seems more helpful to see the systems as placed on a continuum rather than forming a binary opposition. If we write history from after the event, we can see that certain techniques and findings were fruitful and 'reliable', and others not. But at the time the mixture of methods and hypotheses was much more jumbled and it must often have been difficult to know whether an activity was in our terms 'magical' or 'scientific'.

Some of the problems are resolved if we substitute John Ziman's term 'reliable knowledge' for 'science'.[38] That is to say, we think of a continuum from activities and beliefs where the level of 'reliable knowledge' was very low indeed, to modern 'science' where it is much higher. On this continuum, the high or learned magic of the Renaissance lies somewhere in the middle. It strove for roughly the same goal as 'science'—that is, reliable and effective control over nature. But it did so through methods that did not lead to cumulative growth of knowledge, and on the basis of hypotheses about the hidden forces behind natural appearances, the influence of stars, spirits, place, and so on, that have turned out to be incorrect. Yet, if we see magic and science as placed on a continuum, we realize that modern science evolved out of parts of learned magic, as well as having many other roots. This helps to explain the apparently odd fact that it was precisely at the start of the 'scientific revolution' that learned magic reached its highest point. It then becomes easy to see that John Dee, Francis Bacon, and Isaac Newton are among the last of the great magicians, as well as the first great scientists. Of course, this is not to say that magic and science are the same or that the only difference is the quantity of reliable information they generate. The famous characteristics of the scientific method, falsifiability, experimentations, the search for general laws, and so on, do distinguish it from magic, as does the abandonment of the idea of the moving force lying above or outside this natural world. Yet the shift from one world view to another does not need to be seen as a sudden and total transformation. It could partly be seen as the sloughing-off of an old skin, a reordering of the relations between its parts, a shift of emphasis, a tilting in one direction rather than another, almost a change in intellectual taste or fashion. Seen thus, just as the simplest hunter-gatherer sharpening his flints or searching for animals has to be a proto-scientist, so the greatest of scientists, Isaac Newton, spent as much time on his 'magical' activities as on what we approve of as his 'science'.[39]

If this very preliminary account has truth in it, it again simplifies the problem that Keith Thomas addresses. What needs to be explained at the learned level is not a sudden and total revolution from 'magic' to 'science' in 200 years. Rather, we are dealing with a change of emphasis, which occurred

[37] See Geertz, 'Anthropology of Religion'.
[38] J. Ziman, *Reliable Knowledge: An Exploration of the Grounds for Belief in Science* (Cambridge, 1979).
[39] On Newton's magical workings, see e.g. J. M. Keynes, *Essays in Biography* (1951), 313–19.

most dramatically in the famous period 1550–1800, but which is part of a much longer reorientation. The process can, in reality, be dated back to the Greeks, and gathers pace in Europe from about the twelfth century with the revival of Greek–Arabic science and the founding of universities. From that time, the experimentalism, optimism, the search for abstract truths, all were characteristic of work that we can broadly term 'scientific'.

III

Yet even if we make the change much more drawn out and less dramatic, there is still something to explain, and here we may return to Keith Thomas's technological argument. Let us look at this argument again, but in a context where, instead of requiring a sudden dramatic improvement in man's physical environment—for instance, a 'revolution' in medicine, food production, or control of accidents—we would be seeking a long-term and slow improvement from at least the fourteenth century. We would also be looking at the general level—that is to say, whether the improvement was from an already unusually high level of wealth and technology for a 'pre-industrial' society to an even higher one. Finally, we would need to extend our interest outside the rather physical elements of the environment—food, health, fire—to include the political environment.

Let us take first those insecurities on which Thomas himself concentrates. The first is demographic. We have seen that he implies that life was relatively short and uncertain. This is, of course, true if we compare expectation of life at birth in the seventeenth century with the present. Yet the equations look different if we remember that in terms of survival after the age of 1 there was really no secular improvement for most of the population before the late nineteenth century. An Elizabethan villager who had reached the age of 1 had just as good an expectation of life as Robert Koch or Louis Pasteur. This illustrates the second point concerning the general level—that, rather than seeing mortality levels in England as incredibly high before the demographic revolution of the later nineteenth century, we should in cross-comparative perspective see the levels as surprisingly low, a middling plateau that is perfectly compatible with a relatively optimistic and stable attitude towards the future, planning, and achievement.[40] Thomas's second insecurity is food, where he implies that there was widespread shortage, deficiency, and dearth, if not massive famines. Again, of course, there is something in this. But it could be argued that in relative terms the English were an extraordinarily well-fed population and that famine had been banished from all but a corner of the land by the

---

[40] A. Macfarlane, *The Savage Wars of Peace: England, Japan and the Malthusian Trap* (Oxford, 1997), 25–30.

fifteenth century. The light population, efficient agriculture, good communications, early market system, temperate climate, and other factors protected the population from the vagaries of weather that effect so many 'agrarian' societies. It is not at all difficult to argue that the population of England was as well fed in the sixteenth century as in the nineteenth, and in both centuries, apart from Holland, the English in general were probably the best-fed population the world had ever known.[41]

Thomas's third major insecurity is disease. Here again there is a half-truth. It is true that, if we compare an English or American after 1950 with an English woman or man in the sixteenth century, then the latter was subjected to numerous forms of disease that have now been eliminated. But again we need to make at least two qualifications. First, the changes were gradual and complex, with a rise in certain diseases and decline in others. Again, the situation of the later sixteenth century is not notably worse than that of the early nineteenth; old diseases such as plague and leprosy had gone, new diseases such as smallpox and cholera were rampant. Secondly, in comparison to most pre-industrial settled civilizations, the incidence of most diseases was relatively low. It is obviously true that there were widespread illnesses and most people suffered pain with a frequency and intensity that modern Westerners would find difficult to bear. Yet the levels were not usually overwhelming. Furthermore, people could point to some improvements: leprosy had vanished, the sweating sickness disappeared after the sixteenth century, venereal disease declined in virulence, plague become localized in cities and later vanished.[42] Finally, there are accident and misfortune, particularly fire. It is true that fire was a constant hazard, but it is tempting to overplay its importance. In comparison to other misfortunes, it is only of moderate importance. There may even have been early and subtle mechanisms that further reduced the impact of fire. Certainly it was possible for the Japanese, with largely ineffective fire-fighting equipment, no formal insurance, and conflagrations every few years, to face the hazards of fire with some equanimity.[43]

Man's attitude towards the possibility of controlling the external world is affected by many other material, cultural, and political factors. In terms of the material, there is the whole set of protections for his body, particularly housing and clothing. Here the English from at least the fourteenth century, and very markedly from the sixteenth, enjoyed levels of affluence and security that were, with the exception of the Dutch, unprecedented. An average Elizabethan was as affluent, well dressed, housed, and fed as an average inhabitant of England in any period up to the late nineteenth century—and far better than in all other world civilizations in history.[44] When they looked out from this relative warmth and physical security, not over-pressed by long work

[41] Ibid., chs. 5, 6, 8.　　[42] Ibid., pts. III–V.　　[43] Ibid. 233–4.
[44] Ibid., chs. 5, 6, 12, 13.

hours,[45] most people could have some sense of confidence in a reasonably stable, controllable, and ultimately comprehensible external world. They could see the improvements around them—better agriculture, new drinks, better cloth production, better housing, the printing press, gunpowder, and compass. These and other modern improvements, as Thomas argues, gave people a sense of dynamism and progress.[46] Their force was increased because they were based on an already unusually high standard of living.

Furthermore, it was not just the immediate private space of the English that had been domesticated, tamed, brought under control—not merely house, garden, food, and clothing. As Thomas shows, the physical landscape had been tamed and ordered very early. The shape of the fields and hedges, of the roads and paths, of the majority of human settlements, had been laid out by the eleventh century and was to change little over the next 700 years. Dangerous wild animals, which still roamed over much of continental Europe or Scotland until the eighteenth and nineteenth centuries, were destroyed very early. In the sixteenth century William Harrison thought it one of the important blessings of God on England 'that it is void of noisome beasts, as lions, bears, tigers, pards [leopards], wolves, and suchlike, by means whereof our countrymen may travel in safety and our herds and flocks remain for the most part abroad in the field without any herdmen or keeper'.[47] He compared this with the situation beyond the Tweed, where fierce animals abounded. The perceived safety of the countryside went back much earlier. In the early thirteenth century the English monk Bartholomaeus Anglicus noted that in England there were 'few wolves or none' and as a result sheep could be securely left 'without ward in pasture and in fields'. This, he said, went back to Anglo-Saxon times, and had been a phenomenon noted by Bede.[48]

Even more dangerous than animal predators are human ones and it is they who usually make it necessary for armed shepherds to guard the flocks. Thus as important as the control of the physical world of nature was the control of human violence through political and legal means, a subject that Thomas largely omits. Here again it would seem that England had been early tamed. England was a largely unified nation state under the later Anglo-Saxon kings from Alfred onwards and the continuing uncertainties, regional uprisings, and over-mighty subjects were, in the main, eliminated by the strong governments of the Normans and Angevins. Internal warfare and invading armies, which made much of Europe dangerous and led to a weapon-carrying population and the defensive fortifications of nobility and cities up to the nineteenth century, had largely been eliminated by the early medieval period in England. The power of the king's courts, the absence of a standing army, the freedom from foreign invasions provided by sea boundaries, these and other factors

---

[45] Macfarlane, *Savage Wars*, ch. 3.   [46] Thomas, *Religion*, 429–32.
[47] William Harrison, *The Description of England*, ed. G. Edelen (New York, 1968), 324.
[48] Bartholomaeus Anglicus, *On the Properties of Things*, trans. J. Trevisa (1975), ii. 734.

combined to give a very early and continuous peace. The early development of an intricate legal system, monopolization of violence by the State, a high level of participation in the local administration of justice, which are well-known features of England back to the Middle Ages, are all different facets of this stability. The contrast with the devastations of France, Germany, Spain, or Italy through the centuries is instructive.[49]

The differences in political structure would help to explain the curious fact that the English gentry after the fifteenth century were happy to live in unde-fended manor houses in the country, while in most countries they sheltered within huge chateau fortifications or, preferably, within the city walls. Towns and castles were the refuge and the natural home of 'civility' and 'civilization'— that is, of people with urbane, urban, and civilized manners—when times were violent, and hence were far more important on the Continent. It is for these reasons that E. A. Freeman, for instance, when trying to explain the absence of 'capital' cities in England, ascribed it to political factors. The 'princely' and the 'civic' elements show themselves in greater splendour in French rather than English cities 'simply because in England the kingdom was more united, because the general government was stronger, because the English earl or bishop was not an independent prince, nor the English city an independent commonwealth'.[50] Edinburgh or Durham was the nearest British equivalent to such a phenomenon.

A final strand of the explanation of the peculiarities undoubtedly lies in the religious system. Keith Thomas, following Weber, rightly lays considerable stress on this. Christianity in general has a curiously ambivalent attitude towards the relations between man and nature. On the one hand, it stresses an exploitative attitude; all creatures were made by God for man, and can be used for his own good. On the other hand, all creatures were created by God, and man should respect His creation and see His hand in its beauty. The myth of the Garden of Eden is an aspect of the rural emphasis of the religion. Within Christianity, the proto-Protestant and Protestant versions that dominated England stressed an anti-magical, disenchanted attitude towards nature that Weber noted. Long before the Reformation, many of the uncertainties, mys-teries, and extensive ritual interpenetrations had been eliminated. An overlap of the material and spiritual worlds common in many cultures was largely absent. The attack on those popular errors that indicated a fear and awe of nature, the undermining of a belief in divine presences in natural phenomena, had begun long ago under the Anglo-Saxon Church. It was carried to its logical and final limits by Protestantism. An ascetic, anti-magical tendency in Christianity thus fitted with the other forces, political, economic, social, that

---

[49] The differences in warfare are described in Macfarlane, *Savage Wars*, ch. 4; I discuss the wider political and legal differences in more detail in a forthcoming work, titled *The Riddle of the Modern World* (2000).

[50] E. A. Freeman, *Historical Essays*, 4th ser. (1892), 42.

separated the world of man and nature, bringing nature under absolute control, and then allowing a sentimental reintegration on man's own terms. This disenchantment of the world is the central theme of Thomas's work and he summarizes the process thus: 'in place of a natural world redolent with human analogy and symbolic meaning, and sensitive to man's behaviour, they constructed a detached natural scene to be viewed and studied from the outside.'[51]

Other elements of Christianity are also essential. There is the attitude towards time; many have pointed towards Christianity as a historical religion, moving mankind from an original creation through a long series of stages to a final revelation. This gave a sense of openness and progress.[52] Or, again, the theology suggested an omnipotent and omniscient God who had lain down a series of 'laws' that it was man's duty to enquire after. This again was pro-pitious. Thirdly, Christianity took a positive, not to say positivistic, attitude towards the physical world. It existed independently of the observer, it was not an illusion or construct of man's mind, as it tended to become in some forms of Eastern mystical religion, hence precluding serious scientific inves-tigation of the 'natural world'.[53]

All these features were necessary ingredients. Yet, as we can see from the history of certain Catholic countries such as Spain or Portugal, if combined with a different political and social structure these religious beliefs were not enough to lead to the transformation of magic and ritual. It is the total assem-blage—the increasingly high standard of material life and political security as well as the religious tendency that is necessary—in exactly the right mix and over a long period. The roots lie back in north-western Europe from the Middle Ages and we can see them developing, for instance, in England from at least the twelfth century. They are apparent in the work of Bartholomaeus Anglicus, Bracton, Roger Bacon, Occam, and many others. What we see in the sixteenth to eighteenth centuries is not a revolutionary change but a growing confidence and extension of earlier tendencies. By a kind of paradoxical miracle, by the end of the eighteenth century England was both the same and utterly different from the England of Chaucer.

IV

The development was not a steady growth of the kind beloved by Whig his-torians, yet it is, after the event, possible to see a sort of 'progress' in the way in which the balance was tipped. We might, therefore, conclude that in

---

[51] Thomas, *Natural World*, 89.
[52] See e.g. J. B. Bury, *The Idea of Progress* (1921), 23.
[53] See *The Shorter Science and Civilization in China* (Cambridge, 1978), i. 265, an abridgement by C. A. Ronan of Joseph Needham's original text.

England many of the causes of insecurity, war, famine, and most diseases (except plague) had already been brought within reasonable limits by the late fourteenth century. Life was reasonably predictable. The violence of men, weather, and micro-organisms had already largely been brought under control. People felt a reasonable sense of confidence in a relatively stable and predictable world. By the fifteenth century the firm underpinning provided by the reasonably efficient administrative system, the good judicial system, the advanced market economy, meant that there was, for an agrarian economy, already an unusually high level of personal security. Popular magic was needed only at the margins. The learned or intellectual magic described by Stuart Clark was not strongly antithetical to science, but probably a necessary precursor. The area of the 'irrational' was already delimited.

What then happened was that in the sixteenth century all these tendencies were enhanced. The threat of civil war evaporated further. The integrated market economy spread further. Affluence for the middle groups rose. The Poor Law and administration were improved. Plague declined in virulence and there was a relatively healthy period until the 1620s. By the 1590s the balance had been tipped decisively towards a belief in the controllability of the external world, and a sense of optimism and progress was felt, as evidenced by Francis Bacon, for example. Things were improving. Man could raise himself. The setbacks in the 1590s and 1620s momentarily halted this process, but after the 1650s the founding of the Royal Society and other institutions, and the work of Boyle, Hooke, Newton, and others made rapid progress. Confidence rose as conditions improved. The world of Defoe is considerably more complex and sophisticated than the world of Harrison or Camden. As people looked back, they could feel a real sense of discovery and progress, not only over the recent past, but even when compared with the glorious attainments of Greece or Rome.

Standing back from Keith Thomas's work, we see that the problem of the decline of magical and witchcraft beliefs and accusations will be approachable only if we redefine what is to be explained. The strong opposition of 'science' and 'magic' is not helpful. Nor did 'magical beliefs' go through a straightforward secular decline, but rose and fell over time in the period between the fifteenth and eighteenth centuries. Yet, even if we modify the dating and the emphasis put forward in the early formulation by Keith Thomas, there is still something left to explain. Here it is worth exploring the way in which some of the insecurities of life that encourage belief in witchcraft and magic were being eroded from the fifteenth century. The relative affluence, the political and legal security, the relative freedom from the Malthusian ravages of war, famine, and disease, provide a necessary, if far from sufficient, background to what still remains something of a mystery. Keith Thomas posed a real question, and, even if his answer does not fully satisfy either him or us, it characteristically stimulates and challenges us to try and do better.

9

Perceptions of the Metropolis in Seventeenth-Century England

PAUL SLACK

Great towns in the body of a state are like the spleen . . . in the body natural: the monstrous growth of which impoverisheth all the members, by drawing to it all the animal and vital spirits, which should give nourishment unto them.

(Peter Heylyn (1652))[1]

The metropolis is the heart of a nation, through which the trade and commodities of it circulate, like the blood through the heart, which by its motion giveth life and growth to the rest of the body; and if that declines, or be obstructed in its growth, the whole body falls into consumption.

([Nicholas Barbon] (1685))[2]

These contrasting assertions illustrate the two extremes in contemporary perceptions of one of the most important events in seventeenth-century English history: the birth of a metropolis. In 1600 the built-up area of London contained around 200,000 people, 5 per cent of the population of England; in 1700 it had more than half a million people, 11 per cent of the whole. The social and economic repercussions of that development have been described in celebrated articles by F. J. Fisher and E. A. Wrigley.[3] My concern in this essay is to enquire how far, and with what degree of enthusiasm, these repercussions were recognized by contemporaries, and thus to offer a modest contribution to the larger history of man's appreciation of his environment that Keith Thomas has pioneered.[4]

Two preliminary qualifications are necessary. First, I shall be investigating overt public perceptions, whether of applause or condemnation, and not

---

[1] Peter Heylyn, *Cosmographie In Four Bookes* (1652), 270.
[2] [Nicholas Barbon], *An Apology for the Builder* (1685), 30.
[3] F. J. Fisher, *London and the English Economy, 1500–1700*, ed. P. J. Corfield and N. B. Harte (1990), chs. 6, 12; E. A. Wrigley, 'A Simple Model of London's Importance in Changing English Society and Economy 1650–1750', *P&P* 37 (1967), 44–70.
[4] K. Thomas, *Man and the Natural World: Changing Attitudes in England 1500–1800* (1983).

private ones. Private responses to London were often different and must on balance generally have been favourable. If they had not been, there would be no metropolitan phenomenon to be investigated. Nehemiah Wallington's apprentice might say he 'did not like London, and . . . would be gone', and some other immigrants be repelled by the city's noise, stench, and smoke, but all of them had been attracted in the first place by opportunities for betterment.[5] Temporary residents must in general have agreed with Mary Rich, who thought it 'always the saddest thing' to go away again, and with Rebecca Long, who found that time passed more slowly in the country without 'the variety of objects' to be appreciated in town.[6]

Secondly, although I shall be seeking to identify change, it has to be admitted that public attitudes were conspicuously ambivalent throughout the period. London was no different from other great cities in the past in being pictured simultaneously as Babylon and Jerusalem; and the polarity had particular appeal in an intellectual climate where such binary oppositions were familiar rhetorical devices. It was as natural to set urban images of sin, extravagance, dirt, and infection against those of civility, wealth, light, and learning as it was to contrast the notions of London as economic parasite and economic stimulus. Complementary though they were, however, there was a contest between positive and negative views of the city. We will see that the balance of opinion became perceptibly more favourable, particularly in the second half of the seventeenth century; and the reasons for that are not without interest. It was more than a matter of passively accepting an irresistible reality.

I

Physiological metaphors were employed by both sides from the beginning of the public debate about London's growth. The capital 'disperseth foreign wares (as the stomach doth meat) to all the members most commodiously', said an 'Apology (or Defence)' for the city written around 1580 and published by Stow in 1598; that explained the 'flourishing estate' of Norfolk, Suffolk, Essex, Kent, and Sussex. London might well be 'the belly or if you will the head of England', countered Thomas Digges, speaking in Parliament in 1585, but the extremities, 'the legs and hands', also had to live and were being impoverished.[7] These were contributions to an argument initially opened on

---

[5] P. Seaver, *Wallington's World* (1985), 139; D. Souden, 'Migrants and the Population Structure of Later Seventeenth-Century Provincial Cities and Market Towns', in P. Clark (ed.), *The Transformation of English Provincial Towns 1600–1800* (1984), 133.

[6] *Autobiography of Mary Countess of Warwick*, ed. T. C. Croker (Percy Society; 1848), 18; Hants. RO, Jervoise of Herriard collection, 44M69, L31/50 (1616).

[7] John Stow, *A Survey of London*, ed. C. L. Kingsford (2 vols.; Oxford, 1908), ii. 212–13, 387 (the author was probably James Dalton, the City's common pleader); T. E. Hartley, *Proceedings in the Parliaments of Elizabeth I* (3 vols.; Leicester, 1981–95), ii. 112.

somewhat narrower ground: by a royal proclamation of 1580 against new buildings and the creation of new tenements in the city. It was prompted by rising rents, overcrowding, immigration, and the threat of plague in the later 1570s; and it was the beginning of a government campaign waged right down to the Civil War in an effort to maintain a proper balance between country and town, to restore hospitality to the one and health to the other, and so to protect the nation against the multiple threats defined in a Star Chamber prosecution of 1606: 'death, dearth, depopulation, disorder'.[8]

There were soon several voices in contention. In the country the 'natural malice' of 'the gentlemen of England towards the citizens of London' joined with pressure from merchants in the outports for 'the more equal distribution of the wealth of the land . . . even as the equal distributing of nourishment in a man's body'.[9] In the city William Smith drew up a 'Brief Description' of London's fame, antiquity, beauty, good government, and trade in 1588, while an anonymous *Breefe Discourse* of 1584 underlined its role as 'metropolis or mother city', *epitome totius Angliae*, and *totius occidentis emporium*.[10] It is no coincidence that the famous dialogue on *Cyvile and Uncyvile Life*, debating the relative merits of 'civility' and 'rusticity', was published in 1579 and reprinted in 1586, nor that it gave almost equal weight to both sides. If in the end its critic of 'the licentious customs of the city' seems finally persuaded of London's virtues, a similar dialogue thirty years later evened the score. There the 'sweet creatures and civil behaviour' of the Court are ultimately less appealing than the still more 'sweet' country life, 'a simile of heaven upon earth'.[11]

It would be futile to try to estimate which of the contrasting images of London—as a place of 'filth, stench, noise'[12] or of *urbanitas* and 'pleasant walks'[13]—had the greater purchase. In contemporary rhetoric as in reality the two were bound together in a necessary and productive counterpoint. Only 'the head of the empire' could produce the excesses in dress and diet that William Stafford decried in 1581, and the environment of coal and

[8] P. L. Hughes and J. F. Larkin, *Tudor Royal Proclamations* (3 vols.; New Haven, 1964–9), ii, no. 649, pp. 466–8; T. G. Barnes, 'The Prerogative and Environmental Control of London Building in the Early Seventeenth Century: The Lost Opportunity', *California Law Review*, 58 (1970), 1332–63; John Hawarde, *Les Reportes del Cases in Camera Stellata 1593 to 1609*, ed. W. P. Baildon (1894), 319.

[9] George Whetstone, *A Mirrour for Magestrates of Cyties* (1584), sig. Ji; R. Ashton, 'The Parliamentary Agitation for Free Trade in the Opening Years of the Reign of James I', *P&P* 38 (1967), 46.

[10] [William Smith], 'A Breeff Description of The Famous Cittie of London', BL Harleian MS 6363; *A Breefe Discourse, declaring and approuing . . . the laudable Customes of London* (1584), 10, 12.

[11] *The English Courtier, and the Cuntrey-gentleman* (1586), in W. Hazlitt (ed.), *Inedited Tracts* (1868), 15, 92; Nicholas Breton, *The Court and the Country* (1618), sig. A4ᵛ.

[12] Ben Jonson, *Poems*, ed. B. N. Newdigate (Oxford, 1936), 51; I. Archer, 'The Nostalgia of John Stow' in D. L. Smith, R. Strier, and D. Bevington (eds.), *The Theatrical City: Culture, Theatre and Politics in London 1576–1649* (Cambridge, 1995), 22.

[13] Stow, *Survey*, ed. Kingsford, ii. 198; Richard Johnson, *The Pleasant Walkes of Moore-fields* (1607).

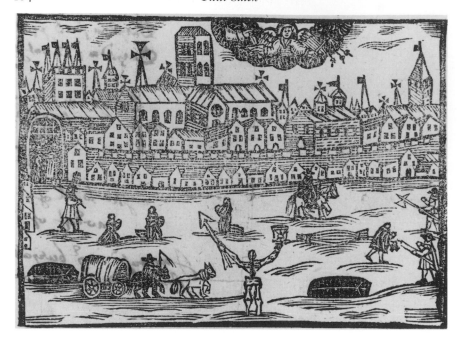

5. Death triumphing over London: from a broadside illustrating the plague of 1636

consumption that Fanshawe summed up in 1630 as 'the smoky glory of the town'.[14] In order to make their moral point about the recurrent plagues that punished the city, Thomas Dekker and his successors had to magnify its status: 'the goodliest of thy neighbours, but the proudest; the wealthiest, but the most wanton';[15] and the woodcut illustrations that decorated broadsheets and plague tracts in the early seventeenth century had impact only because they could show death triumphing over a fine walled city dominated by steeples and the great bulk of old St Paul's. It was an indispensable dialogue in which positive and negative features of London each gave point and meaning to the other.

There is no doubt that the works of the first chorographers and antiquaries boosted the reputation of the city, and hence the power of one particular voice. Camden's summary of London's role—'the Epitome or Breviary of all Britain, the seat of the British Empire, and the King of England's Chamber'—was copied for a century and more, often with the addition of 'Emporium'

[14] William Stafford, *Compendious or briefe Examination of Certayne ordinary Complaints* (1581), ed. F. J. Furnivall (New Shakespere Society; 1876), 65; Richard Fanshawe, 'An Ode', in H. J. C. Grierson and G. Bullough (eds.), *The Oxford Book of Seventeenth-Century Verse* (Oxford, 1934), 451.

[15] Thomas Dekker, *The Seven Deadly Sinnes of London*, quoted in G. K. Paster, *The Idea of the City in the Age of Shakespeare* (Athens, Ga., 1985), 3.

and 'Metropolis' borrowed from the *Breefe Discourse*.[16] English writers also borrowed literary models from abroad, discussing the origins of towns in Aristotelian and Ciceronian terms as places of 'civil life', and enumerating their present attributes.[17] It became usual to describe both the civil aspects of London—its excellent government, religion, arts, and learning—and its economic achievements, its 'merchandise and commerce'. There were accounts not only of London's most famous landmarks, especially London Bridge ('worthily to be numbered among the miracles of the world'), and of the foundation myth of Brutus, with its imperial connotations, but of London's churches and schools, its ships on the Thames, its artificers, and variety of foreign and domestic manufactures.[18] The writers of pageants for the Lord Mayor's Show naturally followed suit. Anthony Munday, busy on his new edition of Stow, presented London as *Metropolis coronata* in 1615, 'the ancient mother of the whole land', admired by figures representing 'learned religion, military discipline, navigation, and homebred husbandry', and as a commercial emporium bringing the fruits 'of all kingdoms, cities and nations' to 'the furthest remote countries' (i.e. counties). Middleton's *Triumphs of Health and Prosperity* of 1626 banished the plague of the previous year and saw London having, 'as in the body, the heart's place, | Fit for her works of piety and grace'.[19]

Yet, in the eyes of the government at least, these celebrations of the city were not wholly at odds with attempts to prevent suburban building, overcrowded tenements, and the flow of migrants. The two went hand in hand in the rhetoric that James I brought to what had previously been more pedestrian Elizabethan statements of environmental intent. Encouraged by Francis Bacon, James determined to refurbish *Augusta*, ancient London, as Augustus had re-edified Rome, transforming it from a city of wood into one of brick. Now that London was 'the greatest, or next the greatest city of the Christian world', it was time for 'an utter cessation of further new buildings' unless they were of 'public use and ornament', like the various embellishments commended in one of his proclamations: Britain's Bourse (Cecil's New Exchange), for instance, Sutton's Hospital (Charterhouse), the New River, and the newly cleared Moorfields. In the hands of Inigo Jones, with his new building regu-

[16] William Camden, *Britannia*, trans. Philemon Holland (1610), 421. Edward Chamberlayne added 'the chiefest Emporium or Town of Trade in the World' in the 1679 and later editions of his *Angliae notitia* ((1679), pt. II, p. 176).

[17] L. Manley, *Literature and Culture in Early Modern London* (Cambridge, 1995), ch. 3. Cf. Adrianus Romanus, *Parvum Theatrum Vrbium* (Frankfurt, 1595), 2–3, on London as *emporium* and *sedes regni*, and a place of wealth and letters.

[18] John Stow, *The Survay of London*, continued by A[nthony] M[unday] (1618), sig. 3ᵛ; Fynes Moryson, *An Itinerary* (1617; 4 vols., Glasgow, 1907–8), iii. 487; Richard Rowlands [Richard Verstegan], *The Post of the World* (1576), 51–2; Heylyn, *Cosmographie*, 5, 270.

[19] D. M. Bergeron (ed.), *Pageants and Entertainments of Anthony Munday* (New York, 1985), 91–2, 129; Paster, *Idea of the City*, 140–1. Cf. Thomas Heywood's *Londini Sinus Salutis, or, Londons Harbour of Health, and Happinesse* (1635).

lations and architectural projects, and of Charles I, with further rhetorical flourishes about 'the seat imperial of this kingdom', the campaign to clean up and control the capital became part of the public programme of early Stuart kingship.[20] Looking to foreign examples, particularly in the greatest city in Christendom, the Paris of Henri IV,[21] it made a great deal of noise, and it undoubtedly sharpened perceptions of what London might be. Yet it was somehow held in balance—in dialogue again—with the view, equally explicit in government statements, that London was a head too big for its body, 'impoverishing and ruining the rest of the kingdom'.[22]

The balance was obviously precarious. There is, therefore, some significance in early hints that there was indeed a tension, even an inconsistency, between what the Crown's left and right hands were doing; and that the arguments of the one might be used against the policies of the other. It must have been with an eye to current concerns that judgements in a remote Elizabethan case about new building were published in 1636. They included Judge Manwood's assertion that 'this city is the greatest city, and most populous in this realm, and the more populous, the more honourable, and the more buildings, the more populous and honourable will it be, and therefore building is to be favoured'.[23] More remarkable still in its anticipation of later argument is a document of *c*.1620 preserved in his 'book of projects' by Robert Cotton, himself a commissioner for London buildings. Not only was new building defended as 'both honourable and utile' in demonstrating the king's 'power' and 'the wealth of his subjects', but, if London was to rival Paris and Madrid, it must be allowed to grow as they were. New houses would improve, not threaten, health, and draw no more people to the capital than would have come anyway. Moreover, if the growth of London raised the price of victuals, as was complained, that could only benefit its suppliers, 'the gentleman, the husbandman, the country farmer, and the grazier'. 'Experience' showed that, when prices rose in London during term, they were accompanied by abundance, not dearth: they might be a stimulus, not a check, to national prosperity.[24]

Experience certainly showed, not only that the growth of London could

---

[20] P. Slack, *From Reformation to Improvement: Public Welfare in Early Modern England* (Oxford, 1999), 70–2; PRO SP 14/165/57; J. F. Larkin and P. L. Hughes, *Stuart Royal Proclamations* (2 vols.; Oxford, 1973–83), i, no. 152, pp. 345–6; ii, no. 9, p. 21. Cf. K. Sharpe, *The Personal Rule of Charles I* (1992), 406–12; J. Newman, 'Inigo Jones and the Politics of Architecture', in K. Sharpe and P. Lake, *Culture and Politics in Early Stuart England* (1994), 229–55.

[21] H. Ballon, *The Paris of Henri IV: Architecture and Urbanism* (Cambridge, Mass., 1991). Cf. also contemporary Madrid: J. Brown and J. H. Elliott, *A Palace for a King: The Buen Retiro and the Court of Philip IV* (New Haven, 1980), 3.

[22] PRO SP 16/533/17, fo. 39ᵛ.

[23] *A Briefe Declaration For What manner of speciall Nusance concerning private dwelling houses, a man may have his remedy* (1636), 23–4; J. H. Baker, *An Introduction to English Legal History* (1971), 240 n.

[24] BL Cotton MS Titus B.V, fo. 213; K. Sharpe, *Sir Robert Cotton 1586–1631* (Oxford, 1979), 122–3, 139, 141.

not in practice be halted, but that it was transforming the metropolis, particularly—and partly by royal licence—in the West End. The credibility of
attempts to restore the balance and distinction between city and country was
visibly undermined by the emergence of 'the Town', which was neither one
nor the other, and where a new style of gentlemanly civility was being
forged.[25] No longer a city defined by its walls and liberties, London was
becoming an amalgam of diverse, socially distinguishable neighbourhoods.
Minority voices apart, however, that did little to make the consequences intellectually acceptable. It is not just 'the increasing fragmentation' of the city that
can be found reflected in late Jacobean and Caroline comedies, for example,
but a profound uncertainty about standards of behaviour in the new environment emerging between Westminster and St Paul's where landed and mercantile notions of honour and respectability collided.[26] The expansion of the
metropolis raised questions about conduct as intractable as those that related
to the management of its physical environment and to the structure of its local
government.[27]

None of these problems had been resolved by 1640. Neither were they to
be in the second half of the century. But they were then pushed into the background, and at last made palatable by two developments: first, by a further
bout of self-congratulation on the glories of the city, better informed and
more persuasive than before; and, secondly, by the elaboration of arguments
designed to show that the whole nation—country as well as town—benefited
from, and should take pride in, the achievement.

II

The impact of the Civil War was as two-edged as most of the rest of our story.
For all the Miltons who saw London as 'the mansion-house of liberty', there
were at least as many more who thought it 'the sink of all the ill-humours
of the kingdom', 'Nodnol', a backwards world, demonstrating, as it did to
Hobbes, that 'the immoderate greatness of a town' was an 'infirmity of a commonwealth'.[28] On the eve of the Restoration, London was still both 'our
kingdom's brightest object, fairest flower', and 'that rebellious city' whose

---

[25] L. Stone, 'The Residential Development of the West End of London in the Seventeenth
Century', in B. Malament (ed.), *After the Reformation: Essays in Honor of J. H. Hexter* (Manches-
ter, 1980), 167–212; A. Bryson, *From Courtesy to Civility: Changing Codes of Conduct in Early
Modern England* (Oxford, 1998), 128–50.

[26] A. Barton, *Essays, Mainly Shakespearean* (Cambridge, 1994), chs. 14, 15, and esp. pp. 345–6,
350–1; M. Butler, *Theatre and Crisis 1632–1642* (Cambridge, 1984), ch. 7; Manley, *Literature and
Culture*, 476–7.

[27] On local government, see V. Pearl, *London and the Outbreak of the Puritan Revolution*
(Oxford, 1961), 31–7.

[28] S. Porter (ed.), *London and the Civil War* (1996), 12; N. G. Brett-James, *The Growth of Stuart
London* (1935), 117; D. Underdown, *A Freeborn People: Politics and the Nation in Seventeenth-Century
England* (Oxford, 1996), 103–4; Thomas Hobbes, *Leviathan*, ed. R. Tuck (Cambridge, 1991), 230.
On Nodnol, see also Manley, *Literature and Culture*, 88.

moral filth meant 'death, plague, sword, fire, vengeance' to come.[29] Yet, when plague, war, and fire did come in the 1660s, London not only survived; it was reborn and rediscovered. The consequences of the Great Fire were wholly positive, providing an opportunity to transform Charles II's 'imperial' city, as his father had been unable to do, into a place of 'uniformity and gracefulness', a capital 'not so much ruined, as refined'. It might not quite prove itself a 'new Jerusalem', but by the 1670s it could better 'dirty Paris' and 'stately Florence', and match recently expanded Amsterdam in environmental improvement.[30]

The Fire thus gave a spur to international comparisons, and particularly to the rivalry between Paris and London, the two urban giants on the European scene. It was a contest determined largely (though not only) by size. The competition was partly about the monuments and ornaments of the two cities, where Louis XIV soon gave Paris the edge. It was partly about relative levels of civility in manners and fashion, on which literary exchanges continued down to 1700 and beyond.[31] But it was also about relative size of population, where assertion was finally, and crucially, replaced by measurement. Until 1670 opinion was divided. Thomas Gainsford thought London more populous as early as 1618. John Finch and Heylyn put Paris first in 1651–2. James Howell's great panegyric on *Londinopolis* of 1657 had London out in front, as well as making it easily the first city of Europe, weighing twenty different criteria for greatness together.[32]

Once bills of mortality had been adopted in Paris in imitation of London in 1670, however, precise calculation could begin. In 1676 John Graunt was able to show that Paris was bigger by a fifth. Three years later Locke was informed that it had 500,000 people to London's 450,000: the difference had narrowed. In 1687 William Petty used the most recent bills to demonstrate to his own satisfaction, and more than once, if probably somewhat prematurely, that London was in the lead.[33] The conclusion was generally accepted by

---

[29] [Dudley, Lord North], *A Forest Promiscuous of Several Seasons Productions*, pt. I (1659), 18; Walter Gostelo, *The coming of God in Mercy, in Vengeance; Begining With fire* (1658), sigs. E1ʳ, D8ᵛ.

[30] 18 & 19 Charles II, c. 8; R. A. Aubin (ed.), *London in Flames, London in Glory: Poems on the Fire and Rebuilding of London 1666–1709* (New Brunswick, NJ, 1943), 55, 141–2, 157; J. I. Israel, *The Dutch Republic: Its Rise, Greatness and Fall 1477–1806* (Oxford, 1995), 863–73.

[31] R. W. Berger, *A Royal Passion: Louis XIV as Patron of Architecture* (Cambridge, 1994), 74 and *passim*. For literary expression of the competition, see e.g. Martin Lister, *A Journey to Paris in the Year 1698* (3rd edn., 1699), 6, parodied in [William King], *A Journey to London In the Year, 1698* (1698).

[32] Thomas Gainsford, *The Glory of England* (1618), 256, 261; M. H. Nicolson and S. Hutton (eds.), *The Conway Letters* (rev. edn., Oxford, 1992), 59; Heylyn, *Cosmographie*, 270; James Howell, *Londinopolis; An Historical Discourse or Perlustration Of the City of London, The Imperial Chamber, and chief Emporium of Great Britain* (1657), 385–91.

[33] *The Economic Writings of Sir William Petty*, ed. C. H. Hull (2 vols.; Cambridge, 1899), ii. 423–4 (Graunt), 505–6, 522–40 (Petty); J. Lough (ed.), *Locke's Travels in France 1675–1679* (Cambridge, 1953), 256. For modern estimates, see A. L. Beier and R. Finlay (eds.), *London 1500–1700: The Making of the Metropolis* (1986), 3.

foreign visitors after 1700, when it had not always been before,[34] and learned debate in the two cities had to turn to the more intricate geometrical issue of which city was the larger in area (with predictable findings on either side).[35] There was still room for disagreement about the precise number of people in London,[36] but there was none about its international primacy in this respect. Thanks to Petty, Chamberlayne's *Angliae notitia* was able to claim in every annual edition from 1687 onwards that London was 'the largest and most populous, the fairest and most opulent city at this day in all Europe, perhaps in the whole world, surpassing even Paris and Rome put together'.[37] Size now came first.

The bills of mortality altered perceptions in other ways too. Published weekly from at least 1603 and in annual summary form regularly from at least 1629, they first cut plague down to size by making its progress measurable and to an extent predictable, and then enabled the whole social demography of the capital to be analysed.[38] The first path-breaking exercise, Graunt's *Natural and Political Observations* of 1662, was in fact notably equivocal in its approach to London's growth. Its hesitant conclusion, that 'the metropolis of England is *perhaps* a head too big for the body and *possibly* too strong', raised questions about old assumptions without resolving the issue; and the passage which seems to argue that the city did *not* consume the population of the country, that both might grow together, is scarcely more decisive.[39] Graunt was far from indulging in Petty's unqualified optimism, his confident projection, for example, that it would be 100 years before London's growth had to cease for lack of resources to sustain it.[40] The bills nevertheless allowed

---

[34] James Beeverell, *The Pleasures of London*, trans. W. H. Quarrell (1940), 16 (1707), 147 (1670); [Samuel Sorbière], *Relation d'un Voyage en Angleterre* (2nd edn., Cologne, 1666), 24; [C. de Saussure], *A Foreign View of England in the Reigns of George I and George II*, ed. Madame van Muyden (1902), 36 (1720s).

[35] *Economic Writings of Petty*, ed. Hull, ii. 522–5; *Histoire de l'Académie Royale des Sciences* (Année 1725) *Avec les Mémoires* (Paris, 1727), 'Mémoires', 48–57; *Philosophical Transactions of the Royal Society*, 35/402 (1728), 432–6.

[36] Estimates of London's population were: based on the bills: 384,000 (excluding Westminster) in the 1660s (Graunt in *Economic Writings of Petty*, ed. Hull, ii. 386); 670,000 or 696,000 in the 1680s (Petty, in ibid. ii. 456, 533–40); 725,903 in 1739 (William Maitland, *The History of London* (1739), 541); based on the number of houses: *c.*530,000 in 1695 (Gregory King in J. Thirsk and J. P. Cooper (eds.), *Seventeenth-Century Economic Documents* (Oxford, 1972), 776); 630,856 in 1716 (*A Computation of the Increase of London* (1719), 5). Earlier estimates had been guesses: e.g. 500,000 in 1584 (*Breefe Discourse*, 15), 600,000 in 1652 (Heylyn, *Cosmographie*, 270); but some later estimates were also inflated: e.g. the often repeated figure of 1.5 million, resting originally on Howell, *Londinopolis* (1657), 403, and Strype's 1,050,000 for 1702: John Stow, *A Survey of the Cities of London and Westminster . . . enlarged . . . by J. Strype* (2 vols.; 1720), i. 3.

[37] Chamberlayne, *Angliae notitia* (1687), pt. II, p. 182, which refers to Petty ('an ingenious gentleman'). The 1684 edn. had deduced from the bills that Paris was more populous: pt. II, p. 182.

[38] On early uses of the bills, see J. C. Robertson, 'Reckoning with London: Interpreting the *Bills of Mortality* before John Graunt', *Urban History*, 23 (1996), 325–50.

[39] *Economic Writings of Petty*, ed. Hull, ii. 320–1 (emphasis added), 370–2; Slack, *Reformation to Improvement*, 95–6.

[40] *Economic Writings of Petty*, ed. Hull, ii. 464–5.

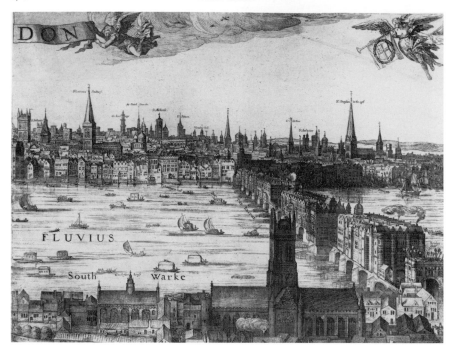

6. Claes Visscher's panorama of London, 1616 (detail)

both authors to show London's qualitative superiority to Paris: it was healthier (plague aside), according to Petty's calculations, and safer, according to Graunt. His finding that 'but few are murthered . . . whereas in Paris few nights scape without their tragedy' endorsed earlier claims that London was, of course, better governed than 'great and populous cities beyond the seas'.[41]

The bills of mortality also helped to mould perceptions of the shape of the metropolis, documenting its shifting centre of gravity as London 'removed westward', and determining its boundaries. As their coverage was extended, notably to include the 'distant parishes' in 1636, the phrase 'within the bills' defined the urban area as effectively as 'within the lines', an equivalent term given temporary currency by the Civil War defences.[42] The construction of mental maps of the metropolis depended also, of course, on some exposure to the real thing. But here too there were new horizons from the 1660s as the number of available images expanded and their quality improved.

---

[41] *Economic Writings of Petty*, ed. Hull, ii. 354, 508, 511, 530–1; Heylyn, *Cosmographie*, 270.
[42] *Economic Writings of Petty*, ed. Hull, i. 41–2, ii. 380; Brett-James, *Growth*, 239 and ch. X.

The 'long view' of London from the south, invented by van Wyngaerde and the originator of the 'copperplate' map in the 1540s and 1550s,[43] had been established as the conventional panorama by Norden and Visscher in 1615–16. We know that it was accessible, since the several sheets of Norden hung at Dulwich College, for example. Yet there were only eleven different 'views' of London before 1640. The great explosion in their popularity came after that date. Between 1640 and *c.*1659 thirty-three different views were printed, and there were another forty-one between 1660 and the end of the century.[44] The production of maps was concentrated still more heavily after the Restoration. Only nine were published before 1640, and another three by 1659, but thirty-one appeared between then and 1690, nine of them in 1666–7 alone.[45] The skills of Dutch printers, the quality of Hollar's productions, and the impetus provided by the Fire, combined to ensure that by the later 1660s Londoners could see—and buy—representations of both the prospect and the street plan of their city.[46]

With proliferation came greater accuracy, notably in the maps of 1676 and 1680–3 showing rebuilt London, which competed with one another in what had become a seller's market. The most remarkable of them was William Morgan's of 1682, 8 foot by 6 foot in size, to a scale of 18 inches to the mile, the first linear ground plan of the whole metropolis.[47] Like the panoramas, they were designed for display. John Overton's of 1676 had marginal illustrations of the chief sights—Guildhall, the Exchange, Charterhouse, the New River—and historical notes.[48] Morgan's, with its calculation of the number of houses (85,000) and inhabitants (an inflated 1,200,000), was commended by the aldermen as 'a very fit ornament and of good use for public places', and sent to the companies to hang in their halls. It hung in country houses too, as at The Vyne in Hampshire, where it still remains, advertising a metropolis 'so rich and populous that no prince in Europe commands the like'.[49]

Accurate maps were also useful. Robert Walton's of 1676 was intended as 'a guide to strangers and such as are not well acquainted herein', and

[43] P. Barber, 'A Glimpse of the Earliest Map-View of London?', *London Topographical Record*, 27 (1995), 100; H. Colvin and S. Foister (eds.), *The Panorama of London circa 1544 by Anthonis van den Wyngaerde* (London Topographical Society, 151; 1996).

[44] I. Scouloudi, *Panoramic Views of London 1600–1666 with Some Later Adaptations: An Annotated List* (1953), 5–6, 19–28, and tables.

[45] J. Howgego, *Printed Maps of London c.1553–1850* (2nd edn., 1978). The numbers here refer to different maps, not (as with the data on panoramas from Scouloudi's list) different editions.

[46] For Pepys's collection, see *The Diary of Samuel Pepys*, ed. R. C. Latham and W. Matthews (11 vols.; 1970–83); vii. 379 n.

[47] Howgego, *Printed Maps*, no. 33; P. Granville, 'The Topography of Seventeenth-Century London: A Review of Maps', *Urban History Yearbook* (1980), 82–3.

[48] John Overton, *A Description of the City of London. The Metropolis of Great Britain* (1676); Howgego, *Printed Maps*, no. 29.

[49] London Corporation RO, Repertory 84, fo. 211[r]; Granville, 'Topography of Seventeenth-Century London', 83. For use of maps in political arithmetic, see *Economic Writings of Petty*, ed. Hull, ii. 385, 542.

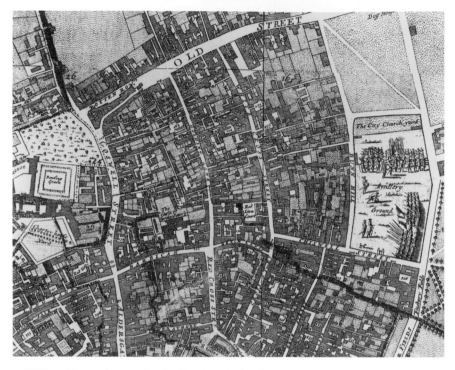

7. William Morgan's map, *London Etc.* (1682) (detail)

the Ogilby and Morgan map of 1676 had a companion *Explanation* with an alphabetical index to streets and lanes. Morgan's listed and documented many alleys, rents, and courts for the first time.[50] Other publications of these years similarly did something to counteract the city's reputation as 'a great vast wilderness'.[51] The first London Directory appeared in 1677, and one of the best of the early guidebooks, Thomas De Laune's *The Present State of London* (1681), included an alphabetical list of carriers, wagoners, and stage-coaches.[52] By the end of the century contemporary London could be known

[50] Howgego, *Printed Maps*, nos. 30, 28; John Ogilby and William Morgan, *London Survey'd: Or, An Explanation of the Large Map of London* (1677), ed. C. Welch (London and Middlesex Archaeological Society; 1895).

[51] D. Maclean and N. G. Brett-James, 'London in 1689–90', *Transactions of the London and Middlesex Archaeological Society*, NS 6 (1929–32), 333. Cf. *A Character of London-Village* (1684) ('some wilderness, or vast meander'); Donald Lupton, *London and the Countrey Carbonadoed* (1632; Aungervyle Society Reprints, Edinburgh, 1884), 60 ('the countryman's laborinth').

[52] C. W. F. Goss, *The London Directories 1677–1855* (1932), 37; Thomas De Laune, *The Present State of London* (1681), 385. Also published in 1681 was Richard Burton [Nathaniel Crouch], *Historical Remarques and Observations Of the Ancient and Present State of London and Westminster*. Cf. D. Webb, 'Guide Books to London before 1800: A Survey', *London Topographical Record*, 26 (1990), 138–52.

as never before. More than that, within a few years its historical topography could also be examined. Edward Hatton's *New View* of 1708 had plans of the city in 1600 and 1707, and other eighteenth-century publications followed his example.[53] The growth of the metropolis could be seen, admired, and measured.

<h1 style="text-align:center">III</h1>

The publishing chronology of maps and guides suggests that the later 1670s and early 1680s may have been as important as the later 1570s and early 1580s for the formation of attitudes towards London; and this conclusion is amply confirmed when we consider published arguments about the role of the metropolis. At the end of Charles II's reign, as in the middle years of Elizabeth's, the issue of new building focused public attention on London, and it then prompted a case for the defence more confident and elaborate than any heard before.

Some of the intellectual and rhetorical ground had been laid earlier. Notions of distribution and circulation were revived in the civil wars when London's 'universal trade throughout the kingdom' was seen also to spread 'civil contagion to all our cities and corporations . . . poisoning whole counties'. Although he had not quite caught up with Harveian physiology, a writer in 1642 was stimulated to describe Manchester as 'the very London' of the north-west, 'the liver that sends blood into all the countries thereabouts'.[54] London could not be ignored either by those writers in the Hartlib circle who looked for means of increasing the nation's agricultural, industrial, and commercial productivity. In 1641 Gabriel Plattes, in his Utopian tract *Macaria*, claimed to be able to show 'how great cities, which formerly devoured the fatness of the kingdom, may yearly make a considerable retribution'. He appears to have had the fertilizing properties of urban waste products in mind, but that provided metaphors of towns 'fructifying' the countryside which had potential for the future.[55] Howell picked up another element in Hartlibean improvement when he asserted that it was 'confessed by all nations, that though the Londoners be not so apt to invent, yet when they have got the invention, they use always to improve it, and bring it to greater perfection'. John Dryden was similarly echoing Interregnum aspirations when he looked to 'our powerful navy' and the 'famed emporium' of London to triumph over

---

[53] [Edward Hatton], *A New View of London* (2 vols.; 1708), i, inserts before pp. i, 1. Maitland's *History* of 1739 contained a view of London *c*.1560, and plans of London in 1643 and after the Fire: frontispiece, opposite pp. 238, 293.

[54] R. C. Richardson, *Puritanism in North-West England* (Manchester, 1972), 12–13.

[55] C. Webster, *Utopian Planning and the Puritan Revolution* (Wellcome Unit for the History of Medicine; Oxford, 1979), 71, 87.

'the British Ocean' in 1667, and (giving Harvey his due) attacked the Dutch for hampering 'trade, which like blood should circularly flow'.[56]

Reflection on the role of London became still more prominent in the economic debates about agricultural depression, low rents, and stagnant population that followed the crises of the mid-1660s. In 1669 one contributor tried to make peace between contending landed, manufacturing, and commercial interests by showing the 'connection of trades one to another'. Labourers gave income to farmers and farmers to the gentry, who employed tradesmen, who in turn consumed country produce, 'as may be witnessed by the building of the city of London, how provision and all consumptive goods are advanced by it'. By this 'circulation, all degrees are either employed, enriched, or both, and hence naturally comes content, harmony, and pleasure, one in another'.[57] On the other side, however, William Coventry found that 'consumption is not well distributed': the decay of country hospitality and the 'luxury' of London living continued to impoverish and depopulate the provinces. The author of *The Grand Concern of England Explained* (1673) agreed. More than 30,000 houses had been built in the 'head too big for the body' since the 1630s; and their inmates, indulging in 'extravagant habits . . . and other debaucheries', would have been more productive 'living an industrious and laborious life' in the country. The country, not London, must be the site of that increase in 'the consumption of the provisions and manufactures of the kingdom, than which nothing can conduce more to the improvement of land'.[58]

These standpoints were voiced in a variety of different contexts, from arguments about the utility of more shops in the rebuilt Exchange in 1668 to parliamentary discussion of interest rates in 1669.[59] But they were articulated with particular relevance to our theme in the renewed debates of the 1670s on whether metropolitan building should be regulated. In 1657 a Protectorate parliament had replaced early Stuart control by proclamation and Star Chamber with a deterrent tax on buildings erected since 1620, but that had collapsed at the Restoration. Against a background of further rapid development in the West End, the question was revived by an uneasy alliance between country interests afraid of a further fall in agricultural rents, on the one hand, and the City corporation, fearful that suburban building might drain away resources needed for reconstruction within the walls, on the other.[60]

[56] Howell, *Londinopolis*, 396; John Dryden, *Annus Mirabilis: The Year of Wonders, 1666* (1667), I, 76.

[57] [William Carter], *England's Interest Asserted, in the Improvement of its Native Commodities* (1669), 14.

[58] Thirsk and Cooper (eds.), *Seventeenth-Century Economic Documents*, 81–3; W. Oldys (ed.), *The Harleian Miscellany*, viii (1746), 549–51.

[59] [Henry Duke], *Londons-Nonsuch, or, The Glory of the Royal Exchange* (1668), in Aubin (ed.), *London in Flames*, 170–84, which defends shops; Thirsk and Cooper (eds.), *Seventeenth-Century Economic Documents*, 68–79. Duke had the support of 'W.P.', probably Petty.

[60] Brett-James, *Growth*, ch. XV; HMC, *8th Report*, app., pt. I (1881), Earl of Jersey, 98–9.

Proposals to prohibit or tax new development were hotly debated in Parliament in 1670, 1674–5, and 1678.[61] There were disputes about whether a tax could be either equitable or effective, an issue on which Petty had already pronounced,[62] about legal mechanisms hampering regulation that were of particular concern to the City,[63] and about the relative weight to be given to agricultural depression and urban improvement. There was no result. The City–Country alliance broke down when a tax seemed more practicable than a blanket prohibition, the London corporation asked for its own citizens to be exempted from it,[64] and backbenchers were suspicious of the uses to which the revenues might be put. Although there were further parliamentary proposals for an imposition or restraint on new building in 1689 and 1709–10, after 1678 this particular debate was effectively over.[65]

What has not hitherto been noticed is the appearance in 1678 of three printed contributions to the argument, all in defence of new building, all anonymous, and the most interesting of them (and possibly the other two) by Nicholas Barbon, son of Praise-God Barbon and the greatest speculative builder of the age.[66] Two of them were broadsheets, no doubt issued together, and probably intended for distribution to MPs. One of these surveyed past history, and concentrated on legal issues and the unconstitutional nature of the proposed tax.[67] The other argued that such a tax would raise very little, since the number of new houses had been greatly exaggerated. It drew on returns from each parish to prove that only 7,500 had been built between 1620 and 1656, and 10,000 between 1656 and 1677.[68] The third publication was a twenty-page tract of striking originality: *A Discourse shewing the Great Advantages That New-Buildings, And the Enlarging of Towns and Cities Do bring to a Nation*. It is clear from its content that it was written by Barbon.[69]

[61] C. A. Edie, 'New Buildings, New Taxes, and Old Interests: An Urban Problem of the 1670s', *Journal of British Studies*, 6 (1967), 35–63. Cf. Thirsk and Cooper (eds.), *Seventeenth-Century Economic Documents*, 687–91.

[62] *Economic Writings of Petty*, ed. Hull, i. 40–2.

[63] For the City's efforts at control and its pressure on parliament up to 1677, see London Corporation RO, Repertory 75, fo. 113, Rep. 78, fos. 126ᵛ, 232ᵛ–233ʳ, Rep. 79, fo. 203ᵛ, Rep. 80, fo. 188ᵛ, Rep. 82, fo. 113.

[64] Rep. 83, fo. 227ᵛ.   [65] Edie, 'New Buildings', 61.

[66] On Barbon's career and other writings, see W. Letwin, *The Origins of Scientific Economics* (New York, 1964), ch. 2.

[67] *Arguments concerning the New-Buildings in the Parishes within the Weekly Bills of Mortality, without the City of London* [1678] (D. Wing, *Short-Title Catalogue of Books . . . 1641–1700* (2nd edn., 1972–88), item A3641).

[68] *A Particular of the New-Buildings within the Bills of Mortality, and without the City of London* [1678] (Wing, item P594B), described in Brett-James, *Growth*, 504–5, who points to similarities with Barbon's arguments elsewhere.

[69] *A Discourse shewing the Great Advantages That New-Buildings, And the Enlarging of Towns and Cities Do bring to a Nation* (Wing, item D1620). In argument and style the *Discourse shewing the Great Advantages* is similar to *An Apology for the Builder* (1685), which has been generally attributed to Barbon, partly because of the circumstances of its publication (Brett-James, *Growth*, 330–1,

Barbon set out to demonstrate that urban development enhanced the wealth and strength of nations and governments, 'increasing their revenue and rendering people more easily governed'. Urban immigrants were no longer the threats to civil order pictured by early Stuart proclamations and royalist tracts, but tradesmen with a necessary interest in the 'peace and quiet of government' that were essential for commerce. In passages reminiscent of the manuscript of *c*.1620 kept by Cotton (and which suggest that Barbon may have had access to the Cottonian library), he compared low prices in the country with high prices in town: the first showed the effects of agrarian improvement not of depopulation; the second were proof of wealth. The rulers of other expanding cities, from classical Rome to contemporary Amsterdam, had set a better example than those who had tried to control London and in consequence deprived a growing population of housing. Figures from the bills of mortality were manipulated to suggest that restrictions on London building had forced 300,000 people to emigrate overseas between 1618 and 1648, and another 100,000 between 1657 and 1664.[70]

Above all there was a 'peculiar happiness and advantage which belongs to the building and enlarging of cities'. It arose from the division of labour, the 'exercise of several arts and callings', and consequently from increasing wealth; and the spur to that was 'emulation': 'the increasing of the inhabitants of a city increaseth the emulation of the people; and emulation increaseth industry, and industry riches.' There were 'two great causes of labour and industry: necessity of food and emulation'. While hunger could easily be assuaged, at least temporarily, however, 'emulation provokes a continued industry, and will not allow no intervals or be ever satisfied'. It was an economic stimulus of infinite potential. 'All men by a perpetual industry are struggling to mend their former condition: and thus the people grow rich, which is the great advantage of a nation.'[71]

Here the argument of the *Grand Concern of England* of 1673 was turned on its head; the urban 'extravagance' castigated by country critics of the metropolis for a century was shown to be a cause of economic growth. It was arguably Barbon's greatest contribution, if not to economic theory, where he has other claims to fame, then to economic history. He was not the only contemporary to defend the consumer against the charge of waste and idleness. But in identifying 'emulation' as the motor of competitive consumption, as he did again in his *Apology for the Builder* (1685) and *A Discourse of Trade* (1690),[72] he provided a model which influenced all later accounts of consumer

339) and partly by comparison with his signed *A Discourse of Trade* (1690). Unlike the *Discourse shewing the Great Advantages*, *An Apology for the Builder* has been much discussed (e.g. by J. O. Appleby, *Economic Thought and Ideology in Seventeenth-Century England* (Princeton, 1978), 137, 176–7, 182).

[70] *Discourse shewing the Great Advantages*, 2, 8, 13–14, 18–19.
[71] Ibid. 4, 5.
[72] [Barbon], *Apology for the Builder*, 33; Barbon, *Discourse of Trade*, 69.

revolutions. The first airing of the case in 1678 had an immediate impact on Petty, as one might expect. Petty's defence of 'the growth of the city of London', written around 1681 and published in 1683, elaborated some of Barbon's arguments, but simply rephrased this particular insight: the 'arts of delight and ornament' were 'best promoted by the greatest number of emulators'—that is, in cities.[73] It is not going too far to suggest that the urban civility that was the *raison d'être* of all towns was here being redefined. The two ancient claims to fame of London and other great cities—that they were centres both of the civilized arts and of flourishing commerce—were firmly yoked together, by consumption; and it was consumption which, by creating wealth, stimulated and justified further urban growth.

In 1678 Barbon had not yet arrived at the metaphor of circulation expounded in the *Apology* of 1685 and quoted at the beginning of this essay.[74] His medical training at Leiden and Utrecht might have been expected to lead him to copy Dryden's analogy with the circulation of the blood, or to take a hint from Edward Phillips's perception in 1676 that that significant duo, 'wealth and honour', were 'distributed' by London's 'prosperous trade . . . to the whole nation'.[75] Perhaps Barbon needed fresh inspiration from publications after 1678. De Laune's guidebook of 1681, for example, explained that London drew provisions from all the counties around and that 'in recompense the country is supplied by the city with all sorts of necessary merchandises wanting there'. In the same year John Houghton concluded from agricultural improvement in the south-east that 'the bigness and great consumption of London doth not only encourage the breeders of provisions and higglers thirty miles off, but even to four score miles', and that, if London's size and consumption increased, its influence would extend still further. Barbon might even have read Alexandre Lemaître's French tract on *The Metropolis* of 1682, which commented that capital cities 'draw their life and glory from all parts of the state, and likewise give them back again to all the provinces'.[76] Three years later Barbon had no doubt that the metropolis gave 'life and growth' to the whole nation, and he now had the coping stone to his argument: metropolitan growth was not only justifiable in itself, but of benefit to the whole. Circulation made it consistent with, even essential to, the health and harmony of town and country.

The *Apology* of 1685 was also unlike the *Discourse shewing the Great Advantages* of 1678 in picking up Dryden's imperial theme: London had opportunity to become 'the metropolis of the world' and to make 'an universal

---

[73] *Economic Writings of Petty*, ed. Hull, ii. 452, 474.

[74] In 1690 (*Discourse of Trade*, 65) Barbon commented on 'fashion' as 'a great promoter of trade': 'it makes a circulation, and gives a value by turns to all sorts of commodities.'

[75] Manley, *Literature and Culture*, 132.

[76] De Laune, *Present State of London*, 298 and cf. p. 305; Thirsk and Cooper (eds.), *Seventeenth-Century Economic Documents*, 176 (Houghton); Alexandre Lemaître, *La Métropolitée ou De l'établissement des villes Capitales* (Amsterdam, 1682), 5 (my translation).

monarchy over the seas, an empire no less glorious, and of much more profit, than of land'.[77] Barbon had been reading in the interim between the two publications. If his images developed afterwards, however, his *Discourse shewing the Great Advantages* was the first attempt to bring something that might be described as socio-economic theory to the defence of urban growth. Its conclusion certainly sounded the death knell of attempts to prevent it. They were evidently absurd

if the employing of the poor makes a nation rich, if the number of people make it strong, if a great city be the glory of a nation, if it renders a people more easily governed, and increases the prince's revenue, and if it be impossible for a nation to be either rich, strong, or great, without increase of buildings.[78]

IV

Barbon and his allies had won the battle over regulation; and although they had not wholly silenced opposing voices, they had also permanently altered the terms in which arguments about London were conducted. While the City, deep in financial crisis, gave up trying to prevent suburban expansion, by 1695 a more cautious political economist than Petty had to acknowledge the strength of his case. Summarizing the two views of the metropolis, Charles Davenant gave greater space to those who thought 'the growth of London not hurtful to the nation', citing both the imperial ambitions that justified metropolitan growth and the redistributive process that made it compatible with a proper balance between town and country. No empire had ever been great without a great and populous city; and it was worth pondering the argument that there was 'not an acre of land in the country, be it never so distant, that is not in some degree bettered by the growth, trade and riches' of the capital. Defoe espoused circulation with less restraint: 'all the several manufactures move in a just rotation from the several countries where they are made to the city of London, as the blood in the body to the heart', and London in return 'circulates all', supplying shopkeepers and tradesmen 'in every part of the country'.[79]

Davenant was right to note that there were still two views. Provincial merchants continued to fear that 'London would swallow up the trade of England',[80] and 'country' opinion to detest metropolitan extravagance and corruption. The moral case against London was now more powerful than the

---

[77] [Barbon], *Apology for the Builder*, 37. Cf. Barbon, *Discourse of Trade*, 40.
[78] *Discourse shewing the Great Advantages*, 20.
[79] Thirsk and Cooper (eds.), *Seventeenth-Century Economic Documents*, 809–10 (Davenant); M. Byrd, *London Transformed: Images of the City in the Eighteenth Century* (New Haven, 1978), 15–17 (Defoe). On Defoe, cf. Appleby, *Economic Thought and Ideology*, 210.
[80] Thirsk and Cooper (eds.), *Seventeenth-Century Economic Documents*, 564.

economic one in sustaining the ambivalence with which this essay began, however. *A Computation of the Increase of London*, published in 1719, merely suggested that 'it may perhaps be found that other parts of England, as well as all North-Britain, are both impoverished and diminished' by 'the increase of London'; but it ended with a resounding assault on the 'atheism, anarchy and confusion' brought by monied men and their political allies.[81] While confirming that the economic case may well have looked stronger from north Britain, Andrew Fletcher's 'Account of a Conversation' of 1703 concluded in similar fashion, advocating twelve cities spread through the three kingdoms as a replacement for 'one great vicious and ungovernable' metropolis.[82]

The simple indictment of metropolitan vice was particularly potent when it was refreshed by the eighteenth-century campaign against the 'luxury' that made London 'the common-sewer of the world'.[83] The fact that luxury was defended in Bernard Mandeville's *Fable of the Bees* (1714) was no help at all to those who wished to advocate the merits of emulation and consumption. Yet even here perceptions were being subtly adjusted, as rhetorical and literary conventions became clichés that could be used cynically, tongue in cheek. Publications like Ned Ward's *The London-Spy* deliberately advertised the 'vanities and vices of the town', its 'continued hurry of vice and pleasure', and proclaimed the manifold attractions of the 'Heaven or Hell' that was London.[84] As Defoe appreciated, the metropolis was both 'great and monstrous', and, as Mandeville more acidly remarked, 'dirty streets are a necessary evil inseparable from the felicity of London'.[85] Much as eighteenth-century moralists and novelists might wish otherwise, they were fully aware that it was impossible to have the town's 'civilities without its vanities'.[86]

Only in the later eighteenth century was there a radical shift of attitude, as the pendulum swung back, away from the attractions of the metropolis. It was pulled by change in the provinces. Perspectives of London were altered by the prospect of urban populations elsewhere now growing faster than that of the capital, and by a provincial 'urban renaissance' advertised by views and maps, histories and guidebooks, as effective as those of the metropolis.[87] In

---

[81] *A Computation*, 6–7, 14–16, 19.

[82] Andrew Fletcher, *Political Works*, ed. J. Robertson (Cambridge, 1997), 211, 213–14.

[83] [Erasmus Jones], *A Trip Through London: Containing Observations on Men and Things* (1728), 1; J. Sekora, *Luxury: The Concept in Western Thought, Eden to Smollett* (Baltimore, 1977), chs. 2, 3.

[84] Edward Ward, *The London-Spy Compleat* (3rd edn., 2 vols., 1706), i. 2; *Hell Upon Earth: Or The Town in an Uproar* (1729), 1; *A Character of London-Village* (1684).

[85] Daniel Defoe, *A Tour through the Whole Island of Great Britain* (2 vols.; Everyman edn., 1962), i. 323; Byrd, *London Transformed*, 29.

[86] J. Barker, *Love Intrigues* (1713), quoted in E. B. Kubek, 'Women's Participation in the Urban Culture of Early Modern London', in A. Bermingham and J. Brewer (eds.), *The Consumption of Culture 1600–1800* (1995), 441.

[87] P. J. Corfield, *The Impact of English Towns 1700–1800* (Oxford, 1982), 10; P. Borsay, *The English Urban Renaissance: Culture and Society in the Provincial Town, 1660–1770* (Oxford, 1989), 80–5, 257–83.

1774 another Scot, Lord Kames, could therefore pick up Andrew Fletcher's speculation, but deal with it more persuasively in a new context. He favoured confining London to 100,000 people and distributing the rest in nine other towns in order to 'diffuse life and vigour through every corner of the island'. Earlier arguments in favour of metropolitan growth were coolly dismissed. Any alleged benefits to agriculture were clearly confined to 'the rich fields round the city'. Circulation was similarly circumscribed: 'a great town is a professed enemy to the free circulation of money', starving the provinces of coin. As for London's international glory, 'it would give one spleen to hear the French and English zealously disputing about the extent of their capitals, as if the prosperity of their country depended on that circumstance'.[88]

No one would have said that 100 years before, when the English were being persuaded that the prosperity of their country and the greatness of its capital were indeed interdependent. By the end of the eighteenth century, however, new centres of merchandise and commerce and a more widely distributed civility had altered the frame of reference created by their metropolitan concentration. International comparisons were still being made, but they were no longer confined to capitals. A 1797 publication presented *A summary view of the present population of the principal cities and towns of France, compared with the principal cities and towns of Great Britain and Ireland*. It was reminiscent of a much earlier tract, the 1549 'Debate of the Heralds', which compared the towns of France and England and listed twenty of the latter against the charge that 'we have never a good town in England, only London'.[89] The fact that that kind of competitive claim could not be made in the intervening two centuries tells us something about the dominance of the metropolis, in perception and in reality, in early modern England.

[88] Henry Home, Lord Kames, *Sketches of the History of Man* (4 vols.; Dublin, 1774), iii, sketch XI, pp. 68–79.
[89] R. H. Tawney and E. Power (eds.), *Tudor Economic Documents* (3 vols.; 1924), iii. 7.

10

Civility and Civic Culture in Early Modern England: The Meanings of Urban Freedom

JONATHAN BARRY

> [Freeholders] and those [that] are the freemen of corporations, were looked upon by the former constitution to comprehend the permanent interest of the kingdom. For [*first*], he that hath his livelihood by his trade, and by his freedom of trading in such a corporation, which he cannot exercise in another, he is tied to that place, [*for*] his livelihood depends upon it. And secondly, that man hath an interest, hath a permanent interest there, upon which he may live, and live a freeman without dependence.
>
> (Henry Ireton, Putney, 29 October 1647)[1]

Embedded in the heart of Anna Bryson's recent study of civility in early modern England is a paradox. The codes of civility recommended to the gentry and those aspiring to gentility sought to inculcate modes of behaviour that were, in many cases, those practised by servants and tradesmen, as well as other inferiors, in their dealings with their masters, customers, and superiors.[2] If the essence of civility lay in mastering techniques of self-presentation that would encourage self-control and accommodation to others, then such values, voluntarily adopted by the gentry, were simple necessity to much of the rest of the population. Of course, to the contemporary élite (and to many historians) there is all the difference in the world between the voluntary adoption, as a matter of virtue and good manners, of a code of conduct, and its practice as a social necessity by others. It is curious, however, that so much attention has been devoted to the former and so little to the latter. The aim here is to redress the balance somewhat by considering the meaning of civility for a particular group among the non-gentry of early modern England—namely, urban freemen—especially those in the larger or more established towns with a strong civic culture. In so doing, I hope to extend Keith

---

[1] A. S. P. Woodhouse (ed.), *Puritanism and Liberty: Being the Army Debates (1647–9) from the Clarke Manuscripts with Supplementary Documents* (1974), 57–8.

[2] A. Bryson, *From Courtesy to Civility: Changing Codes of Conduct in Early Modern England* (Oxford, 1998).

Thomas's mission of taking seriously those 'popular beliefs' that intelligent people of the past took seriously but which we now tend to deride.[3]

In this respect the civility of towndwellers has suffered from a double derision, with the mockery of contemporary gentry echoed and reinforced by the condescension and implicit rebuke of modern historians. Both traditions have assumed that civility belonged naturally to the gentry (even if they had to learn it) and that it could reach the rest of society only once it had triumphed among the élite, through the example they offered, which would breed emulation and diffusion of good manners. This model has underpinned most recent work on the social history of manners and cultural change, and has been taken as the implicit message of Norbert Elias's influential studies, given their focus on conduct books and the taming of court society. However, this may be to miss the deeper message of Elias's work. Given that he was building on the work of Weber and others on the culture of capitalism, it appears that Elias was taking for granted the civilizing effects of commerce and the forms of self-control associated with the interdependence implicit in trading relationships. Indeed, in the context of his work as a whole, it appears that civility was for Elias a particular manifestation of the broader phenomenon of social and psychological interdependence (as experienced by historical actors and worked out in historical processes) whose growing intensification was the core feature of social change.[4] It is this broader sense of civility, rather than specific forms of conduct, that will be considered in this essay.

In this context, urban freemen form a particularly significant group amongst the non-gentry for the study of civility. If, as suggested above, it was the voluntary adoption of codes of civility, rather than the forms of conduct themselves, that marked out the gentry, then the notion of independence, or freedom, in choosing this form of behaviour, becomes crucial. Yet the gentry were not the only class in early modern England to characterize themselves as independent, or free. At one level, English national culture embodied the notion that all Englishmen (excluding, more or less explicitly, women and children) were freeborn and that this independence was a national birthright to be cherished and defended. It is not practicable here to analyse how far this ideology prevailed against alternative modes of deference and hierarchy, and how far it affected regular social encounters, as opposed to stylized political debate and occasional collective action (riots, elections, etc.), though this is an important debate. But within this broader rhetoric, and providing its most vociferous core support, in the lively political culture of London and other towns, lay the urban freemen whose status embodied this

---

[3] K. Thomas, *Religion and the Decline of Magic: Studies in Popular Beliefs in Sixteenth and Seventeenth Century England* (1971), p. ix.

[4] The best introduction to Elias's work as a whole remains S. Mennell, *Norbert Elias: Civilisation and the Human Self-Image* (Oxford, 1989). I am grateful to Prof. Mennell for discussion of Elias's assumptions about commerce.

claim in a sharply defined form. Furthermore, urban freedom, it will be argued, offered a very specific solution to the problem of how to reconcile the notion of an English inheritance of freedom with the daily realities of hierarchy and social necessity. I will argue that urban freedom provided an alternative education in the modes of civility, one embodied not in books so much as in institutions and practices embedded in urban life, but all the more effective for that.

A further advantage of studying urban freemen is that it reminds us that civility not only had a political dimension but, in its Renaissance form at least, was closely associated with the civic politics of the city states and urban federalism of Italy, Germany, and the Low Countries. It is historiographically unfortunate that the many studies of this 'civic humanist' tradition, in which active political participation was a key attribute of civility, have not, in general, been integrated with the sociocultural studies of civility. Where they have, it has been to present civility as an alternative to such participation, bred in courts and associated with aristocratic rather than civic modes of politics. In the English context this trend has been even more marked, because it has been widely assumed that such civic humanist values were a learned import from the Continent appealing to an educated élite (which they were) and not also an indigenous tradition bred out of the practices and ideology of English urban life.[5] This neglect is the more curious (and serious), because studies of English imperialism, both in the British Isles and overseas, have noted the crucial importance of the term 'civility' as a justification for the destruction of Celtic or native Indian ways of life. The characteristic form of such English civility was the plantation of urban commercial settlement, complete with the common law and the privileges of urban freedom, as the cornerstone of the civilizing process. Unfortunately, there is not scope here to discuss this international dimension of urban freedom, but it remained important in the rest of the British Empire, especially in Anglo-Irish Dublin, Edinburgh, and the American colonies, until the late eighteenth century.[6]

[5] This has been an unfortunate effect of the magisterial influence of J. G. A. Pocock (notably in *The Machiavellian Moment* (Princeton, 1975) and *Virtue, Commerce and History* (Cambridge, 1985)) and of the 'Cambridge School', whose approach has remained resolutely textual, though for an interesting analysis of how this might apply to the politics of late Tudor Tewkesbury, see M. Peltonen, *Classical Humanism and Republicanism in English Political Thought 1570–1640* (Cambridge, 1995), 54–73. L. Klein ('Liberty, Manners and Politeness in Early Eighteenth-Century England', *Historical Journal*, 32 (1989), 583–605) firmly links liberty, civility, and civic humanism, but in an aristocratic context, while N. Phillipson ('Politics and Politeness in the Reigns of Anne and the Early Hanoverians', in J. G. A. Pocock (ed.), *Varieties of British Political Thought 1500–1800* (Cambridge, 1993), 211–45) is typical of many in setting the 'politics of manners' against that of civic virtue.

[6] M. E. James, *Family, Lineage and Civil Society* (Oxford, 1974); A. Laurence, 'The Cradle to the Grave: English Observations of Irish Social Customs', *The Seventeenth Century*, 3 (1988), 63–84; J. Leerssen, 'Wildness, Wilderness and Ireland', *Journal of the History of Ideas*, 56 (1995), 25–39; J. C. D. Clark, *The Language of Liberty 1660–1832* (Cambridge, 1994); J. Hill, *From Patriots to Unionists: Dublin Civic Politics and Irish Protestant Patriotism 1660–1840* (Oxford, 1997).

This growing importance abroad was matched by a growing significance in domestic politics. The House of Commons, concerned at the manipulation of electorates and able from 1604 to decide electoral franchises, often selected a broad parliamentary electorate in boroughs, to match the 40-shilling freeholder electorate of the counties. During the Putney Debates Ireton assumed, as my epigraph shows, that the borough franchise was precisely a freeman franchise and none of his more radical opponents pointed out his error— perhaps they assumed the same. As a result, by 1689 or so, the largest single category of borough franchise, covering almost 100 seats and returning 200 MPs, was that based on the urban freemen, though sometimes supplemented by others such as urban freeholders. After 1688, and especially after 1715, the Commons began to prefer more manageable electorates, but freemen franchises remained the largest category and, furthermore, they increasingly dominated the publicly visible world of electoral politics. Most of the larger seats and a rising proportion of the regularly contested seats were those with freemen franchises and the electoral culture of the country revolved around these, at a time when the county freeholders were participating less and less often in actual elections. Moreover, a divided élite drew heavily on the language of freedom to legitimate its own political behaviour and to rally support from the parliamentary electorate, notably the urban freemen. One simple, but often neglected, consequence of this is that more people were officially identified as urban freemen in the late seventeenth and early eighteenth centuries than ever before, both absolutely and relative to national urban population, certainly if one excludes London, although there too the City of London's freemen population included about 75 per cent of the adult males, numbering about 50,000 in 1675. During the eighteenth century the relative proportions almost certainly fell, not least due to urban growth outside corporate towns, but the absolute numbers involved probably grew, if only gradually.[7]

Despite this, there have been few studies of urban freemen, especially outside London, and almost no consideration of them as a social and cultural

---

[7] The freeman boroughs can be traced in the volumes of the History of Parliament Trust and in J. H. Philbin, *Parliamentary Representation 1832 England and Wales* (New Haven, 1965). For summaries, see W. A. Speck, *Tory and Whig: The Struggle in the Constituencies 1701–15* (1970), 126–31; D. Hirst, *Representative of the People?* (Cambridge, 1976), 213–15; J. A. Phillips, *Electoral Behaviour in Unreformed England* (Princeton, 1982), 61; F. O'Gorman, *Voters, Patrons and Parties: The Unreformed Electoral System of Hanoverian England 1734–1832* (Oxford, 1989), 44–5, 180–1 (where he suggests an electorate of about 65,000 in various freeman boroughs in the mid-eighteenth century, rising to *c.*72,000 in the later eighteenth century and just over 90,000 by 1831). I have documented the arguments in this and following paragraphs in J. Barry, 'I significati della libertà: La libertà urbana nell'Inghilterra del XVII e XVIII secolo', *Quaderni storici*, 89 (Aug. 1995), 487–513. Space here does not permit reproduction of all the references contained there. R. Sweet ('Freemen and Independence in English Borough Politics *c.*1770–1830', *P&P* 161 (Nov. 1998), 84–115) reinforces many of the points made here and develops them in detail for the period covered.

grouping.[8] Although the latter is most directly relevant to the theme of civility, it is thus necessary first to consider the economic and political aspects of urban freedom. As I have suggested above, these were not divorced from notions of civility in this period. They provided the key legal and institutional meanings of urban freedom, although I shall argue that these were saturated with sociocultural assumptions as well. Furthermore the historiographical neglect of the subject is largely explained by the dominant approaches of economic and political historians. Urban freemen have been marginalized within each tradition and study of them has fallen between the two stools. Their assumptions need to be understood and corrected.

To economic historians, who have dominated urban historiography, urban freemen have been of interest on two counts. One, methodological, has been the use of freemen records as a guide to urban occupational structure. While this has generated interesting debates about how far freemen were representative of urban society, it has not encouraged much work on the freedom as such, and most such studies have focused on the seventeenth century or before, on the assumption that thereafter the freedom became politicized and hence lost its connection with economic benefits. Logically this need not make it a less useful guide to occupations; indeed, arguably it becomes a better one, but this point has not been pursued. This is perhaps because of the other economic issue. Since Victorian debates between free-trade and corporatist economic historians, the question of the urban freedom has normally been viewed as a subset of the debate about the timing, causes, and desirability of the decline of guild and corporate restrictions on trade. While this has been variously dated, most economic historians have argued (or assumed) that it was well under way by the mid-seventeenth century, and that urban freedom was less and less valued as an economic advantage thereafter. Implicitly, at least, England as a land of free trade is often contrasted with the continued corporatism of continental economies. Finally, the labour history perspective on the eighteenth century has led to a neglect of institutions like urban freedom, which was shared by a range of urban social groups, in favour of nascent working-class collectivities.

Historians of urban politics have also devoted little specific attention to urban freemen, with some notable exceptions. The emphasis on oligarchy in urban government has led urban freedom to be seen as merely a charade or irrelevance in municipal politics. With a few exceptions, such as Norwich and London, freemen's political rights are viewed as resting increasingly on their

---

[8] Sweet ('Freemen and Independence') focuses on the political aspect, while bringing out admirably the connections of that with civic identity and the sense of history. The same is true of the rich analysis, for an even later period, of P. Searby, 'Chartists and Freemen in Coventry, 1838–1860', *Social History*, 2 (1977), 761–84. See also the essays on Bristol citizenship by J. Barry and S. Poole in M. Dresser and P. Ollerenshaw (eds.), *The Making of Modern Bristol* (Bristol, 1996), 25–47, 76–95.

parliamentary franchise. Until recently, the exercise of this franchise has been dismissed as unthinking or cynical, with freemen voters either supporting local leaders regardless of national issues or offering their votes for sale through corrupt practices—rendering urban freedom little more than a gravy ticket. Most recent work has shown this to be profoundly misleading, but, despite the prominent place often taken by freemen electorates in such studies, historians have been reluctant to explore the specific contribution of urban freedom. Instead, the conceptual model used has been of 'popular' politics, with urban freemen as merely one variant of a popular dimension to urban politics challenging its oligarchical features. Although such work, especially that of Brewer, Rogers, and O'Gorman, has highlighted the issue of independence as central to such urban electors, no sustained attempt has been made to relate this to the category of urban freedom. This reflects the pull of nineteenth-century models in which new forms of popular urban association are ever being looked for and the radical potential of traditional modes, such as the freedom, played down. But, by revealing urban politics as a complex matter of negotiation, propaganda, and ideological debate, such work has laid the foundations for a reconsideration of the place of the urban freemen.[9]

How can we define urban freedom? In the broadest sense, urban freemen were the citizens, the bourgeois, of English towns. They were intended to represent, as Ireton assumed, the 'permanent, fixed interest' of each specific town, because they were tied to its fortunes as a town by their juridical and economic privileges and duties as town inhabitants. Urban freedom could be gained in various ways, depending on local custom or charter, but was most often earned by apprenticeship, claimed by inheritance, or paid for by fine (often called redemption): town corporations controlled this last method of entry and, by extension, could usually create freemen gratis. The original features of the freedom most often stressed were economic, relating to trading and employment benefits and duties. Some occupations were restricted to freemen, while the freemen of different towns had reciprocal exemptions from the duties or tolls placed on 'foreigners'—that is, on the non-free. Eighteenth-century Londoners and provincial townsmen were still travelling England armed with such exemption certificates—and corporations such as Leicester were still taking legal action when their freemen's rights were denied in the 1750s.[10] Freemen swore oaths not to connive at breaking these rules and could

---

[9] J. Brewer, *Party Ideology and Popular Politics at the Accession of George III* (Cambridge, 1976); Phillips, *Electoral Behaviour*; O'Gorman, *Voters, Patrons and Parties*; N. Rogers, *Whigs and Cities: Popular Politics in the Age of Walpole and Pitt* (Oxford, 1989); J. E. Bradley, *Religion, Revolution and English Radicalism: Nonconformity in Eighteenth-Century Politics and Society* (Cambridge, 1990); J. A. Phillips, *The Great Reform Bill in the Boroughs* (Oxford, 1992); K. Wilson, *The Sense of the People* (Cambridge, 1995). The historiographical shift is critically surveyed in J. Innes, 'Representative Histories', *Journal of Historical Sociology*, 4 (1991).

[10] G. A. Chinnery (ed.), *Records of Borough of Leicester*, v. *Hall Books and Papers 1689–1835* (Leicester, 1965), nos. 498, 522, 609, 644, 702. There is no systematic modern study of the varying

sue and be sued only in the town's own courts for cases connected with these rights. The freemen also formed the town's broadest political community or commonalty, and the electorate for some town offices, while most town offices were open only to freemen. By 1600 many such elections were either notional or closely restrained by prior nominations, but in some towns key offices like the mayorship were still open contests. As we have seen, in many corporate towns freemen formed part or all of the parliamentary electorate. Urban freedom was thus inherently both economic and political: more precisely, it reflected an urban society in which the distinction between economic and political was neither desirable nor practical.

The conventional wisdom is that during the early modern period the economic and the political separated and that as part of this process urban freedom moved inexorably from being primarily an economic status to a largely political one. While there is a fundamental truth in this, it is a truth that conceals a lot of other interesting truths, and above all the necessary dialectic between economic and political aspects of freedom. The real story is one of a constantly changing balance between the economic and political aspects of urban freedom and the perceived ability of freemen to represent, in various senses, urban society. Indeed, both the economic and political dimensions of the freedom can be understood only in terms of a deeper set of assumptions about urban society and its relationship to the broader social order. Urban freedom represented an ideal type of the form in which civility could be both transmitted and represented within an 'ancient-constitution' model, in which the measure of citizenship was a historical category: those who had qualified for membership by undergoing one or more of a series of processes that should guarantee that they were aware of and committed to

freedom rights in different towns, but the basic information for the 1830s can be gleaned from *Appendix to Report from Commissioners on Municipal Corporations in England and Wales (Parliamentary Papers*, 1835 (116), xxiii–xxvi). Extensive discussions of freemen's rights in particular parliamentary boroughs can be found in S. Lambert (ed.), *House of Commons Sessional Papers of the Eighteenth Century: Reports and Papers* (Wilmington, Del., 1975), xxx (1774–1782 elections), esp. that for Preston, 321–50, and lxxxix (1792–3), esp. for Grimsby, 71 *et seq*. The classic study remains S. and B. Webb, *English Local Government from the Revolution to the Municipal Corporations Act: The Manor and the Borough* (2 vols.; 1908). Freemen's rolls have been published only for the larger towns of Chester, Exeter, Gloucester, Lancaster, Leicester, Newcastle-upon-Tyne, Norwich, Preston, and York. Recent examples with good introductions include M. M. Rowe and A. M. Jackson (eds.), *Exeter Freemen 1266–1967* (Devon and Cornwall Record Society, Extra Series I; Exeter, 1973) and A. D. J. Jurica (ed.), *A List of the Register of the Freemen of the City of Gloucester 1641–1838* (Bristol and Gloucestershire Archaeological Society, Gloucestershire Records Series, 4; 1991). *The Eighteenth-Century Short-Title Catalogue* reveals the English towns with published appeals to or concerning freemen or free burgesses: Alnwick, Bath, Bedford, Bristol, Canterbury, Carlisle, Chester, Christchurch, Colchester, Coventry, Derby, Durham, Exeter, Hereford, Ipswich, Kings Lynn, Lancaster, Leicester, Lincoln, Liverpool, Maidstone*, Newcastle-under-Lyme, Newcastle-upon-Tyne*, Norwich, Nottingham, Oxford, Richmond, Rochester, Saint Albans, Shrewsbury, Sudbury, Warwick, Worcester, York (those with largest surviving corpus of literature are asterisked). I have not undertaken the close study of these texts that is long overdue.

the collective values of the place, but also capable of independent judgement and action in the exercise of their representative function. This ideal type was to be replaced, in the nineteenth century, by an alternative image of (local) citizenship—namely, qualification by the ownership of property or payment of rates, as measured at the time of qualification. I have explored elsewhere how this transition might have occurred in the political sphere, suggesting that one reason was the pressure put on the definition of urban freedom by the very importance of urban freedom in parliamentary elections. This led to ever-increasing demands for the tight definition of freedom, which in turn both encouraged people to exploit the loopholes in those definitions (notably non-resident and 'honorary' freemen) and led to polemical focus on those whose technical qualification stood in clear contrast to their inability to represent, at election time, the ideal type of the virtuous, independent resident urban householder. Hence the attractions of the alternative model, with its instant test of who was suitably qualified.[11]

Yet this political explanation does not seem sufficient, either to account for the immense durability of urban freedom or to explain why it was finally eclipsed. To do this one needs to offer an explanation of why the ideal type itself lost conviction. One feature of this is certainly economic change, but another, on which I shall focus here, is a changing sense of urban civility, not merely in the sense of urban manners (in the modern sense), but more profoundly in terms of the values and processes necessary to sustain urban society—that is, urban manners in the early modern sense.

To understand the socio-economic meaning of the freedom during the seventeenth and eighteenth centuries we need to understand how urban freedom had been used by urban communities to regulate competition. As recent work on medieval and early modern towns has shown, there was no 'golden age' when all townsmen had been freemen or when towns had sought to regulate all of the economy through the freedom. Instead, the freedom, like the guild system, had always been a legal fiction employed flexibly to stabilize urban society. There were a number of reasons why towns had not insisted on a legal monopoly. One was the legal and political difficulty in enforcing such rules, which ran against some free-trade principles in law and powerful vested interests outside. But even within the town there could be mixed feelings. The economic privileges of freedom were more relevant to certain trades than others, dealing in particular with retail businesses and craftsmen who sold their own products. Other occupations, such as the professions, many service trades, certain types of manufacture and labouring occupations had never been systematically integrated, although some of their members might be free and particular towns might seek to control sensitive occupations through this

---

[11] Barry, 'I significati della libertà', 503–8. This builds on the analysis by P. Langford, *Public Life and the Propertied Englishman 1689–1798* (Oxford, 1991), ch. 4, esp. pp. 282–7.

mechanism. The high point of such efforts would appear to be in the late six-teenth or early seventeenth centuries, rather than earlier, but this was not uni-versally the case. As Walker's research on guilds makes very clear, moreover, such efforts at regulation remained at a high level into the early eighteenth century, and fell away only gradually and piecemeal thereafter. Such regula-tion was always seeking to balance the advantages of innovation and open trade with the need to offer protection to a core group of traders identified as an essential part of urban society.[12]

Two key considerations were involved here. One was that the benefits of urban life should be enjoyed primarily by those who had contributed their time and money to maintain urban government and society and who could be held to account to the rest for their behaviour. There was therefore an explicit trade-off, reflected in the freeman's oath, between gaining the advan-tages of freedom and being able and willing to pay taxes, participate in town government, and subject oneself and one's property to the town's courts. Given the delicate networks of credit and financial interdependency that char-acterized town life and the dependence of urban government on unpaid work and civic self-rule, such a trade-off was fully rational.[13] Moreover, the system was being worked largely by those who stood to gain from such preferential treatment. This group was not necessarily just an urban oligarchy, narrowly defined, however, for such notions also appealed to the middling sort more generally and indeed were enforced by the town's leaders partly to win the support of this wider community.

Even in tightly regulated places and periods, however, the rules of freedom, like guild ones, were applied flexibly. Many towns, for example, contained areas, such as their so-called liberties, where regulations did not apply; sub-urban areas outside corporate jurisdiction were increasingly important. Town authorities, and even freemen, were ambivalent about such places, reflecting more general reasons for not enforcing monopolies. Producers in a particu-lar trade, especially the larger ones who often dominated town government, might not want to restrict totally the flow of cheap labour or subcontracting

---

[12] M. J. Walker, 'The Extent of the Guild Control in Trades in England *c*.1660–1720', Ph.D thesis (Cambridge, 1985). Other key studies include: P. J. Corfield, *The Impact of English Towns 1700–1800* (Oxford, 1982), 86–93; H. Swanson, 'The Illusion of Economic Structure: Craft Guilds in Late Medieval English Towns', *P&P* 121 (1988), 29–48; P. J. Corfield and D. Keene (eds.), *Work in Towns* (Leicester, 1990); I. Archer, *The Pursuit of Stability* (Cambridge, 1991); C. Brooks, 'Apprenticeship, Mobility and the Middling Sort 1550–1800', in J. Barry and C. Brooks (eds.), *The Middling Sort of People* (Basingstoke, 1994), 52–83; J. P. Ward, *Metropolitan Communities* (Stanford, Calif., 1997); M. Pelling, *The Common Lot* (Harlow, 1998). My ideas here are much indebted to M. Sonenscher, *Work and Wages: Natural Law, Politics and the Eighteenth-Century French Trades* (Cambridge, 1989), a work sadly without a parallel in the historiography of Britain.

[13] J. Brewer, 'The Commercialization of Politics', in N. McKendrick *et al.*, *Birth of a Consumer Society* (1981), 197–262; D. H. Sacks, *The Widening Gate: Bristol and the Atlantic Economy, 1450–1700* (Berkeley and Los Angeles, 1991); C. Muldrew, *The Economy of Obligation* (Basingstoke, 1998).

skills, while mercantile groups might welcome such alternative supplies. As consumers, townspeople knew the dangers of a closed shop, especially in sensitive products such as food, and often invoked competition in times of scarcity or dispute. On the other hand, they also accepted the need to ensure the stable business conditions and trading standards of a core trading group. The two needs could often be reconciled by offering *de facto* recognition without full freemen's rights to a peripheral class, who could be taxed for the privilege as and when convenient and, in times of pressure, either compelled to accept the freedom or expelled to improve the chances of the core group. During the unstable economic circumstance of much of the seventeenth century, such flexibility was crucial to urban strategies. In the eighteenth century, it could be argued, market expansion and slightly more stable economic conditions, together with the emergence of new forms of capital formation and insurance, made reliance on these older forms of regulation less essential, but their decline was very gradual.

There is, in short, plenty of evidence to suggest that the economic privileges of the freedom were still relevant in many towns into the eighteenth century, and that stereotyped images of monopolistic customs giving way to rational competition are unrealistic. This should encourage us to consider other, arguably equally important, ways in which urban freedom was related to urban stability. Trading privileges were only one way in which freemen had priority access to urban resources in times of need. Many towns had common lands, usually for pasture, access to which was reserved for freemen, thus providing a vital cushion against price fluctuations or trade downturn. Equally important were charities reserved for those in life-cycle crises, such as impoverished freemen or their orphans and widows. Another bonus to the family budget was the so-called free school, which was 'free' only in that it offered free entry to its resident freemen and often university scholarships for its brightest sons thereafter. For the urban middling sort such apparently marginal benefits lessened the dangers of urban trading and in particular the burdens of family provision. It is perhaps not entirely fanciful to view the way in which many freemen exacted a price for their vote, especially in the smaller freemen boroughs, as a further development of such an insurance mentality. In Grampound, for example, the hapless candidates and their agents found themselves taking on all sorts of responsibilities for debts, family crises, and the like, as well as providing regular annuities and gratuities to their established supporters.[14]

In this respect being an urban freeman was in itself a bulwark against the blows of urban fortune and the permanent risk of 'dependence'. As such, the

---

[14] I owe the Grampound point to the research in progress of John More. This theme is well explored for the nineteenth century by Searby, 'Chartists and Freemen'. The wider picture is the subject of J. Barry, 'Bourgeois Collectivism', in Barry and Brooks (eds.), *Middling Sort*, 84–112, especially 95–100.

freedom, like the guilds, provided the crucial model for the new forms of association, such as friendly societies and freemasons' lodges, which mushroomed after 1700 for this same purpose. Note, for example, the regular use of the term 'free member' in friendly societies to designate those who had paid the initial premiums necessary to gain benefits; the terminology of the freemasons is self-evident.[15] Becoming free was thus part of a continuing strategy of self-defence, of the reproduction of independent trading households in urban society. Freeman status helped to make you free and keep you free. But at the same time freedom was a condition of becoming and remaining a freeman. To become a freeman one had to demonstrate an a priori case that one could maintain an independent trading household; moreover, in many towns, one could lose one's freeman status if one failed to maintain this degree of independence—for example, by requiring poor relief or leaving the urban community. In pursuing these features, we come up against a crucial ambiguity of the very term 'free man'. The ideology is one of male independence, but, as we have seen, the purposes of the freedom were often household centred and equally the resources needed to become a freeman depended less on the individual than on a household and, in some cases at least, on women.

Let us look again at how the freedom was obtained. Purchase was usually the most expensive. Such fines have normally been regarded as a useful boost to civic finances, but their legitimation, surely, was to purchase a share in existing urban amenities and to demonstrate one's financial standing. In practice the hefty fines may have been paid in instalments. However, purchasing freedom was never regarded as an ideal method of entry. The fully legitimate forms were inheritance (or patrimony), apprenticeship (or, as it was often termed, significantly, servitude) and, thirdly, in some towns, marriage to the widows and/or daughters of freemen. Patrimonial entry reflects an ideology of male birthright, with the town as an extended family with property rights descending in the male line, and such sons were usually charged the lowest entry fees of all. Indirectly, such rights could be transmitted in some towns through widows and daughters, but could be exercised only by a male who took over such a free household—and thus established a presumptive claim to the independence it supported. This provision reflected the common urban problem of sustaining population, as well as giving a further advantage to native women over immigrant ones in the marriage stakes. The final method of entry, apprenticeship, was also a way of bringing new blood into the urban

---

[15] See Barry, 'Bourgeois Collectivism'; P. Clark, *Sociability and Urbanity in the Eighteenth-Century City* (Leicester, 1986); J. Money, 'Freemasonry and the Fabric of Loyalism in Hanoverian England', in E. Hellmuth (ed.), *The Transformation of Political Culture in Britain and Germany in the Late Eighteenth Century* (Oxford, 1990), 273–90; R. J. Morris, 'Clubs, Societies and Associations', in F. M. L. Thompson (ed.), *The Cambridge Social History of Britain, 1750–1950*, iii (Cambridge, 1990), 395–443. I am grateful to Martin Gorsky for his advice regarding friendly societies.

family, but on strict terms. Only by a period of servitude to urban society in general, and an urban household in particular, could the apprentice, like the child, inherit freedom out of servitude, when of an age to set up his own household. During the sixteenth and seventeenth centuries the apprenticeship route into the freedom had become both more dominant and more carefully regulated. Despite this, many, perhaps most, apprentices before the Civil War never took out urban freedom, but it seems that this pattern changed after the mid-century, with a much higher take-up of freedom by the 1670s onwards and into the early eighteenth century. This was surely due to the much greater incentive for those qualified to take up the freedom. By the eighteenth century, as apprenticeship began a slow decline in many urban occupations, though not all, patrimony and marriage grew once more as routes into the freedom. This trend may also reflect shifting urban demography, as greater dynastic continuity and a female bias to immigration changed the profile of potential freemen.[16]

Urban freedom thus systematically tempered the full effects of the market, not merely or even primarily by constituting a cartel, but by offering freemen (one is tempted to call them 'stakeholders') ways of establishing their claim to a stake in civil society and a number of forms of assistance to ensure that they could sustain this position and pass it on to the next generation. In doing so it laid heavy emphasis on the household, both as the means of gaining that claim and as the organization to be protected. In this respect, once again, I would argue that urban freedom represented a much wider trend in early modern urban society, and urban freemen were the ideal types of the urban middling sort. I have called this culture 'bourgeois collectivism' to underline the divergence from our stereotype of market-oriented possessive individualism.[17] But it might be equally appropriate (and less anachronistic) to call it 'civility'. The remainder of this essay will consider urban freedom as an example of such civility and how it might have given place, gradually, to an alternative urban civility.

How did urban freedom as a form of civility differ from that associated with the gentry and how did it negotiate that fine line between necessity and independence identified at the start of this essay? The main answers will already be clear. It was explicitly collective in its nature and it emphasized, rather than concealing, the economic and political dimensions of social interaction. But, at the same time, it removed such economic and political dimensions from the realm of necessity and reconciled their force with independence, by presenting them as the rules of an association to which the freeman had voluntarily adhered for the collective as well as his individual

---

[16] I. K. Ben-Amos, 'Failure to Become Freemen: Urban Apprentices in Early Modern England', *Social History*, 16 (1991), 154–72; Brooks, 'Apprenticeship'.

[17] Barry, 'Bourgeois Collectivism'. See also J. Barry, 'Identité urbaine et classes moyennes dans l'Angleterre moderne', *Annales ESC*, 48 (1993), 853–84.

good. The ultimate form taken by this reconciliation was that of the law: the law seen not as a form of servitude (as it would be for slaves or in a tyranny), but as the embodiment and guardian of freedoms and liberties, which could not otherwise exist.

The freeman was thus 'civilized' by undergoing an education that was not primarily in books or formal education, but rather in the institutions of the household, either as a child within a freeman household and/or as an apprentice within one (the latter crucial for the many migrants into town). Schooling might also serve to distinguish the urban freeman: most urban occupations expected some level of literacy and, as we have seen, access to urban 'free schools' could be an important privilege, offering a higher standard than the parental purse might have been able to afford unaided, and subject to the public scrutiny of city authorities.[18] But greater emphasis was laid on education within and for work, and hence on the educative value of work itself, not just for the apprentice or child but throughout life. The values instilled would be all those qualities, such as thrift, respectability, and industry, often labelled the Protestant work ethic and seen as the foundation of individualism. But their success was assumed not only to depend on collective rather than individual action, but also to be accompanied by a set of overtly collective virtues, of sociability and good fellowship.

These values were to be expressed both within the household and in a wide range of other public settings. Just as much as any gentleman, the urban freeman's civility was both developed and tested in the public sphere. This would have included the dense urban world of alehouses, inns, and, later, coffee houses and other places of entertainment. But it would also have included the many meetings in the dense network of associations, secular and religious, political and business, corporate and unofficial, to which urban freemen characteristically belonged. While there were, of course, crucial differences between these many kinds of association (and rivalries between them), they shared many of the same elements of civility, once again in the form of dialectic tensions. These include those between self-control and obedience to others, between competition and cooperation, between restraint and liberality. We may see the practice of associational life as providing the bourgeoisie with a constantly renewed experience and representation of how to manage their lives in accordance with these values, and in particular how to balance their apparently contradictory requirements. The central notion here, one often evoked by contemporaries as they extolled the virtues

[18] See L. Stone, 'Literacy and Education in England 1640–1900', *P&P* 42 (1969), 69–139; W. B. Stephens, 'Illiteracy and Schooling in Provincial Towns 1640–1870', in D. Reeder (ed.), *Urban Education in the Nineteenth Century* (1977), 27–48; R. A. Houston, *Scottish Literacy and Scottish Identity* (Cambridge, 1985); J. Barry, 'Popular Culture in Seventeenth-Century Bristol', in B. Reay (ed.), *Popular Culture in Seventeenth-Century England* (1985), 59–90; and other works discussed in J. Barry, 'Literacy and Literature in Popular Culture', in T. Harris (ed.), *Popular Culture in Early Modern England* (Basingstoke, 1995), 69–94, 232–41.

of life in the 'middle station', was of the 'golden mean'. To be a member of the middling sort you had to learn how to practise moderation, but the middling sort were seen as uniquely placed to achieve this ideal state, if properly trained.

The role of associations in this process of training was twofold. On the one hand, the values preached by the sermons, toasts, insignia, recitation of rules, and the like at associational events provided a prudential code for the urban freeman seeking to maintain his freedom. Its messages were, however, also embodied in the actual practices needed to carry off such occasions successfully. For example, he learnt to balance the demands of sociability, expressed most commonly in expenditure on proper clothes, food, and drink, with appropriate restraint, such as limits on expenditure and drunkenness and insistence on correct clothing for one's position within the association. Plaudits for order and decency followed correct performance; criticism and penalties followed infractions. Both the group and the individual were thus under permanent scrutiny for the adequate expression of bourgeois self-management, itself the prerequisite for genuine freedom. Association thus succeeded apprenticeship as the proving ground for the urban freeman.

Finally, urban freemen had a third setting—namely, the exercise of political responsibility. Here, too, the same dialectic can be observed, between the model of the virtuous freeman exercising an independent choice and the public world of ritual, festivity, and collective sociability with which that process was often associated. It is all too easy for us to associate the latter aspect with corruption (as many contemporary critics also did) and judge the political world of the freeman by the standards of a modern secret voting process—forgetting both the public world of political sociability still found today and the assumption then that such public display was an integral part of the freedoms of the urban electorate. Hence, of course, the outrage often expressed by urban freemen at electoral deals or other élite stratagems to prevent freemen from exercising their vote: this was to impugn their civility while removing the opportunity for its exercise.[19]

Alongside the elaborate rituals involved in much of this civility, there was an elaborate social vocabulary to express these values, in which words such as fellowship, benevolence, decorum, and respectability were quite as important as the term 'gentility' (on which historians have lavished such attention). One crucial vocabulary pointed to civic benefits and social utility, in particular the complex language of charity and mutual benefit. As noted above, one might regard urban freedom as a form of mutual benefit association, yet the forms such benefit took, including the support of families, allowed this to be pre-

[19] J. Epstein, 'Understanding the Cap of Liberty: Symbolic Practice and Social Conflict in Early Nineteenth-Century England', *P&P* 122 (1989), 75–118; F. O'Gorman, 'Campaigns, Rituals and Ceremonies: The Social Meaning of Elections in England 1780–1860', *P&P* 135 (1992), 79–115; Sweet, 'Freemen and Independence'.

sented as unselfish measures for the public good, allowing even the humbler freeman to feel a supporter of charity, not, as the poor, a humble dependent upon it. A second cluster of terms concerned antiquity, honour, and precedence. Like other bourgeois associations, urban freemen could claim for their towns and their privileges, and hence for themselves, precisely those qualities, associated with continuity, that the gentry claimed, as individuals, from their relationship to land and family.[20] Finally, of course, there were the notions of freedom, citizenship, and independence themselves. These too had their balancing requirements, such as loyalty, obedience, unity, and impartiality. It is worth remembering here that, while urban freedom was often employed in a radical critique of oligarchy, it had its own inherent conservatism. It often expressed patriarchal and paternalistic sentiments towards women, children, and the dependent poor and it often involved unequal responsibilities and power within the urban freemen, while excluding many others from its privileges. It also involved a complex mixture of the highly local and particularistic (the specific civility of a particular town), and the national and universal (urban freedom as a nationally defined category linked to Crown, law, and Parliament and part of a national constitution of freedoms).[21] It is misleading, therefore, to present this culture as a localist, provincial culture, in contrast to the national metropolitan civility of the gentry and urban élites, because this culture was in its own way national (and found its fullest expression, of course, in the metropolis among the London freemen).[22]

Underlying all these aspects of civility was the urban obsession with regulating citizens' behaviour to ensure order and decency, two of the highest terms of praise, though, as we have seen, they also sought to provide conditions in which sociability and communal solidarity could safely be expressed. Hence the constant urban efforts to ensure the 'reformation of manners', a movement through which the middling sort were imposing civility on themselves as much as on those above and below them, and which offered them yet another associational setting in which to practise their civility. Many of the characteristic features of gentry civility can be understood only in terms of their interaction, in London and elsewhere, with such urban regulation, whether it took the form of new standards of genteel self-regulation or, as often, in the assertion of a form of counter-civility in the persona of the rake or fop.[23]

---

[20] As Sweet notes, 'Freemen and Independence', 112–13.

[21] Barry, 'I significati della libertà', 493–5.

[22] *Pace* D. Wahrman, 'National Society, Communal Culture', *Social History*, 17 (1992), 43–72. See J. Barry, 'Provincial Town Culture 1640–1780', in J. Pittock and A. Wear (eds.), *Interpretation and Cultural History* (Basingstoke, 1991), 198–234.

[23] M. Ingram, 'The Reformation of Manners in Early Modern England', in P. Griffiths *et al.*, *The Experience of Authority in Early Modern England* (Basingstoke, 1996), 47–88; Bryson, *From Courtesy to Civility*, ch. 7. I explore the centrality of the reformation of manners in urban society in J. Barry, 'Begging, Swearing and Cursing', in Barry, *Religion in Bristol* (Bristol, forthcoming).

During the early modern period these forms of civility were in constant contact, above all in London. There is no space here to debate how far one civility conquered the other: clearly they intermingled to produce some peculiarly English forms of civility. In the context of urban freedom, the remaining question is how far this produced a new form of urban civility, different from that sketched above, whose dominance helped to break the hold of the urban freeman as an ideal type for urban civility. My brief answer would be that such a change did occur, but gradually and in a very complex way. If, as I have argued elsewhere, one can see many of the features of the polite society of the urban renaissance as deeply indebted to this earlier civic culture in forms and values, and supplementing rather than replacing the older forms, it becomes harder to see why the growth of polite society should, in itself, have undermined urban freedom.[24] However, it is possible to see a change in the civilizing process embodied in these forms of civility, compared to the process typified by urban freedom. Both the education for such civility and the public expressions of that civility came to owe less and less to rites of passage through collective institutions associated with the household and the town, and had more and more to do with schooling and possession of specific cultural attributes at a particular moment of time. Like the political right of representation, civility ceased to be defined by continuity over time and became defined by meeting a contemporary standard of performance. In that respect, perhaps, the codes of civility elucidated by Anna Bryson were finally to win the day. While it is tempting to consider this transition as that from community to class, or regard it as the commodification of culture within a consumer society, I believe it is valuable to retain the specific reference to a change in the evaluation of time. Not only does this retain the political as well as economic dimension, mirroring the shift away from an ancient-constitution model, but it also correlates with that fundamental shift in attitudes to knowledge (away from tradition as the ultimate source of legitimacy) and in social experience (towards a greater confidence in impersonal techniques for overcoming the risks posed by the natural and social environment) that Keith Thomas identified as crucial in *Religion and the Decline of Magic.*[25]

---

[24] P. Borsay, *The English Urban Renaissance* (Oxford, 1989); J. Brewer, *The Pleasures of the Imagination* (1997). For my criticism of these approaches, see Barry, 'Provincial Town Culture', and also J. Barry, 'Consumers' Passions', *Historical Journal*, 34 (1991), 207–16.

[25] Thomas, *Religion*, 428–32, 576–9, 602–6, 644–7, 662–3. For this, see my discussions in J. Barry, 'A Historical Postscript', in D. Castiglione and L. Sharpe (eds.), *Shifting the Boundaries: Transformation of the Languages of Public and Private in the Eighteenth Century* (Exeter, 1995), 220–37, and in J. Barry, 'Introduction: Keith Thomas and the Problem of Witchcraft', in Barry *et al.* (eds.), *Witchcraft in Early Modern Europe* (Cambridge, 1996), 1–45, esp. 25–30.

11

Arson, Threats of Arson, and Incivility in Early Modern England

BERNARD CAPP

The notebook of the Norfolk Justice Robert Doughty contains a specimen oath administered to those asking to have an enemy bound over for threatening behaviour: 'You shall swear that you require not the peace against AB for any private malice, hatred or evil will, but for that you are afraid (he or she) will burn your houses, kill, maim, or otherwise do you some bodily harm, and so help you God'.[1] The oath reminds us that the campaign for the reformation of manners was waged across a very broad front, its targets ranging from vulgarity and profanity to behaviour that posed a direct threat to life and property. Recognisances played a key role in keeping the peace and curbing these grosser forms of incivility.[2] What is striking is to find arson placed first in Doughty's list of reasons for binding someone over, and this essay sets out to fill a gap in the historiography of crime by investigating the social history of arson (and of threats and suspicions) in the context of the civilizing process.

I

John Archer's important studies of arson in the nineteenth century focused on the dramatic wave of attacks by desperate farm labourers on the stacks, barns, and sometimes houses of wealthy landowners.[3] Such attacks have tended to overshadow the much wider role that arson played in early modern society. In Tudor and Stuart times, as Keith Thomas observed in a pioneering survey in 1971, arson was 'a common means of revenge for those who felt themselves injured by their neighbours'.[4] Though most familiar as a weapon

---

[1] *The Notebook of Robert Doughty 1662–1665*, ed. J. M. Rosenheim (Norfolk Record Society, 54; 1989), 15.

[2] S. Hindle, 'The Keeping of the Public Peace', in P. Griffiths, A. Fox, and S. Hindle (eds.), *The Experience of Authority in Early Modern England* (1996), 213–48.

[3] J. E. Archer, *By a Flash and a Scare* (Oxford, 1989); J. E. Archer, 'Under Cover of Night: Arson and Animal Maiming', in G. E. Mingay (ed.), *The Unquiet Countryside* (1989), 65–79.

[4] K. Thomas, *Religion and the Decline of Magic: Studies in Popular Beliefs in Sixteenth and Seventeenth Century England* (1971), 531.

of the poor and marginal, it was also employed in disputes between neighbours of roughly equal standing, initially at all social levels, and sometimes
by the strong against the weak. Professional criminals too used arson to
further or conceal their crimes. In 1700 a gang unable to break into Dr
Hans Sloane's house in Bloomsbury set fire to it, and posing as rescuers then
exploited the ensuing confusion to carry away his valuables.[5]

Fire was one of the most terrifying threats facing our ancestors, in an age
of timber and thatch and with no insurance companies to offer financial protection.[6] It followed that arson was one of the most horrific crimes imagin-
able, for it threatened both life and property. The Great Fire of London in
1666, widely seen as deliberate, served as a terrifying reminder of the scale of
the arsonist's power. The law was correspondingly severe. Arson was a major
felony, punished by hanging (and in earlier times, appropriately, by burning),
and one of the first to deny offenders benefit of clergy, in 1532.[7] Sir Matthew
Hale laid down that even a child below the age of criminal responsibility
(14) could be hanged for arson, 'if by circumstances it can appear he knew it
to be evil', and he noted with equanimity the execution of an 8-year-old boy
in 1630.[8] Acts of 1550 and 1553, passed in a period of economic distress and
political tension, extended the felony to cover rick-burning by groups of
more than twelve persons.[9] To call someone an arsonist was itself actionable
as slander, and labels such as 'incendiary' and 'firebrand' carried a powerful
resonance.[10]

Yet arson is almost totally absent from studies of early modern crime, and
the reason quickly becomes evident when we turn to the criminal records. Only
one of the 1,631 crimes recorded in East Sussex between 1592 and 1640 concerned arson.[11] Assize records tell a similar story. Elizabethan Sussex saw only
five people indicted for the offence, three being acquitted and one found insane;
in Elizabethan Essex seven were indicted, of whom four were acquitted, while
only one of the four people indicted in Jacobean Kent was convicted and condemned.[12] How should we interpret this paucity of evidence? It could be that
the crime was so universally detested, and the penalty so severe, that it was rarely
committed, especially as arson in an urban environment was such an indiscriminate and uncontrollable weapon. It might also be that the 'dark figure' of
unrecorded crime was particularly high in this instance, for rudimentary foren-

[5] *A full and true Account, of the Behaviours . . . of the Condemn'd Criminals . . . executed at Tyburn*
[on 24 May] (1700); *An Account of the Apprehending . . . of John Davis* (1700).
[6] Thomas, *Religion*, 15–17.
[7] 23 Hen. VIII, c. 1; 1 Mary, c. 12; Sir M. Hale, *Historia Placitorum Coronae* (1736), i. 570–4.
[8] Hale, *Historia*, i. 25, 569–70.   [9] 3 and 4 Ed. VI, c. 5; 1 Mary, c. 12.
[10] W. Sheppard, *Action upon the Case for Slander* (1662), 36, 43, 132.
[11] C. Herrup, *The Common Peace: Participation and the Criminal Law in Seventeenth-Century
England* (Cambridge, 1987), 27.
[12] J. S. Cockburn (ed.), *Calendar of Assize Records: Sussex Indictments, Elizabeth I* (1975), 189,
226, 314, 389; J. S. Cockburn (ed.), *Calendar of Assize Records: Essex Indictments, Elizabeth I* (1982),
224, 231, 253, 354, 494, 523; J. S. Cockburn (ed.), *Calendar of Assize Records: Kent Indictments, James
I* (1980), 16, 37, 147.

sic skills made arson extremely difficult to distinguish from accidental fires. The felony was also defined in highly restrictive terms, excluding many acts we would today classify as arson. It applied only to burning occupied dwelling houses or adjacent outbuildings, and barns full of corn. Moreover, the building had to be seriously damaged or destroyed; a fire quickly extinguished was not felonious. In enclosure disputes we often find protesters burning hedges and fences, but they were prosecuted for riot, not arson.[13] And when arson served to conceal other major crimes, usually house-breaking or murder, offenders were generally prosecuted under these other headings.[14]

Despite the paucity of court records, contemporaries knew that a candle and wisp of straw were enough to give any disgruntled individual a terrifying power of life and death. Their fears were well founded. In 1631 three people were hanged for destroying forty houses at Walberswick (Suffolk), while two embittered naval seamen were executed after they burned their ship ('the old bitch') at Malta in 1676, with fatal consequences.[15] Some attacks had still more terrible effects. In November 1641 one Simon Man, nursing a grudge, started a fire in the hold of the *Bonaventure* at Blackwall that killed the master and fifty-seven members of the crew, and destroyed the ship with its cargo of Malaga wine worth £40,000.[16] There was even greater carnage in 1727 at Barwell, near Newmarket, when a barn where 100 people had assembled to watch a puppet show 'was set on fire on purpose by a man who was displeased because he might not see the show for nothing'. At least seventy-eight people died in the flames.[17]

II

It is impossible now to quantify the 'dark figure' of unrecorded arson. A far more rewarding approach is to explore the variety of contexts in which threats and fears of arson, as well as the crime itself, figured in the lives and discourse of contemporaries. We need to create a typology of arson in early modern England, one that looks beyond the statutory definition and gives full weight to individual as well as collective action.[18]

Our first category of arson, as a weapon of collective rural protest, needs

[13] R. B. Manning, *Village Revolts: Social Protest and Popular Disturbances in England 1509–1640* (Oxford, 1988), 43, 47, 128, 277.

[14] See e.g. N.B., *A Compleat Collection of Remarkable Tryals* (1718), i. 60–1, 192–224; G. T. Crook (ed.), *The Complete Newgate Calendar*, ii (1926), 7–8, 79, 176, 194–5.

[15] Thomas, *Religion*, 532; Bodl. MS Rawlinson C972, fos. 9–16.

[16] *Sad Newes from Black-Wall* (1641).

[17] 'The Journal of John Hobson', ed. C. Jackson, in *Yorkshire Diaries and Autobiographies* (Surtees Society, 65; 1877), 274.

[18] For parallels, see P. Roberts, 'Arson, Conspiracy and Rumour in Early Modern Europe', *Continuity and Change*, 12 (1997), 9–29; A. Abbiateci, 'Arsonists in Eighteenth-Century France: An Essay in the Typology of Crime', in R. Forster and O. Ranum (eds.), *Deviants and the Abandoned in French Society* (1978), 157–79.

no further elaboration here; its familiar image as a crime of the dispossessed and weak is well founded. We might, however, note the occasional urban parallels, such as the weavers' riots of August 1675 when hundreds of looms were rifled and burned in and around the capital.[19] Urban attacks could also function as a political weapon, as in 1595 when a London crowd threatened to kill a hated mayor and burn his house, or in 1640 when there was talk of firing Lambeth Palace and burning the despised Archbishop Laud.[20]

The second category has received rather less attention: attacks or threats by disgruntled individuals against their superiors. Offenders were often vagrants or other marginal figures, such as the Kent labourer sentenced to hang in 1607 for firing a gentleman's house with a candle and a stack of broom.[21] Their motives are usually impossible to determine; few arsonists left any recorded explanation for their action, while the motivation of those making threats of arson has usually to be surmised from very brief court minutes. The London Bridewell court, which exercised wide-ranging jurisdiction over petty offenders, dealt with a steady trickle of such cases. Winifred Knight was whipped in 1610 as a lewd woman who had threatened to burn her neighbours' houses, while Elizabeth Raunce was described as 'an idle young woman and one that will not follow no honest calling but disturbs her neighbours with outrageous speeches and threatens to fire their houses'.[22] The courts tried to distinguish between anti-social, maladjusted people and genuine 'lunatics', who featured in a significant number of cases.[23] A few individuals resist easy categorization, such as John Heuce, 'a vile and stout vagabond', who in 1562 was moved by the holy spirit to give away all his goods and beg for a living, but also threatened to fire his neighbours' houses—perhaps finding them unwilling to give him relief.[24]

Marginal individuals who fell foul of the law might also threaten arson to intimidate parish officers or magistrates, hoping thus to evade punishment. In 1617 a bogus cripple threatened to fire the house of the London constable who had arrested him, while a Leicester man, bound over in 1630 for threatening to fire the town, warned the mayor darkly 'that if he sent him to prison he were best not to let him out again'.[25] In 1642 Elizabeth Lawrence, a London

---

[19] Hale, *Historia*, i. *143; T. Harris, *London Crowds in the Reign of Charles II* (Cambridge, 1990), 196.

[20] Manning, *Village Revolts*, 209; *CSPD 1640*, 88, 377.

[21] Cockburn (ed.), *Calendar: Kent, James I*, 37.

[22] Guildhall Library, Bridewell court book (hereafter BCB) (on microfilm) 5, fo. 415, 7, fo. 302; cf. 7, fo. 86, 8, 22 Sept. 1641, 25 Feb. 1642; 11, fo. 51. (I have cited Bridewell court books by folio number where available, and otherwise by date.)

[23] Cockburn (ed.), *Calendar: Sussex, Elizabeth*, 314; J. C. Jeaffreson (ed.), *Middlesex County Records* (1886–92), iii. 291; n. 99 below; cf. Abbiateci, 'Arsonists', 159–63.

[24] BCB 1, fo. 186ᵛ.

[25] BCB 6, 26 July 1617; Leicestershire RO, Hall Papers (hereafter LRO), BRII/18/17, p. 551; G. R. Quaife, *Wanton Wenches and Wayward Wives* (1979), 28; W. Le Hardy (ed.), *Hertfordshire County Records*, v (Hertford, 1928), 199, 246.

prostitute who had unwisely 'attempted to entice the beadle to lewdness', threatened to burn down his house when he tried to carry her to Bridewell.[26] If such threats failed, as they often did, vagrants might vow to return and burn down the town where they had been whipped, a satisfying if self-defeating fantasy of revenge that offered some illusory sense of power and control over their own destiny.[27] In 1690 a highwayman told the magistrate who committed him 'that if ever he came out of prison, he would fire his house'.[28] Most such threats were empty, but it was unwise to ignore them. Even prisoners sometimes started fires, to effect an escape or more often to vent their impotent rage and despair. Conspiracies were detected to burn down Newgate in 1601 and again in 1683, while in 1618 a man was charged with firing the Gatehouse.[29]

The third category of arson is domestic: a weapon employed in disputes between members of the same household. Here too we often find a pattern of subordinates, especially servants, striking back at those in authority. Ill-treated servants had very few means of redress, but if driven beyond endurance they had plentiful opportunities for lethal retribution, with arson offering one of the readiest means. Delinquent servants enjoyed similar opportunities. When a Southampton baker turned out his apprentice for 'lewdness' in 1608, his wife feared the youth would steal back and burn down their house in revenge.[30] Such fears might be well grounded. Mary Benson, a London maid-servant, was condemned to death in 1687 for robbing and firing her master's house, which she had fled after locking the doors and taking the key, leaving the household still asleep in their beds.[31] Anne Selby, aged 18, hanged the same year for burning her employers' house, confessed she had done so at the instigation of a man with a grudge against the family, who had promised to marry her and take her to Ireland.[32] Lowly servants were the most likely to be seduced by such temptations, but rebellious adolescents too might view arson as a powerful weapon against parents or elder siblings. Robert Huffer, 'a notorious rogue', threatened to burn his brother's house in London in 1625, and stabbed his sister with a knife, while in 1642 Henry Kitchen was charged with threatening to fire his father's house and stabbing the Bridewell porter. He claimed to have been drunk.[33] Other attacks were triggered by desperation,

[26] BCB 8, 30 Sept. 1642.
[27] J. C. Atkinson (ed.), *Quarter Sessions Records* (North Riding Record Society; 1884–92), ii. 101–2.
[28] *The Proceedings . . . in the Old Bailey . . . 15 and 16 January 1690* (henceforth *Proceedings in the Old Bailey*, with dates) (1690), 1; Thomas, *Religion*, 531.
[29] BCB 7, fo. 211ᵛ; N.B., *Compleat Collection*, 278–87; Jeaffreson (ed.), *Middlesex County Records*, ii. 134.
[30] *The Assembly Books of Southampton*, i. *1602–1608* (Southampton Record Society, 1; 1907), 77.
[31] *Proceedings in the Old Bailey*, 31 Aug., 1, 3 Sept. 1687 (1687), 2.
[32] Ibid., 12–13 May 1687 (1687), 4; *The True Account of the Behaviour . . . of the Criminals* (1687), 3.
[33] BCB 6, 16 Apr. 1625; 8, 25 Feb. 1642; cf. 7, fo. 171.

sometimes with tragic results. In 1705 one John Davis of Launceston, 'having caused a person to be press'd with whom his daughter was engag'd, she, out of revenge, one night set the house on fire, whereby her father, mother and her self were burnt'.[34] Though the circumstances were unusual, the combination of revenge and suicidal despair was not uncommon.

Domestic arson was not necessarily, however, a crime of subordinate members of the household. When we turn from actions to threats, we find that in marital disputes they were almost always made by the husband, which we can probably interpret as both a terrifying form of intimidation and an expression of frustrated rage at his failure to maintain 'proper' control over the household. In 1648 a profane Essex man, irritated by his wife's habit of frequenting sermons, swore either to drown or to burn her.[35] Threats were more often directed against the house itself, or its contents. John Voak of Portsmouth, drunken and disreputable, allegedly threatened to fire his own house in 1660 in an incident almost certainly bound up with his marital problems; he was later also accused of smashing open the door, beating his wife, and railing at her as whore and bitch.[36] A Dorset man also accused of beating his wife, repeatedly, threatened to burn down his mother-in-law's house, perhaps holding her to blame for his marital problems.[37] Sometimes the desperate behaviour triggered by marital breakdown could anticipate the modern crime of murder followed by suicide. In 1626 William Boules of Reading, threatening to kill his wife and fire his house, drew his sword on the constable and swore to kill anyone who tried to resist him.[38] Desperate wives were much less likely to threaten arson or violence, for such words would simply trigger a beating. A man in Douglas, Isle of Man, had his wife bound over on the grounds that he feared she 'would burn his house upon him', but the accusation may have been part of his devious legal manœuvres to win control of her property.[39]

So far we have considered arson as a weapon of the weak, and in a domestic context. The fourth major category is in quarrels between persons of roughly equal standing.[40] Categories might easily overlap, of course, for

---

[34] *Remarks and Collections of Thomas Hearne*, i. *1705–1707*, ed. C. E. Doble (Oxford Historical Society, 2; 1885), 38.

[35] J. A. Sharpe, 'Domestic Homicide in Early Modern England', *Historical Journal*, 24 (1981), 31; BCB 7, fos. 25ᵛ, 233.

[36] M. J. Hoad (ed.), *Portsmouth Record Series: Borough Sessions Papers 1653–1688* (1971), 15, 20, 23, 161.

[37] *The Casebook of Sir Francis Ashley JP, Recorder of Dorchester 1614–35*, ed. J. H. Bettey (Dorset Record Society, 7; 1981), 60; *Notebook of Robert Doughty*, 68.

[38] J. M. Guilding (ed.), *Reading Records: The Diary of the Corporation*, ii. *1603–1629* (Reading, 1895), 327.

[39] M. Blundell (ed.), *Cavalier: Letters of William Blundell to his Friends 1620–1698* (1933), 160.

[40] W. Le Hardy (ed.), *County of Middlesex: Calendar to the Sessions Records*, NS i. *1612–1614* (1935), 46, 96, 232, 314; LRO BRII/18/26A, p. 216.

domestic quarrels sometimes developed into disputes between neighbours. A Somerset woman threatened to fire three neighbouring houses, alleging that the women living there were her husband's whores, 'all of them'.[41] In a fevered sexual triangle in London in 1605, Agnes Browne allegedly threatened to cut the throat of her lover's wife and set fire to her house, while one Richard Ward was charged in 1642 with 'setting his [own] house on fire with intent to burn his neighbours'.[42] Threats of arson between neighbours were most common among the 'lower sorts' and habitual offenders might be among the marginal figures discussed earlier. Neighbours complained that Alice Rashforth, who had threatened to fire their houses, 'was a common brawler and disturber of them'. True to form, she threatened and railed at the constable who arrested her.[43] Sometimes threats were clearly drink related. In 1607 John Jones, a common drunkard, admitted threatening to fire the house of Goodwife Denys, probably an alehouse, after she refused to let him be alone with a woman there.[44] Another importunate customer told an alewife in 1630 that 'if she would not give him drink he would burn the house'.[45] But we also find seemingly respectable artisans turning to such threats when tempers boiled over. In 1621 Robert Botham of Leicester demolished a wall he resented, and threatened to kill one neighbour and to burn the house of another.[46] In 1633 an angry London woman who threatened to burn a neighbour's house even sent for a link, while John Blackwell, who assaulted a midwife with a knife, threatened to kill her and to fire her house.[47] Similar outbursts can be found throughout the century and the country. A Warwickshire carpenter beat an alehouse-keeper in 1691 and threatened to fire his house, while three years later an angry woman allegedly railed at a Kenilworth weaver: 'Damn you for a dam'd pocky dog, you have built an house but by God's wounds you shall see that I will set it all in a flame.'[48]

It was not only lowly artisans, however, who used or threatened arson in pursuit of their grievances. David Palliser notes that four of the first six men to be bound over in Tudor York on suspicion of intended arson were aldermen or future aldermen.[49] Well into the sixteenth century we can also find members of the landed élite ready to employ this as well as other forms of violence in feuds with neighbouring landowners. In a Star Chamber case, a Yorkshire gentleman charged Sir William Gascoigne with sending forty of his servants to attack his house in April 1530, with orders to take it by storm 'and if they could not do so, they should fire the house and

---

[41] Quaife, *Wanton Wenches*, 159.   [42] BCB 5, fo. 8ᵛ; 8, 27 May 1642.
[43] BCB 8, fo. 128.   [44] BCB 5, fo. 182ᵛ.   [45] BCB 7, fo. 166ᵛ.
[46] LRO BRII/18/14, p. 79; cf. BRII/18/18, p. 206.   [47] BCB 7, fo. 312ᵛ; 8, fo. 149.
[48] Warwickshire RO (hereafter WRO), CR 103, Justice's Notebook of William Bromley, 23, 59–61.
[49] D. Palliser, 'Civic Mentality and the Environment in Tudor York', *Northern History*, 18 (1982), 93–4.

burn it'.[50] A contemporary Gloucestershire feud ended in farce when Sir Maurice Berkeley and his men raided the deer park of Anne, dowager Lady Berkeley, and attempted to fire a hayrick close to the manor house, hoping the flames would spread to it; by chance, a rival band of poachers were hiding inside the rick, and leaped out to save themselves, whereupon both groups fled in terror from the other.[51] In *As You Like It*, Orlando learns that his malevolent brother is planning 'To burn the lodging where you use to lie, | And you within it'.[52] Aristocratic habits of violence were slow to change, and at the close of the sixteenth century there was still nothing implausible in such a scenario.

The use of arson in disputes over enclosure or common rights, generally seen as a weapon of the weak, needs in some instances, to be reinterpreted, for it could also occur in situations where the opposing parties were relatively equal in strength. At Chepping Wycombe (Buckinghamshire), an enclosing yeoman complained that rioters who cut down and burned his hedges by night in 1542 had been set on by the mayor and burgesses.[53] In northern riots, gentlemen often played a significant role throughout the sixteenth century. In 1601 a band of 40–50 men and fifteen women, led by a local gentleman, burned 3,000 feet of quickset hedging on Selby Moor. Such an episode belonged, at least in part, to the world of gentry feuding.[54] The balance between local communities and improving landlords was also relatively even in the West Country struggles chronicled by Buchanan Sharp, despite the social inequality between the rival parties. When 3,000 rioters marching with drums and banners smashed enclosures in the Forest of Dean in April 1631, the occupants of the houses they fired must have seen the rioters, not the landowners, as the stronger party.[55]

Such episodes herald our fifth category, one rarely noticed by historians: the use or threat of arson by the strong against the weak. It should hardly surprise us. In time of war commanders frequently used arson as a weapon against military and civilian targets alike, with the 1640s no exception. Ordinary soldiers sometimes followed their lead. A soldier in the Bishops' Wars in 1639, piqued when a man he had plundered dared to complain, took revenge by firing his haystacks.[56] Soldiers might also be tempted to use such weapons in their private concerns. Shortly after Marston Moor, for example, a 'bloody-

---

[50] H. B. McCall (ed.), *Yorkshire Star Chamber Proceedings*, ii (Yorkshire Archaeological Society, 45; 1911), 50; cf. Hale, *Historia*, i. 135–6.

[51] R. B. Manning, *Hunters and Poachers* (Oxford, 1993), 139–40.

[52] II. iii. 24–5; cf. R. Cust, 'Honour and Politics in Early Stuart England. The Case of *Beaumont v. Hastings*', *P&P* 149 (1995), 75.

[53] Manning, *Village Revolts*, 43.

[54] C. M. Fraser (ed.), *Durham Quarter Sessions Rolls, 1471–1625* (Surtees Society, 199; 1991), 125–6; Manning, *Village Revolts*, 276–7.

[55] B. Sharp, *In Contempt of All Authority* (1980), 96.

[56] 'The Journal of John Aston, 1639', in J. C. Hodgson (ed.), *Six North Country Diaries* (Surtees Society, 118; 1910), 12–13.

looked' Scottish officer quartered in Yorkshire pressed marriage on the young Alice Wandesford, and finding himself rebuffed threatened that his country-men would return to burn down her mother's house and 'all she had'.[57] Arson by the powerful as a weapon of intimidation and retribution had a very long history, and lived on in popular memory.[58] Following the violent protests in Devon in 1549 over the new prayer book, the firing of two barns at Crediton and some threatening words by Walter Raleigh to an old woman at St Mary Clyst were sufficient to send rumours sweeping through the countryside that 'the gentlemen would burn them out of their houses and spoil them', while some of Monmouth's nervous supporters in Wiltshire in 1685 spread reports that the king's forces had burned the town of Frome.[59] At the other end of the country, the notorious Westmorland gang of robbers chronicled by Alan Macfarlane were able to frighten local inhabitants into silence by threatening to burn their houses.[60]

We can also find arson employed by the strong against the weak in far more mundane circumstances, in particular to drive away poor families thought likely to burden the parish poor rates. In 1602 a Worcestershire villager and his friends smashed timber and furniture that a poor man had assembled to build a cottage, warning 'that if ever the house be erected he will fire and burn the same'.[61] In 1625 Sir Charles Berkeley's tenants burned down a cottage he had erected for a poor family on the manorial waste, justifying their action by saying the family was lewd and, with small children, likely to burden the poor rates.[62] The following year we find the inhabitants of Knowle (Warwickshire) objecting when a man from nearby Balsall intruded his wife and four children into an empty cottage there and abandoned them; the villagers warned her to leave and threatened to burn down her house if she refused.[63] Gentlemen, too, occasionally resorted to similar tactics. At Stathern (Leicestershire) there was deep resentment in 1627 when Robert Rowse settled a number of poor tenants in his houses in Rotten Row: 'Thou dost bring them to the town to make beggars of them,' complained Anthony Greenwood, gentleman, 'but if thou wilt not take an order with them we will take an order with them and fire them down.'[64] Even more striking was the behaviour of the Presbyterian minister and lord of the manor of Cobham, John Platt, who sent fifty men to attack the Diggers' settlement in 1650, burning six cottages and furniture,

---

[57] *The Autobiography of Mrs Alice Thornton*, ed. C. Jackson (Surtees Society, 62; 1875), 44–6.
[58] Hale, *Historia*, i. 567.
[59] F. Rose-Troup, *The Western Rebellion of 1549* (1913), 144–6; B. H. Cunnington (ed.), *Records of the County of Wilts* (Devizes, 1932), 272.
[60] A. Macfarlane, *The Justice and the Mare's Ale* (Oxford, 1981), 80, 167.
[61] J. W. Willis Bund (ed.), *Worcestershire County Records: Calendar of the Quarter Sessions Papers, 1591–1643* (Worcester, 1900), 52.
[62] Manning, *Village Revolts*, 178.
[63] S. C. Ratcliff and H. C. Johnson (eds.), *Warwick County Records*, i (Warwick, 1935), 39–40, 44–5.
[64] LRO, Archdeaconry of Leicester instance cause papers, 1 D 41/4, Box 3/30.

clothing, and household goods. Platt succeeded in driving out a band he viewed as dangerous and persistent squatters, not idealistic visionaries.[65] Communities employed pressure and intimidation in a wide variety of forms to drive away unwanted newcomers, and probably turned to arson only when less draconian methods had failed, as at Stathern, Cobham, and probably Knowle. As a threat it was likely to prove highly effective, even if it might also attract the magistrate's attention, and it was sometimes used against other 'undesirables' too. In 1658 a Somerset woman called her neighbour Thomas Bartlett, cobbler, a witch, and allegedly threatened to burn his house and all his conjuring books. Burning a witch's thatch was widely regarded as a means to undo her *maleficium*, and, however implausible as counter-magic, must have been a highly effective form of intimidation.[66]

Our final category comprises arson employed against any person, group, or object seen as likely to divide or contaminate the community. Such contamination might be literal: the women who burned down the pesthouses of Salisbury (1627) and Colchester (1631) did so partly because they feared contagion.[67] More often the targets were religious. From the early days of the Reformation there were attacks on images and other 'popish' symbols, sometimes with official blessing, which reached a peak in the bonfires of altar rails in the early 1640s. In the Restoration period Nonconformists frequently faced threatening language and behaviour designed to intimidate or drive them away. A mob at Wincanton burned the Nonconformist minister in effigy, while a profane Suffolk man allegedly burned an old hog trough on a large bonfire, dubbing it 'the Phanaticks Pulpit'.[68] The preacher Oliver Heywood reported that a Yorkshire farmer, objecting to the local meeting house, had declared 'that if the house were his he would burn us out'; Heywood noted smugly that the farmer's own barn burned down soon afterwards.[69] Some Nonconformists faced more serious attacks. In 1677 Quakers in Plymouth, forced to worship in the street, were harassed by soldiers from the garrison throwing 'squibs of fire, and hot burning coals' on them from a window.[70] Attacks on meeting houses erected after the Toleration Act of 1689 culminated in a night of wild rioting in London in 1710 during the Sacheverell trial, when High Church mobs (including some 'gentlemen mobsters') sacked meeting houses and made bonfires in the street of their furniture and fittings. One

[65] G. H. Sabine (ed.), *The Works of Gerrard Winstanley* (New York, 1965), 433–5.

[66] E. H. Bates Harbin (ed.), *Quarter Sessions Records for the County of Somerset*, iii. *Commonwealth 1646–1660* (Somerset Record Society, 28; 1912), 362; Thomas, *Religion*, 544.

[67] P. Slack, *The Impact of Plague in Tudor and Stuart England* (Oxford, 1990), 299.

[68] M. Aston, *Faith and Fire* (1993), 231–313; *Mirabilis Annus. Or the Year of Prodigies and Wonders* (1661), 54–6, 73–6 (*recte* 77–8).

[69] *The Rev. Oliver Heywood, BA, 1630–1702: His Autobiography, Diaries, Anecdote and Event Books*, ed. J. H. Turner (Brighouse and Bingley, 1882–5), iii. 186.

[70] *A Brief Account of some of the late and present sufferings of the . . . Quakers* (1680), 24.

group of rioters even marched to sack and burn the Bank of England, which they identified with hated Whigs and Dissenters.[71]

III

The acts and threats of arson discussed above were mirrored by popular fears and suspicions, and it is to these that we now turn. In the event of a fire, when was arson suspected, and why? Who was likely to fall under suspicion? How close are the parallels with witchcraft, another 'invisible' crime of the malevolent?

Most fires were regarded as accidental, just as most deaths were assumed to be natural. Rumours and suspicions of arson flourished most in periods of national tension, as we might expect. The 'Annals of Coventry' record in 1553 that, when the stunning news arrived of Lady Jane Grey's proclamation as queen, a cry went up that the town had been fired in four places, and the walls were manned in case of attack.[72] Similarly, tension in London over Strafford's fate and the revelation of the 'Army Plot' in May 1641 triggered a panic that papists had set the House of Commons on fire, while news of the Irish rebellion in November sparked further alarms.[73] In more normal periods, victims of fire might suspect arson where there were unusual circumstances, such as a blaze starting in the middle of the night or in a room with no hearth or other obvious source. As with witchcraft, a victim suspecting arson nearly always had a likely culprit in mind, someone he already distrusted or believed held a grudge. When Henry Stempe of Upper Beeding (Sussex) lost 13d. in August 1614, and a sheet in October, he suspected Margaret Botting, spinster, possibly his servant, on both occasions, and when his house burned down in December he had no doubt that Margaret was again to blame. An Assize jury disagreed.[74] In some cases marginal and unpopular people might find themselves suspected of both witchcraft and arson. In 1572 Cecily Silles, a labourer's wife from Clacton (Essex), was accused of bewitching a child and firing a barn; her husband was also charged with arson, and later accused of firing it again.[75] Suspicions of witchcraft sometimes festered for years before resulting in a formal accusation, and again (if much less often) the same applies to arson. Such cases

[71] G. Holmes, *The Trial of Doctor Sacheverell* (1973), 156–76; G. Holmes, 'The Sacheverell Riots', *P&P* 72 (1976), 64–7, 75–81.

[72] F. Burbidge, *Old Coventry and Lady Godiva* (Birmingham [1952]), 229.

[73] R. Clifton, 'The Popular Fear of Catholics during the English Revolution', *P&P* 52 (1971), 25–6, 29; B. Manning, *The English People and the English Revolution* (1978), 27; *Bloody Newes from Norwich* (1641), sig. A2ᵛ.

[74] Cockburn (ed.), *Calendar: Sussex, James I*, 63; cf. Thomas, *Religion*, 546–60.

[75] Cockburn (ed.), *Calendar: Essex, Elizabeth*, 224, 231; Thomas, *Religion*, 533–4, 559–60; C. L. Ewen, *Witchcraft and Demonianism* (1933), 159–60, 302, 362–3, 403.

might even be connected. When Judith Sawkyns of Aylesford (Kent), a widow described revealingly as a 'common witch', was indicted at Maidstone Assizes in 1657 for bewitching a child to death, fifteen women and three men were ready to testify against her. But the jury threw out a further charge of firing a barn a year earlier, which was supported by only three witnesses, and it would probably never have reached the courts but for the passions roused by the witchcraft allegations.[76]

Allegations were generally made against individuals viewed as suspicious on account of their uncivil language and behaviour, or marginal status, such as servants, foreigners, and vagrants. The examinations of Margaret Byx and her friends, executed in 1615 for burning down Wymondham (Norfolk), exposed a range of contemporary assumptions, associating the accused with witchcraft, gypsies, vagrants, Scots, and popery.[77] Religious minorities were potentially the most threatening of all marginal groups, for they possessed organization and structure, and could be seen as driven by a sinister ideology. From the late Elizabethan period Catholics, increasingly identified with England's foreign enemies, became extremely vulnerable in periods of political tension, such as 1640–2. The deluded French Catholic executed after confessing to the Great Fire in 1666, Robert Hubert, fitted the popular stereotype admirably. In the weeks following the Fire, a wave of panics spread across the country, many of them involving alleged papist designs.[78] Similar panics occurred later in the reign, as fears mounted over a Catholic Succession. Titus Oates 'revealed' that a serious fire in Southwark in 1676 was the work of a Jesuit agent and three Irishmen, adding that Jesuits were planning to plunder and fire all the major English urban centres.[79] In 1679 Elizabeth Oxley confessed to firing her employer's house in Fetter Lane, blaming a man who had converted her to Rome and promised £5.[80] Margaret Clark, hanged a few months later for burning her master's house in Southwark, said she had been offered the huge sum of £2,000 by three unknown gentlemen, quickly suspected to be 'agents of the Popish Firing Plot'.[81] It remains unclear how far such 'confessions' were extracted by interrogators determined to expose a conspiracy, or reflect a pathetic bid for notoriety; in many cases, perhaps, both.[82] Wild rumours circulated. At Royston (Hertfordshire), a labourer's wife reported that a serious fire in Southwark had been started by servants of the

---

[76] J. C. Cockburn (ed.), *Calendar of Assize Records: Kent Indictments, 1649–1659* (1989), 271.

[77] H. W. Saunders (ed.), *The Official Papers of Sir Nathaniel Bacon of Stiffkey* (Camden Society, 3rd ser., 26; 1915), 31–3.

[78] W. G. Bell, *The Great Fire* (1923), 32–3, 191–209; J. P. Kenyon, *The Popish Plot* (1974), 11–14; *CSPD 1666–7*, 103, 110, 116, 127, 148, 168.

[79] T. Oates, *A True Narrative of the Horrid Plot* (Dublin, 1679), 23, 40.

[80] *Londons Flames* (1679), 15–17.

[81] *The True Narrative of the Proceedings at the Assizes . . . of Surrey*, 12–17 Mar. 1680 [1680], 2; *Warning for Servants* (1680), *passim*.

[82] *The True Narrative of the Proceedings at the Sessions for London and Middlesex*, 5 June 1679 (1679), 4–5.

duke of York.[83] Bizarre stories surfaced of sheep found with their bellies ripped open to remove the fat for incendiary devices. One such report at Bristol was investigated by the mayor and aldermen, and a printed account urged readers to take due warning and elect MPs vigilant in resisting the popish menace.[84] Even fires that had clearly originated in household tensions were now interpreted as popish conspiracy. The wretched story of Elizabeth Owen, a maidservant of 'sullen, dogged temper' who fired her employers' house in Fleet Street in 1680 after a 'falling-out, over the dressing of the dinner', was published under the title, *The Jesuites Firing-Plot Revived: or, a Warning to House-Keepers in the many Firing Plots the cunning Jesuites have of late Contrived; in which for the most part they Employ Silly Servant-Maides*. Contemporary prejudices were equally obvious in the case of another London servant, charged with setting fire to her employers' house in 1679 but acquitted after the court heard she was 'well educated in the Protestant religion, so far from a papist, that she had been that day with her master and mistress at church'.[85] A reporter describing a huge fire at Wapping in 1682, which destroyed almost 700 houses, thought it necessary to remind readers that fires could sometimes be caused by negligence rather than popish malice.[86] Alarms of popish arson predictably resurfaced in the tense weeks at the close of 1688.

Though Catholics were the most feared, other religious minorities also fell under suspicion. A libel thrown one night into the mayor of Canterbury's house in 1643 accused the militant Puritan minister Richard Culmer of planning to round up local royalists, lock them in a house, and burn it.[87] In June 1659 an anonymous leaflet scattered in the streets of London warned that the Fifth Monarchists were poised to burn the city and massacre its inhabitants. 'Beware Tuesday next', it urged.[88] Roger L'Estrange claimed in December 1659 that the army itself, despairing of the Good Old Cause, was planning to fire the city and had laid in stocks of fireballs at St Paul's and Gresham College.[89] Such fears survived the king's return, with Major White allegedly vowing in December 1660 to fire the city and pull the king from his throne.[90] Some contemporaries blamed the Great Fire on Nonconformists as well as, or instead of, Catholics.[91] A generation later Titus Oates linked Fifth Monarchists with Jesuits in his revelations, while a Rye House plotter was accused of planning to fire London and blame it on papists.[92]

[83] W. Le Hardy (ed.), *Hertfordshire County Records*, vi (Hertford, 1930), 342.

[84] *Strange and Wonderful News from Bristol* [1679], 2–4; cf. *CSPD 1666–7*, 105, 110, 116, 127.

[85] *The True Narrative of the Proceedings at the Sessions for London and Middlesex*, 30 Apr. 1679 (1679), 5.

[86] *A Modest Account of that most dreadful Fire, which happened at Wapping* (1682), 2.

[87] R. Culmer, *A Parish Looking-Glasse* (1657), 10.

[88] *An Alarum to the City and Souldiery* (1659), broadside.

[89] R. L'Estrange, *A Short View of some remarkable transactions* (1660), 41.

[90] *CSPD 1660–1*, 413.   [91] Bell, *Great Fire*, 190; *CSPD 1666–7*, 116.

[92] T. Oates, *Oates's Manifesto* (1683), 10; Harris, *London Crowds*, 149.

In our own century we are familiar with society's tendency to project its worst nightmares onto minorities of whatever kind, and we rightly see Catholics, Nonconformists, and other persecuted groups as the victims of such a process. But we should also bear in mind that contemporary discourse could make minority groups the agents, in part, of their own misfortunes. Many early Quakers were fond of inflammatory language, predicting with relish how divine wrath in the shape of burning towns and cities would consume their enemies. In 1650 the Ranter Abiezer Coppe depicted God himself as an arsonist. His aptly titled *A Fiery Flying Rolle* predicted terrible fires, and detected God's hand in a number of recent conflagrations. 'I the Lord fired the barning and ricks of a miser in Worcestershire this year,' he noted complacently, 'the very same day that he brought in his own, as he accounted it.'[93] Coppe's practice of speaking with God's voice must have aroused suspicions that he was the instrument as well as eyewitness of this event. At the other end of the religious spectrum, some Catholics allegedly pronounced the Great Fire of 1666 to be God's punishment for heretics.[94] Such rash language reflects the uncivil discourse also evident in the neighbourhood quarrels surveyed earlier. It did not take an overt threat to arouse suspicions of arson (or witchcraft). Malevolent wishes, wild predictions, and rash outbursts, all familiar features of alehouse and street conversation, could easily be misinterpreted as declarations of intent. In 1561 a Frenchman was whipped 'for talking foolish words of the burning of Paul's church', while Somerset villagers became understandably nervous in 1656 when a troublesome neighbour wished the squire's house was on fire, with the squire inside.[95] Loose talk was even more likely to provoke alarm when it touched on contemporary politics in a period of tension. When a man grumbled at the dinner table of a Laudian minister in 1641 that he would like to see several MPs hanged and the City of London burned down, his words were quickly in print and heightened the prevailing mood of crisis.[96] Similarly, a Middlesex woman was prosecuted in 1657 for saying she would like to see Whitehall on fire around the Lord Protector's ears.[97] A contemporary discourse in which curses, malevolent wishes, threats, and predictions were freely bandied about in public was a fertile breeding ground for fears, suspicions, and repression.

IV

This essay has argued that fears, threats, and acts of arson played a significantly larger role than historians of crime have traditionally allotted them. It remains

---

[93] N. Smith (ed.), *A Collection of Ranter Writings* (1983), 110–11.
[94] Bell, *Great Fire*, 198, 325–6; Kenyon, *Popish Plot*, 13.
[95] BCB 1, fo. 137ᵛ; Bates Harbin, *Quarter Sessions Records for Somerset*, iii. 305.
[96] *Englands Ioyalty* (1641), 2–3.
[97] Jeaffreson (ed.), *Middlesex County Records*, iii. 271; cf. 260.

the case that prosecutions remained few, and that courts appear to have been reluctant to convict when there was any element of doubt. Despite temporary panics, notably in 1666, there was no resulting wave of indictments, convictions, and executions. The contrasts between arson and witchcraft are as intriguing as the parallels. Both involved hidden malice and threatened life, with arson arguably the greater threat, for few suspected witches of aspiring to destroy whole cities. Given the terrible losses occasioned by fire in early modern England, the refusal of magistrates or juries to give way to panics is striking. People who threatened arson were generally bound over, and if necessary detained until they could produce satisfactory sureties; some were subsequently fined, and vagrants were likely to be whipped.[98] Offenders judged to be insane escaped punishment, though they might be detained in a House of Correction if they appeared to pose an immediate threat. In 1659 the London Bridewell court ordered one man to be released as soon as the churchwardens of his parish could produce a medical certificate attesting his lunacy.[99] The courts occasionally allowed convicted arsonists to escape the gallows by claiming benefit of clergy, against the statute, where there were extenuating circumstances.[100] They also exercised discretion within the law by imposing non-capital sentences when a fire had been quenched before doing serious damage. An apprentice who tried to burn his master's house in 1689 was transported, not hanged, while a woman convicted of firing a house in Edmonton in 1700 was sentenced to be whipped through the streets.[101] Juries exercised both caution and independence in weighing evidence, and they were sometimes even prepared to acquit servants charged by their employers.[102] An Old Bailey jury that cleared an alleged arsonist in December 1689 was scolded by the Recorder, who railed that 'they did not act like true English-men' in freeing 'such pernicious and base fellows, as would burn them all in their beds'.[103]

The apparently judicious conduct of arson trials remains puzzling. Though witchcraft cases also had a relatively high acquittal rate, several hundred 'witches' were sent to the gallows on the strength of extremely circumstantial evidence.[104] Why did the fears and suspicions surrounding arson not lead to

---

[98] BCB 8, fo. 13; S. A. Peyton (ed.), *Minutes of Proceedings in Quarter Sessions . . . in the county of Lincoln, 1674–1695* (Lincoln Record Society, 25–6; 1931), ii. 363; Le Hardy, *Hertfordshire County Records*, vi. 391; Atkinson, *Quarter Sessions Records*, vi. 274.

[99] BCB 8, fo. 105ᵛ; 10, fo. 128ᵛ; Cockburn (ed.), *Calendar: Essex, James I*, 96; Cockburn (ed.), *Calendar: Sussex, Elizabeth*, 314; Atkinson, *Quarter Sessions Records*, vii. 194; Jeaffreson (ed.), *Middlesex County Records*, iii. 291.

[100] Cockburn (ed.), *Calendar: Sussex, Elizabeth*, 226; Cockburn (ed.), *Calendar: Kent, Elizabeth*, 184.

[101] *Proceedings in the Old Bailey*, 11–14 Dec. 1689 (1689), 4; W. J. Hardy (ed.), *Middlesex County Records: Calendar of the Sessions Books, 1689 to 1709* (1905), 222.

[102] *Proceedings in the Old Bailey*, 12–13 Oct. 1687 (1687), 2.

[103] Ibid. 11–14 Dec. 1689 (1689), 1–2.

[104] J. Sharpe (*Instruments of Darkness* (1996), 113) notes that only 32% of those accused of witchcraft on the Home Circuit suffered any punishment.

many more indictments and executions, especially as suspected arsonists, like witches, were often poor and marginal? One obvious and perhaps key difference was the absence of any satanic element in most cases of arson. A man who threatened to burn his neighbour's house was still perceived as a rational agent, however malevolent; a recognisance provided a 'cooling-off' period and a satisfactory deterrent. The witch, by contrast, was not viewed as rational. Her malevolence, inflamed by Satan and executed through his 'familiars', was of a different order. No one believed that binding over a suspected witch could provide satisfactory protection. In the aftermath of a fire, the victim might suspect malice, but neighbours knew how easily accidents could occur, and there was unlikely to be any conclusive evidence among the smouldering remains. They were also aware that the *victim* of fire might be the malicious party, using an accident to bring a false charge of arson against an enemy, a device that might result in the execution of an innocent person for a non-existent crime.[105] By contrast, witchcraft was usually suspected when neighbours and even medical practitioners had proved unable to explain the symptoms afflicting the victim by any other means.

Early modern arson has a history as well as typology, with changes as well as continuities in both targets and perpetrators. The Henrician felony was closely tied to behaviour that threatened life, and excluded most fires that damaged property alone. Legislation in the late seventeenth and early eighteenth centuries witnessed a significant and familiar shift towards the greater protection of property, and there is some evidence for an increase in the number of prosecutions for malicious damage. In 1671 the felony was redefined to include firing stacks of hay or corn at night.[106] A bill introduced in 1698 would have made parishes liable for the damage incurred by an arson attack if the offenders were not discovered. Its originator, one Reading of Epworth (Lincolnshire), was engaged in a bitter local dispute over common rights; his opponents, who were eventually able to block the bill, accused him of using an accidental fire at his own house to smear them as arsonists.[107] Other bills succeeded. In 1702 it became a felony to burn or destroy a ship to defraud the owners or insurers, reflecting the arrival of the modern crime of insurance fraud, while in 1723 the notorious Waltham Black Act extended the law to protect game in the wake of arson attacks by poaching gangs.[108]

The evolution of the law reflected broader social and cultural shifts. Arson seems to have been an acceptable weapon for feuding members of the landed classes in the sixteenth century, especially in the north. It was no longer accept-

[105] For a Warwickshire man in 1687 suborning a labourer to perjure himself against his employer after a haystack fire, see WRO CR103, Bromley's Notebook, 8–9.

[106] Thomas, *Religion*, 533; 22 & 23 Charles II, c. 7.

[107] *Commons Journals*, xii (1803), 38, 47, 96; *A True Account how Mr Reading's House at Santoft happened to be Burnt* (?1700).

[108] 1 Anne, c. 9; N.B., *Compleat Collection*, ii. 8–11; 9 Geo. I, c. 22; E. P. Thompson, *Whigs and Hunters* (1977), 42–3, 147, 166; cf. 225–6.

able by the later seventeenth century, as newer codes of civility persuaded the élite to curb their traditional violence or channel it into more structured forms, notably the duel. The newly respectable 'middling sorts' adopted a similarly hostile view. Arson had become, for the most part, a crime of the uncivil poor, in quarrels among themselves or as a weapon against their superiors. Arsonists were now likely to be poor, alienated, and marginal, which remains largely the pattern today. But modern insurance fraud, and ideologically motivated attacks on ethnic minorities, furriers, and similar targets, remind us that arson is still a hydra-headed and vigorous beast.[109]

[109] A Home Office report notes that an average of 3,500 fires are started deliberately each week in the UK: *The Times*, 24 May 1999, 16.

12

Civility, Civilizing Processes, and the End of Public Punishment in England

J. A. SHARPE

Amidst all the present-day concern about crime, nobody in a position of any influence in either western Europe or North America has so far called for the reintroduction of that best known of historical penal sanctions, the public execution: even the most retributionist of politicians would baulk at that. Changed attitudes to public execution are commonly held to mark off the barbaric, inhumane, and uncivilized past from our more civilized, sensitized, and refined present. The history of punishment is usually portrayed as a simple record of progress away from the horrors of Newgate, the pillory, the convict ship, and above all the public execution. This widely diffused popular model of penal history provides hardliners and liberals alike with a mythologized past upon which to draw.

Until recently, historians endorsed such an outlook. For J. H. Plumb, in the eighteenth century 'violence, crime, cruelty, dirt, disease . . . were accepted by the majority of mankind as a part of the nature of life, like the weather or the seasons'. It was, therefore, unsurprising that the English should be a 'callous people', or that 'the popular sights of London were the lunatics at Bedlam, the whipping of half-naked women at the Bridewell, the stoning to death of pilloried men and women, or the hangings at Tyburn where a girl and a boy might be seen dangling between a highwayman and a murderer'.[1] Likewise Dorothy Marshall, evoking the dreadfulness of the period, pointed out that 'men were hanged for food rioting: children were hanged for petty thefts. The old proverb that one might as well be hanged for a sheep as a lamb was bitterly true'.[2] For V. H. H. Green, it was 'against this background of strong drink and violence, odorous sanitation, poor health and even more unpleasing vices, that crime and poverty established themselves', and with W. E. H. Lecky he saw the penal code of the period as 'a mere sanguinary chaos'.[3] The consensus about the eighteenth-century public execution that

---

[1] J. H. Plumb, *The First Four Georges* (1956), 20, 16.
[2] D. Marshall, *Eighteenth-Century England* (1962), 243.
[3] V. H. H. Green, *The Hanoverians 1714–1815* (1948), 254.

these quotations illustrate helps explain the potency and pervasiveness of such descriptions of Tyburn hangings as that offered by Bernard de Mandeville,[4] or such visual images as the famous print by Hogarth showing Tom Idle's execution there.[5]

The pervasiveness of these images of *ancien régime* punishment should not obscure the existence of a number of academic studies devoted to the subject.[6] Michel Foucault's work on punishment,[7] despite some trumpeting by his acolytes, has not had much impact upon students of the history of punishment in England,[8] but was valuable at least in questioning the existing Whiggish interpretation of penal history. As is perhaps not so widely realized, Foucault's analysis of these changes constitutes only one of a number of rival interpretations. And Foucault was not the first in the field: perhaps the earliest were Georg Rusche and Otto Kirchheimer, who, despite their crudely Marxist approach, did try to link changing penal methods and broader socio-economic change.[9] This framework was taken further by a number of later, subtler, writers, among then Michael Ignatieff, whose study of the origins of the penitentiary prison in England appeared in 1978.[10] More recently Vic Gatrell, in a massively documented book, has analysed the significance of a key incident in English penal history, the abolition of public executions in 1868.[11] The historians of public execution in the Netherlands[12] and Germany[13] have also avoided a Whiggish approach.

[4] Bernard de Mandeville, *An Enquiry into the Causes of the Frequent Executions at Tyburn: and a Proposal for some Regulations concerning Felons in Prison, and the good Effects to be Expected from them* (1725), 18–37.

[5] For a commentary on this print, see R. Paulson, *Hogarth's Graphic Works* (2 vols.; New Haven, 1965), i. 200–1.

[6] D. Garland, *Punishment and Modern Society: A Study in Social Theory* (Oxford, 1990), is a very effective overview. J. A. Sharpe (*Judicial Punishment in England* (1990)) provides a brief introduction to developments from *c*.1500 onwards.

[7] M. Foucault, *Discipline and Punish: The Birth of the Prison* (1977).

[8] Thus L. Radzinowicz and R. Hood (*The Emergence of Penal Policy in Victorian and Edwardian England* (1986)) feel it necessary to make only two passing references to Foucault in their 778 pages of text.

[9] G. Rusche and O. Kirchheimer, *Punishment and Social Structure* (New York, 1939; rev. edn., 1968). This work is contextualized by the 'Introduction' to its French edition, *Peine et structure sociale*, ed. R. Lévy and H. Zander (Paris, 1994). For a more recent statement of the broadly Marxist position on the history of punishment, see D. Melossi and M. Pavarini, *The Prison and the Factory: The Origins of the Penitentiary System* (1981).

[10] M. Ignatieff, *A Just Measure of Pain: The Penitentiary and the Industrial Revolution* (1978). For a broader statement of Ignatieff's views, which includes an autocritique of his book, see M. Ignatieff, 'State, Civil Society and Total Institutions: A Critique of Recent Histories of Punishment', in S. Cohen and A. Scull (eds.), *Social Control and the State* (Oxford, 1983).

[11] V. A. C. Gatrell, *The Hanging Tree: Execution and the English People 1770–1868* (Oxford, 1994).

[12] P. Spierenburg, *The Spectacle of Suffering: Executions and the Evolution of Repression: From a Preindustrial Metropolis to the European Experience* (Cambridge, 1984).

[13] R. J. Evans, *Rituals of Retribution: Capital Punishment in Germany, 1600–1987* (Oxford, 1996). This should be read in conjunction with R. van Dulmen, *Theatre of Horror: Crime and Punishment in Early Modern Germany* (Oxford, 1990).

Yet even these historians share something of the earlier outlook: 'our subject-matter', writes Gatrell, 'can hardly be dissociated from the processes through which a brand of civility has been fragilely attained in the West', and he goes on to say of the year in which public execution was discontinued in England that 'we cannot deny that 1868 was a civilizing moment in British history'.[14] A more direct connection between changing attitudes to public punishment and the spread of civility has been postulated by the Dutch historian Pieter Spierenburg, whose study of scaffold punishments in early modern Amsterdam was heavily influenced by Norbert Elias's concept of a civilizing process. Spierenburg claims that by the middle of the eighteenth century new thresholds had been reached in the amount of mutual identification that human beings were capable of, so that by about 1800 members of the crowd at public executions 'could feel the pain of the delinquents on the scaffold'.[15]

The abandonment of public execution was undoubtedly a shift of major importance: but there is a danger that focusing upon it may 'flatten' the early modern period into a vast, featureless, unchanging plateau of public execution whereby the various reforms of the late eighteenth and early nineteenth centuries are preceded by an unvarying resort to what now seems a barbarous practice. Yet, for England at least, things are more complicated.

I

The image of the eighteenth-century Tyburn public execution is a potent one, reinforced as it is by the widespread knowledge that parliamentary legislation in the century after 1688 created a 'Bloody Code', which meant that by about 1800 over 200 capital offences, most of them crimes against property, existed on the English statute book.[16] What is less familiar, and rather surprising, is that actual levels of execution over the eighteenth century were far lower than they had been in the later Tudor and early Stuart periods. Gaps in the appropriate court archives preclude the drawing-up of national statistics, but such records as do survive are unequivocal. The issue is well illustrated by the archives of the Court of Great Sessions of the Palatinate of Chester, which form the most continuous run of indictments for felony surviving for early modern England. Before that court, capital sentences were being awarded at an average rate of about eight a year in the 1580s, slightly higher in the difficult 1590s, and then, after a fall over the first twenty years of the seventeenth century, at an average rate of about sixteen a year in that other difficult decade, the 1620s. This level of executions was halved in the 1630s, and

[14] Gatrell, *Hanging Tree*, pp. ix, 590.   [15] Spierenburg, *Spectacle of Suffering*, 184.
[16] For the classic account of the operation of the criminal law in the period of the Bloody Code, see L. Radzinowicz, *The Movement for Reform 1750–1833* (1948).

then the cessation of meetings of the Court of Great Sessions over much
of the 1640s, when Cheshire was immersed in the Civil Wars, produced a
yet lower level. But the return of stability in the 1650s, and of the Stuart regime
in the 1660s, did not re-establish the levels of execution existing in, say,
the 1630s. They remained low: the 166 capital sentences handed out by the
court in the 1620s contrast with the ten awarded in the first decade of the
eighteenth century. And, lest this pattern should be written off as a regional
aberration, it should be noted that something very like it occurred on the
Home Circuit of the assizes (comprehending Essex, Hertfordshire, Kent,
Surrey, and Sussex), and, admittedly on the strength of rather more frag-
mentary evidence, the south-western county of Devon. Thus it would seem
that levels of execution were much lower in the late seventeenth and early
eighteenth centuries than in the decades around 1600, while the proportion
of those accused of felony who were executed also fell markedly. In the 1590s
a person accused of felony before the Court of Great Sessions at Chester or
before the Home Circuit assizes stood a one in four of five chance of being
executed: by the early eighteenth century, the chance had dropped to about
one in ten.[17]

These figures demonstrate that the mid-seventeenth century experienced
one of the most remarkable shifts in the punishment of criminals in English
history, away from a penal regime that experienced very high levels of capital
punishment to one that, while accepting the use of hanging as the standard
penal option, employed it with much less frequency. The reasons for this
development are very difficult to discern: unlike the years following 1750, the
seventeenth century apparently experienced infuriatingly little debate about
crime and punishment, and our explanations must for the present remain
conjectural. Perhaps the surest, if least easily demonstrable, line of argument
would be to see this transition as a symptom of a more general shift: that
demographic growth, which had been one of the basic facts of English social
life for a century before the 1630s, slackened after that decade. There was thus
less pressure at the base of society, so that, for example, the run of bad harvests in the 1690s did not produce the social crisis that a run of bad harvests
had precipitated in the 1590s. And, on at least an initial reading of comments
from well-placed observers, there was less tension at the top of society in the
years around 1700 than there had been a century earlier.[18] But other factors
may have been at work. The 1640s and 1650s experienced a desire for legal
reform that included disquiet about the use of the death penalty for property
offences. This was an important aspect of Leveller critiques of the legal system,
expressed perhaps most forcefully in the writings of Samuel Chidley.[19] But

[17] For a fuller discussion of these issues, see J. A. Sharpe, *Crime in Early Modern England
1550–1750* (1984), 63–6, and Sharpe, *Judicial Punishment in England*, 28–36.

[18] This theme is developed in J. A. Sharpe, *Early Modern England: A Social History 1550–1760*
(2nd edn., 1997), 355–7.

[19] D. Veall, *The Popular Movement for Law Reform 1640–1660* (Oxford, 1970), remains the standard introduction to the subject.

there may have been a more general sense of the need to curb the severity of the law in this matter: even Oliver Cromwell, in his speech at the opening of Parliament on 17 September 1656, advised Parliament that there were 'abominable laws that will be in your power to alter', adding that the 'ill framing' of the laws made it possible 'to hang a man for sixpence, threepence, I know not what'.[20] Concern over the high incidence of capital punishment may be an issue where the reforming programmes of the Interregnum coincided with the wider culture of the political nation.

Whatever its cause, analysis of the relevant court archives makes the mid-seventeenth-century drop in levels of execution incontrovertible. What is much harder to demonstrate is another important shift over the mid-sixteenth century. It is difficult to discover much about changes in the punishment of criminals in that most uncharted of historical frontier zones that lies between the late medieval and the early modern periods. There appears to have been even less by way of social debate than there was in the mid-seventeenth century, good secondary works are few, and the relevant archival base is much weaker than for the later period. But it seems that the fifteenth century witnessed relatively low levels of capital punishment,[21] while the scaffold ceremonies that were to be such a feature of Stuart and Hanoverian public execution were as yet very undeveloped. The increased levels of execution were essentially the product of the Tudor Age, perhaps not unconnected with that creation of a 'Tudor Bloody Code' that commenced in the second half of the reign of Henry VIII.[22] The concept of the 'Tudor Revolution in Government' is not one that enjoys much currency among historians at present, but there was certainly a tightening of government over the second third of the sixteenth century, a tightening that had an as yet under-researched impact on law enforcement. As we have hinted, few documentary sources exist upon which relevant research might be based, but one such is constituted by the archives of the assizes in the Palatinate of Lancaster. A preliminary survey of the records of this court in the 1530s and 1540s suggests that levels of execution, although still fairly low in absolute terms, rose appreciably in the 1540s. Evidence for a 'Tudor Revolution in Government' may have been available dangling from the end of ropes in at least one northern county.[23]

But reassembling the statistics of execution can only be part of the story. We are concerned not only with the totals of capital punishment, but also with the fact that this penalty was inflicted in public. An attempt to assess how

[20] *The Writings and Speeches of Oliver Cromwell*, ed. W. C. Abbott (4 vols.; Cambridge, Mass., 1937–47), iv. 274.
[21] See e.g. the remarks on the low levels of capital punishment made by E. Powell, *Kingship, Law and Society: Criminal Justice in the Reign of Henry V* (Oxford, 1989), 82.
[22] For a discussion of the relevant legislation, see Sharpe, *Judicial Punishment in England*, 27–8.
[23] This conclusion is based on a preliminary survey of the Palatinate of Lancaster Clerk of the Crown Assize Rolls (PL 25), and Indictments (PL 26). Documents consulted are: PRO PL 25/5–7; 25/11; 25/14; 25/22–4; 26/14/1; 26/296/3–4.

such executions relate to a history of civility must, therefore, take into account the reactions of the crowds attending these spectacles of suffering. Historical myth would have such crowds demonstrating attitudes and reactions appropriate to the callous, brutalized, and gin-sodden denizens of a less civilized age. Contemporary accounts, however, suggest that this was not always the case. Consider, for example, the Yorkshire Nonconformist Ralph Thoresby, then aged 24, describing the execution near Leeds of a man named Holroyd in 1682. Holroyd had murdered three people, among them his mother, and a crowd of 'many thousand spectators' had gathered. These were, however, 'alas! frustrated exceedingly in their expectations'. Holroyd, so Thoresby recorded, died

> In the most resolute manner that ever eye beheld, wishing (upon the top of the ladder) he might never come where God had anything to do if he was guilty, and so threw himself off in an anger as it were, without any recommendation of himself to God that any could observe, which struck tears into my eyes, and terror into my heart for his poor soul, earnestly imploring, while I saw any signs of life, that God would give him repentance for his crying sins, and be better to him than his desires.

Thoresby was one of the godly, and his reaction was undoubtedly especially appropriate to a member of that group. But this account of a provincial public execution raises some important questions. Thoresby himself was not brutalized or callous, but clearly read the theatre of punishment in religious terms. His wording suggests that this was a general reaction: it was not just he, but the thousands of other spectators who were 'frustrated exceedingly in their expectations': and those expectations were that the convicted murderer would behave penitently on the scaffold, and leave them with an edifying speech rather than with a resolute renunciation of the Almighty.[24] Those attending this execution were evidently not the desensitized and gin-sodden mob of historical myth, but rather adherents to the ideal of a Christian Commonwealth.

This conclusion receives considerable reinforcement from most descriptions of the execution of felons, and especially murderers, in the seventeenth century. There are, of course, problems of interpretation here: we are being presented with at best a sample of those executed, while the heavily formulaic descriptions of how these criminals behaved on the scaffold induces some suspicions. The pamphlet accounts of 'last dying speeches' are indeed very stereotyped, and obviously in some measure represent an idealized version of how officialdom wanted people to interpret the public execution. Yet corroborative evidence helps support the overwhelming impression that these men and women undergoing execution were expected to spend their last few moments reinforcing the moral universe that the spectators at the

---

[24] *Diary of Ralph Thoresby, F.R.S.*, ed. Joseph Hunter (2 vols.; 1830), i. 131.

execution described by Ralph Thoresby clearly inhabited.[25] The object, as a pamphlet of 1609 put it, was that, for felons on the scaffold, if 'the course of their lives had not taught them to live well: yet the care of their soules remembered them to dye well'.[26] As I have argued elsewhere, the origins of all this appear to have resided in that great Tudor innovation, the show trial and public execution for treason.[27] The ceremonies and conventions adopted for dealing with the upper-class traitor gradually became adapted to the punishments inflicted on the lowly felon. As the seventeenth century progressed, the rituals surrounding the executions of felons became more ornate and, in particular, the speeches made by the condemned on the gallows assumed a central importance. Those speeches became very conventional, with the sufferers telling the audience how their sad fate had its origins in youthful sinfulness, which, unchecked, led the offender into an ever-escalating series of misdeeds that ended with the crime for which the death penalty had been awarded. The condemned usually ended their speech by accepting their fate, stressing the importance of obedience to the laws of the monarch and of God, and advising their listeners to take heed of the end they had come to. Those awaiting execution were frequently worked upon by clergy, who, indeed, became only marginally less important participants than the condemned man or woman in the theatre of execution: even the eminent William Perkins involved himself in talking convicted felons through their last moments.[28] Contemporary thinking on death, of course, emphasized the desirability of making a 'good end', and thus with these scaffold ceremonies the history of punishment converges with the wider cultural history of death. But it becomes evident that, here as elsewhere, the history of 'civility' in England needs to address the fact that Christianity was a vital factor for many of that society's inhabitants.

The far richer and more varied evidence available for the eighteenth century suggests that crowd reactions were becoming less stereotyped, or that possibly, as we have hinted, the evidence made available to us from the seventeenth century presents a more restricted picture. Research on the Tyburn crowd, for

[25] These are discussed in J. A. Sharpe, 'Last Dying Speeches: Religion, Ideology and Public Execution in Seventeenth-Century England', *P&P* 107 (1985), 144–67. For different interpretations of public executions in this period, see T. W. Laqueur, 'Crowds, Carnival and the State in English Executions, 1604–1868', in A. L. Beier, D. Cannadine, and J. M. Rosenheim (eds.), *The First Modern Society: Essays in English History in Honour of Lawrence Stone* (Cambridge, 1989); and P. Lake and M. Questier, 'Agency, Appropriation and Rhetoric under the Gallows: Puritans, Romanists and the State in Early Modern England', *P&P* 153 (1996), 64–107.

[26] *The Araignement and Burning of Margaret Ferne-seede, for the Murther of her late Husband Anthony Ferne-seede, found deade in Peckham Field neere Lambeth, having once before attempted to poyson him with Broth, being executed in S. Georges-Field the last of Februarie 1608* (1609), sig. B2.

[27] Sharpe, 'Last Dying Speeches'. The early stages of this process are sketched in L. B. Smith, 'English Treason Trials and Confessions in the Sixteenth Century', *Journal of the History of Ideas*, 15 (1954), 471–98.

[28] I. Breward (ed.), *William Perkins* (Abingdon, 1969), 17–18.

example, demonstrates that this was a much more heterogeneous entity than might have been imagined, and one capable of a spectrum of responses to the spectacle it witnessed.[29] Thus we find execution crowds cheering the high-wayman who died game, booing the heinous murderer to his or her grave, or weeping with the offender who died in a contrite or godly fashion, with sections of the crowd showing workforce solidarity when the convicted person was a member of one of London's trades or racial solidarity when the convicted person was one of London's Irish. Sections of the crowd were not so brutal or callous as to be happy when the corpse of their executed relatives or friends was taken off to be dissected by the surgeons.[30] The image of the public execution that comes to us from the seventeenth century, of the crowd at an execution and the convicted felon on the gallows sharing an experience of religious theatre, may have fragmented in the eighteenth century, although this experience clearly remained as one of the major possible variants.[31]

Thus one of the most urgent items on the agenda of historians of punishment in early modern England is the reconstruction and analysis of the reactions of crowds attending public executions between, let us say, 1600 and 1868: only when this is completed will we be able to say with any precision how much 'civility' was on display at the public execution, or how that phenomenon can help inform us of the onward march of any 'civilizing process'. Such a reconstruction must take into account provincial executions: our views are perhaps still too affected by what happened at Tyburn, and by the reactions of large crowds in what was already in many ways an anonymous metropolitan area. And such an investigation might also look beyond the execution proper to those broader aspects of the folklore, or what might almost be described as the cultural anthropology, of capital punishment. Readers of Thomas Hardy will recall the therapeutic properties attributed to 'the withered arm' of an executed person, and the suspicion that here as elsewhere Hardy got his folklore right is reinforced by the account of an executioner at Bodmin in Cornwall who, after a hanging in 1845, sold lengths of the rope at a shilling each, these being employed by the local populace for healing purposes. This folklore may not tell us much about 'civility' as practised by the gentry, but it does remind us that the public execution was part of a rich and complex popular culture: once more the phenomenon defies being written off as a simple exercise in barbarism or callousness.[32]

[29] Gatrell, *Hanging Tree*, pt. I, 'The Scaffold and the Crowd'; P. Linebaugh, *The London Hanged: Crime and Civil Society in the Eighteenth Century* (1991).

[30] P. Linebaugh, 'The Tyburn Riot against the Surgeons', in D. Hay *et al.*, *Albion's Fatal Tree: Crime and Society in Eighteenth-Century England* (1975).

[31] For the continued importance of religion in Hanoverian attitudes to the death penalty, see R. McGowen, 'The Changing Face of God's Justice: The Debates over Divine and Human Punishment in Eighteenth-Century England', *Criminal Justice History*, 9 (1988), 63–98.

[32] Thomas Hardy, 'The Withered Arm', which first appeared in *Blackwood's Magazine* (Jan. 1888); T. Deane and T. Shaw, *The Folklore of Cornwall* (1975), 120; for some wider evidence, see Radzinowicz, *Movement for Reform*, 190–4.

II

But in our search for elements of 'civility' in the history of punishment in early modern England we must confront another problem: the attention that has, understandably, been devoted to that central drama of the early modern penal system, the public execution, has tended to obscure the fact that that system possessed a wide variety of other methods of punishing criminals. Indeed, it seems likely that, if the records of all courts with a 'criminal' jurisdiction were to be consulted, it would be revealed that the most common form of punishment inflicted on criminals in the period in question would be fining: whatever the early modern criminal justice system was doing to the body or souls of offenders, it was certainly damaging their purses. There was also, in the house of correction, from the Elizabethan period a penal institution that, on the strength of some historical interpretations at least, seems to have prefigured a number of the elements of the nineteenth-century penitentiary prison.[33] And, of course, as well as these, to the modern mind, rational ways of punishing offenders, there existed that extensive repertoire of penal practices—whipping at the cart's tale or at a whipping post, the pillory, the stocks, the ducking stool, the scold's bridle, penances ordered by the ecclesiastical courts, the parading of offenders against sexual morality on carts through the streets of borough towns—which were as public as public executions, but have so far received relatively little sustained analysis from serious historians. But here, too, even a preliminary investigation suggests the existence of a complex and shifting pattern, and of a set of popular attitudes that makes it difficult to employ these penal practices as evidence of a 'barbaric' early modern penal system.[34]

One obvious point of entry into attitudinal issues, if we may begin with the non-capital punishment of felons, is that provided by what might be termed, perhaps a little anachronistically, 'sentencing policy'. The overwhelming impression here is of a draconian penal code that was constantly being adjusted to the advantage of accused or convicted persons. Benefit of clergy, that 'pious perjury' that enabled first offenders for some felonies, notably grand larceny and manslaughter, to escape with a branding rather than being hanged, was used from the late sixteenth century to save many offenders from the noose.[35] By the same period many persons accused of theft benefited from the courts' downward adjustment of the value of the goods

---

[33] The fullest discussion of this institution is J. Innes, 'Prisons for the Poor: English Bridewells, 1550–1800', in F. Snyder and D. Hay (eds.), *Labour, Law and Crime: An Historical Perspective* (1987).

[34] M. Ingram, 'Juridical Folklore in England illustrated by Rough Music', in C. W. Brooks and M. Lobban (eds.), *Communities and Courts in Britain 1150–1900* (1997), 69.

[35] See the evidence gathered by J. A. Sharpe, *Crime in Seventeenth-Century England: A County Study* (Cambridge, 1983), 145–6, and J. G. Bellamy, *Criminal Law and Society in Late Medieval and Tudor England* (Gloucester, 1984), ch. 6, 'Benefit of Clergy in the Fifteenth and Sixteenth Centuries'.

they had allegedly stolen to below the value of a shilling, thus reducing their offence from grand larceny, a capital offence, to petty larceny, normally punished by whipping.[36] It seems likely that many of those women escaping execution on a plea of pregnancy were not in fact with child, while many of those who were did not, as the law directed, suffer execution after their infant was delivered.[37] From 1718 early experiments in transporting convicted felons to the American colonies were codified in an important piece of legislation, and by the outbreak of the American War of Independence some 30,000 English felons had been sent across the Atlantic after conviction.[38] In the eighteenth century those who *were* executed at the end of a typical assize were a group who had been carefully selected from a much larger pool of those at risk of being hanged.[39] The Elizabethan and Stuart periods are much less well documented than the Hanoverian in this matter, but an earlier version of the same pattern is discernible.[40] Execution was not just a brainless, knee-jerk reaction on the part of the authorities: throughout the early modern period official willingness to bend the law to help save large numbers of felons from hanging suggests that the courts employed a complex, and by no means barbaric, rationale when dealing with the serious offender.

The deliberations of assize judges, and especially eighteenth-century assize judges, have attracted some scholarly attention. So far, with a few exceptions, comparatively little has been devoted to the history and significance of the more community-based public punishments, many of them symbolic or shaming, inflicted by the inferior courts. Such punishments were, perhaps, most frequently awarded when the ecclesiastical courts ordered those before them to perform penance. Consider Agnes Wright of Chipping Barnet, performing penance in 1606 after committing fornication with Edward Fisher, a Londoner. The certificate returned by the minister and churchwardens of the parish recounted how she

at the beginning of the second lesson in Morning Prayer did present herself in the middle alley of the church of Chipping Barnet, near the seat of the minister, covered in white and there like a penitent . . . sinner stood till the end of the second lesson, at which time kneeling down upon her knees she confessed that she had grievously offended Almighty God . . . praying to God to forgive her and the congregation to

---

[36] Sharpe, *County Study*, 91–2, 146.

[37] See the discussion of this topic in J. S. Cockburn, *A Calendar of Assize Records: Introduction* (1985), 117–21.

[38] A development described by A. R. Ekirch, *Bound for America: The Transportation of British Convicts to the Colonies, 1718–1775* (Oxford, 1987).

[39] D. Hay, 'Property, Authority and the Criminal Law', in Hay *et al.*, *Albion's Fatal Tree*; P. King, 'Decision Makers and Decision Making in the English Criminal Law, 1750–1800', *Historical Journal*, 27 (1984), 25–58.

[40] J. Samaha, 'Hanging for Felony: The Rule of Law in Elizabethan Colchester', *Historical Journal*, 21 (1978), 763–82.

pray for her, that neither she nor any of them might hereafter be tempted to commit the like grievous offence.[41]

Despite the familiarity of such penances, it should be remembered that this type of ritual was not restricted to the punishments meted out by the ecclesiastical courts. In 1529, for example, five women were convicted by the City of London's courts for 'continually using the abominable custom of the foul and detestable sin of lechery and bawdry to the great displeasure of almighty God and to the great nuisance of their neighbours'. They were ordered, 'according to the old and ancient laws and customs of this city', to be conveyed from their prison to Newgate, wearing hoods and holding white rods 'in token of common bawds', and to be accompanied on their journey 'with minstrelsy, that is to say with pans and basins ringing before them'. They were to be thus paraded through the streets of London to Aldgate, where they were to be banished from the City of London for ever.[42] The significance of such punishments, many examples of which are to be found in the records of English borough courts, has so far received little attention. Yet they hold as many clues to the uncovering of the logic of past penal practices as does the relatively much studied public execution.

It is, as yet, very difficult to be anything other than tentative about changes in non-capital punishment over the three centuries that preceded 1868. There do seem to have been some early signs of a shift in emphasis in the secondary punishments awarded for serious crime by the assizes and quarter sessions in the early eighteenth century, with benefit of clergy being largely superseded by transportation to the Americas, and the emergence of early forms of that imprisonment with hard labour, which was to form the staple of nineteenth-century punishment.[43] What is less certain is how far changes were taking place in the charivari-like community-based 'shaming' punishments to which we alluded in the previous paragraph. Officialdom, of course, still made use of the pillory. Use of penance by the ecclesiastical courts may well have survived in some areas: numerous certificates of penance, for example, many of them recorded on specially printed forms, survive for the Archdeaconry of Berkshire over the eighteenth century.[44] But there does seem to have been a decline in officially ordered and enforced shaming punishments. In 1478, for example, one William Campion was found guilty in London of tapping a conduit and diverting the water into his

---

[41] P. Hair, *Before the Bawdy Court: Selections from Church Court and Other Records Relating to the Correction of Moral Offences in England, Scotland and New England, 1300–1800* (1972), 44–5.

[42] Ingram, 'Juridical Folklore', 69.

[43] See J. Beattie, *Crime and the Courts in England 1660–1800* (Oxford, 1986), ch. 9, 'The Impact of Transportation'.

[44] Berks. RO, D/A2/c. 176–9.

own well. He was ordered to be paraded through the streets of the city on a horse, 'with a vessel like unto a conduit full of water upon his head, the same water running by small pipes out of the same vessel and when the water is wasted new water to be put in the said vessel again'.[45] It is a little difficult to imagine the London authorities ordering this sort of punishment in the eighteenth century. The charivari became an element in popular culture, but declined as an element in officialdom's penal sanctions: 'the framework of penal ideas and social values that had sustained both popular ridings and official shame punishments slowly altered in ways that gradually diminished the communal element in the detection of offenders and the infliction of punishments.' An important aspect of this process was growing concern by civic authorities over the public-order dimensions of allowing crowds to gather.[46]

We return, therefore, to the problem of crowd reactions. The official ideal was, of course, that the crowd should be impressed by the shamefulness or heinousness of the offence being corrected, and that it should be reminded of the wages of sin and crime. On occasions, of course, this reaction did take the form of popular brutality: a case of 1618 from Burton on Trent, for example, shows a shaming punishment being eagerly inflicted by a crowd against a couple suspected of sexual immorality, in which there is considerable difficulty in distinguishing between the 'official' and the 'popular' elements.[47] An illustration to a pamphlet describing the riding of projectors and patentees of 1641 shows men and women (possibly adults of the better sort) watching the punishments from a window, while others (possibly boys) throw missiles at a hapless man riding a horse backwards.[48] But it is perhaps with the pillory that the documentation does help us trace variations in crowd attitudes, although here again such evidence seems strongest for the eighteenth century. Indeed, we even have the first-hand reports of some of those experiencing the punishment. In 1703 William Fuller, condemned by the House of Lords for publishing false and malicious books, told how, while he stood in the pillory, 'never was man amongst Turks or Barbarians known to be worse used . . . I was stifled with all manner of dirt, filth and rotten eggs . . . I was all over bruised from head to heel', and, of course, occasional deaths occurred when those in the pillory were handled too roughly.[49] Others fared better. The best-known example came again in 1703, when Daniel Defoe stood in the pillory as part of his punishment for allegedly libelling the Church of England in his *The Shortest Way with the Dissenters*. On

---

[45] Ingram, 'Juridical Folkore', 71.   [46] Ibid. 81.

[47] J. R. Kent, '"Folk Justice" and Royal Justice in Early Modern England: A "Charivari" in the Midlands', *Midland History*, 8 (1983), 70–85.

[48] Reproduced in Ingram, 'Juridical Folklore', 73.

[49] Cited in P. A. Backscheider, *Daniel Defoe: His Life* (Baltimore, 1989), 118. For a brief account of Fuller's crowded career, see *DNB*.

this occasion the mob, doubtlessly stage-managed by Defoe's political backers, formed a guard around the pillory, covered it with flowers, and drank his health while he stood there.[50] It is not, perhaps, surprising that the Act of 1816 abolishing the use of the pillory for all offences other than perjury should justify this step by claiming 'the punishment of the pillory has in many cases been found inexpedient and not fully to answer the purpose for which it was intended'. It is also fairly typical that the Act does not inform us what that purpose was.[51]

Mention of the abolition of pillory punishments, of course, leads us to the problem of the timing of the abolition or falling into disuse of the old penal repertoire. What is clear is that the abolition of the public execution in 1868 was preceded by about a century in which the range of punishments inflicted became more limited, and, possibly, the punishment of criminals became more 'civilized'. The burning of women convicted of treason (which included the murder of husbands) went in 1789,[52] while the whipping of females was abolished in 1817,[53] reminders that, here as elsewhere, civility was gendered. The old, colourful, charivariesque punishments had, we have argued, largely disappeared by 1700, and perhaps the frequency with which they were inflicted has in any case been overestimated. Thus references to cucking-stools occur most often on occasions when it was reported to local courts that they were out of repair.[54] Similarly, a jury presentment to the court leet of Manchester in 1591, which noted that 'the boothes, the cage and the couc-stoole' were 'in greate decaye', while 'the watter diche course of the same cookestoole is taken awaye and inclosed', evinces a generally pessimistic impression of the upkeep of the instruments of local, community-based punishment.[55] Other local punishments died out: the use of the stocks ended in the early nineteenth century, and that of the scold's bridle perhaps a little before this. By the end of the Victorian era educated observers were treating such punishments as quaint and folkloric evidence of a bygone, and perhaps more primitive age. Still, the onward march of progress in penal matters should not be oversimplified. As we have noted, the whipping of women was abolished in 1817, and the public whipping of men went in 1868. But this latter development was accompanied by a ferocious hardening of attitudes towards crime, which followed the 'garrottings' of that year, when a series of well-publicized street robberies set off a moral panic. One element in this panic

---

[50] Backscheider, *Daniel Defoe*, 118–19.

[51] 56 Geo. III, c. 168.

[52] A. D. Harvey, 'Research Note: Burning Women at the Stake in Eighteenth-Century England', *Criminal Justice History*, 11 (1990), 193–5.

[53] 57 Geo. III, c. 57.

[54] J. W. Spargo, *Juridical Folklore in England Illustrated by the Cucking-Stool* (Durham, NC, 1944).

[55] *The Court Leet Records of the Manor of Manchester*, ed. J. P. Earwaker (12 vols.; Manchester, 1884–90), ii. 52.

was an insistence that men convicted of these and related offences should be severely flogged: the floggings, however, like hangings, were now to take place within prison walls.[56]

III

Many explanations have been put forward for the massive shift in penal strategies, which led, in the decades around 1800, to the replacement of capital punishment by the penitentiary prison as the normal method of dealing with criminals. What the previous pages have aimed to show is that these explanations must take account of the complexity of the system of punishment in the two or three centuries before that date, and the fact that considerable changes had occurred over that period. Thus there was the sixteenth-century transition to more frequent use of capital punishment; the drop in the use of capital punishment over the seventeenth century; the apparent elaboration of scaffold ceremonial and ritual over that century; shifts in official attitudes to lesser forms of shaming punishment; and the continued search for secondary punishments over the eighteenth century. Equally, any discussion of the long-term history of capital punishment has to take into account that remarkable, and as far as can be seen judicially driven, flexibility in sentencing policy, a flexibility that, even in the late-Elizabethan period, was ensuring that many convicted felons were escaping the noose.

How, then, can we fit notions of 'civility' into the story of the decline of the public execution? The term itself, as this volume demonstrates, was open to a number of meanings in the sixteenth, seventeenth, and eighteenth centuries, but it was, of course, already being used in ways similar to its modern sense. 'Civility' was a term used to described the condition of being civilized, of being recognizably distanced from barbarity. This usage was extended (a process that perhaps became more marked in the eighteenth century) to include the behaviour appropriate to civilized people, and was perhaps most properly to be expected among those who had received what the age regarded as a polite or liberal education. Even people who had not received such an education, however, might demonstrate 'civility' in the form of everyday politeness, courtesy, or consideration for others. Obviously, such notions had a bearing on the growing sense of the 'barbarity' of the public execution, and on the supposedly 'civilized' nature of those individuals who found themselves opposed to the phenomenon. But one suspects that, when seventeenth- or eighteenth-century observers used the term 'civility' in their discussions of punishment, it was as frequently applied to isolated acts of courtesy or polite-

---

[56] For the background to this development, see Radzinowicz and Hood, *Emergence of Penal Policy*, ch. 21, 'The Mentality of the Cat and the Birch'.

ness on the scaffold as it was used in opposition to any perceived 'barbarity' inherent in public execution. Moreover, most refined observers, of course, would have regarded the bulk of those who were executed, men and women from the labouring classes, as people who existed outside the place of 'civility' and civilized behaviour. It is, perhaps, instructive that the only regular use of the term 'civility' in connection with the criminal justice system comes with 'civility money', a tip or *douceur* that gaolers, bailiffs, and other petty officials expected from those passing through their custody.[57]

There are, perhaps, some other major considerations that need to be mentioned. First, it is now generally accepted that one of the changes in attitudes to public execution occurring in the years around 1800 was that an increasingly genteel élite was coming to regard being a spectator at a public execution as a decidedly plebeian activity. Not just those suffering on the gallows, but also those watching them suffer, were the sort of people who would have been excluded by the élite from the world of 'civility'.[58] Secondly, the great change of 1868, which made execution a private rather than a public matter, made the whole business of capital punishment more acceptable to the sensitive: civility was enhanced by removing the barbarous from public view, and also rendering it inaccessible to the uncivilized lower orders. There were strong abolitionist stirrings in the 1860s, and there is little doubt that the decision to remove executions from the public gaze, and thus render them less obtrusively unpleasant events, did much to ensure that capital punishment survived.[59] And, of course, as we have hinted, the abolition of public execution in 1868 came as the culmination of a lengthy period of reforms and rationalization. The decline in executions that we have traced from the later seventeenth century was reversed temporarily in the late eighteenth, but by the early nineteenth century, as Peel's programme of reform lessened the number of capital felonies, the totals of those executed fell drastically, and continued to do so as the nineteenth century progressed.[60] The history of public execution, we must reiterate, cannot be divorced from the context of the wider history of the punishment of criminals.

---

[57] Thus Henry Fielding, *Amelia* (1751), bk. 8, ch. 10, has the hero, Booth, imprisoned in Newgate, having a bailiff asking him for 'civility money'. Booth, being unwilling to pay, is advised to do so by a lawyer who is present, who explains that it is 'a present or fee' that the prison officials 'expect as in a manner their due, tho' in reality they have no right'.

[58] A point explored and contextualized by Gatrell, *Hanging Tree*, esp. 601–11.

[59] See ibid. 610–11 for some pithy comments on Victorian sensitivity and the shift of executions to within the prison walls. For a good discussion of the debate on capital punishment in this period, see Radzinowicz and Hood, *Emergence of Penal Policy*, ch. 20, 'The Equation between Murder and the Death Penalty Maintained'.

[60] A brief summary of execution statistics over the relevant period is provided by C. Emsley, *Crime and Society in England 1750–1900* (2nd edn., 1996), 271, table 10.5. The 'standard approach' to Peel's reforms is given in N. Gash, *Mr Secretary Peel: The Life of Sir Robert Peel to 1830* (1961), ch. 9, 'Legal Reform'. For a less approbatory treatment of this theme, see Gatrell, *Hanging Tree*, ch. 21, 'Mercy and Mr Peel'.

Yet this leads to a final observation. 'Civility' or terms like it may not have been used much in early modern comments on penal policy, but any easy notion that the arrival of a 'civilizing process' in the late eighteenth century led to a retreat from capital punishment needs to be informed by the many scraps of evidence that suggest that at least a few people in the sixteenth and seventeenth centuries were unhappy with the high levels of capital punishment that obtained. Perhaps the strongest, if implicit, evidence on this point is the apparent ease with which the courts felt able to remove large numbers of convicted felons from capital punishment through the varied processes of benefit of clergy, pleas of the belly, undervaluing of stolen goods, and transportation to the Americas. And there is that body of adverse comment on capital punishment that emerged as an aspect of a wider desire for law reform in the 1640s and 1650s, and that is in urgent need of further investigation. But, even outside these reforming decades, individuals can be found expressing disquiet at the widespread use of capital punishment in England. More's *Utopia*, to take a well-known example, contained a passage in which the numerous executions of thieves were commented on adversely, and hanging castigated as a harsh and ineffective punishment.[61] Less predictably, Sir Edward Coke, in his *Institutes*, commented on 'what a lamentable case it is to see so many Christian men and women strangled on that cursed tree of that gallows', adding that, if any man should see all of those hanged in one year in England gathered together, 'if there were any spark of grace, or charity in him, it would make his heart to bleed for pity and compassion'.[62] And, if we may return to that Renaissance humanism that animated Sir Thomas More, we find Thomas Starkey, in a work written around 1530, putting forward the idea that 'the ordur of our law also in the punnyschment of theft ys over strayte . . . for wyth us for every lytyl theft a man ys by & by hangyd without mercy or pyte', a state of affairs that, he opined, 'faylyth much from gud cyvylyte'.[63] Detailed research might reveal that the frequent, and public, use of the gallows was not accepted as uncritically in the early modern period as has been supposed.

---

[61] Thomas More, *Utopia*, ed. G. M. Logan and R. M. Adams (Cambridge, 1989), 16.

[62] Sir Edward Coke, *The Third Part of the Institutes of the Laws of England* (1644), sig Kk.

[63] Thomas Starkey, *A Dialogue between Pole and Lupset*, ed. T. F. Mayer (Camden Society, 4th ser., 37; 1989), 80. Interestingly, this work also puts forward the idea that convicted thieves should be sentenced to hard labour on public works, 'wych payne schold be more grevuse to them then deth' (ibid. 131).

13

From the German Forests to Civil Society: The Frankish Myth and the Ancient Constitution in France

ROBIN BRIGGS

At three séances of the Académie des Inscriptions in November and December 1714 the young antiquarian Nicolas Fréret read a paper 'De l'origine des français et de leur établissement dans la Gaule'.[1] He argued—rashly, as it turned out—that the supposed Trojan descent of the Franks was no more than a myth, and that they had been a confederation of German tribes, long-time allies of the Romans who finally moved to fill the void left by the collapse of Roman power in Gaul. Not obviously seditious stuff, one might think, so it is rather startling that Chancellor Voysin issued a *lettre de cachet* on 26 December consigning Fréret to the Bastille, whence he emerged six months later, at the end of June 1715. He seems to have been the victim of a petty act of spite, a denunciation from a much older scholar, the abbé Vertot. The Chancellor's letter ordering the arrest suggested that Jansenism was as much the issue as dangerous views about the French past, but there was a sense in which they went together.[2] Fréret's criticism of the standard national history by the Jesuit Father Gabriel Daniel was implicitly a much wider attack on the monarchy and its traditional defenders. It can be associated with Marc Fumaroli's telling antithesis between two cultures, the one puritanical, Gallican, and *parlementaire*, the other more sensual, Jesuitical, and absolutist.[3] Fréret was a friend of the comte de Boulainvilliers, who took a rather different view of the Franks, and is often, somewhat misleadingly, represented as a racist who believed the nobility to derive their pre-eminence from that conquest by their Frankish ancestors long ago.

---

[1] A revised and expanded version was finally published 150 years later, in *Mémoires de l'Institut Impériale de France, Académie des Inscriptions et Belles-Lettres*, xxiii (1868), 323–559.

[2] The letter is printed in C. Grell and C. Volpilhac-Auger (eds.), *Nicolas Fréret, légende et vérité* (Oxford, 1994), 26 n. 6.

[3] D. A. Bell, *Lawyers and Citizens: The Making of a Political Elite in Old Regime France* (New York, 1994), 46, summarizing M. Fumaroli, *L'Âge de l'éloquence: Rhétorique et 'res litteraria' de la Rénaissance au seuil de l'époque classique* (Geneva, 1980), 585–622.

I

Shortly before Fréret's misfortunes began, between 1709 and 1712, the British government, in its attempts to reach a peace settlement with France, had raised major constitutional issues. The duke of Marlborough and some of his Whig allies thought that only the re-establishment of the Estates-General as a regular feature of French government could prevent further aggression against the rest of Europe. Even Henry St John, perhaps inadvertently, tied to the essential demand that Philip V of Spain renounce his right of succession to the French throne a request that Louis XIV should summon an Estates-General to ratify this decision.[4] Did this betray an understandable anxiety to secure binding guarantees for a commitment that even foreigners could see might contravene the so-called fundamental laws, in this case as they affected the succession? The foreign minister Torcy was alarmed by a possible congruence with the ideas of the noble dissidents at court. The problems over the succession raised quite enough difficult issues to excite these critics with or without external pressure. There was a flurry of activity in the group recently associated with the duc de Bourgogne, and both the duc de Noailles and the duc de Saint-Simon wrote treatises on the problem. The latter argued that the ultimate legislative and constitutive power lay with the peerage, so advocated the calling of an assembly in which they would be joined by the simple dukes and the officers of the Crown. To justify this unlikely proposal he wrote a lengthy history of French government, claiming that it had followed a consistent pattern back to the Merovingian kings, and that the assemblies of the ancient Franks had been composed only of great lords. The ducs de Beauvillier and de Chevreuse bravely tried to press these views on Louis XIV, with predictable lack of success.[5]

Such an appeal to history was a clever way of asserting alternative values, when the Crown itself had so often backed its territorial and political claims with some distinctly partisan interpretations of the past. This essay will seek to show how opponents of absolutism were able to construct a distinctive form of civil history, whose effectiveness had little to do with accuracy. The obvious comparison is with the Norman Yoke theories deployed against the Stuarts in England. The two were linked through Tacitus' *Germania*, with its picture of primitive freedoms in the Teutonic forests, but of course the French version long stressed the benefits of a conquest (or for some a fusion) that was also a liberation from Roman rule. It was a myth of legitimation, whereas the English version depicted the invaders as destroying the ancient constitution, yet both ultimately looked back to lost freedoms. There was some

[4] J. Klaits, *Printed Propaganda under Louis XIV: Absolute Monarchy and Public Opinion* (Princeton, 1976), 260–72.

[5] H. A. Ellis, *Boulainvilliers and the French Monarchy: Aristocratic Politics in Early Eighteenth-Century France* (1988), 94–101; Saint-Simon, *Traités politiques et autres écrits*, ed. Y. Coirault (Paris, 1996), 137–306.

interaction between the two. Hotman's *Francogallia* became a popular text for the later seventeenth-century Whigs, and was published in translation in 1711.[6] The *Vindiciae contra tyrannos* was published in English in 1648 and again in 1689. The Norman Yoke theory, on the other hand, made no discernible impact on pre-revolutionary France, unless one counts the bizarre attempt to circulate a translation of the *Agreement of the People* among the Bordelais rebels in 1652–3.[7] It was in the early nineteenth century that Scott's *Ivanhoe* seems to have helped persuade French romantic historians that they needed a racial conflict of their own to act as an organizing scheme for national history, at a time when this also fitted into the developing antagonisms of right and left. This emerged with the versions offered by the brothers Amédée and Augustin Thierry, by Guizot, and numerous others, leading into much measuring of skulls and pseudo-scientific absurdities.[8]

As many commentators have pointed out, appeals to the French past suddenly went out of favour once the Revolution was properly under way. References now became distinctly unfavourable, as with Sieyes's famous suggestion that the nobles might be sent back to their Franconian forests. Marat's unpublished essay in praise of Montesquieu, written for the Academy of Bordeaux, had earlier included a declaration of hatred for the feudal laws, 'bloodthirsty laws carried into the whole of Europe from the German forests which so long caused the human race to groan under the oppression of a multitude of little tyrants'.[9] A certain M. Ducalle went to the extreme of demanding that the very name of the French should be abandoned 'now that we have at last thrown off our shackles? While they repudiate the offer of brotherhood, we make a show of extravagant servility in calling ourselves by their name. Are we really the offspring of their impure blood? God forbid, citizens! We are descended from the pure-blooded Gauls . . .?.[10] In his violently hostile *Histoire critique de la noblesse* (Paris, 1790) Jacques-Antoine Dulaure wrote: 'Ah, unhappy people, you were under the feet of the barbarians, whose progenitors massacred your ancestors. They are all foreigners, savages who escaped from the forests of Germany and the icy wastes of Saxony . . .?.[11] In such writings the doctrine of racial supremacy, which had never in fact generated any real enthusiasm among the nobles themselves, was being used to powerful effect against them; paradoxically this was probably the most significant long-

[6] F. Hotman, *Francogallia*, ed. R. E. Giesey and J. H. M. Salmon (Cambridge, 1972), 121–5.

[7] P. A. Knachel, *England and the Fronde* (Ithaca, NY, 1967), 198–200.

[8] L. Poliakov, *The Aryan Myth: A History of Racist and Nationalist Ideas in Europe* (1971), 29–36 and *passim*; K. Pomian, 'Francs et Gaulois', in P. Nora (ed.), *Les Lieux de mémoire*, III. *Les France*, i. *Conflits et partages* (Paris, 1992), 41–105.

[9] E. Carcassonne, *Montesquieu et le problème de la constitution française au XVIIIᵉ siècle* (Paris, 1927), 170–1.

[10] Poliakov, *Aryan Myth*, 29.

[11] K. F. Werner, 'La "Conquête Franque" de la Gaule: Itinéraires historiographiques d'une erreur', in O. Guyotjeannin (ed.), *Clovis chez les historiens* (Paris, 1996), 7–45, citation p. 11 n. 15.

term effect of Boulainvilliers's 'racial' theories, as a means of isolating and discrediting the traditional nobility.

Outside observers who had been reading French political literature were also capable of reading the Revolution in these terms; Catherine the Great wrote a celebrated letter to Grimm stating that 'The Gauls are driving out the Franks', then predicting a bloody revenge by the latter.[12] Of course, when the Restoration finally came it was not very bloody, but the ideological battle was still intense, helping the whole subject to acquire a salience it had not really possessed before 1789. The role of the Aryan myth for the French right of this century is well known, while in the 1990s M. Bruno Mégret of the National Front has been associated with the ingeniously titled GRECE, the Group for European Civilization Research and Studies, peddling a combination of neo-paganism with admiration for the Aryan forebears of warrior Europe.[13] In this light Tacitus, Hotman, Boulainvilliers, and many others can be linked to some very dubious modern theories. Not only is the very idea of such posthumous guilt by association always very dubious, however; there is a serious risk that it will lead to anachronism and misunderstanding about the role of ideas in their own time. This may well have happened with Boulainvilliers, since his views about the Frankish conquest look very different in their proper context. It is important to step outside these modern connotations in order to see what was really being argued about under the *Ancien Régime*.

II

Modern historians still have to admit to large areas of ignorance or doubt about the Franks and Merovingian Gaul; between the sixteenth and the eighteenth centuries the problem was of course much greater. With so little hard fact to go on, there were great open spaces that could be filled by fantasy, while genuine documents were often subjected to systematic misinterpretation, based on what now seem some very rash philological and historical principles. François Furet plausibly claimed that French writing on the history of France went into quite a serious decline, after its very promising beginnings in the sixteenth century. The greatest weakness was probably the split between the learned antiquarian tradition and the literary one, which meant that the very real advances made by the former were never really carried over into the public sphere, or incorporated into broader interpretations.[14] Nor were the various partisan versions of the past subjected to very much serious criticism, so that they competed more on their rhetorical skill and their appeals

---

[12] Poliakov, *Aryan Myth*, 29.
[13] W. Pfaff, 'The Presentable Face of France's Extreme Right', *International Herald Tribune*, 13 Feb. 1997, 8.
[14] F. Furet, *In the Workshop of History* (Chicago, 1984), 80–7.

to particular interests than on their accuracy. Leading interpreters in this style included Boulainvilliers, Voltaire, and Mably, all of whom mixed lively insights with highly suspect methodology.

Modern commentators have often identified noble racism as a rather pathetic fiction developed by a class in decline, acting as a compensation in fantasy for what they had lost in reality. This is certainly the general vision of André Devyver's invaluable study, which collects up a huge mass of evidence on the subject.[15] As the whole notion of the aristocracy being subjugated by the monarchy comes into question, however, so must this analysis. More recently Harold Ellis has demonstrated how much it distorts the true situation of Boulainvilliers, who was far nearer to the centre of power than had been generally understood, and cannot be seen as an excluded country squire.[16] Such misunderstandings are largely associated with a dismissive attitude to the nobles as predestined losers, doomed by the march of history, and capable only of sterile obstructionism—just the view that the post-1815 mythology of Franks and Gauls was frequently used to support. It fits very well with the modern version of the *thèse royale*, as expounded by such historians as Michel Antoine and François Bluche. They imply that, if only the Crown had shown sufficient determination to brush these selfish reactionaries aside, or the nobles themselves had foreseen the effects of their behaviour, then the disaster of the Revolution could have been averted. The way in which the Crown and its advisers bungled every chance to move in this direction, down to and including the first year of the Revolution, suggests there were more serious obstacles to be overcome.

In truth the idea of a society levelled out to form a single mass of subjects, ruled by a benevolent monarch, was completely foreign to early modern thinking. If the Crown did in practice exploit social divisions and help to multiply categories, this did not imply any deliberate long-term policy, merely an expediency that was primarily driven by financial concerns. There was a huge amount of double-think and double-talk involved, as the monarchy undermined traditional values by selling privileges and rights that were supposedly attached to virtue, then invoked those same values when it tried to take away or diminish what it had sold. It is now plain that venality of office, far from becoming a relatively minor issue in the eighteenth century, had continued the same sorry pattern of false promises, extortion, and the like right to the end.[17] Kings and ministers were not necessarily cynical; the evidence suggests rather that they shared a set of assumptions with the privileged groups as a whole, and took them so much for granted that they thought local or minor infractions were merely matters of convenience, with no implications

---

[15] A. Devyver, *Le Sang épuré: Les Préjugés de race chez les gentilshommes français de l'Ancien Régime (1560–1720)* (Brussels, 1973).

[16] Ellis, *Boulainvilliers, passim.*

[17] W. Doyle, *Venality: The Sale of Offices in Eighteenth-Century France* (Oxford, 1996).

for principle. The attitude of Richelieu or Colbert to the nobility is permeated by this kind of ambiguity, yet in the end it would seem absurd to deny that these ministers saw the *ducs et pairs* as the rightful summit of French society, and conducted their own familial policies accordingly. There is a splendid sentence in the *Testament politique*, in which Richelieu complains that the rich financiers 'marry into the great houses of the kingdom, which are bastardised in this fashion, and now only produce half-breeds, as far removed from the generosity of their ancestors as they often are from any resemblance to their features'.[18] One wonders what his niece's unwilling husband the Prince de Condé would have thought about that. What runs through the literature is a conviction that men are unequal in talents and virtue as well as in fortune, and that such inequalities are transmitted by heredity. This was not incompatible with the notion that men were originally free and equal in rights, which underlay so much contractualist thinking; on the other hand, it explained by historical argument how those shared rights had been transformed into a hierarchical society. More liberal or realistic thinkers found little difficulty in developing the notion of a permeable élite, renewing itself through selective recruitment. The revolutionary debates on suffrage would reveal just how far the French radicals, like their English predecessors of the seventeenth century, still thought in terms of a natural ruling class marked off from the common herd.[19]

In such a context the notion of the Frankish conquest and the truly ancient nobility ceases to have particularly dramatic implications in social terms. If it had already become a *lieu commun* by the later sixteenth century—so that it crops up with fair frequency in the debate over noble status traced by Arlette Jouanna, then reappears in the *Mazarinades*, before its reworking under Louis XIV by Le Laboureur, Boulainvilliers, and Saint-Simon—most of these evocations are just part of a much wider rhetoric.[20] In practice everyone agreed that only suitable élites should enjoy privileges and a share in power, while a range of arguments were deployed to defend the specific claims of subgroups. The same individuals often adopted different postures within a single work. Since virtue, valour, and nobility were supposed to go together, there was bound to be a constant friction between theory and observed reality, and most of those concerned had every interest in blurring the boundaries. The royal government discovered this rather painfully when it tried to exploit the apparent detestation of *anoblis* among the supposedly ancient nobility, only to find that these denunciations had not been meant so literally, and that there was

---

[18] L. André (ed.), *Testament politique du Cardinal de Richelieu* (Paris, 1947), 251. Devyver (*Sang épuré*, 157 n. 3) is obviously right to replace André's meaningless 'motifs' by 'mestifs'.

[19] M. Crook, *Elections in the French Revolution: An Apprenticeship in Democracy, 1789–1799* (Cambridge, 1996).

[20] A. Jouanna, *L'Idée de race en France au XVIᵉ siècle et au début du XVIIᵉ siècle* (2 vols.; Montpellier, 1981), and *Ordre social: Mythes et hiérarchies dans la France du XVIᵉ siècle* (Paris, 1977).

great dislike of its clumsy intervention. Another example might be La Roque's treatise on the nobility, which began with the classic assertion that there was some indefinable virtue in the seed, then later said that marriage with a roturier always left a stain in the blood, and that 'the *anobli* acquires nobility but not *race*'. Despite frequent references of this type to doctrines of blood and race, and an eloquent exposition of the claims of the *gentilshommes de nom et d'armes*, La Roque's work is very largely a legal tract explaining the innumerable ways in which nobility can be validated or acquired, which could be regarded as an elaborate defence of *anoblissement*. All nobles are not equal, but they are all nobles.[21]

Boulainvilliers himself did not draw many striking conclusions from his Germanist theories where the nobility was concerned. He did want there to be a catalogue of French noble families, in which the respective doses of Frankish blood would be assessed, without actually suggesting how this mystical calculation was to be performed.[22] DNA testing would presumably have struck him as a dream come true in this respect. The true purpose of his 'racism' was surely not to prove that the nobles could draw any inalienable right from a conquest some 1,300 years earlier, or that his beloved feudalism should be restored; rather it was to prove to their modern successors that they had a duty to match the standards set by their ancestors and stand up against the abuses of royal power. On the other hand, he was not apparently much interested in suggesting systematic policies for the future. This would have been almost superfluous, when so many people agreed—at least in principle— that more respect for traditional social divisions was desirable, and would strengthen the French state. Obviously the classic area where this operated was that of military service, a vast subject that goes beyond the remit of this essay. In this area one can accept all David Bien's subtle analysis of the Ségur ordinance of 1781, and recognize the numerous practical reasons for such a reform, while noting the highly traditional assumptions and values it espoused.[23] Bien's more recent work on the corporate structure of French society, powerfully reinforced by royal fiscal and borrowing policies, does in fact confirm this approach. Because there were no effective national bodies, he argues, the royal debt could be managed only through an infinity of smaller self-governing corporations, engaged in perpetual bargaining in which privileges were traded off against sections of the state's obligations.[24]

What was really at the heart of the discussions about the medieval past, then, was not an argument about social divisions that were disputed more in

---

[21] G. A. de la Roque, *Traité de la noblesse, de ses différentes espèces* (Paris, 1678).

[22] Devyver, *Sang épuré*, 376–7.

[23] D. Bien, 'The Army in the French Enlightenment: Reform, Reaction, and Revolution', *P&P* 85 (1979), 68–98.

[24] D. Bien, 'Old Regime Origins of Democratic Liberty', in D. Van Kley (ed.), *The French Idea of Freedom* (Stanford, Calif., 1994), 23–71.

detail than in principle. It was a long-running political debate about the nature of the French state, and the proper relationship between the monarchy and its subjects; in other words, was there a French constitution? The crucial advantage of the Frankish conquest theory was that it established the rights of the French as a free people, independent of any previous servitude to Rome. It was for such purposes that the *literati* in the service of the medieval monarchy had already used the theme, to reject universalist claims on behalf of both Empire and papacy.[25] From this aspect there were great advantages in the various modifications that united Franks and Gauls, the most ingenious being that adopted by Bodin among others, according to which the Germans were actually Gauls who had fled from the Roman conquest, then returned to reclaim their lost rights and reunite their nation.[26] Hotman's Francogallic state was another variant on this theme, however different his political conclusions. This was truly present-centred history, and for most of its existence it was a relatively marginal form of rhetoric, used to diverse ends, and apparently impotent to divert the inexorable advance of royal power. Here too this mode of argument needs to be understood against the background of a conventional wisdom.

France, according to this view, was a monarchy governed by fundamental law, which the king himself was bound to respect. The idea of fundamental law was deeply ambiguous, and was in many ways little more than a metaphor to express vague yet powerfully held notions about the essentially mixed nature of the state. Good kings were defined by their instinctive understanding of this unwritten constitution, which went well beyond the very scanty group of fundamental laws a jurist might have identified. There were just three of these, the Salic law governing the succession, the inalienable status of the royal demesne, and the royal duty to eradicate heresy; however ingeniously these were interpreted, they plainly fell far short of being a constitution. The good king would add to these, as a minimum, respect for and enforcement of the law, protection of his subjects' property rights, and the taking of good council on major issues of policy. Those kings who managed to play their role in general conformity to this image, or at least to project the idea that they did, were able to mobilize a formidable degree of support; whatever their individual defects, those who ruled between 1483 and 1559 just about managed to do so. The century between 1559 and 1661, on the other hand, was one of persistent crisis and instability, broken only by a short interlude under Henri IV. Religious division, combined with civil wars, then a massively expensive foreign war, forced the Crown to pursue divisive policies and extract taxes by

---

[25] J. Krynen, *L'Empire du roi: Idées et croyances politiques en France XIIIᵉ–XVᵉ siècle* (Paris, 1993), 101–3 and *passim*.

[26] Although Bodin is often cited as the originator of this notion in his *Methodus* of 1566, according to C. Volpilhac-Auger (*Tacite en France de Montesquieu à Chateaubriand* (Oxford, 1993), 311), it appears in a 1557 work by the jurist Jean Connan.

force and fraud. First the Protestants, then the Catholic zealots of the League, were driven to denounce the kings as tyrants, and develop constitutional theories intended to rein in their powers. The ministries of Richelieu and Mazarin generated a new wave of opposition, which identified the Cardinals and their cliques as the agents of tyranny, illegitimate usurpers of power from naïve or youthful kings.

Despite the intensity of these crises, they had an ironic result, which was to demonstrate the hopeless inability of the opposition to formulate a position that would rally general support, and the mere opportunism of most of their claims to constitutional principle. It is easy to read into Hotman, for example, an attempt to justify the intervention of German Protestants in French affairs, alongside his unrealistic view of the Estates. He seems to have thought the latter would support the Protestant challenge to royal authority, when in reality there was no chance at all of this happening. Then there was the abrupt volte-face he and other Huguenot writers performed once Henri of Navarre had become the heir to the throne, matched by the audacity of the League in appropriating the old Protestant arguments. These apparently cynical switches of position can perhaps be partly explained in terms of wider intellectual practices among French lawyers, who seem to have cited their authorities in a strangely piecemeal fashion that does not fit with modern ideas about coherence and consistency.[27] When one adds the murders of Henri III and Henri IV, and the debate over tyrannicide, it is easy to see how any defence of ancient liberties looked like a threat to civil peace in the kingdom. If there were some echoes of these ideas at the Estates of 1614, the general tenor of the debates was unambiguous in its support for royal authority. Condé and other noble malcontents found themselves isolated, having apparently believed (just like Hotman) that any such assembly must naturally support what they saw as their unanswerable claims.

The experience of 1614–15 did not wholly discourage the middling and lesser nobility from seeing the Estates as a way of challenging misgovernment, as is shown by the repeated demands for their convocation during the Fronde. While there are many reasons to believe that this crisis had no real prospect of derailing royal authority, it is surely a sign of real panic that the government even contemplated calling the Estates in 1649 and 1651, when such a step might have had explosive consequences. While the *Mazarinades* may contain relatively little that aspires to the status of political thought, they do betray a widespread belief that the Crown and its ministers were subverting the proper forms of the state. The more serious pamphlets contain relatively frequent references to the Franks and the supposed ancient constitution, amidst their central concern with tyranny and despotism as a perversion of true kingship,

[27] D. R. Kelley, *The Beginning of Ideology: Consciousness and Society in the French Reformation* (Cambridge, 1981), 206–10.

which threatened the whole state with ruin. In 1649 the marquis de Clanleu wrote passionately in this vein, drawing a comparison with the Turks when he claimed:

France has never been under a despotic government, unless it has been during the last thirty years when we have been subject to the mercy of the ministers, and exposed to their tyranny . . . the kings of our time cannot pretend to any other rights over France than those possessed by Merovée . . . so that one may draw this conclusion, that since France is not a conquered territory, she cannot be treated like a slave . . .

He went on to tell the Regent what she should teach her son:

It is true that here we find a science unknown to us today, when we are so accustomed to slavery that we cannot believe our fathers were ever free; but let her teach him if it please her that the safe way for a king is not to keep his subjects pinned down by the violence of extortions; for in thinking to deprive them of the means of rebellion, one does not thereby remove their will, and sooner or later, at the least hope of relief, they choose to throw off the yoke, with no regard for either oaths or respect.[28]

Another writer put some remarkable if unlikely words into the mouth of the late king Louis XIII:

Do you think that France is necessarily obliged to remain under the yoke of kings? Do you not know that they came from Germany to live here, and that to be worthy of the name she bears, France must needs recover the freedom she lost several centuries ago? She bears a natural love to her kings: but Rome loved hers too, yet did not fail to drive them out, when she saw they believed the name of king dispensed them from recognizing any other law than that of their desires. All that which has begun may come to an end, and if those who came from Germany with the kings have left descendants who love them, the blood of the Gauls, over whom they usurped their power, is their natural enemy. It is true that the Gauls were previously subject to the Romans, but those Romans did not treat them with such harshness as the kings who rule them presently . . .[29]

As so often, these ostensibly radical noises did not develop into anything resembling a programme of political action. The ultimate result of all this sound and fury was probably something in the vein of the disabused realism of Arnauld D'Andilly's *La Vérité toute nue* of 1652, in which he excoriated the selfish politics of all sides, then concluded that, if the King truly wished to reinstall Mazarin, that might be deplorable, yet it would be much better to obey than to prolong the horrors of civil war.

This claim to be the only guarantor of public order was of course the trump card, which the monarchy repeatedly played, and which always seemed to work, at the cost of intermittent bouts of anarchy as a form of inoculation. Richelieu and his publicists not only put forward their *raison d'enfer*, but also

[28] *Lettre d'avis à Messieurs du Parlement de Paris escrite par un provincial* (Paris, 1649), 21–2, 25.
[29] *L'Esprit du feu Roy Louis le Juste a la Reyne* (Paris, 1652).

developed an astonishingly autocratic divine right line. Among Dupuy's papers is a piece on 'The obedience due to kings even if they are tyrants and heretics', while a 1631 pamphlet declared 'it is a kind of sacrilege to question the judgement of the prince, and to raise the question whether he has treated someone well or badly'.[30] Kings possessed special abilities conferred by God, which placed them above any criticism. Although these are fairly extreme cases, they are not really out of line with the language of absolute monarchy down at least to the end of Louis XV's reign. This was echoed in the big general histories of France, in which authors such as Mezeray and Daniel sedulously avoided potentially controversial discussions of politics and institutions; for them, royal power was inherently mysterious and secret, not accessible to scholarly investigation.[31] Linguet would eventually take the Machiavellian argument to self-parodic lengths with his defence of oriental despotism and his claims that injustice and cruelty could secure peace and security for the majority.[32] In a less openly provocative style the Crown had come to rely on a remarkably stark doctrine, which simply treated any dissent as incipient treason. The personal rule of Louis XIV seemed to demonstrate that this approach could work, if handled with the appropriate mixture of tact and firmness. When John Northleigh visited France in the 1680s he remarked of his hosts:

They themselves thought their monarchy the best, because the most absolute; and tho' they are slaves for it, pride themselves in the Chains they wear: They will call this Absolute Power a just one, tho' it reduce the subject to just nothing; and tho' they groan under it, will hardly suffer a stranger to whisper against it.[33]

Other British travellers recorded similar attitudes, even at the end of the reign. Boulainvilliers himself deplored the blindness of his contemporaries to what had happened, and to the abuses of despotic kingship visible all around them. He condemned most intendants for their inability 'to recognize any principle of government other than the pure despotism of a prince and his ministers'.[34]

III

The history of the Franks and the three successive races of French kings was therefore commonly portrayed as a tragic tale of the loss of political freedom

---

[30] E. Thuau, *Raison d'état et pensée politique à l'époque de Richelieu* (Paris, 1966), 244, 248 n. 4.

[31] C. Grell, 'L'Histoire de France et le mythe de la monarchie au XVIIᵉ siècle', in Y.–M. Bercé and P. Contamine (eds.), *Histoires de France, Historiens de la France* (Paris, 1994), 165–88.

[32] R. I. Boss, 'Linguet: The Reformer as Anti-"Philosophe"', *Studies on Voltaire and the Eighteenth Century*, 151 (Oxford, 1976), 333–51.

[33] J. Lough, *France Observed in the Seventeenth Century by British Travellers* (Stocksfield, 1984), 154.

[34] *État de la France* (3 vols.; 1727), preface, p. xx.

and the rise of despotism. For most authors Charlemagne stood out as the great hero, who had restored political rights as well as public order, but since his time decay had resumed.[35] The writers who took this line did not argue crudely for an impossible restoration of past structures; they tried to apply the central principle of using institutions to safeguard political liberty, adapting it to the circumstances of their own time. At first their efforts appeared to have fallen on stony ground, at least in the sphere of political action. The regent Orléans and Cardinal Fleury followed the kind of moderate policies that made talk of despotism seem unreasonable. Between 1712 and 1718 concern about the succession, coupled with the problems of Philip V's renunciation and Louis XIV's attempt to legitimize his bastard sons, did create a temporary effervescence, in which questions about fundamental law and the need for consent from the élites came to the fore. The Regent dealt with the crisis skilfully, temporizing for long enough for irreconcilable divisions to emerge among the noble factions, then imposing an authoritarian solution.[36] Such tactical adroitness became ever harder to repeat, however, in the much more testing circumstances after 1750. During the interim, constitutionalism had succeeded in attracting growing intellectual interest, which culminated in the work of Montesquieu. As a *parlementaire* he personified the strong eighteenth-century tendency to see the *parlements* as the one relic of the old freedoms, however imperfect, and as the only check on arbitrary government. In 1732 a powerful Frondeur pamphlet by Louis Machon was reprinted under the title *Judicium Francorum* to hammer home this point, possibly under Jansenist auspices. The links between political and religious opposition pointed up how far eighteenth-century fears of despotism centred on the Church, but also how readily all issues were assimilated into a general struggle between 'justice' and 'arbitrary despotism'.[37]

The relative quiet of the three decades between John Law's System and the conflicts between Crown and *parlement* in the 1750s is deceptive, for this period saw some crucial developments. Defenders of the monarchy ceased to rely so heavily on biblical sources and divine right, in the increasingly unfashionable style of Bossuet, moving instead to develop their own version of French history. The abbé Du Bos, who like Boulainvilliers had worked for the Regent, became the count's most formidable critic, at least where the alleged Frankish conquest was concerned. Du Bos sought to replace this violent takeover of power with its antithesis, a peaceful transfer of authority, which allowed Franks and Gauls to merge into one nation. Since he also claimed that Justinian had formally ceded his rights to the Frankish kings in 537, for him it was the kings of France rather than the German emperors who were the true heirs of the Caesars, and drew their authority directly from this

---

[35] R. Morrissey, *L'Empereur à la barbe fleurie: Charlemagne dans la mythologie et l'histoire de la France* (Paris, 1997).

[36] Ellis, *Boulainvilliers*, 94–106, 112–92.   [37] Bell, *Lawyers*, 205.

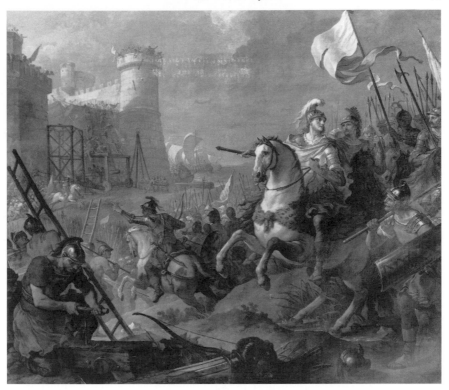

8. Charles-Joseph Natoire, *Le Siège de Bordeaux* (1735). Eighteenth-century history painters generally ignored the Franks, the one exception being a commission to Natoire from contrôleur-général Orry in the 1730s, for a series on Clovis. *The Siege of Bordeaux* is the most striking of the artist's six canvases; he apparently made a serious effort at historical authenticity.

source. Despite the serious merits of some of his historical arguments, Du Bos took them to extremes that laid him open to damaging criticism.[38] His 'Romanist' stance actually illustrates the trap in which the monarchy found itself; while it could hardly abandon the field to its opponents, engaging in controversy was dangerous in itself, exposing what were potentially damaging aspects of its own position. As Lombard pointed out long ago, his views were those of a bourgeois of the 1730s, content to shelter behind the Crown for protection against noble arrogance without demanding political rights. By placing a supposedly perfect system at the outset of the monarchy, he froze the future as well as the past in an immobile despotism, which was precisely what a growing number of Frenchmen would come to regard as

[38] A. Lombard, *L'Abbé Du Bos: Un initiateur de la pensée moderne (1670–1742)* (Paris, 1913).

the central defect of their polity.[39] They were, therefore, drawn to a largely mythical past, which challenged the atemporal and self-justifying rhetoric of absolutism.

From the later seventeenth century, once the Crown had established an effective monopoly of force, political action was restricted to the spheres of court intrigue and public or private debate. The royal court was increasingly identified with the corruption of the monarchy, which one historian has linked to the haunting of the French imagination by the image of oriental despotism, with its sinister cortège of janissaries, eunuchs, and dumb servants.[40] David Bell has pointed to the vital role played by the barristers in opening up debate; as one group that was not a formal corporation, but that excelled in glossing written texts, they also enjoyed the right to publish briefs without censorship. Bell identifies them with a 'darkly Augustinian vision', in which royal and papal authorities were regularly blamed for moves that threatened 'arbitrary despotism' and the ruin of the kingdom. The apparently secondary Jansenist crises of the Council of Embrun (1727) and the curés of Orléans (1730–1) saw these criticisms redoubled, the emergence of *mémoires judiciaires* as a regular form of opposition pamphleteering, and a strike by the barristers that paralysed the Parisian courts so effectively that Fleury was forced to climb down. These events are directly linked to the much more dangerous symbiosis between a renewed Jansenist crisis and the sudden flowering of the rhetoric of Frankish liberties in the mid-1750s. The Jansenist barrister Le Paige was the central figure at the outset, reviving and adapting the views of both the sixteenth-century writers and Boulainvilliers to develop a political argument from the ancient constitution. Within a few years his doctrines had become assimilated into the standard language of *parlementaire* protests against government legislation, as one confrontation followed another.[41] The *Grandes remontrances* of April 1753, with their trenchant tone and erudite apparatus, were in striking contrast to their predecessors; they were also printed, against all precedent, and established a position from which the *parlement* would scarcely diverge for many years.[42]

There was an obvious formal affinity between a movement like Jansenism, which idealized the primitive Church, and a political theory posited on the corruption of ancient virtues.[43] When they coalesced in the 1750s, however, there was nothing inevitable about the process, and the *parlement* was certainly not driven by some mysterious intoxication with fantasies about the

---

[39] Lombard, *L'Abbé Du Bos*, 458.

[40] B. Barret-Kriegel, *Les Historiens de la monarchie*, i. *Jean Mabillon* (Paris, 1988), 247–8.

[41] Bell, *Lawyers*, *passim*.

[42] J. M. J. Rogister, *Louis XV and the Parlement of Paris, 1737–1755* (Cambridge, 1995), 173–81; J. Flammermont, *Remontrances du parlement de Paris au XVIIIe siècle* (3 vols.; Paris, 1888–98), i. 506–614.

[43] D. K. Van Kley, *The Religious Origins of the French Revolution: From Calvin to the Civil Constitution, 1560–1791* (1996).

Merovingian past. Bungling and contradictory government policies, coupled with the malign effects of court intrigue and Louis XV's irresolution, were much more important.[44] The other great problem for the government stemmed from its crippling obsession with the imposition of order within the Church, which exacerbated the very divisions it was supposed to eliminate. The appointment of an archbishop of Paris whom the king could not control was enough to set off a major political crisis, which then interlocked with a range of other issues. From the disputes over the sacraments, through the financial crises of the Seven Years War, to the Brittany affair and the *parlement Maupeou*, the government repeatedly appeared arbitrary and tyrannical. In this light Maupeou's revolution did indeed look like the final unveiling of full-blown despotism, whose agenda had already been heard in the *discours de la flagellation* a few years earlier.[45] Someone—perhaps Calonne, who is reputed to have been the chief draftsman—enjoyed writing that harangue, and Louis XV probably enjoyed himself delivering it; in the short term it produced some effect, partly because it was coupled with relatively lenient treatment of the opposition. It remained a major strategic error for the monarch to be drawn into an uncompromising declaration of absolutism, when this subverted many of the unstated assumptions on which government actually worked.

The 'Maupeou revolution' of 1771–4 was just the most dramatic example of a growing tendency for the Crown to resort to arbitrary methods, in order to break out of the multiple restraints on its power. The humiliations of the Seven Years War clearly played a major role in persuading ministers and others that a major effort for rational reform was needed. Unfortunately much of this necessarily took the form of an attack on privileges, when nearly all holders of wealth and power saw such inherited rights as the only restraint on ministerial despotism. The 'coercive liberalization' offered even by reforming ministers was also seen by many as part of a wider European trend towards authoritarian government, exemplified by Frederick the Great, Struensee, Gustavus III, and others, but most clearly incarnated by Maupeou and Terray.[46] Among the disastrous results of the royal *coup* of 1771, furthermore, was the disillusionment of those who backed the Crown, with whatever reservations, only to be disavowed and humiliated three years later. Many others concluded that fundamental constitutional change was the only way forward, like those Parisian barristers who now modelled themselves on the ancient Romans, and missed few opportunities to parade their principles.[47] Further

---

[44] Rogister, *Louis XV*; J. Swann, *Politics and the Parlement of Paris under Louis XV, 1754–1774* (Cambridge, 1995).

[45] Flammermont, *Remontrances*, ii. 554–60 (3 Mar. 1766).

[46] D. Echeverria, *The Maupeou Revolution: A Study in the History of Libertarianism. France 1770–1774* (1985), 63–4. For coercive liberalization, see D. Gordon, *Citizens without Sovereignty: Equality and Sociability in French Thought, 1670–1789* (Princeton, 1994), 209–12.

[47] Swann, *Politics*, 367–8; Bell, *Lawyers*, 202–10.

evidence for the way the government had boxed itself into a corner can be found in the various writings that supported its position. Some of these were astonishingly inept restatements of divine right absolutism, while others found it necessary to fight on the dangerous ground of Frankish history. Among the problems that might arise from an excessively thorough probing of the past was that of justifying the changes of dynasty; although the usurpations of Pepin le Bref and Hugues Capet could be seen as partly validated by their desire to restore the original order of the state, such notions had their own unwelcome implications.

One reforming minister, Bertin, sponsored the curious figure of Jacob-Nicolas Moreau, a known enemy of the *philosophes* who now built up a great arsenal of documents to defend royal claims, while publishing prolific but often maladroit works on French history. Moreau asserted that 'the despotism of our first kings came from the marshes of Germany. It was in Gaul that our ancestors discovered liberty, beyond the Rhine they had known only despotism or licence.'[48] This was all part of an attempt to demonstrate that absolute power was the true protection for personal liberty, and that all France's problems in the past had been the result of petty noble tyrants usurping royal authority. The more stridently such views were expressed, the more they encouraged opponents to controvert them, in an argument that could never be settled by scholarly means, even had the disputants tried harder to be impartial. A largely illusory ancient constitution had become an important symbol of the demands of the emerging political nation, and the Germanic liberties would be one of the most powerful themes of the pamphlets of 1787–9. They are part of that strange medley of disparate ideas that contributed to the revolutionary crisis, although it would be rash to attribute too grand a causal role to them. Their own metaphorical role was twofold. First, they provided a respectable historical cover for the central issue of French political life from Louis XI (execrated by the great majority of commentators as a tyrant, sometimes as the French Nero) to Louis XVI; where did one find the boundary between legitimate kingship and despotism?[49] Secondly, they fostered a liberalism that actually emerged from ideas of privilege, and that could temporarily reunite a nation so long divided by more or less deliberate royal policies.[50]

[48] D. Gembicki, *Histoire et politique à la fin de l'ancien régime: Jacob-Nicolas Moreau (1717–1803)* (Paris, 1979), 275; see also K. M. Baker, 'Controlling French History: the Ideological Arsenal of Jacob-Nicolas Moreau', in his *Inventing the French Revolution: Essays on French Political Culture in the Eighteenth Century* (Cambridge, 1990), 59–85.

[49] For Louis XI, see A. Bakos, *Images of Kingship in Early Modern France: Louis XI in Political Thought, 1560–1789* (1997).

[50] D. Richet, 'Autour des origines idéologiques lointaines de la Révolution française: Élites et despotisme', *Annales ESC*, 24 (1969), 1–23.

IV

One writer who played with such themes was Louis-Sébastien Mercier, that indefatigable scribbler who was best known for his subversive *L'An 2440, rêve s'il en fut jamais* (1771). This curious utopia in the style of the *philosophes* results from the act of a king who voluntarily relinquished absolute power, possibly an oblique reference to Charlemagne. Mercier's journalistic connections won him some favour with Marie Antoinette, not necessarily the way to her husband's approval.[51] He picked up the mood of the moment, greeting the ascension of Louis XVI by going back instead of forward with an excruciating play entitled *Childeric*. In this the hero is a despotic king (the father of Clovis) who incurs the just indignation of a free people, and is duly deposed by his Frankish warriors. He then goes on his travels to undergo the philosophical amendment that will render him worthy of the crown, and returns to be reinstated. Childeric addresses his restored subjects with an oath 'to respect the liberty of the fatherland, to defend it, to be the chief of warriors and the vigilant eye of the laws, while being the first to submit myself to their inviolable authority, because when one has the misfortune of total power, one has no more shame in daring to do anything'.[52] Whatever Louis XVI made of this bizarre lesson in kingship, he did restore the *parlement*, provoking Maupeou to grumble that after he had won a conflict that had been going on for 300 years the king wanted to lose it again. A more plausible view would be that the kind of overt ministerial despotism embodied by the Chancellor had been a disaster. Crucially, the Maupeou revolution had demonstrated that the Crown did not accept the legitimacy of any other power in the state; as far as the kings were concerned, the ancient constitution was indeed a dusty myth, to be brushed aside at will.

After this episode even the *parlement* of Paris, itself much cowed by its experience, was inclined to look to the Estates General as the only hope for constitutional reform. Such a meeting might, it was hoped, allow a benevolent king to strike a new contract with the nation, emulating the great restoration of Frankish liberties by Charlemagne. One of the most percipient of all the political writers of the time, Mably, was sceptical of this possibility, noting how many of the vested interests created by the Crown itself would now oppose such a reforming king, who was in any case a rare creature seen only three or four times in the history of the world. He also considered that the *parlement* had been a totally inadequate defender of liberty, and that its historical pretensions were false; the only remedy for the vices of French government was the restoration of the Estates General, 'not as they actually

---

[51] N. R. Gelbart, *Feminine and Opposition Journalism in Old Regime France: The Journal des Dames* (Berkeley and Los Angeles, 1987), 196–8, 213–21.
[52] L.-S. Mercier, *Childeric premier, roi de France* (1774), 79.

were, but as they should have been'. His vision of the absolute monarchy as an innovation included a comparison of the great Ordinances of 1355–7 to Magna Carta, but unlike the English the French had followed the way of royal power rather than that of liberty.[53] Louis XVI was so alarmed at the news of the imminent publication of Mably's *Observations sur l'histoire de France* in October 1788 that he wrote in his own hand: 'I know that an incendiary and dangerous work has been brought into my kingdom. I order you to use every means to prevent its receiving any publicity.'[54]

This reaction was more evidence for the instinctive authoritarianism that would repeatedly wreck the king's political chances, even if he and Calonne thought that they were attempting a true recasting of the state in 1786–7, when the eagerly awaited Assembly of Notables proved a fiasco. This episode confirmed both that the ministers and their advisers were dimly aware of the need to find a new way of legitimating royal authority, and that they would cling tenaciously to all their old powers in a self-defeating fashion. In this twilight period of half-hearted reform the various plans for provincial or other assemblies also betrayed the government's unease, at the same time as they displayed a familiar refusal to envisage any genuine devolution of power. The real objective, apparent to everyone, was the creation of docile and easily controlled bodies, intended to aid the Crown in fleecing its subjects more efficiently. This type of blinkered thinking was all too evident in the disastrous attempt of May 1788 to create a *cour plenière* to take over the review functions of the *parlement*. Government claims that this was a revival of the ancient Curia Regis cut little ice against the 'general outcry' described by Besenval, who noted how the plan 'was seen as a despotic idea, a veil intended to cover up tyranny'.[55] In the face of such provocative ineptitude, which we should perhaps see as stemming from the Crown's own central myth of indispensability, tales about lost liberties were bound to prove attractive, however flimsy their historical basis. No doubt they were less important than notions about classical republican virtues, or about the potential application of scientific method, both of which were being widely inculcated by the educational system.[56] Nevertheless, the powerful image of a free nation that had fallen into a kind of slavery played its part in undermining the legitimacy of a monarchy whose ancestry had once been traced back to Pharamond or even the legendary Trojan Francion, on whom Fréret had rashly poured his bucket of cold water. In this fashion some of the paths to civil society were opened

[53] G. Bonnot de Mably, *Œuvres complètes* (15 vols.; Paris, 1794–5), iii. 302–3; J. K. Wright, *A Classical Republican in Eighteenth Century France: The Political Thought of Mably* (Stanford, Calif., 1997), 152–3.

[54] B. Grosperrin, *La Répresentation de l'histoire de France dans l'historiographie des Lumières* (2 vols.; Lille, 1982), 186.

[55] Carcassonne, *Montesquieu*, 577.

[56] L. W. B. Brockliss, *French Higher Education in the Seventeenth and Eighteenth Centuries: A Cultural History* (Oxford, 1987).

up by an ingenious vision of the primitive virtues of the ancestors, exponents of a virile style of citizenship whose revival was widely seen as the only hope for escape from servitude. There was no real difference between the values attributed to the Germanic invaders and those of republican Rome, as glorified in David's *Oath of the Horatii*, so that they could readily combine in an unusual yet potent form of civil history as political critique.

14

Music, Reason, and Politeness: Magic and Witchcraft in the Career of George Frideric Handel

IAN BOSTRIDGE

If there was an Age of Enlightenment in the eighteenth century, then the naturalized Englishman George Frideric Handel—baptized Georg Friederich Händel—was one of its ornaments, quite literally. The famous marble of the composer by Louis François Roubiliac, now in the Victoria and Albert Museum, shows him as the apotheosis of laid-back civility. No wild-eyed creator of transcendent sounds, he is presented instead as an urbane genius, the calm strummer of soothing harmonies, playing on Orpheus' lyre, a cupid at his feet, in a state of emphatic relaxation. Lounging wigless in cap, loose clothes, and half-relinquished slippers, his elbow rests on a pile of musical scores.[1] The statue, the first public statue of a British artist, was intended for Vauxhall Pleasure Gardens, a 'Scene . . . of the most rational, elegant, and innocent kind'.[2]

Rationality and elegance were at the heart of eighteenth-century culture—in literature, in architecture, in garden design, and in music too. Those polite ideals had, inevitably, a political complexion, and political uses. They were vital players in the Whig project to lower the temperature of English politics and to reconfigure the frontiers of the sacred and the secular in public life. Changes in attitudes to witchcraft—an amphibious crime, a diabolical felony, grounded in religious conceptions of the Reformation state—were part of this process. This essay looks at the theme of enchantment, both in discussions about Handel and in Handel's works themselves, to investigate how, as public figure and as composer, he fitted into the Whig project. If the marble Handel was a symbol of the reign of reason and elegance, in what ways did the flesh-and-blood Handel engage with the new politics of politeness?

---

[1] On the Roubiliac marble, see D. Bindman, 'Roubiliac's Statue of Handel and the keeping of Order in Vauxhall Gardens in the Early Eighteenth Century', *Sculpture Journal*, 1 (1997), 22–31.

[2] J. Brewer, *The Pleasures of the Imagination: English Culture in the Eighteenth Century* (1997), 376; J. Lockman, *A Sketch of Spring-Gardens, Vaux-Hall, In a Letter to a Noble Lord* (1752), 28.

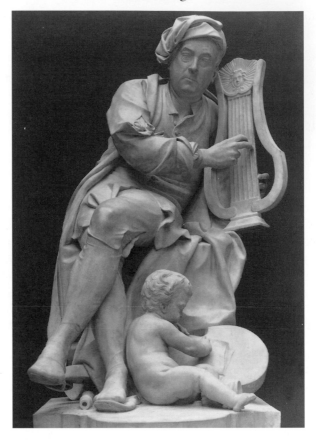

9. George Frideric Handel by Louis François Roubiliac, 1738

The flesh-and-blood Handel was born into a very different world from his marble effigy, in 1685. He enrolled as a student at his home university of Halle (nicknamed Hölle, or hell) on 10 February 1702, most likely as a law student.[3] Here in Halle one of the last great debates on the reality of witchcraft and of magic was conducted, at much the same time as the young Handel was studying. It started with a moderately sceptical inaugural disputation in October 1701,[4] swiftly followed by Christian Thomasius's notorious and thoroughly sceptical *De crimine magiae*, which opened the floodgates to furious controversy, drawing in university officials, theologians, lawyers, judges, and pastors.[5] It was here that the work of the English sceptic John Webster

[3] D. Burrows, *Handel* (Oxford, 1994), 9–10.
[4] Felix Braehm, 'De Fallicibus Iudiciis Magiae', 22 Oct. 1701.
[5] Christian Thomasius, *Dissertatione de crimine magiae* (Halle, 1701).

was first published in German in 1719; and an acceptable thesis for the law doctorate at Halle, as late as 1700, had catalogued the different species of apparitions sent by Satan to buffet and injure mankind.[6]

Handel himself, with pastors on his mother's side of the family, was a Lutheran conformist, taking communion at the *Marktkirche* for the first time in April 1701. If he was indeed a lawyer, he would have been taught by Thomasius, and he did manifest early on a Thomasian penchant for religious tolerance, deciding to take up a post as organist at the reformed, Calvinist cathedral in Halle.[7] Whatever his own views, he was raised in a world yet to be disenchanted, in which the power of magic remained a contentious business, not a hackneyed superstition.

In 1706 Handel went south—to Venice, Florence, Rome, Naples. Away from 'the cold, primitive lands where the people have nothing to do and no means of amusing themselves, where they drink beer and milk,' to the land of orange blossom, 'a civilized country with an agreeable climate'. These are the words of an Italian contemporary of Handel's, the scholar Girolamo Tartarotti of Rovereto, in the Venetian Republic. But civilized, agreeable Italy was free neither from learned nor judicial superstition, neither while Handel was there (a number of witches were executed in the year he left, 1709) nor when Tartarotti wrote his *On the Nocturnal Gatherings of Witches*, published in 1749.[8]

Tartarotti's book was the occasion of another one of those learned debates about magic and witchcraft that indicate that the Enlightenment was not so simple. This was not only because Tartarotti raised a storm of protest from theologians and others who wanted, in the middle of the eighteenth century, to maintain the reality of witches, satanic pact and all. From the other camp, fellow illuminati accused Tartarotti of not going far enough; for, while banishing the old wives' tales of hags and midnight sabbaths, he had main-

---

[6] John Webster, *Untersuchung der vermeinten und sogenannten Hexereyen* (Halle, 1719); Andreas Becker, *Disputatio Judica de Jure Spectrorum* (Halle, 1700).

[7] W. Braun, 'Beiträge zu G. F. Händels Jugendzeit in Halle (1685–1703)', *Wissenschaftliche Zeitschrift der Martin-Luther-Universität Halle-Wittenberg*, 8/4 (1959), 851–62. Thomasius was teaching in the law faculty in the summer semester of 1702 and the winter of 1702–3, during Handel's time at the university. John Hawkins, who knew Handel, records that the mature composer, based in London, though 'of the Lutheran profession . . . was not such a bigot as to decline a general conformity with that of the country which he had chosen for his residence'. Indeed Handel was naturalized in 1727, a process that required religious conformity. Handel 'would often speak of it as one of the great felicities of his life that he was settled in a country where no man suffers any molestation or inconvenience on account of his religious principles', an optimistically Whiggish view (John Hawkins, *A General History of the Science and Practice of Music* (5 vols., 1776; 1853 edn. in 2 vols.), ii. 911).

[8] G. Tartarotti, *Del congresso notturno delle lammie libri tre . . . S'aggiungono due dissertazioni epistolari sopra l'arte magica* (Rovereto, 1749). On Tartarotti, see F. Venturi, 'Enlightenment versus the Powers of Darkness', in Venturi, *Italy and the Enlightenment: Studies in a Cosmopolitan Century* (1972), 103–33, quotation from Tartarotti at 108.

tained the reality of magical operations, of spirits and of magi.[9] This is an important distinction—between what was known as 'modern' witchcraft, the supposed practice of impoverished and malicious old women in out-of-the-way villages, and the old-fashioned sorcery of the highborn, of learned philosophers or scheming damsels, John Dee at the court of Queen Elizabeth or Elizabeth's own mother, Anne Boleyn, at her father's court. It is the latter sort of love magic in which Alcina, denizen of the Renaissance imaginings of Ariosto, eponymous enchantress of Handel's spectacle of an opera, was immersed; utterly different from the nefarious practices of the choppy-fingered witch of Endor, who plays a cameo part in another work Handel wrote in the 1730s, the oratorio *Saul*.

On 21 June 1749 Maria Renata Singerin was beheaded as a witch at Würzburg. Much to Tartarotti's horror, she had been convicted of having had carnal relations with the devil from childhood to the age of 73. Her body was burnt while a Jesuit railed against those 'people in our age who do not believe in witches or magicians, nor in the devil, nor even in God himself'. The debate over witchcraft remained muddy, as some accused Tartarotti of insufficient daring in countering superstition; of having, in effect, weakened his argument against witchcraft by refusing to dismiss the possibility of magic. Tartarotti himself remained convinced that those who dismissed magic altogether were dangerous extremists who rejected the supernatural and risked alienating ordinary God-fearing folk.[10] It is well worth remembering, if we want to understand the world in and for which Handel wrote, that even the *Encyclopédie*, fount of enlightened righteousness, did not, in its article on sorcerers, deny the reality of magic. 'To believe all these stories, or to reject them absolutely—these are two equally dangerous extremes.'[11]

The London that Handel visited in 1710–11 and where he settled in 1712 was far from an oasis of politeness or the politics of reason. He arrived, on the contrary, at the height of the 'rage of party' and the furious struggle between Whigs and Tories for the control of the Queen's government. In the midst of all this there occurred a most notorious witchcraft case: not the last execution (that had been in 1685, the year of Handel's birth), but the last conviction in England, of one Jane Wenham, a spinster of Walkern in Hertfordshire, and a media event at that. 'Thousands of people flock'd in from all Parts of the Country to see her in Gaol; but when she came to her Tryal, so vast a Number of People have not been together at the Assizes in the memory of Man.'[12]

---

[9] Tartarotti, *Del congresso* in Venturi, 108.   [10] Ibid.

[11] 'Ajouter foi trop légèrement à tout ce qu'on raconte en ce genre, & rejetter absolument tout ce qu'on en dit, sont deux extrêmes également dangereux' (Denis Diderot et al., *Encyclopédie* (Neufchâtel, 1765), xv, entry under *sorciers*). This entry was probably by Diderot himself.

[12] *An Account of the Tryal, Examination and Condemnation of Jane Wenham* (1712), BL 515.1.6 (28).

Pardoned at the instance of the assize judge, she was the occasion for a furious political storm in which a Tory pamphleteer, Francis Bragge, used Wenham's guilt and the reality of witchcraft as a rallying cry for disaffected traditionalists, 'highfliers', with their theme of 'the church in danger'. Against Bragge was ranged a variety of Whig and Whiggish writers, more or less progressive, more or less sceptical of the possibility of witchcraft, but all convinced of Wenham's innocence. Not long afterwards, the Tories were definitively routed, the Whigs ascendant with George I on the throne in 1714, and the Tory party and its ideology damned by its supposed association with the failed Jacobite revolt of 1715. Witchcraft, before the Wenham trial, had been a marginal but moderately sensible belief, something a down-to-earth hack journalist like Daniel Defoe could safely espouse in a 1711 article in his *Review*. Now it was laughed out of existence as just the sort of crazy thing you would expect Tories—those beaten, fanatical, unfashionable, and excluded Tories— to believe. And so it remained right up to the repeal of the laws against witchcraft in 1736.[13]

A long-standing belief like that in witchcraft was not, however, so easily to be hooted out of the world. In England, lynchings of suspected witches continued to be reported throughout the eighteenth century, into the nineteenth and beyond. Moreover, at the fringes of the lower clergy, among dissatisfied priests or Methodist preachers, the polite world's rejection of traditional witchcraft beliefs was a source of disquiet. Giving up witchcraft is giving up the Bible, thought John Wesley. In the polite world itself, some remained confused, like Boswell's Dr Johnson: 'He did not affirm anything positively upon a subject which it is the fashion of the times to laugh at as a matter of absurd credulity. He only seemed willing, as a candid enquirer after truth, however strange and inexplicable, to shew that he understood what might be urged for it.'[14]

Beyond this marginal existence at the fringes of intellectual life, the language of witchcraft cropped up in new areas of social existence, becoming increasingly a metaphor but retaining nevertheless some element of literal force that it is difficult to quantify. Witchcraft lurked beneath the polite veneer of Handel's London. When, in a sermon of 1723, Bishop Gibson of London complained of 'Loose and Atheistical Assemblies', fashionable masquerades whose sexual and social licence enlarged 'the Empire of Sin and Satan upon earth', we are not quite clear how literal he was being, especially since another

---

[13] For the ideological history of witchcraft in this period see I. Bostridge, *Witchcraft and its Transformations c.1650–c.1750* (Oxford, 1997): 109–32 and 136–8 on Defoe; 132–6 on Wenham; 155–70 on highflying.

[14] See Henry Moore, *The Life of the Reverend John Wesley* (Leeds, 1825), 323; also John Wesley, *The Journal of Rev. John Wesley* (4 vols.; 1906), iii. 412, entry for 4 July 1770; James Boswell, *Boswell's Life of Johnson. Together with Boswell's Journal of a Tour to the Hebrides and Johnson's Diary of A Journey into North Wales*, ed. G. B. Hill and L. F. Powell (6 vols.; Oxford, 1934), v. 178–9. Wesley's and Johnson's Tory, even Jacobitical, roots are noteworthy here.

critic of 1724 spoke of masqueraders 'entering into a League with the World, the Flesh and the Devil'. Masquerades, masked balls at which classes and sexes mixed in promiscuous anonymity, were organized by Handel's partner, the Swiss impresario Heidegger, and he too was condemned, with more obviously satirical intent, as one of Satan's first ministers for being 'so wicked to let in the Devil'.[15]

The line between the literal and the metaphorical is difficult to draw in a period like this, when categories of truth and fiction (as in Defoe's narratives), or the boundaries between the natural and the supernatural, are being redrawn. This is certainly striking in Hogarth's satirical print, the bogus *Masquerade Ticket*. One element of the picture is thoroughly literal, though also apparently disengaged from any belief in witchcraft proper—the fancy-dress witch in the foreground. But another portion points towards the threat of diabolism at work in a new social arena—what appears to be a picture of a witches' sabbath, which presides, brooding, at the back of the assembly hall. As Daniel Defoe had it, if you cannot find witches at work in villages any more, turning the milk sour or making children cough up rusty old nails, that is because the Devil has found new places to make his influence felt. He goes to the masquerade; he works in the City, with its stockjobbers and diabolical money worship, as in Hogarth's *Emblematical Print on the South Sea Scheme*; he presides as the genius of Walpole's diabolical party politics in Defoe's *Political History of the Devil*; and, in another Hogarth print of 1724, he is in the market for masquerades and operas.[16]

Witchcraft *was* at the opera, of course, in the form of Italian 'magic' operas, five of which Handel wrote in the course of his London career: *Rinaldo* (1711), *Teseo* (1712), *Amadigi* (1715), and, in a second burst, *Orlando* (1733) and *Alcina* (1735).[17] Apart from the magical machinery that such entertainments involved, music itself was associated with enchantment. This was a theme with which Handel's contemporaries often played, in conversation and printed satire. In 1735, for example, Mrs Pendarves wrote to her mother, Mrs Mary Glanville, describing a rehearsal of Handel's latest magic opera, *Alcina*: 'Whilst Mr Handel was playing his part, I could not help thinking him a necromancer in the midst of his own enchantments.'[18] This is standard stuff, comparable to Handel's Orpheus-like pose on the Roubiliac monument.

---

[15] Edmund Gibson, *A Sermon Preached to the Societies for the Reformation of Manners* (1723), 19, 5; *Of Plays and Masquerades* (1719), 28; 'A Strange and Wonderfull Relation how the Devill Appeared last night At the Masquerade in the Hay-Market' (?1718), in P. J. Croft, *Autograph Poetry in the English Language* (1973), i. 64–7.

[16] *Hogarth's Graphic Works*, ed. R. Paulson (3rd rev. edn., 1989), plate 113, cat. 109, and plate 12, cat. 10; Daniel Defoe, *The Political History of the Devil* (1726), 388–9. For a fuller account of the afterlife of witchcraft theory and its metaphors, see Bostridge, *Witchcraft*, chs. 6–8.

[17] On these, see W. Dean, *Handel and the Opera Seria* (Oxford, 1970).

[18] 12 Apr. 1735, printed in O. E. Deutsch, *Handel: A Documentary Biography* (1955).

More difficult to understand, in its dogged insistence on the witchcraft metaphor, is a satire of 1734 from the *Daily Post*, entitled 'Harmony in an Uproar'. A satirical attack on Handel, it was evidently written by a Handelian unhappy with spiteful opposition to the composer's dominance of the London music scene. 'You are charg'd', he writes, 'with having bewitch'd us for the Space of twenty Years past; nor do we know where your Inchantments will end, if a timely Stop is not put to them.' The standard comparison to Orpheus or Apollo is, however, given a diabolical twist:

nothing was ever looked upon more proper to carry on Inchantments by than Harmony; it was always made use of by Antients and Moderns upon such Occasions, at all solemn Sacrifices, Invocations of Ghosts or Devils, calling up Spirits from the Earth, or down from the Air, Musick was held the only Lure to entice them; nay Belzebub himself has a great Command that Way, and constantly entertains his Votaries at their Installations, Festivals, and Nocturnal Meetings, with Operas, Symphonies, Voluntaries, and Madrigals in the Air, and I fear, Sir, has but too often lent a helping Hand to you.

The satire pushes conspiracy theories about the German-born court favourite to a ridiculous diabolical extreme:

If at any Time the Magick of your Opera lost its Force, by being too often us'd, away went the D-l and you to work in a Vizard, to hide your evil Designs, and then out comes an Oratorio, or a Serenata; and just as we had begun to recover our Senses, all of a sudden we run as mad as ever; and hoity toity, away went we, like so many Witches on Broomsticks and Hobby-Horses, to the Prince of Darkness's Midnight Revels. If this is not downright Witchcraft, I never knew a Conjuror in my Life.[19]

More than mere professional envy at the sheer diversity and appeal of Handel's work, there is a hint here that his highly successful religious oratorios are a blind for theatrical diabolism, a way of insinuating the carnivalesque revelry of the operatic stage into religious devotion. It had been Handel's *Esther; an Oratorio or Sacred Drama* that had brought the new hybrid form before the London public. One contemporary called that work an 'oratoria or religious opera', and the new form certainly opened up possibilities for mingling edification and entertainment, and a long tradition of using theatre performers within a religious framework.[20]

Anxiety about this mixing of the sacred and profane reached its peak with the *Messiah*, but it must have been uncomfortable for some religious spectators from its very outset, given the continuing currency of notions of the theatre as diabolical in itself. An example is Arthur Bedford's tract of 1719,

---

[19] Published in the *Daily Journal*, 18 Mar. 1734, and reprinted in *Händel-Handbuch: Dokumente zu Leben und Schaffen*, iv (1985), 230, 233.

[20] A. Hicks, 'Handel and the Idea of an Oratorio', in *The Cambridge Companion to Handel*, ed. D. Burrows (Cambridge, 1997), 145–63, citing Viscount Percival at 152. See also the classic account of Handel's oratorios, W. Dean, *Handel's Dramatic Oratorios and Masques* (Oxford, 1959).

A Serious Remonstrance In Behalf of the Christian Religion, Against The Horrid Blasphemies and Impieties which are still used in the English Play-Houses, to the great Dishonour of Almighty God, and in Contempt of the Statutes of this Realm. Shewing their plain Tendency to overthrow all Piety, and advance the Interest and Honour of the Devil in the World. For Bedford, with his epigraph that 'to compliment Vice is but one remove from Worshipping the Devil', one of the evils of the theatre was to 'encourage . . . Witchcraft and Magick' by representing them on the stage, just as in all Handel's magic operas performed in London, from *Rinaldo* in 1711 to *Alcina* in 1735:

> Another Method, made use of at the Play-Houses, is to entertain their Followers with magical Representations, conjuring, or consulting the Devil. This surely can be no great Diversion, at least no proper one for *Christians*, and may be apt to fill the Heads of raw and ignorant Persons with false and dangerous Notions, as if the Devil's Power and Knowledge was much greater than it is; insomuch that they may come in time to think it their Interest to be upon good Terms with him; as we hear of many in our own Country, who have been so wicked, as to make Compacts with him, and as some of the Indians are said to worship him for fear lest he Should hurt them: and thus the Worship of God is of course laid aside, and all hope of his Favour and Blessing is renounced and forfeited.

This is a very serious matter for Bedford, who cautions those 'tempted to go to the Play-house, [to] consider your Baptismal Vow'. 'Such Places and Entertainments as these', he concludes, 'must be a disservice to our King, our Church, and our Constitution.'[21]

   Opera was viewed in itself as diabolical in the same way. The mixed genre of oratorio was, perhaps, even worse. The satirist of 'Harmony in an Uproar' is well aware of the accusations, and ridicules them while at the same time praising Handel's skill: 'It has in many Particulars been made manifest to the religious Part of your Audiences, that for these twenty Years past (as was well observed in your Trial) you have practis'd Sorcery in this Kingdom upon his Majesty's Liege Subjects, and often bewitched every Sense we have.'[22] The 'religious Part of your Audiences' seems very much like ironic code for the backswoodsmen and bigots who after the secured Hanoverian succession of 1714 were lumped together as disaffected to the regime. After the 1715 revolt, in the writings both of Whig churchmen and freethinkers, belief in witchcraft came to be seen as the prerogative of such superstitious stick-in-the muds, the sort who believed equally in the Royal Touch or the Royal Martyr of 1649. In such writings, the real 'crime' of witchcraft, that condemned in the Bible, was divorced from modern-day pacts with the Devil and the felonies of the Elizabethan and Jacobean legislation, coming to be seen instead as

---

[21] Arthur Bedford, *A Serious Remonstrance* (1719), ch. III (heading), 9, 377–8.
[22] *Händel-Handbuch*, iv. 233.

superstition itself, rebellion, and, by extension, the growth in faction that accompanied the development of party government.[23]

Handel had already been used, by the opposition, as a proxy for Walpole's administration. At the height of the Excise Crisis, on 7 April 1733, an issue of the most prominent opposition publication, the *Craftsman*, attacked Walpole via Handel. It is quite clear in that piece that, for Handel's opera management, the reader should understand Walpole's management of state, and, for oratorio, a controversial new entertainment with controversially high ticket prices, he should understand the excise, a more than controversial new tax.[24] 'Harmony in an Uproar', then, is best interpreted as a reply to the *Craftsman*, from a friend of Handel's and, it would seem, an adherent of the regime. The running joke about witchcraft is part of a whole tradition in which church-in-danger opposition to the Whig regime was portrayed as old-fashioned superstition.[25] Another joke is specifically directed against the Patriot opposition. Their table-turning claims that Walpole's Whigs were attacking liberty, the traditional preserve of Whig ideology ever since the Glorious Revolution, are reduced to the absurd accusation that Handel is 'threatning us with an entire Destruction of Liberty, and an absolute Tyranny in your Person over the whole Territory of the Haymarket'. But, to return to the climax of the witchcraft joke: 'And if the Statute for burning Witches and Wizards was in full Force, I know who should soon be whipp'd into the Middle of a Bonefire of his own Works, and like a Swan die to some Tune.'[26] The statute was, of course, no longer 'in full Force'; it remained on the statute book, only to be repealed some two years later, in 1736.

Music was part of the political process in eighteenth-century England. Not only did Handel encounter, as Ruth Smith puts it, 'a strong tradition of political allusion in music theatre works';[27] the front of house was an important arena for social display and political posturing. 'It is requisite', opined the *Weekly Journal* in 1725, that 'every one, who has the Pleasure of thinking himself a fine Gentleman, should, being first laden with a Competency of Powder and Essence, make his personal Appearance every Opera Night at the Haymarket'.[28] This was partly a matter of social display, but it was also an intensely political concern, never more so than in the 1730s, when two rival

---

[23] See Bostridge, *Witchcraft*, 155–70.   [24] Reprinted in Deutsch, *Handel*, 310–13.
[25] See Bostridge, *Witchcraft*, 155–70.   [26] *Händel-Handbuch*, iv. 234.
[27] R. Smith, *Handel's Oratorios and 18th Century Thought* (Cambridge, 1995), 200. See also R. Strohm, 'Handel and his Italian Opera Texts', in Strohm, *Essays on Handel and Italian Opera* (Cambridge, 1985), 35: 'It is no secret, for example, that contemporary political events played an important part in determining the choice of an opera's subject. The question is how the artist translated such subjects, whether he played them down or accentuated them, removed or actually restored their topicality.'
[28] *Weekly Journal: or, Saturday's Post*, 18 Dec. 1725, quoted in W. Weber, 'Handel's London— Social, Political and Intellectual Contexts', in *The Cambridge Companion to Handel*, 47–8.

opera companies struggled for existence and for patronage. The Opera of the Nobility was a creature of the Prince of Wales, determined to pique his own sister and, ultimately, the King and his first minister. Lord Hervey described the effect of this opera war. It 'may seem a trifle', he wrote, but 'the effects of it were no trifles':

The King and Queen were as much in earnest upon this subject as their son and daughter . . . they were both Handelists . . . The affair grew as serious as that of the Greens and the Blues [chariot teams] under Justinian at Constantinople. An anti-Handelist was looked upon as an anti-courtier, and voting against the Court in Parliament was hardly a less remissible or venial sin than speaking against Handel or going to the Lincoln's Field Opera.

The Princess Royal expected 'in a little while to see half the House of Lords playing in the orchestra in their robes and coronets', while the King complained that 'he did not think setting oneself at the head of a faction of fiddlers a very honourable occupation for people of quality'.[29] If 'Harmony in an Uproar' shows us a public Handel, with his reputation a matter of partisan political debate, Hervey's account shows us that, beyond Grub Street, Handel as operatic icon was, in the 1730s, co-opted into the very highest of high politics as well. Given the political colouring of the operatic scene in the 1730s, is there anything to tie together Handel's work in the 1730s and the political maelstrom into which he was drawn?

The 1730s saw contentious religious issues—so disturbing during the rage of party, and which the post-1715 regime had kept out of politics—returning to the political arena. An alliance emerged between hitherto opposition Whigs and their ministerial colleagues, reacting against attempts to advance ecclesiastical influence on the part of Walpole's 'pope', Edmund Gibson, bishop of London. This Whig coalition was evident in the promotion of quintessentially Whiggish schemes concerning Quaker tithes, mortmain, and, around the same time, witchcraft. These were unambitious projects in many senses, but they redefined the relationship between secular and religious jurisdictions, and could usefully consolidate the Whig 'project', helping to focus a 'progressive' allegiance that could draw waverers back to the ministry, redefining the centre of political gravity.[30] Handel's last magic opera, *Alcina*, was a product of this period of Whig redefinition.

It is striking in the first place that Handel's magic operas—Italian operas, but with libretto books in English widely distributed—cluster in two groups into the years in which witchcraft was a matter for public debate: 1711–15, at the time of the rage of party, and the expulsion of witchcraft from polite discourse; and the 1730s, the years of Whig enlightenment and the repeal of the witchcraft legislation. *Orlando* (1733) is a return, as Donald Burrows writes,

---

[29] *Lord Hervey's Memoirs*, ed. R. Sedgwick (1963), 42–3.
[30] See Bostridge, *Witchcraft*, 180–4.

'to the sort of drama that Handel had developed 20 years before, involving a supernatural dimension and transformation scenes: this contrasts with the operas that had been his concern since the start of the Academy in which the characters, however much fired by jealousy or passion, generally behave rationally'.[31] In *Orlando*, the magician Zoroastro wishes to establish reason through magic; all the while, the commonsensical Dorinda 'has no use for his astrology, his flying geniuses, or stage-craft in producing enchanted palaces, temples, statues, magic rings and grottos'.[32] By the time of Handel's farewell to magic, *Alcina* (1735), the ideological point is much clearer, and magic is cast out by reason.

Handel was brought up in a world in which witchcraft and magic were still serious matters of debate; he moved to England at a period of heightened political tension in which witchcraft was one occasion of ideological dispute. He reached the height of his cultural, indeed political,[33] influence in the 1730s, when religious dispute flared up after a ten-year lull. Once again, the criminal law of witchcraft was part of this, however marginal: as a symbol of triumphant Reason, orderliness, and the unity of the Whig project, the old laws against witchcraft were repealed. As Rogero puts it in the English of the *Alcina* wordbook, 'my reason has subdu'd the Force | Of Foul Inchantment'. The triumph of rationality has its visual metaphor in this spectacular opera, 'an Urn rais'd in the Middle which incloses the whole Power of the Inchantment', which Rogero 'throws down and breaks', at which 'the Scene wholly disappears'.[34]

That scene disappeared for ever: Handel wrote no more magic operas.[35] Serious debate about witchcraft was finally expelled from polite discourse.

---

[31] In A. Holden (ed.), *The Viking Opera Guide* (1993), 435.

[32] R. Strohm, 'Comic Traditions in Handel's *Orlando*', in Strohm, *Essays*, 253.

[33] Handel's immersion in the political world was long-standing. The father was a member of the Hanoverian court; the son may well have acted as a Hanoverian agent in relaying news about the state of Queen Anne's health back to the Elector in the last year or so of her life: Burrows, *Handel*, 72–3.

[34] *The Librettos of Handel's Operas*, ed. E. T. Harris (1989), vii. 178, 201, 206.

[35] Handel's position from the late 1730s on became more complex. The texts and themes of his English oratorios show anti-deistical, even non-juring associations, religious in the partisan sense that 'Harmony in an Uproar' parodied, and a world away from Whig ideology. Handel's most prominent oratorio librettist, Charles Jennens, was indeed a non-juror, and his *Messiah* a specifically anti-deistical work, designed to underline the prophetic truth of the Old Testament. Jennens's comments on his working relationship with Handel in his letters to Edward Holdsworth are justly taken by Ruth Smith to suggest that Handel was, in some sense, being used: R. Smith, 'The Achievements of Charles Jennens, 1700–1773', *Music & Letters*, 70/2 (1989), 184. As a sophisticated musical entrepreneur, however, he was also, perhaps, using Jennens. The case of *Saul*, another Jennens libretto, is the most intriguing. Part III starts with the witch of Endor. There is a strong presumption that this could be read as an anti-Catholic text: Romanism was long associated with witchcraft in the pamphlet tradition, and Saul's descent into witchcraft was easily paralleled by James II's descent into Popery. On the other hand, the text of *Saul* was written at the time of the repeal of the witchcraft legislation or just after. Serious discussion of witchcraft theory, which briefly revived early in 1736, usually involved some discussion

The 'Reason' that achieved this, which we associate with the eighteenth century, which the governing élite embraced, and which foreigners admired, was not there to be discovered, but had to be constructed. Reason had to be created and fought for piecemeal. The system of thought that was being dismantled had immense resources and tremendous resilience. Its rhetoric was powerful, its partisans intelligent, its language enchanting. For the audiences of Handel's earlier magic operas, even for its composer, magic was not dead and buried. *Alcina* itself may have had its part to play in the process of enlightenment. The evil enchantress of 1735 might represent, not so much sorcery, as the enchantment that superstition itself could weave. When at the end of the opera Rogero smashes the 'infamous urn', a complex metaphor is at work. Alcina's magical realm, summoned from the power of the urn, active force of all the enchantment, disappears. In the world of the opera, the evil sorceress has been overcome; in the world of the composer, the spectacle of opera and the enchantment of music, the suspension of disbelief, has reached its preordained end. In the world of politics, in which eighteenth-century opera undoubtedly played, enlightenment has been achieved. A supernatural nightmare has been banished and human intellect restored.

To underline this ideological strain in the opera, we need only look at the finale. *Alcina* ends, as Handel operas typically do, with a brief and simple chorus performed by the principals:

> Who has redeem'd us from our senseless State,
> From Night's dark Horrors,
> And brought us back to Life and Liberty . . .
> Who has again reviv'd our Reason, and thrown off
> The Veil that cover'd us?
> After the bitter Torments past,
> Our Souls find Peace and smiling Joys at last . . .
> How blest this Day,
> That brings such Ease;
> And now forgetting what we bear,
> Our Hearts know nought but present Peace.[36]

Here is the tell-tale association of the expulsion of magic, the triumph of rationality, and the achievement of (social) peace. The keywords are those of Whig ideology: under the current dispensation reason is revived, the horrors of dark night are forgotten, liberty has been restored, and nothing but peace is known, peace and ease.

of the hermeneutics of the Endor incident, reality, or fraud. The treatment, in the earlier part of the oratorio, of conflict between a just son, Jonathan, and his envious father, Saul, might also have had an oppositional resonance in a decade in which the relations between the King and the Prince of Wales were profoundly troubled.

  [36] *Librettos of Handel's operas*, vii. 206.

Handel, as Whig emblem, did symbolize social peace. His music was viewed as an agent of social, even political harmony, an antidote to the divisiveness that the Hanoverian élite anathematized. Here is Handel's erstwhile librettist, Aaron Hill, in the 1730s:

> Teach us, undying Charmer, to compose
> Our inbred Storms, and 'scape impending Woes . . .
> And since thy Notes, can n'er, in vain implore!
> Bid 'em becalm unresting Faction o'er;
> Inspire Content, and Peace, in each proud Breast,
> Bid th'unwilling Land be blest.[37]

As for ease, we have seen that on display in Vauxhall Pleasure Gardens, and Handel with his slipper dangling off. The management of Vauxhall Pleasure Gardens 'thought it proper, that his Effigies should preside there, where his Harmony has so often charm'd even the greatest Crouds into the profoundest Calm and most decent behaviour . . . the whole composition is in a very elegant taste'.[38] In the course of the 1730s, Handel's music and public reputation were closely associated with the ambitions of the Whig ascendancy—with the rejection of highflying superstition, the cause of order, and the advancement of politeness and reason in government. Music was deeply implicated in the politics of politeness.

---

[37] Reprinted in Deutsch, *Handel*, 306–7. This ode was written 'on Occasion of Mr Handel's Great Te Deum at the Feast of the Sons of the Clergy', a feast at which the main protagonist of the church-in-danger crisis of Anne's reign, Henry Sacheverell, had preached, to highflying and divisive effect, in 1711. See also Daniel Prat, 'Ode to Mr Handel, on his Playing the Organ' (1722), reprinted in Deutsch, *Handel*, 139–44: 'See! DISCORD of her Rage disarm'd, / Relenting, calm, and bland as PEACE; / Ev'n restless noisy FACTION charm'd'.
[38] John Lockman in *Daily Post*, 18 Apr., 2 May 1738, cited in Bindman, 'Roubiliac's Statue', 28.

15

Wild Wales: Civilizing the Welsh from the Sixteenth to the Nineteenth Centuries

PRYS MORGAN

Edward Williams 'Iolo Morganwg' (1747–1826), antiquarian, mythologist, and inventor of the Gorsedd of Bards, whose birthplace lies just across the valley from the childhood home of Keith Thomas, said 'The Welsh, with their language, retain in its words and phrases . . . a tolerable history of their progress in arts, literary knowledge, and civilization. They are, I believe, the most tenacious, the Jews, perhaps, excepted, of ancient customs and usages and national peculiarities, of any civilized people in Europe, and the English the least so.'[1] Iolo also believed that the courtesy, civility, and cleanliness of his own native Vale of Glamorgan were superior to those of any part of Wales, a view generally shared by contemporary English travellers, describing it as 'rich and pleasing', in contrast to many other parts.[2] Iolo Morganwg's was a confident view of the superiority of Welsh culture at the time of Romanticism, when English sympathy for things Welsh rose to a high point. But the theme of this chapter is to show that in previous centuries the Welsh were considered wild and uncivil, and that, once the Romantic aura had been shattered in the second quarter of the nineteenth century, the image of barbarism and incivility returned.

Keith Thomas in his *Man and the Natural World* concentrates on the changing attitudes in England towards the natural world from 1500 to 1800, but, since the Welsh were the nearest neighbours, and inhabited the wilds, they were subject to the same changes of attitude as those towards beasts, plants, or landscape. The Welsh lived 'very beastly and rudely in respect of civility'.[3] Because the Welsh were housed under the same roof as their animals, their dwellings comically resembled Noah's Ark.[4] William Camden, who kept a

---

[1] National Library of Wales, NLW MS 13097B, fo. 207, quoted in G. H. Jenkins (ed.), *The Welsh Language before the Industrial Revolution* (Cardiff, 1997), 399.

[2] P. Jenkins, *The Making of a Ruling Class: The Glamorgan Gentry, 1640–1790* (Cambridge, 1983), 6.

[3] K. Thomas, *Man and the Natural World: Changing Attitudes in England 1500–1800* (1983), 94.

[4] W.R. (possibly W. Richards of Helmdon), *Wallography or the Briton Described* (1682), 110–11.

Welsh servant to tutor him in the language, admired in 1586 the fine buildings within the walls of Caernarfon, and the neatness and civility of the townspeople, but hated the rough and craggy landscape.[5] The urge to tame and
civilize Nature is paralleled in this period by plans to civilize the Welsh. The
underlying theme of *Man and the Natural World*, the pre-Romantic fear and
suspicion of the wilds being replaced by a Romantic admiration for all that
was close to Nature, can also be applied to the changing attitudes of the
English towards the Welsh.

This chapter is concerned only with the early modern period, but it goes
without saying that the English in the sixteenth century inherited a long tradition of defining themselves as a civilized people, superior to the neighbouring Welsh.[6] Even in the twelfth century Giraldus Cambrensis remarked
that the Welsh did not live like other peoples in towns or villages or castles,
but led a solitary existence deep in the woods. It was often observed that they
lived hardily, going barefoot and barelegged in the harshest weather, spoke a
barbaric language, and had their own peculiar laws and customs. Bringing
them into the fold of civilization was one justification for conquering them.
The question of military conquest did not arise in the sixteenth century, but
the image of the Welsh had not greatly changed.

The absorption of the Welsh into the English state system in the early sixteenth century was justified by English administrators such as Rowland Lee,
bishop of Lichfield, and President of the Council of Wales on the eve of the
Acts of Union (1536, 1543), on the grounds that the Welsh were murderous,
barbarous, thieving rogues, civility in the eyes of such men being equated
with law-abiding orderliness. Lee objected to Thomas Cromwell that John
Scudamore was unsuited to public office because he was a 'gentleman living
nigh the Welshry, and kindred and allied to the same'.[7] Some of the Welsh
were already desirous of being anglicized even before the Acts of Union:
William Jones of Newport directed in his will in 1529 that his children were
to be sent to Bristol to be 'browght up accordyng to the manerez and condi-
cionez of the norture of Inglonde'.[8] The gentry of mid- and north Wales were
considerably anglicized by frequenting such towns as Chester and Shrewsbury, but Lee (equating incivility, as so many did, with poverty) warned
Cromwell in March 1536 that it would be impossible to find Welsh gentlemen

---

[5] E. Gibson (ed.), Camden, *Britannia* (1696), 666, quoted in Thomas, *Man and the Natural World*, 258.

[6] For a recent account of medieval attitudes, R. R. Davies, 'The Peoples of Britain and Ireland, 1100–1400: i, Identities', *TRHS* 6th ser., 4 (1994), 1–20; R. R. Davies, 'The Peoples of Britain and Ireland, 1100–1400: ii. Names, Boundaries and Regnal Solidarities', ibid. 5 (1995), 1–20; R. R. Davies, 'The Peoples of Britain and Ireland, 1100–1400: iii, Laws and Customs', ibid. 6 (1996), 1–23.

[7] J. G. Jones (ed.), *Class, Community and Culture in Tudor Wales* (Cardiff, 1983), 7.

[8] PRO, Early Chancery Proceedings 831/60, quoted in E. A. Lewis, *Early Chancery Proceedings (Wales)* (Cardiff, 1937), 222.

suitable to be JPs, 'for there be very fewe Welshmen in Wales above Brecknock
that maye dispende ten pounde lande, and to say truthe, their discretion lesse
than their landes'.[9] The coming almost simultaneously of the Acts of Union
and the Henrician Reformation opened the threat (never realized) of a Welsh
Catholic reaction, which justified dignitaries, such as the reforming Bishop
Barlow of St David's, in using ecclesiastical revenues to establish English-lan-
guage grammar schools. Barlow told Cromwell in March 1538 that he intended
to establish one 'whereby God's honour preferred, the Welsh rudeness
decreasing, Christian civility may be introduced to the famous renown of the
King's supremacy'.[10] Barlow in August of that year wrote again to Cromwell
about his school: 'the Welshe rudeness wolde sone be framed to English cyvil-
itie and their corrupte capacyties easily reformed with godly intelligens'.[11] It
was notable that, at Ruthin School, the statutes encouraged Latin and Greek
in the upper forms by banning English, while encouraging English in the
lower forms by banning Welsh.[12] Welsh humanists and Anglicans created a
distinctive Anglican culture through the medium of Welsh, but others wished,
in the long term, to civilize the Welsh by introducing them to English ways
and manners through evangelizing them. The tradition continued into the
seventeenth century, as in 1622 John Brinsley the educational reformer hoped
to anglicize the Welsh, Irish, Virginians, and Bermudans, reducing them all
to 'a loving civility'.[13] The Puritan writers in the mid-seventeenth century,
however, still saw Wales as one of the dark corners of the land, the metaphor
of light and darkness having replaced the earlier ones of wildness and barbarism. John Lewis of Glasgrug, who tried to interpret the parliamentary propaganda to the Welsh during the Civil Wars, thought the Puritan tendency to
harp on about Welsh darkness and backwardness objectionable.[14]

The triumph of Protestantism and the advance of English were all very well,
but it was the good order coming as a result of the Acts of Union of 1536 and
1543 that seemed to be the greatest help in forwarding civility. This was the
view of outside observers such as William Gerard, who told Walsingham in
1576: 'At this daie it is to be affirmed, that in Wales vniversallie, are as civille
people and obedient to lawe, as are in England.'[15] Gerard in Ireland compared
that country with Wales, noting that Edward I had thought he had conquered

---

[9] Quoted by J. G. Jones, in G. H. Jenkins (ed.), *Welsh Language*, 181; also J. G. Jones (ed.),
Class, Community and Culture, 167.
[10] From T. Wright (ed.), *Three Chapters of Letters Relating to the Suppression of the Monasteries*
(1843), 184–5, quoted in T. Herbert and G. E. Jones, *Tudor Wales* (Cardiff, 1988), 120.
[11] PRO SP 1/ 113/ fo. 114, quoted by P. R. Roberts, in G. H. Jenkins (ed.), *Welsh Language*,
136.
[12] Quoted by W. P. Griffith, in G. H. Jenkins (ed.), *Welsh Language*, 298.
[13] J. G. Jones (ed.), *Class, Community and Culture*, 108.
[14] A. H. Dodd, *Studies in Stuart Wales* (Cardiff, 1952), 5: and for Puritanism in Wales in the
Interregnum, see G. H. Jenkins, *The Foundations of Modern Wales, 1642–1780* (Oxford, 1987),
43–86.
[15] Quoted in *Y Cymmrodor*, 13: 148–9.

Wales, but the 'Walshe disorders' continued until Henry VIII established justices itinerant 'by which travell onely I saye Walles was brought to knowe civilitie the same as in at this daye'.[16] It was even suggested to Lord Huntingdon
that he should use in the north of England the methods successfully employed
to pacify Wales.[17]

Gentry commentators of the period, such as Sir John Wynn, Rice Merrick,
and, above all, George Owen, made use of the word 'civility' in their praise
for the new order after the Acts of Union. They believed that the political confusion, the variety of legal systems, and the 'colonial' divisions of Welsh natives
and English settlers had prevented the Welsh from progressing towards
what they felt was a superior English civility. Owen, a Welsh-speaking
Pembrokeshire lawyer and landowner, particularly emphasized civility in his
'Dialogue of the Government of Wales' written in 1594. 'Butt sithence the
tyme of *H7* and *H8* that wee weare emanncipated as it weare and made free
to trade and trafficke through England, the gentlemenn and people in wales
have greatly encreased in learning and civilltye for nowe great numbres of
youthes are contynewally brought vpp and mayntayned at the Uniuersityes of
Oxford and Cambridge'.[18] Wales had even begun to look more like a civil
country because its houses now flourished instead of being burned down once
a year, as used to happen in lawless times.[19] Barthol, Owen's imaginary inter-
locutor in 'The Dialogue', noted that it was the new laws brought in under
Henry VIII that had caused this revolution—'surely these lawes have brought
Wales to great Civilitie from yt evill government that was here in ould
time'[20]—but also noted that not all parts of Wales shared this new civility
equally, Pembrokeshire being specially blessed as a 'happy Cyvill country',
being 'mere Englishe', where the towns closely resembled English towns.
Tenby's people were 'so full of courtesy and kyndnesse', Pembroke's people
'very cyvill and orderly', and Haverfordwest had such 'very civil people I could
not imagine that I was then in Wales'.[21] Owen in another work recognized
that the men of the south looked down on the Welsh of the north of the
county as 'mountain men'.[22] He contrasts the way in which gentlemen dine
frequently together in a courteous way in inns and taverns in the highly developed parts of Wales, with the pockets of banditry still surviving in remote wild
areas on the borders of Radnorshire and Cardiganshire.[23] Owen's desciptions
of the people of other Welsh counties could be unflattering, most being
described as 'unruly', or quarrelsome and given to legal disputes, the only ones

---

[16] Quoted by R. Suggett, in G. H. Jenkins (ed.), *Welsh Language*, 153.
[17] G. Williams, *Recovery, Reorientation and Reformation: Wales, c.1415–1642* (Oxford, 1987),
356–7.
[18] H. Owen (ed.), *The Description of Pembrokshire*, iii (1906), 1–119, esp. 56. The 'Dialogue',
which is printed as part of Owen's collected works, is an imaginary conversation between a
Pembrokeshire man, obviously George Owen, and a German lawyer called Barthol.
[19] Ibid. 57.   [20] Ibid. 91.   [21] Ibid. 16.   [22] Ibid. i (1892), 41–4.
[23] Ibid. iii. 98, for dining together, and iii. 92–3 for the mid-Wales brigands.

who were 'veary ciuile withall' being the inhabitants of Flintshire; even Carmarthenshire people were 'vnruly' and given to 'brawles and other disorders', the town of Carmarthen having 'vnruly and quarelous people there'.[24] Yet several observers regarded Carmarthen as the best town in Wales, a royal commission during Edward VI's reign stating it was 'the ffarest Towne in all South Waills, and of most Scevillytie'.[25]

The work of recent scholars on the gentry in the Tudor and early Stuart periods shows that the Welsh native gentry had their own tradition of politeness, with its emphasis on patronage of Welsh poetry and music, and on keeping open house, but that, by the early seventeenth century, this had been replaced by standards of Renaissance gentlemanliness, with a tradition of public service replacing that of the local armed chieftain, and it also entailed gradual anglicization, as the gentry more and more frequently attended Inns of Court and the universities and intermarried with English families.[26] Sir John Wynn of Gwydir spent much of his time in England and sent his son to school at Bedford.[27] John Williams of Conwy, Archbishop of York in the Civil War period, was so mocked by his fellow undergraduates at St John's, Cambridge, for his broken English that he went into purdah until he had polished and perfected his speech. Welsh students coming to the universities were mocked for believing that even the animals in the fields around Oxford and Cambridge bleated and lowed in Latin and Greek.[28] Cadwaladr Wynn in the early seventeenth century was told by his father, a Merioneth gentleman, to 'praise God that thou hast careful parents to place thee in Oxford, a famous university, the fountain and well-head of all learning', adding 'I had rather that you should keep company with studious, honest Englishmen than with many of your own countrymen, who are more prone to be idle and riotous than the English'.[29] That the Welsh were feckless and workshy was a common jibe in the Tudor period, to be found in the descriptions of Wales by John Leland and Thomas Churchyard; clearly, in this period, hard work and reliability formed part of the English notion of civility.

The Welsh were no longer seen by the English as foreigners in the

[24] Ibid. iv (1936), 401, 544, 584, 691.

[25] J. R. Daniel-Tyssen, *Royal Charters . . . of Carmarthen* (Carmarthen, 1876), 38–41.

[26] G. E. Jones, *The Gentry and the Elizabethan State* (Llandybie, 1977); J. G. Jones, *Concepts of Order and Gentility in Wales, 1540–1640* (Llandysul, 1992); J. G. Jones, *The Morgan Family of Tredegar: Origins, Growth and Advancement, c.1340–1674* (Newport, 1995); J. G. Jones, *The Wynn Family of Gwydir: Origins, Growth and Development* (Aberystwyth, 1995); J. G. Jones, *Law, Order and Government in Caernarfonshire, 1558–1640: The Justices of the Peace and the Gentry* (Cardiff, 1996); J. G. Jones, *The Welsh Gentry 1536–1640: Images of Status, Honour and Authority* (Cardiff, 1998); and H. A. Lloyd, *The Gentry of South West Wales, 1540–1640* (Cardiff, 1968), *passim*.

[27] G. D. Owen, *Elizabethan Wales* (Cardiff, 1962), 206.

[28] W. P. Griffith, *Learning, Law and Religion: Higher Education and Welsh Society, c.1540–1640* (Cardiff, 1996), 93.

[29] T. Jones Pierce (ed.), *Calendar of Clenennau Letters and Papers, National Library of Wales Journal*, 4/1 (1947), suppl. 126–7.

seventeenth century, although Sir Benjamin Rudyerd in 1628 said 'Wales is scarce in Christendom',[30] but rather as strange poverty-stricken neighbours with odd customs and manners, who lived in a repellent landscape of hills and mountains. They also flocked into England to look for work, and provided the cannon fodder of the Royalist armies during the Civil Wars. One way to civilize them was to supply them with good Protestant preachers, another to provide them with free schools, teaching them English if possible. The Welsh humanist scholars of the sixteenth and early seventeenth centuries had tried to argue that Welsh was not as barbarous a tongue as the English thought,[31] but the historiographer royal, James Howell (a native of Llangammarch), stated in his dictionary of 1660 that English was 'the Civill'st Tonge of Christendom', portraying in the frontispiece the Welsh (or 'British') language as a wild warrior maiden beyond the pale of polite languages.[32] Another was to persuade them to change their ways by ridicule, the literature of Welsh caricature from the mid-sixteenth to the mid-eighteenth centuries, in the form of ballads, woodcuts, and satires, bearing witness to the image the Welsh had in English eyes.[33] This is the period of 'Poor Taffy', the barefoot, barelegged Welshman, who, not affording a horse, always rode a billy goat, and, unable to buy meat, would then eat 'Welsh Rarebit'. Taffy used a 'Welsh Comb' (running his fingers through his unkempt hair), hugged himself in a 'Welsh Embrace' (scratching himself for numerous lice), was shiftless, sticky-fingered, spoke in hilariously broken English, yet at the same time boasting his ancient lineage. The Welsh themselves found the taunts depressing and disheartening, the balladist Matthew Owen of Llangar in the mid-seventeenth century complaining that the Welsh endured the scorn of the English up in their moors and mountains.[34] The infamous *Wallography or the Briton Described* of W.R. (probably William Richards of Helmdon) about 1682 is only one among many full-length satires, remarking not only on the filth and ugliness of Wales and the Welsh, but also on the uncouthness of their language and the wilderness in which they lived—Wales was an 'excellent place in which to breed a famine'. The Welsh 'splutter forth a kind of loathing for our English language, the native Gibberish is usually prattled throughout the whole Taphydome', but W.R. prophesied it would soon be Englished out of Wales.[35] The genre had

---

[30] Quoted in C. Hill, *Society and Puritanism in Pre-Revolutionary England* (pbk. edn., 1966), 58.

[31] e.g. William Salesbury to Richard Colyngbourne in 1550, in R. B. Jones, *The Old British Tongue: The Vernacular in Wales, 1540–1640* (Cardiff, 1970), 47.

[32] J. Howell, *Lexicon Tetraglotton: An English–French–Italian–Spanish Dictionary* (1660), sig. A1r; the frontispiece by W. Faithorne is 'La Ligue des Langues'. An extensive collection of Welsh proverbs is given as an appendix to the lexicon.

[33] W. J. Hughes, *Wales and the Welsh in English Literature from Shakespeare to Scott* (Wrexham, 1924); E. D. Snyder, 'The Wild Irish: A Study of Some English Satires against the Irish, Scots and Welsh', *Modern Philology*, 17 (1920), 702–10; P. Lord, *Words with Pictures: Welsh Images and Images of Wales in the Popular Press, 1640–1860* (Aberystwyth, 1995), the last lavishly illustrated.

[34] Quoted in P. Morgan, *The Eighteenth-Century Renaissance* (Llandybie, 1981), 15.

[35] W. R., *Wallography*, 121–4.

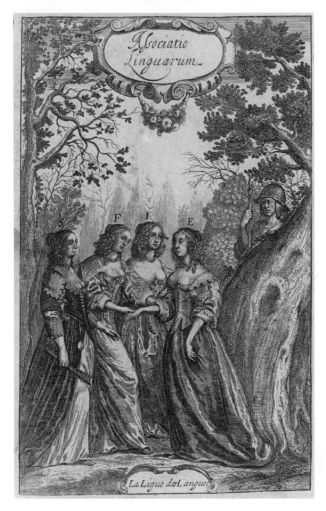

10. The 'League of Languages' as seen by James Howell, *Lexicon Tetraglotton* (1660), frontispiece, Welsh being an embattled warrior maiden beyond the pale of courtly tongues

been created, and Ned Ward's *Trip to North-Wales* in 1701 appears to echo W.R.: Wales was 'the Fag-end of Creation; the very rubbish of Noah's Flood', and, as for the people, 'They live lazily and heathenishly; they Eat and Drink nastily; Lodge hardly; snore profoundly; Belsh perpetually; shift rarely; louse frequently; and smoke Tobacco everlastingly.'[36] It may be that some of the remotest Welsh mountains did resemble the satire: one of the correspondents of Edward Lhuyd, then at the Ashmolean in Oxford, reported on Llanberis

---

[36] Ned Ward, *A Trip to North-Wales* (1701), 6.

in 1683 that in that Snowdonian parish there 'was neither a miller, fuller nor any other tradesman but one tayler lives; there's not a cock, hen or goose, nay n're any oven in ye Parish'.[37]

Edward Lhuyd and his friends helped to launch a cultural revival during the eighteenth century, one aspect of which was a great development in Welsh lexicography.[38] Enough grammars and dictionaries had been published by the end of the century to enable the historian of language to measure the semantic changes in the Welsh words for 'civility'.[39] The Anglo-French 'courteous' was borrowed by Welsh as *cwrtais* as early as the thirteenth century, but from the same period there were native words such as *boneddigaidd* (gentle, or polite) derived from the word *bonedd*, meaning 'gentry'. Walters in 1773 used the noun *boneddigeiddrwydd* for 'genteelness'. But the main Welsh word for civility or politeness comes from a native word *moes*, which in thirteenth-century sources meant behaviour that is usual or customary.[40] By the four-teenth century it had spawned several adjectives such as *moesgar*, which clearly indicated politeness or courtesy. *Moes* also had the meaning of the act of curt-seying. In Renaissance Welsh several abstract nouns with the meaning of 'politeness' were derived from *moes*, which Davies in 1632 translated as 'urban-itas'. Davies also gives *moes ac anfoes* (literally 'courtesy and discourtesy') to indicate the fault of addressing the same person as 'thee-and-thou' and 'you'. The derivative noun *moesgarwch* is given in a manuscript of 1604–7 as 'human-itas' but by Davies in 1632 as 'civilitas'. The eighteenth-century lexicographers, such as Walters, built on those definitions, expressing them in English as 'courteous', 'mannerly', 'civil', and 'genteel'. But all was not plain sailing, because, by the late seventeenth century, Puritan moralists, such as Stephen Hughes in 1688, were using words derived from *moes* critically, to indicate a mere 'external decency' as he put it, glossing it, in order to drive the point home, with a transliteration from English—namely, *sifil*. This was worldly civility as contrasted with inner godliness. Several eighteenth-century Puritans and Evangelicals gave this pejorative acceptation to 'mannerliness', but it grad-ually disappeared during the early nineteenth century, as the Welsh came to accept that outward respectability could be a reflection of inner godliness. The conclusion that may be drawn from this semantic examination is that the Welsh, whatever the misgivings the English had about them, were certainly

---

[37] F. E. Emery, 'A New Account of Snowdonia', *National Library of Wales Journal*, 28 (1974), 409.

[38] G. H. Jenkins, 'The Cultural Uses of the Welsh Language, 1660–1800', in G. H. Jenkins (ed.), *The Welsh Language before the Industrial Revolution* (Cardiff, 1997), 369–406.

[39] The essential source is the almost completed University of Wales Dictionary, *Geiriadur Pri-fysgol Cymru: A Dictionary of the Welsh Language* (Cardiff, 1950–), based on historical prin-ciples, two particularly good dictionaries being the Humanist one of Dr John Davies, *Antiquae Linguae Britannicae . . . Dictionarium Duplex* (1632), and John Walters, *A Dictionary of the Welsh Language* (Cowbridge, in parts from 1770 to 1795).

[40] *Geiriadur Prifysgol Cymru*, i (1950–67), 2476–7.

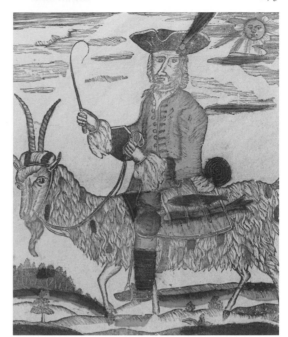

11 (*right*). Shon-ap-Morgan, caricature of about 1747 of the threadbare Welsh gentleman on goatback

12 (*below*). A late example of the Welsh caricature, one of the goat-riders carrying a proverbial Welsh pedigree dating 'from before the Flood': Richard Newton, *On a Journey to a Courtship in Wales* (1795)

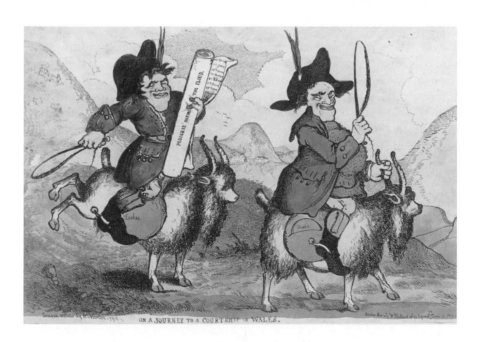

aware from the thirteenth century onwards of politeness and civility, and had developed their own vocabulary to express them.

A recent work on Welsh caricatures, Peter Lord's *Words with Pictures*, makes it clear that the savagery of the satire is gradually diminished by the middle of the eighteenth century, disappearing before its end.[41] This is the period of one of the greatest shifts in the stereotyping of Wild Wales, away from the hostile image of incivility to one of admiration. This change came about for many complex reasons, some arising from the great cultural changes lumped together under the heading of Romanticism, with its admiration for the primitive, peripheral, remote, and close to Nature, especially wild or mountainous nature, and its simultaneous rejection of that which was metropolitan and rootlessly international.[42] An aspect of this was the so-called Celtic Revival in English literature;[43] another was the English discovering the early history and archaeology of Britain, a past that they realized they had to share with the Welsh.[44] In the words of a recent historian, the eighteenth-century English began to admit that 'Welshmen were a kind of living archaeology of Englishmen'.[45] Another factor causing change, happening more or less simultaneously with the discovery of a common past, was the political need for the English to build up a Britain-wide solidarity with the Scots and the Welsh, the better to fight the interminable wars against France.[46] As early as 1746 Shenstone in a poem apostrophized Wales's 'bleak, joyless regions' as refuges of Liberty.[47] The Welsh, who had so long resisted conquerors, came to be a commonly shared symbol of Britain's determination 'never to be slaves'. The Welsh, reciprocating warmly, jumped at the opportunity to show that they deserved respect as the 'Earliest Natives' (*Cymmrodorion*) of Great Britain, the anthem of the Honourable Society of Cymmrodorion, the foremost Welsh cultural association, founded in 1751, being as anti-French as 'Hearts of Oak'.[48] The Welsh bestirred themselves into producing pictures, engravings, collections of literature, music, and history, dictionaries of inordinate length, to show that they, too, had a worthy past, and a copious living language and

---

[41] This confirms the argument of W. J. Hughes, *Wales and the Welsh in English Literature*, ch. V, pp. 62 ff. on Romanticism, and ch. VI, pp. 84 ff. on tourism.

[42] G. A. Williams, 'Wales', in R. Porter and M. Teich (eds.), *Romanticism in National Context* (Cambridge, 1988), 9–36.

[43] E. D. Snyder, *The Celtic Revival in English Literature, 1760–1800* (Cambridge, Mass., 1923), *passim*.

[44] S. Smiles, *The Image of Antiquity: Ancient Britain and the Romantic Imagination* (New Haven, 1994), *passim*.

[45] Lord, *Words with Pictures*, 26.

[46] L. Colley, *Britons: Forging the Nation 1707–1837* (New Haven, 1992), *passim*.

[47] W. Shenstone, Elegy xxi (1746) on a rumoured tax on luxuries, quoted in I. B. Rees, *The Mountains of Wales* (Gregynog, 1987), 51.

[48] R. T. Jenkins and H. Ramage, *History of the Honourable Society of Cymmrodorion, 1751–1951* (1951), 239–40.

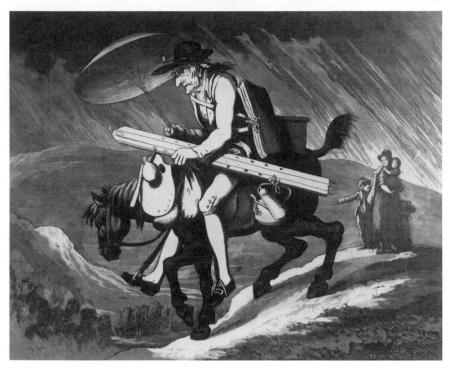

13. *The Artist Travelling through Wales* (1799), after Thomas Rowlandson

culture, all in a uniquely beautiful landscape setting.[49] The hoary old stereotypes of incivility survived with greater difficulty in the warmth of the sun of
Britannic unity and Romantic appreciation.

The Romantic travellers who came into Wales in floods from the 1770s to
the 1830s, however, took a very ambiguous view of the country, delighting as
they did in the picturesque valleys and ruins, thrilling to the vast mountains,
but grumbling about the wretched inns and dwellings, and uncertain as to
what to make of the raw new industrial developments that were beginning to
transform the face of the country in the last decades of the eighteenth century.
Valentine Morris, MP for Monmouthshire, told a parliamentary inquiry in
1754 that there were no roads in his county, but that they travelled in ditches.[50]
Yet by 1800 Wales was served at least in part by a network of roads and canals
that enabled the tourists to reach deep into the wilds. In the mountains,

[49] P. Morgan, 'From a Death to a View: The Hunt for the Welsh Past in the Romantic Period',
in E. Hobsbawm and T. Ranger (eds.), *The Invention of Tradition* (Cambridge, 1983), 43–100
passim.
[50] D. J. Davies, *Economic History of South Wales prior to 1800* (Cardiff, 1933), 91.

however, the peasants still used primitive wheelless carts even in the early nine-teenth century. The travellers were all aware of this paradoxical situation, and that Wales was divided into two ill-defined zones, an 'outer Wales', which was in a state of rapid industrialization and modernization, and an 'inner Wales'— the real object of Romantic expeditions—which was unchanged. Wales's own *philosophe*, David Williams, remarked of south Wales in 1796 that the devel-oped areas had only very recently changed, and had been transformed by a decade or two of industry more than they had for fifteen centuries.[51] Despite the large number of enclosure acts at the end of the eighteenth century, there were still over one million and a half acres of Wales as unenclosed waste in 1795.[52] Despite the development of major industries during the late eighteenth century, Wales still lacked towns of any size.[53] Many travellers noted the great contrasts between different areas: Joseph Cradock, for example, in 1770 found Wrexham highly civilized, while the peasants in the hills to the west were wild and untamed, and Nathaniel Spence in 1771 contrasted the 'very polite and hospitable' nature of lowland Montgomeryshire with the 'ferocious rusticity' of the hill country.[54] The vocabulary used to describe the Welsh greatly changed in the later eighteenth century. In place of 'backwardness', the term 'simplicity' was used—for example, by William Jones of Llangadfan—to describe the inhabitants of mid-Wales,[55] and Battista Angeloni (John Shebbeare) admired the 'greater simplicity of manners' of the Welsh peasants in 1756.[56] Sir Thomas Gery Cullum admired the Welsh acceptance of their poverty without complaint.[57] S. T. Coleridge and Joseph Hucks toured Wales in 1795, remarking on 'simplicity of nature' and 'lack of artificial manners' of a people they also called 'unpolished'.[58] Some English travellers found 'Welsh civility' lacking in decorum, the Welsh over-friendly, garrulous, and inquisi-tive.[59] John Byng (later Lord Torrington), the most ambiguous of all the trav-

---

[51] D. Williams, *History of Monmouthshire* (Monmouth, 1796), 328–9.

[52] D. J. Davies, *Economic History*, 88; G. H. Jenkins, *Foundations of Modern Wales, Wales 1642–1780* (Oxford, 1989), 112.

[53] H. Carter, *Towns of Wales* (Cardiff, 1965), *passim*; H. Carter, 'Growth and Decline of Welsh Towns', in D. Moore (ed.), *Wales in the Eighteenth Century* (Llandybie, 1976), 47–62; and H. Carter, *National Atlas of Wales* (Cardiff, 1989), map. 8.6. for towns.

[54] Nathaniel Spence, *The Complete English Traveller* (1771), 399, quoted by M. Humphreys, *The Crisis of Community: Montgomeryshire 1680–1815* (Cardiff, 1996), 6.

[55] National Library of Wales, NLW MS 13221E, fo. 343, quoted by Humphreys, *The Crisis of Community*, 254. Jones complained bitterly of the scorn for Welsh culture among the gentry, who regarded the common Welsh as mere brutes.

[56] Battista Angeloni, *Letters to the English Nation* (2nd edn., 2 vols., 1756), 27, 33, 34, 35, on the Welsh.

[57] H. M. Vaughan (ed.), 'The Travel Diary of Sir Thomas Gery Cullum', *Y Cymmrodor*, 38 (1927), 49, for poor but decent Carmarthenshire peasants in 1775.

[58] A. R. Jones and W. Tydeman (eds.), *A Pedestrian Tour of Wales 1795* (Cardiff, 1979), 18, 61. They also appreciated the 'wild and irregular genius' of the Welsh, though Coleridge in retro-spect thought the Welsh did not appreciate the beauty of their own country.

[59] P. Langford, 'British Politeness and the Progress of Western Manners: An Eighteenth-Century Enigma', *TRHS* 6th ser., 7 (1997), 53–72, esp. 67.

ellers of the period, adored the Welsh landscape, but disliked the people: 'To me the Welsh appear'd as inferior to the common English in civility, as they are in stature and comeliness; particularly the women, who are very ugly and dwarfish.'[60] The paradox is that the Romantic Wales that was the creation of Welsh propagandists and publicists, and the object of English Romantic travel, was, at least after 1800, being gradually confined to certain regions, while other parts of Wales were being developed, modernized, and, in a material sense, civilized. Indeed the ever-contrary John Byng complained that, because of an 'alteration in the manners of the people' between 1784 and 1793, half the curiosity of travel into Wales was undone.[61]

The alteration in the manners of the people was part of a gradual process of modernization of Wales during the century, greatly accelerated towards its end, of which only a few instances will be noted here. Welsh traditional and oral culture had been replaced by that of the printed book, and printers and publishers proliferated after 1718 through Wales.[62] Professional artists began to settle in various towns, such as Swansea, late in the century.[63] The growing prosperity of the middle class is evidenced by the rapid spread of clockmakers and furniture-makers in the middle of the century.[64] Towns began to have music rooms, libraries, assembly rooms, and theatres, with polite dance music specifically written for the routs and balls at places such as Tenby and Swansea.[65] Even the depths of the Welsh countryside were penetrated by the game of cricket by 1783, and Swansea had a club by 1785.[66] The 'uncivil' image of poverty combined with indolence, which had so long been part and parcel of the English view of the Welsh, was just beginning to retreat, in the face of agrarian improvements, and the exploitation of hitherto untapped sources of raw materials, copper in Anglesey, slate in Caernarfonshire, coal in the north-east, and iron in Glamorgan.

For the Welsh the mountains had become after 1815 a literal 'moral high ground', because, as a result of the Romantic movement, they had been able to revalue their despised topography, and, with that, most other aspects of their life, so that their popular culture had come to be admired and studied. But, simultaneously, the Welsh had also created for themselves a

---

[60] *Torrington Diaries*, ed. C. B. Andrews (4 vols.; 1934–6), i. 291 (south Wales, 1787).

[61] Ibid. iii. 254–5.

[62] I. Jones, *History of Printing and Printers in Wales to 1810* (Cardiff, 1925), and E. Rees, *Libri Walliae: Catalogue of Welsh Books and Books Published in Wales, 1546–1820* (2 vols.; Aberystwyth, 1987), esp. ii, app., pp. 1–69.

[63] P. Joyner, *Catalogue of Artists in Wales*, c.1740–1850 (Aberystwyth, 1997), *passim*.

[64] A. Davies and W. T. R. Pryce, *Samuel Roberts Clockmaker* (Cardiff, 1985), and A. Davies, *The Welsh Dresser and Assorted Cupboards* (Cardiff, 1991), *passim*.

[65] C. Price, *The English Theatre in Wales* (Cardiff, 1948), *passim*; P. Jenkins, 'The Spread of Metropolitan Standards', in *The Making of a Ruling Class*, 239–71; see also R. H. Bowen (ed.), *The Cambrian Trifles: The South Wales Repertory of Polite Country Dances for 1812 by W. Burton Hart* (Welsh Folk Dance Society, n.p., 1994), *passim*.

[66] A. Hignell, *A Favourit' Game: Cricket in South Wales before 1914* (Cardiff, 1992), *passim*.

metaphorical 'moral high ground', in a way, a new kind of civility. Although eighteenth-century evangelists were concerned with salvation and spirituality rather than morality, in practice they quickly threw themselves into a moral and ethical crusade: Howell Harris, for example, in 1740 (only five years after the start of the Methodist revival) attacked in Monmouth the races, balls, assemblies, whoring, and drinking of all classes.[67] John Wesley preached at Newport in 1739 to a stone-throwing rabble 'wild as bears', but returned there in 1775 to a wholly transformed population.[68] Several of the early Methodist preachers were reformed pugilists.[69] Thomas Charles of Bala, who dominated Methodism at the end of the eighteenth century, prided himself in having entirely destroyed the merriment of harping, singing, and dancing, and all the licentiousness that went with it in 1791, delighting in the 'decency of conduct and sobriety of countenance of our country people' that resulted.[70] Edmund Hyde Hall noted the disappearance of traditional rough sports in Caernarfonshire in the years before 1809, attributing the decline of 'rowdiness' and 'savageism' partly to the 'sour spirit of Methodism', but partly to the 'rapacious character of the age', which made employers encourage a tightly disciplined workforce.[71] During the French Revolutionary wars, and in the period of reaction in the early nineteenth century, the Welsh Methodists were anxious to show they were quiet and loyal.[72] Outward sobriety and civility were signs of political quiet as well as godliness. The artist Hugh Hughes, a fervent Methodist before he became a radical stormy petrel, attended the vast open-air Methodist meetings at Bala in 1820, observing the effects of preaching upon congregations of seventeen or eighteen thousand:

I felt highly pleased and delighted here with the appearance and conduct of this multitude of my countrymen, decent in their dresses and clean in their persons, with scarcely an exception, civil and quiet and serious. . . . 'Tis as clear as noonday that this preaching does not only effectively render more strictly moral those who value and believe it, but that it has changed the whole face of our country, by raising, humanising, taming, enlightening, and moralising the mass of the population.[73]

[67] P. Jenkins, *The Making of a Ruling Class*, 270.

[68] A. H. Williams, *John Wesley in Wales* (Cardiff, 1975), 5, 92.

[69] e.g. George Heycock was known as 'Bruiser Heycock': see the English synopsis of two early Victorian biographies by Matthews of Ewenny, A. L. Evans, *Siencyn Penhydd and George Heycock* (Port Talbot, 1989).

[70] D. E. Jenkins, *Life and Letters of Thomas Charles of Bala* (3 vols.; Denbigh, 1908), ii. 88–91, quoted in P. Morgan, *The Eighteenth Century Renaissance* (Llandybie, 1981), 28–9. Cf. G. H. Jenkins, *Foundations of Modern Wales* (Oxford, 1987), 368, for Methodist ethical and moral improvement.

[71] *A Description of Caernarvonshire by E. H. Hall, 1809–11*, ed. E. G. Jones (Caernarfon, 1952), 315, 321.

[72] R. Jones, *Drych yr Amseroedd* (Trefriw, 1820; ed. G. Ashton, Cardiff, 1958), 28; also J. Roberts, *Pregethau a Homiliau* (Dolgellau, 1817), p. viii.

[73] Quoted by P. Lord, *Hugh Hughes: Arlunydd gwlad* (Llandysul, 1995), 35–6, and P. Lord, *Gwenllian: Essays in Visual Culture* (Llandysul, 1994), 48.

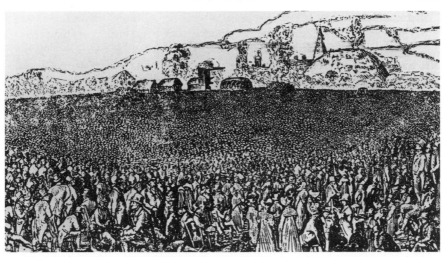

14. Hugh Hughes described the Methodist Association at Bala in his diary for 1820, but made this wood engraving while attending a similar one in 1816: Jonathan Jones, *Cofiant Thomas Jones, Dinbych* (Denbigh, 1897), 364

As a result of missions, educational efforts, Methodist revivalism, and perhaps because industrialists needed a more disciplined workforce, the Welsh were rapidly becoming a more sober and orderly people in their social life. From 1836 onwards the temperance and total abstinence movements came to play a prominent part in the life of the working classes.[74] Throughout the first half of the nineteenth century a chapel opened somewhere in Wales at the rate of one per fortnight, or even oftener. It was in a sense a 'nonconformist revolution'.[75] A good indicator of the 'new civility' of the Welsh is the rapid spread of choirs, choral meetings, and festivals in the middle decades of the nineteenth century.[76] Just as Iolo Morganwg in the late eighteenth century had considered the Welsh a superior people to the English because they had a greater sense of continuity and history, so the Welsh by the 1830s and 1840s saw themselves as a superior people in the religious sense, more pious, sober, and godly than any other European people, the Scots perhaps excepted. It became a commonplace of mid-nineteenth-century Welsh journals that the Welsh were a new Israel, specially chosen by God, 'The Land of Great

[74] W. R. Lambert, *Drink and Sobriety in Victorian Wales c.1820–c.1895* (Cardiff, 1983), 35–6, on rapid growth of respectability amongst Welsh workers and peasants in the early nineteenth century.

[75] R. Tudur Jones, *Hanes Annibynwyr Cymru* (Swansea, 1966), 221–51, on 'nonconformist civilization' and its rapid domination of Welsh life by the mid-nineteenth century.

[76] P. Morgan, 'Mid-Victorian Wales and its Crisis of Identity', in L. Brockliss and D. Eastwood (eds.), *A Union of Multiple Identities* (Manchester, 1997), 105–6, and G. Williams, *Valleys of Song: Music and Society in Wales, 1840–1914* (Cardiff, 1998), *passim*.

Privileges', the 'Land of the Revivals', curiously echoing the self-righteous Protestantism of Puritans in seventeenth-century England.[77]

One reason for this new kind of 'chapel civility' (as it might be termed) replacing the older Romantic pride in Wild Welshness was that by the 1830s and 1840s the older Romantic indicators of Welshness were wearing threadbare. The often fantastic or mythological theorizing about things Welsh began to be shown up as false, as new sciences arose, with philologists, anthropologists, and archaeologists, especially in the 1830s and 1840s, weighing, and often finding wanting, so much of the paraphernalia of Welsh culture, such as its Celticism and Druidism. The Welsh found themselves more and more drawn into the materialism and progressivism of early Victorian England, enticed by vast opportunities as they joined the Workshop of the World. Yet, by a curious twist of fate, the English were to return once more to the old attack on Wild Wales, bringing the wheel to full circle by the mid-nineteenth century.

The Welsh found themselves, as did all the Celtic peoples, the victims of various types of racism or racial theories in the mid-nineteenth century, some downright hostile, others, such as the 'visionary Celt', merely patronizing.[78] The Welsh had become a highly industrialized people by this epoch, with the population rapidly expanding, even doubling in the fifty years from 1801 to 1851, and with that becoming a difficult and volatile society. Not only had there been frequent food riots since the 1790s, but after 1816 there were also extremely violent industrial strikes, which had to be suppressed by troops, and serious risings such as those in Merthyr in 1831, and in Newport in 1839, together with rural rioting, ostensibly over toll gates (the Rebecca Riots), from 1839 to 1843. The Chartist uprising of 1839 in Newport pricked the conscience of the local middle classes, who began a programme of educating and civilizing the local population with cultural activities—a series of art exhibitions began in 1841, for example.[79] The gradual expansion (in absolute terms) of Welsh speakers in this period, together with the explosion of nonconformity, and the sporadic violence in various parts of Wales, had attracted a great deal of hostility from outside Wales, raising fears that once again Wales had become a restless, barbaric society, flying rapidly out of the reach of the forces of order, in dire need of civilization. The government report of 1844 on the Rebecca Riots in south Wales had pressed for rapid anglicization of the Welsh, but, when no new government proposals were forthcoming after two years' delay, William Williams, MP for Coventry, called for a Royal Commission to examine ways of introducing English to the Welsh masses, saying that it was

[77] See e.g. the journal *Yr Adolygydd*, 3 (1850), 19, on the incomparable religiosity of Wales.
[78] P. Sims-Williams, 'The Visionary Celt: The Construction of an Ethnic Preconception', *Cambridge Medieval Celtic Studies*, 2 (1986), 71–96.
[79] J. Wilson, *Art and Society in Newport: J. F. Mullock and the Victorian Achievement* (Newport, 1993), esp. 33–51.

'the only road to knowledge . . . the road to improvement and civilisation', and, further, that it would bring a knowledge of 'the arts and comforts of civilised life among the poor Welshmen'.[80] In the event the government appointed three commissioners, R. R. W. Lingen, J. C. Symons, and H. V. Johnson, to report on Wales to the Privy Council Committee on Education, and these produced their famous reports in 1847.

The Blue Books on Welsh Education,[81] which also dealt with the social mores of the Welsh working classes, were only the most famous of several government reports on the working classes in Wales from 1839 onwards that emphasized the wild and uncouth nature of the Welsh, ignoring many of the improvements of what we have called 'chapel civility'. The Blue Books emphasized the dirt and filth of Welsh dwellings, the slatternliness and lack of chastity in Welsh women, the want of order and methodicality in behaviour, the backwardness caused by the limitations of the Welsh language, and many other features that seem to hark back to a much earlier period in Welsh history—for example, the caricaturists of the 'Poor Taffy' school or Anglo-Norman critics in the Middle Ages. The aim of several of these reports was to bring in a system of free education to teach them all English language and English ways. H. V. Johnson found Flint wretched, squalid, and ragged (much as Celia Fiennes had found it 150 years before), and, as though the Romantic admirers of Wales had left no legacy, they wound their weary way through a Wales that was bleak, barren, dreary, desolate, and wild, where, in villages always straggling and dilapidated, there lived primitive peasants who, disgustingly, lived under the same roof as their animals, and rude industrial workers who were dangerous. The feature of the reports that gave most offence was the short personal reports of the three commissioners. They do not use the word 'civility' but constantly harp on 'civilisation'. The Welsh were not greatly given to serious crime: Lingen was surprised that the infamous criminal quarter of Merthyr, called 'China', was so peaceful, and that the Welsh in general were so religious, but, even so, they were impulsive, lacking in methodicality, temperance, chastity, and fair-dealing, and had recently displayed 'wild fanaticism'.[82] They were unacquainted with any 'superior civilisation', the widespread premarital

---

[80] G. T. Roberts, *The Language of the Blue Books: The Perfect Instrument of Empire* (Cardiff, 1998), 23.

[81] The 'Blue Books' are *The Report of the Commissioners of Inquiry into the State of Education in Wales* (*Parliamentary Papers*, 1847) (870), xxvii. See also D. Salmon, 'The Story of a Welsh Education Commission', *Y Cymmrodor*, 24 (1913), 189–237; P. Morgan, 'From Long Knives to Blue Books', in R. R. Davies *et al.* (eds.), *Welsh Society and Nationhood* (Cardiff, 1984), 119–215; P. Morgan, 'Pictures for the Million of Wales, 1848: The Political Cartoons of Hugh Hughes', *Transactions of the Honourable Society of Cymmrodorion for 1994* (1995), 65–80; I. G. Jones, *Mid-Victorian Wales: The Observers and the Observed* (Llandysul, 1991), 103–65; and G. E. Jones, *The Education of a Nation* (Cardiff, 1998), 12–33. G. T. Roberts, *The Language of the Blue Books: The Perfect Instrument of Empire* (Cardiff, 1998), is an examination of the Blue Books text in the light of recent sociolinguistics.

[82] *Report on the State of Education in Wales* [Blue Books], I. 6.

intercourse was a vice 'unchecked by any instrument of civilisation'. Johnson talked of 'The germs of the barbarous and immoral habits which disfigure Welsh civilisation'.[83] The language, he said, was a sign of 'imperfect civilisation', adding a few pages later: 'The minds of our common people are becoming thoroughly and universally depraved and brutalised.'[84] Later in his report he remarked on 'the imperfect nature of indigenous civilisation if isolated and unaided'.[85] J. C. Symons made similar remarks about the Welsh of his area (the south-east), that the Welsh 'are but slightly acquainted with the common observances of civilised life', their language being a terrible drawback because it 'dissevers the people from intercourse which would help advance their civilisation'.[86] He was amazed at the prevalence of beliefs in magic: 'Superstition prevails. Belief in charms, supernatural appearances, and even in witchcraft, sturdily survive all the civilisation and light which has long ago banished these remnants of the dark ages elsewhere.'[87] In south-east Wales, at least, religion had not led to the decline of magic.

The publication of these reports led to an unprecedented furore in Wales, hence the sobriquet 'Treason of the Blue Books', which delayed for several decades the introduction of compulsory English education. Some of the critics of the Blue Books, such as Evan Jones 'Ieuan Gwynedd', accused the commissioners of trying to prove the Welsh total barbarians.[88] The general reaction in the late 1840s was a furiously nationalistic one of wounded pride, and not a little shame; but about 1853–4 the Nonconformists came to feel that they were the victims of the slings and arrows of the three commissioners, and accused the government, in league with the Anglican minority, of hatching a plot against the Welsh people, gradually creating for themselves in the 1860s and 1870s a new kind of nationality, expressed through religion.[89] A third reaction that gradually became more important was a conviction of the need to listen to the criticisms of the commissioners, and to bring hygiene, chastity, and all the trappings of Victorian respectability to the Welsh, including English language and culture.[90]

In fact, the great fears and alarms of the authorities in the 1830s and 1840s were unfounded, because the high noon of Victorian prosperity lay immediately ahead, and Wales became one of the most successfully industrialized parts of the British Empire, the Welsh turning their energies towards self-improvement and involvement in radical politics,[91] their country spreadeagled

[83] *Report on the State of Education in Wales* [Blue Books], III. 8.   [84] Ibid. III. 59, 68.
[85] Ibid. III. 64–5.   [86] Ibid. II. 65, 66.   [87] Ibid. II. 64.
[88] Ieuan Gwynedd, ballad in *Almanac y Cymry* (1849), 55–8.
[89] P. Morgan, 'Mid-Victorian Wales and its Crisis of Identity', 93–109.
[90] G. H. Jenkins, *Language and Community in the Nineteenth Century* (Cardiff, 1998), esp. the preface by G. H. Jenkins, pp. 1–20, on the rapid decline of Welsh from the 1840s to 1900.
[91] I. G. Jones, *Explorations and Explanations: Essays in the Social History of Victorian Wales* (Llandysul, 1981), I. G. Jones, *Communities: Essays in the Social History of Victorian Wales* (Llandysul, 1987), I. G. Jones, *Mid-Victorian Wales: The Observers and the Observed* (Cardiff, 1992), *passim*, for the great shift towards nonconformist and radical culture.

with canals, railways, hotels and tourists, mines and quarries, until the Wild Wales survived only in the interstices of the world of Progress.[92] It is true that the defensive and reactive Welshness of the mid-nineteenth century wished to emphasize how central to nationality the mountains were, and some of the most popular poems and songs of the period in Welsh make great play of wild mountain landscape—for example, the Welsh National Anthem written in 1856, or the Prince of Wales's anthem (God Bless the Prince of Wales) written in 1862. But this was not a dominant feature for Welsh life. It is striking how George Borrow, who toured Wales in 1854 and wrote up his travels in his classic *Wild Wales* in 1862, had to select carefully the parts of Wales that would serve his thesis, and he scampered with embarrassment through the industrial parts of south-east Wales. Borrow wanted continuity with the distant past of ancient Welsh history and literature. The spell had been broken by generations of improvers, cultivators, and civilizers, critics, preachers, and propagandists, the wildness retreating in the face of industrialization. Borrow's title *Wild Wales* comes from a late medieval prophetic rhyme, foretelling that the Welsh would 'praise their Lord, keep their language, and lose their land, save Wild Wales'. By this period they were praising their Lord more than ever, it was true, and still to some extent keeping their language, but the wildness of their Wales had been truly lost.

[92] For language change see D. Jones, *The Coming of the Railways and Language Change in North Wales* (Aberystwyth, 1995), *passim*, and D. Jones, *Statistical Evidence Relating to the Welsh Language, 1801–1911* (Cardiff, 1998), *passim*.

16

The Moral Economy of Business: A Historical Perspective on Ethics and Efficiency

LESLIE HANNAH

I

When the cold war ended, policy-makers' prescriptions for the post-Soviet economies stressed the need to spread property rights, individualism, and competitive markets. The extreme triumphalism of the Chicago school of economics, at least in its populist versions, treated the free market as all-sufficing. Yet markets need a web of constraints, both on the state and on private individuals, if they are to function effectively. All systems require rules and, where they are routinely accepted with few enforcement costs, there is an enormous potential social benefit, not (as in the simplistic free marketeer's model of regulation) a deadweight social cost.

All this is familiar enough; as Adam Smith perfectly well understood, morality is the necessary foundation of economic behaviour[1] without which the 'invisible hand' of markets simply cannot work. Even Chicago economists now make a routine bow to the role of law, morals, or cultural norms in creating effective markets. Many economists go further and see altruistic or cooperative, as well as self-regarding and competitive, behaviour as sometimes necessary for efficient economic outcomes.[2] Some economic processes require reciprocity, trust, and commitment between the parties, rather than the opportunistic and selfish utility maximization of rational-choice models. The importance of reputation and commitment in generating business success is emphasized in normative textbooks of late-twentieth-century business strategy, as well as in historical analyses of the road to bourgeois affluence in the

I am grateful to Stephan Epstein and Adrian Seville for rescuing me from many errors and infelicities of style, though they may not have completely succeeded.

[1] Smith has often been presented as not understanding this: see e.g. A. Oncken, 'Das Adam-Smith Problem', *Zeitschrift für Sozialwissenschaft*, 1 (1898); but cf. Adam Smith, *The Theory of Moral Sentiments*, ed. D. D. Raphael and A. L. Macfie (Oxford, 1976), 20–5.

[2] F. Hirsch, *The Social Limits to Growth* (1977); R. H. Frank, 'If *Homo Economicus* could Choose his own Utility Function would he Want One with a Conscience?', *American Economic Review*, 77/4 (Sept. 1987), 593–604; see also A. Offer, 'Between the Gift and the Market: The Economy of Regard', *EcHR* 50 (1997), 450–76.

early eighteenth century.[3] Moreover, as other countries equalled or overtook the economic performance of Britain and America in the twentieth century, the alleged Anglo-American commitment to markets and amoral individualism was often compared unfavourably with alternative cultural norms in Japan and Germany. These allegedly stress cooperative, coordinated, and non-litigious business strategies and communitarian respect for equity and mutual expectations, even where they are not explicitly specified in the formal contracts of commercial exchange.[4]

Sociologists and historians are beginning to analyse how societies have attempted to reconcile the conflicting virtues of individual self-interested striving with the social civility on which its success paradoxically rests.[5] Government guarantees of property rights and freedom of contract are neither necessary nor sufficient conditions for the creation of efficient market capitalism. Many small-scale pre-industrial societies have developed self-enforcing cooperative solutions because their dense social network of inter-action rapidly perceives and penalizes opportunistic individualism. For more complex societies, where exchange is more anonymous, it becomes more difficult to enforce cooperative behaviour. The State can then in principle be usefully invoked, but at the risk of enhancing regulatory costs through extending political corruption or enhancing the influence of outside rent-seeking interests.[6]

In practice, governments always leave much of the necessary regulation to others. Anthropologists include religion or mythologized history among the ways in which a society can ensure that contracts are fulfilled and civility upheld. Religious sanctions—effectively enforcing behaviour by posting the afterlife as a bond—can be seen as an advance on primitive, cooperation-enforcing institutions, such as mutual hostage-taking, much discussed by game theorists.[7] However, all these methods are in tension with the plural-

---

[3] J. Kay, *The Foundations of Corporate Success* (Oxford, 1993), esp. chs. 3, 6; P. Earle, *The Making of the English Middle Class* (1989).

[4] See e.g. C. Crouch and D. Marquand (eds.), *Ethics and Markets: Cooperation and Competition within Capitalist Economies* (Oxford, 1993).

[5] For pre-modern examples, see A. Greif, 'Reputation and Coalitions in Medieval Trade: Evidence from the Maghribi Traders', *Journal of Economic History*, 49 (1989), 857–82; P. R. Milgrom, D. C. North, and B. W. Weingast, 'The Role of Institutions in the Revival of Trade: The Law Merchant, Private Judges and the Champagne Fairs', *Economics and Politics*, 2 (1990), 1–23.

[6] Analysis is particularly difficult because rent-seeking may still be compatible with positive developmental outcomes: it is not always part of a zero-sum or negative-sum game. See, generally, D. C. North, *Institutions, Institutional Change and Economic Performance* (Cambridge, 1990), esp. 54 ff.

[7] D. T. Campbell, 'The Two Distinct Routes of Kin Selection to Ultrasociability for the Humanities and Social Science', in D. L. Bridgeman (ed.), *The Nature of Prosocial Development: Interdisciplinary Theories and Strategies* (New York, 1983), 11–41; E. R. Constant II, 'The Cult of Mer: Or Why There is a Collective in Your Consciousness', *Business and Economic History*, 22 (1993), 127–37.

ism of successful modern societies. Other 'private-order'[8] regulatory institutions include medieval guilds or modern professional associations (including stock exchanges or the Lloyds insurance market), which can monitor the quality of products or behaviour of members, though these too may be subject to corruption or the abuse of monopoly privileges.

There is no reason—other than misty-eyed wishful thinking—to believe that moral behaviour will always be economically efficient; nor is there any reason to believe that some forms of enforcement mechanism (e.g. guild rules) are always better than others (e.g. internalized religious values). Hence, it seems likely that in pluralist societies a variety of 'private-order' regulatory institutions will be a source of economic strength. Competition will then ensure that regulators do not survive if they offer protection at a greater cost than customers are willing to pay for the benefits.[9] Yet, private-order regulators that do provide such benefits may gain such prestige that their natural monopoly will be used to exploit the consumer and restrict economic growth; politicians will then be tempted to intervene with legal regulation. The state is, however, merely the last in a line of potential villains: *quis custodiet ipsos custodes?* In wrestling with such problems, different cultures have reached very different solutions in this difficult area.

One of the most promising economic approaches to the evolution of trust and reciprocity has come through applying game theory, especially the theory of repeated games, in which experience of earlier cooperation or non-cooperation can influence future behaviour. The game theorist's classic one-period prisoner's dilemma postulates criminals who are separated for interrogation. They each know that if neither confesses they will go free, but if both confess they will go to jail; however, if one confesses and the other does not, the one who confesses will get a lighter sentence. In this situation, the chance of confession is high: the normal result is non-cooperation and both go to jail. But if the game is repeated, the chance of achieving the cooperative solution of neither confessing is considerably enhanced. In the repeated game (which approximates more closely to real life), the political scientist Robert Axelrod[10] showed that the most successful strategy is neither consistent cooperation nor consistent self-interested competition, but rather a 'tit-for-tat' strategy with a bias to cooperate. The optimal rule is to cooperate in the first period and then to mimic the rival, so that, if the rival cooperates, continue cooperation; if the rival does not, punish him by non-cooperation. This rule shows two elements of what might be thought of as conventional Christian morality: it is nice (it starts by being cooperative) and it is forgiving (if

---

[8] The phrase is owed to O. E. Williamson, *The Economic Institutions of Capitalism: Firms, Markets and Relational Contracting* (New York, 1985), 164–6.

[9] J. Kay, 'The Forms of Regulation', in A. Seldon (ed.), *Financial Regulation or Over-Regulation?* (London: Institute of Economic Affairs, 1988), 33–42.

[10] R. Axelrod, *The Evolution of Cooperation* (New York, 1984).

cooperation is reinstated, earlier non-cooperation is forgotten). But it is also firmly retaliatory and has no element of 'turning the other cheek': unco-operative behaviour is punished. In mathematical simulations of populations pursuing both 'tit-for-tat' and *any* alternative strategies (for example, consistent rivalry, consistent cooperation, random variations), those pursuing a 'tit-for-tat' strategy normally come to dominate a population.

Such formal models of how constructive,[11] cooperative behaviour evolves are suggestive, but they lack empirical content. It is perfectly possible for such evolutionary processes to generate 'successful' behaviour from a quite random set of initial attributes; indeed, that is one of the strengths of Axelrod's result. Yet, by the same token, such models cannot rule out the possibility that distinctive economic developments in the real world have actually been promoted by more deliberative processes. The fact that some societies are richer than others *could* be the result of random forces producing randomly different outcomes, but it could also be that successfully cooperative forms of behaviour were either more widespread in the initial population or more selectively encouraged in the 'successful' societies. Finally, the dichotomy between such extreme characterizations of economic developmental processes may be a misleading one: societies that successfully generate variety (and permit selection among varieties based on market competition) may also be the ones that discourage dysfunctional behaviour and reward the right mix of cooperation and competition, even if the perception of the process is intuitive and *post hoc* rather than planned and deliberative.

II

The classical historical paradigm of economic growth, Britain's Industrial Revolution, provides the backdrop for a case study. The seventeenth-century world out of which these industrial changes grew has been characterized by the historian of its business community as one in which the word 'business' was 'synonymous with corruption, opportunism and deceit' (though, as today, such views were not universally shared).[12] It was a seamy world in which milk and wine were watered, packaging was deceptive, weights and measures were manipulated against the consumer, and greed overwhelmed integrity in many dealings with government or by monopolists. Con men, fraudulent bankrupts, and broken merchants clogged the courts with tales of bribery, corruption, cheating, and lying, while moralists excoriated the market

---

[11] It is, of course, ironic that game theory's classic dilemma is of two criminals trying to cheat justice: their cooperation makes society a worse place. But the *logic* is identical for cooperative actions with positive results.

[12] R. Grassby, *The Business Community of Seventeenth-Century England* (Cambridge, 1995), 293.

as a battlefield controlled by the Devil. Yet, at the same time, reputation and credit were fundamental for business success; and so suitably controlled and presented moral behaviour brought potential rewards.[13] Here then was a wide canvas of varied human behaviour, out of which successful strategies could be selected. In eighteenth-century England, many types of religious, social, or economic experiments were feasible. Among many that emerged was the distinctive Quaker approach.

Not that the Quakers initially behaved in ways that were at all obviously 'civil'. However, by the 1670s they had ceased to be gratuitously offensive during other people's worship and were more straightforwardly concerned to plead for their toleration by others. They suffered continued persecution for a time, but after the Glorious Revolution they shared the grudging acceptance granted to Nonconformists generally. In temporal, as in spiritual affairs, the years that followed provided ample incentive to create the conditions for a settled and godly life.[14]

Quaker values have often been linked to their economic success; and the sect certainly had an unusually demanding and relevant set of spiritual and moral requirements. Yet many religious groups promoted similar values. Furthermore, then as now, aggressive signs of religiosity and morality could all too often conceal skullduggery. As Groucho Marx later put it: 'What you need to succeed in business is honesty. Fake that and you've got it made.' Quakers were no doubt as frail as most contemporary businessmen, and were at least as tempted as others by the South Sea Bubble.[15] The Quaker inventor and industrialist Dr Edmund Wright ruined a distinguished career by using the resources of the mainly Quaker-dominated London Lead Company to speculate in the Bubble frenzy. Most speculators were immediately exposed when the markets fell in 1720, but he and a group of corrupt Quakers managed to conceal their losses from other shareholders for nearly a decade. Only when Wright died was the Quaker banker John Freame able fully to investigate and expose the conspiracy (a detail discreetly omitted from the sanitized accounts by later Quaker historians). Freame then prosecuted the fraudsters and successfully reconstructed the finances of the company.[16]

That such a successful reconstruction occurred is itself symptomatic of Quaker peculiarity: the intervention of bankers to restructure companies is

[13] An aspect given greater emphasis in Earle, *The Making of the English Middle Class.*

[14] W. C. Braithwaite, *The Second Period of Quakerism*, ed. H. J. Cadbury (new edn., Cambridge, 1961); N. C. Hunt, *Two Early Political Associations* (Oxford, 1961).

[15] [Elias Brocket] 'Damon', *The Yea and Nay Stockjobbers or the Change Alley Quakers Anatomised* (1720), 7; 'Temple-Mills', *The Quakers' Dialogue*, (n.d. [1720?]). See also the 1714 printed list of South Sea Company subscribers in BL 1887 b.63.

[16] Cf. the London Lead Company records (Tyne & Wear RO) with the sanitized account by the Quaker historian Arthur Raistrick, in his *Two Centuries of Industrial Welfare: The London (Quaker) Lead Company 1692–1905* (1938), reissued as supplement no. 19 to *Journal of the Friends' Historical Society* (1977).

not a general eighteenth-century phenomenon. The Quakers were quite distinctive in their social organization. Their efficient nationwide and international information networks, familial credit relationships, and the like secured a collective enforcement of personal morality in business dealings that could supply a competitive advantage. What distinguished the Quakers was not simply their unusually comprehensive application of Christian principles in everyday commercial practice, but also the extent and effectiveness of their internal disciplinary procedures and their control of Quaker membership. The peculiarities of Quakers, which they deliberately accentuated in the eighteenth century, in themselves constituted a powerful safeguard against false members: it took some strength of mind to wear Quaker garb (which became increasingly archaic as well as plain), or to use Quaker forms of address such as 'thee' and 'thou' (whether, as initially, they were rudely over-familiar, or, as later, merely archaic). Frugality and abstention from luxurious dress and other expensive conceits may have been conducive to capital accumulation, but they were not practices that recommended themselves to the majority of rich men.

Quaker discipline had its roots in the movement's history during the period of the 'sufferings'. From the 1670s onwards, it became common for members of a local meeting to be visited and advised on their behaviour, including their business behaviour where appropriate. 'Disorderly walkers' were supposed initially to be directly admonished by individual Friends, but, if this did not work, questions about members' breaches of commercial morality could be raised formally at monthly meetings. A visit by a deputation of two or three Friends would be authorized, and if, after diligent enquiry and discussion with the alleged miscreant, they reported continuing delinquency, the meeting would normally offer the sinner the option of accepting a written condemnation as an earnest of his intentions to reform. If he refused, he was 'disowned'—that is, expelled from their Society. Migration was no escape from the discipline: a written certificate of 'clearness' was required for a traveller to be admitted to a new meeting, as well as for Friends entering into marriages. The system extended to transatlantic migration, and needed to do so, given that in the 1680s out of 50,000 or so Friends, for example, 6,000 went to Pennsylvania and 1,500 to East Jersey.[17]

Quaker discipline was direct, relentless, comprehensive, and intrusive. Yet it was tempered by self-discipline and restraint of possible abuses. The fact that formal procedures for resolving disputes were available reinforced the Quaker distaste for tittle-tattle. 'Be no busybodies,' William Penn wrote in 1682; 'meddle not with other folks' matters but when in conscience and duly pressed, for it procures trouble, and is ill-mannered, and very unseemly

---

[17] For such certificates of removal, see A. C. Myers, *Quaker Arrivals in Philadelphia 1682–1750* (Philadelphia, 1902).

to wise men.'[18] Members were encouraged to condemn wrongdoing openly, but gossip behind the backs of alleged miscreants was strongly discouraged: baseless and slanderous speculation of the kind that could ruin innocent contemporary businessmen was thereby generally avoided.

To outsiders, Quakers sometimes seemed absurdly scrupulous. Thus the Quaker merchant James Pembleton of Philadelphia, whose ship, the *Hannah*, was seized by French pirates in the Caribbean in 1758, kept a promise extorted under duress to pay the ransom. He maintained his position despite a clear legal ruling that agreements made under duress were not binding and in the face of the strong indignation of his fellow merchants.[19] In Britain, Quaker bankers like Samuel Gurney of Norwich sometimes refused to prosecute dishonest clerks or forgers to avoid the outcome of hanging (of which they disapproved), even to the extent of risking criminal charges for compounding a felony.[20] The immediate effect of such behaviour was what their critics said: it allowed pirates and forgers to escape with impunity, thus presumably obstructing economic growth. Yet it also reinforced the Quaker reputation for integrity, without actually requiring all Quakers to behave in such an extreme way.

The Quakers also took their well-known lead in advancing contemporary moral standards, most notably in relation to one of the most profitable eighteenth-century businesses, the slave trade. The Quakers were among the earliest unequivocal abolitionists, when many of their clients and competitors were profiting from slave-trading and slave-owning.[21] Quakers had earlier been shareholders in such slave-trading companies as the Royal Africa Company and the South Sea Company; Caribbean Quakers in the early eighteenth century had themselves been slavemasters, though some Quakers found such activities disquieting even then.[22] By the 1770s opinion against slavery had hardened and Quakers who owned or traded slaves were disowned in both England and Pennsylvania.[23] In 1795 David Barclay the younger (who became a partner in the London bank of Barclay, Bevan & Co. in 1774) called in a debt due in Jamaica and thus became the owner of Unity Valley Pen, with thirty-two slaves on a grazing farm. His agent initially refused to release the slaves, considering it would make him unpopular on the island, so Barclay

[18] Letter dated 4 Aug. 1682, repr. in J. Soderland (ed.), *William Penn and the Founding of Pennsylvania, 1680–1684: A Documentary History* (Philadelphia, 1783), 171.

[19] F. B. Tolles, *Meeting House and Counting House: The Quaker Merchants of Colonial Philadelphia, 1682–1763* (Chapel Hill, NY, 1948), 59–60.

[20] P. H. Emden, *Quakers in Commerce: A Record of Business Achievement* ([1939]), 111; H. R. Geldart, *Memorials of Samuel Gurney* (1857), 35–7; and see generally W. H. Bidwell, *Annals of an East Anglian Bank* (1900).

[21] J. E. Inikori, 'The Credit Needs of the African Trade and the Development of the Credit Economy in England', *Explorations in Economic History*, 27 (1990), 197–231.

[22] M. R. Watts, *The Dissenters* (Oxford, 1978), 479; G. S. De Krey, *A Fractured Society: The Politics of London in the First Age of Party 1688–1715* (Oxford, 1985), 97.

[23] R. W. Fogel, *Without Consent or Contract* (1989), ch. 7.

transported them to Philadelphia, where he had acquaintances in the Abolition of Slavery Society, and freed them there. The upshot was that he got
£5,000 rather than the £8,000 that was his commercial due from his
security. Quakers like David Barclay thus believed in the moralization of
wealth, long before 'ethical' investment was an issue for others. This belief
derived from the Quaker view that wealth was a conditional trust, not an
absolute possession: the wealthy could not use their wealth to oppress their
fellow men. It is also perhaps no accident that in one of Paul Johnson's case
studies of nineteenth-century attempts to enforce moral behaviour on the
Stock Exchange, the leading prosecuting counsel was a Quaker.[24] (Quakers
were then no longer disqualified—by themselves or the state—from being
lawyers.)

The strength of an individual's conviction in the face of worldly disapproval
in the more extreme Quaker 'testimonies' was a source of unQuakerly pride,
admired and noticed, but not necessarily emulated, even by punctilious
Friends;[25] it was also a highly effective form of advertisement for Quaker
trustworthiness, honesty, and reliability as an absolute commitment, not to
be conveniently readjusted for an individual's own short-term self-interest. A
contract with a Quaker would have legal form and specific content, but the
unspecified, implicit contract was frequently just as important.

Not all such extreme testimonies had a negative economic impact. The most
obvious positive outcome of Quaker commitment to fulfil contracts beyond
what the law required could be seen both in bankruptcy proceedings and in
their frequent resort to arbitration rather than the courts. Bankrupt Quakers
were not permitted to settle with their creditors or go bankrupt and leave it
at that: there would, both before and after such decisions, be careful enquiry
and supervision by delegates of the meeting to ensure that the creditors were
satisfied as fully as possible beyond the law.[26] Even after a formal bankruptcy,
relatives would sometimes even seek to rescue the family reputation by paying
more than the creditors had accepted on a voluntary basis.[27]

Legal proceedings to enforce formal contracts were costly and protracted;
sensible men—both Quakers and non-Quakers—tried to avoid them. But
Quakers particularly disliked conflict with their fellow men and their pacifism

---

[24] D. Barclay, *Account of the Emancipation of the Slaves of Unity Valley in Jamaica* (1801); Johnson,
below, p. 310.

[25] Cf. the Backhouses (northern Quaker bankers) demanding the full death penalty prescribed
by law: M. Phillips, *A History of Banks, Bankers and Banking in Northumberland, Durham and
North Yorkshire* (1894), 139 n.

[26] Although the minutes of the Gracechurch Street Monthly Meeting (which probably
contained the more interesting examples of the behaviour of the greatest London merchants
towards each other) were destroyed by fire in 1821, the flavour of their proceedings can be gauged
from the surviving minutes of the London and Middlesex six-weeks meeting, *passim*, in Friends'
Library.

[27] Register of Commissioners in Bankruptcy, PRO IND 22640 B4/7, p. 212; *London Gazette*,
no. 7163, 20–23 Jan. 1732, no. 7170, 13–17 Feb. 1732, no. 7401, 10–13 May 1735; *Gentleman's
Magazine*, 3 (1733), 48, for the case of Thomas Gould, the bankrupt Quaker banker in Cornhill.

extended to a strong distaste for legal conflict. Seventeenth-century Quakers had a strong distaste for legal actions, not least because their unwillingness to take oaths often disqualified their evidence. After the 1696 Affirmation Act this inconvenience was removed, but Quakers refusing oaths could still not become lawyers (nor, of course, MPs, university students, military men, or clerics) and their distaste for the law was if anything intensified. Quakers were from 1697 forbidden to take a fellow Quaker to court: before doing so they had first to seek arbitration from delegates of the monthly meeting; only if a Quaker failed to respond to their admonitions was another Quaker permitted to prosecute. In 1737 the London Yearly Meeting extended the injunction to use arbitration to Quakers' dealings with others.[28] Thus anyone in a contractual dispute with a Quaker could expect that he would submit to arbitration rather than go to law. This was only on a 'tit-for-tat' basis, however; anyone—Quaker or non-Quaker—who trifled with such 'nice' behaviour could quickly find himself in Chancery.

The power to enforce implicit contracts through the discipline of the meeting gave a special competitive advantage in banking or long-distance colonial trade, which differed in crucial respects from the more common requirements of spot-trading.[29] Non-Quakers—even those with a poor reputation—could benefit from business contact with the Quakers' moral economy. In the bill of exchange, for example, the relationship between payer and drawer required trust in only one direction, while that between drawee and payee was essentially a spot transaction, requiring no trust. The crucial relationship was that between drawer and drawee:[30] it could prosper only on the basis of long-term relations of trust and reciprocity, where the implicit Quaker contract gave an especially powerful competitive advantage. The economic innovation of the bill of exchange—its role strengthened by legislation in the 1690s—did not require all participants in trade to act with exemplary honesty, but rather enabled a range of averagely competent and honest (and even some dishonest) merchants to benefit (for a fee) from the hyper-honesty of a few others. That this service was valuable was clear from the rates of return achieved by the reputable Quaker transatlantic merchants and Quaker goldsmith bankers: their return on capital of well above 30 per cent was substantially higher than the norm in London trade and was essentially a premium for reputation in issuing, endorsing, or accepting bills of exchange, requiring trust over both time and distance.[31]

---

[28] *Extract from the Minutes and Advices of the Yearly Meeting of Friends* (1822), 5–6.

[29] The Quaker preference for fixed prices over dishonest haggling and their reputation for refusing to adulterate goods differentiated their approach in many retail spot markets and may also have been a competitive advantage in other spot trades also.

[30] Of course, endorsing and accepting bills of exchange implied further levels of trust.

[31] M. Ackrill and L. Hannah, *Barclays Bank: A History* (forthcoming). Of course other non-Quaker merchants could also achieve high reputation in these trades and gain substantial market shares: see e.g. J. M. Price, *Perry of London: A Family and Firm on the Seaborne Frontier, 1617–1753* (Cambridge, Mass., 1992).

The Quakers were the first dissenters to hold meetings in every English county, and Quaker bankers in Lombard Street thus had ready access to a nationwide network of correspondents providing financial intelligence: the nearest thing the eighteenth century had to a credit reference agency. Quaker networks were also, perhaps, one reason why the complex features of the three-way trade between the Caribbean, the American colonies, and Britain prospered in Quaker Philadelphia and indeed why Philadelphia soon became the largest city in the Americas.[32] Similar processes may have helped to establish the position of leading Quaker merchants in London, as well as the network of Quaker bankers in Lombard Street and their Quaker country banking correspondents. In East Anglia, for example, the Gurneys, Peckovers, Birkbecks, and Buxtons formed marriage alliances and partnerships that created the largest, and largely Quaker, banking network of the nineteenth century. Their branches in these agricultural centres generated surpluses, which they invested through the intermediation of the Barclay, Bevan & Co. partnership in Lombard Street (giving them access to the London money markets) and the Backhouse banking network in the north-east (providing outlets for their surplus capital in developing new industries). By the late eighteenth century at least 15 per cent and perhaps as many as a quarter of English banks had been founded by Quakers. Some of the major investment projects of the Industrial Revolution—from the large-scale London breweries of the later eighteenth century, through the canal building projects of the Regency period, to the first modern railway between Stockton and Darlington—were financed with Quaker capital.[33]

III

The spread of 'civil' behaviour throughout eighteenth-century British society may have been encouraged by observing the success of Quaker behaviour.[34] That was, of course, only one of many sources of growing civility, but it is perhaps no accident that the two most celebrated business moralists on either side of the eighteenth-century Atlantic—Daniel Defoe and Benjamin Franklin—were admirers of and deeply influenced by the Quakers they

[32] M. Balderston (ed.), *James Claypoole's Letter Book: London and Philadelphia 1681–1684* (San Marino, Calif., 1967); J. M. Price, 'The Great Quaker Families of Eighteenth Century London: The Rise and Fall of a Sectarian Patriciate', in R. S. Dunn and M. Dunn (eds.), *The World of William Penn* (Philadelphia, 1986).

[33] W. H. Bidwell, *Annals of an East Anglian Bank* (Norwich, 1900); Phillips, *History of Banks, Bankers and Banking*; L. Pressnell, *Country Banking in the Industrial Revolution* (Oxford, 1956); D. H. Pratt, *English Quakers and the Industrial Revolution* (New York, 1985); J. R. Ward, *The Finance of Canal Building in Eighteenth Century England* (Oxford, 1974).

[34] For a practical assessment of the influence of Quaker reputation, see K. Morgan (ed.), *An American Quaker in the British Isles: The Travel Journals of Jabez Maud Fisher 1775–1779* (Oxford, 1992).

encountered.[35] Nor was Voltaire slow to recognize the peculiarity of the Quakers as one source of Anglo-Saxon progress.[36] One did not, however, have to be a Quaker to develop a good reputation as a merchant or to conclude that arbitration might be better for all parties to a business dispute than legal confrontation. Even if Quakers did not influence others, they could have influenced economic growth in the alternative way postulated in the game-theoretic model of the spread of 'tit-for-tat' behaviour. This allows for the spread of cooperative behaviour and other-regarding actions that reinforce reputation simply because they multiply in number while those pursuing less successful strategies disappear.

One complication needs, however, to be allowed for. There were around 60,000 Quakers in 1680, making them the largest of the sects. Yet by 1800 they numbered less than 20,000, and by 1860 less than 14,000.[37] If they had merely kept pace with the rest of the population,[38] there would in 1860 have been nearly 225,000 Quakers. Their impact stemmed less from their number than from advances in their livelihood and influence.

The early Quakers included every class from servants and apprentices to landed gentry. In one study of Lancashire, Gloucestershire, Wiltshire, Bristol, Buckinghamshire, London, and Middlesex up to 1688 both the very wealthy and day labourers were under-represented among Quakers, but the rural and urban petty bourgeoisie and artisans were over-represented. They were not generally in the heavily capitalized trades in which they later became strong, but were strongly represented in trades quite hard pressed by competition and economic change such as textiles.[39] Vann's attempt to argue for higher Quaker social status in the early period is unconvincing.[40] One cannot unambiguously equate contemporary status descriptions directly with income levels, but seventeenth-century Quakers do not seem to have been substantially richer than the average contemporary Englishman. Yet eighteenth-century Quaker registers in London show a decline in the proportion of artisans and a rise in

[35] Daniel Defoe, *The Compleat English Tradesman* (1727); C. Van Doren, *Benjamin Franklin* (1939).

[36] See Voltaire, *Letters on England* (1733), chs. 1–4, for his observations on the Hampstead Quaker Andrew Pitt.

[37] E. Isichei, *Victorian Quakers* (1970), 112.

[38] For population growth between 1680 and 1860, see E. A. Wrigley and R. Schofield, *The Population History of England 1541–1871: A Reconstruction* (Cambridge, 1981), 532–5.

[39] A. Cole, 'The Social Origins of the Early Friends', *Journal of the Friends' Historical Society*, 48 (1957), 99–118. These include the main concentrations of Quaker strength in England and Wales, except for Westmorland, Yorkshire, and Norwich, where literary evidence is also compatible with a similar social structure of Quakerism.

[40] R. T. Vann, 'Quakerism and the Social Structure of the Interregnum', *P&P* 43 (1969). See also B. Stevenson, 'The Social and Economic Status of Post-Restoration Dissenters, 1660–1725', in M. Spufford (ed.), *The World of Rural Dissenters 1520–1725* (Cambridge, 1995), 332–59; L. D. Schwarz, *London in the Age of Industrialisation* (Cambridge, 1992), 132; R. T. Vann and D. Eversley, *Friends in Life and Death: The British and Irish Quakers in the Demographic Transition 1650–1900* (Cambridge, 1992).

the proportion of merchants,[41] and, by the mid-Victorian period, Quaker incomes were perhaps eight times the national average.[42]

Does this change indicate the overall upward social mobility of the group, rather than social exclusion of its poorer members? The discipline of monthly meetings enforced by the London merchant élite may have excluded some and discouraged others. More than 7 per cent of early London Quakers were mariners: useful to the merchants, certainly, but also well known as members of the London rabble and unlikely to welcome the early meetings' rulings of the 1690s that they should not carry arms when French or Caribbean privateers threatened their ships and livelihoods. It is in principle easier to conduct studies of family reconstitution and inter-generational social mobility for eighteenth-century Quakers than for any groups other than the aristocracy. Though the records before 1730 are sketchy, they are consistent with the view that some exclusion of the poor occurred then.[43] But this is unlikely to be the only source of rising average Quaker affluence.

We are left, then, with strong circumstantial evidence that hyper-morality— provided it was plausibly enforced by disciplinary mechanisms superior to those provided in civil and criminal law—could be a source of competitive advantage and resulted in very high Quaker incomes. This is not, of course, to say that the Quakers adopted it for this reason. We do not trust the moralist who argues that honesty is the best policy; we are more likely to respect the one who argues that honesty is right. However, like the Quakers, we might note that it is wise to require more than an aura of honesty and to enforce disciplined adherence to moral rules. Moreover, like the historian, we can also observe that, while honesty does not always pay, the reputation it creates will, in the right circumstances, produce a competitive advantage.

Quakers were only one among several influences helping to create a climate conducive to rapid economic growth. Such influences were not necessarily integral to a firm's long-run survival. Though many enterprises of Quaker origin—including, for example, Barclays and Lloyds among the four largest clearing banks—continued to prosper into the twentieth century,[44] they did so for changed reasons. The first half of the nineteenth century saw the

---

[41] W. Beck and T. F. Ball, *London Friends' Meetings* (1869), 90. For a similar trend in the seventeenth century, see also Cole, 'Social Origins', 114–15.

[42] *The Friend* (1863), 208, estimates total annual income of Friends at £2m.–£3m., i.e. a maximum of, say, £220 per head. National income per head was then £26: C. H. Feinstein, *National Income, Expenditure and Output of the United Kingdom 1855–1965* (Cambridge, 1972), T42.

[43] Beck and Ball, *London Friends' Meetings*, 90; J. Landers, *Death and the Metropolis: Studies in the Demographic History of London 1670–1830* (Cambridge, 1993), 133–4.

[44] Many business families were no longer Quakers, but even in the twentieth century a higher proportion of Quakers than any other religious group were active in business: see D. J. Jeremy, *Capitalists and Christians* (Oxford, 1990), and T. A. B. Corley, 'How Quakers Coped with Success: Quaker Industrialists 1860–1914', in D. J. Jeremy (ed.), *Business and Religion in Britain* (Aldershot, 1988).

majority of the richer Quaker bankers defect to evangelical Christianity or Anglicanism, though they often maintained an austere and highly moral public and private demeanour even in their new religion.[45] More importantly, the business world was changing. The international bill business, for example, no longer gave the same competitive advantage to reputation after the mid-Victorian innovation of the international telegraph. This reduced the value of their trust networks for long-distance settlement by creating what were, in effect, spot markets with immediate transmission of settlement moneys if traders required it. Trust in the broader sense is, of course, integral to banking, but, as overall levels of wealth multiplied, the practice of taking security became an effective substitute in many banking transactions for the local networks of trust and information that had given Quaker bankers such a marked advantage. The special economic value of a reputation for hyper-morality may be crucial only at particular moments in a firm's history.

IV

The Quakers were by no means alone among religious or ethnic groups in finding a commercial advantage in reciprocity and trust. Long-distance medieval trade also prospered where reciprocity could be reinforced by ethnicity or other means of group solidarity.[46] Pre-colonial African traders used letters of credit or bills of exchange underwritten by ethnic-cum-religious diasporas controlling long-distance trade and credits.[47] The Huguenot refugees in Britain of the late seventeenth century strengthened an already existing set of banking and trading links through the centre of international Calvinism in Geneva, though the disciplinary function of their elders in the Consistory was applied very lightly and many Huguenots were rapidly assimilated by the Anglican establishment.[48] The Scots diaspora in London and America has played a parallel role in banking and trade;[49] there are parallels, too,

---

[45] Ackrill and Hannah, *Barclays Bank*, ch. 1.

[46] A. Greif, 'The Organisation of Long Distance Trade: Reputation and Coalitions in the Geniza Documents and Genoa during the Eleventh and Twelfth Centuries', *Journal of Economic History*, 51 (June 1991), 459–62.

[47] G. Austin, 'Indigenous Credit Institutions in West Africa *c.*1750–1960', in G. Austin and K. Sugihara (eds.), *Local Suppliers of Credit in the Third World* (1993), 93–159.

[48] F. Crouzet, 'The Huguenots and the English Financial Revolution', in P. Higonnet, D. S. Landes, and H. Rosovsky (eds.), *Favorites of Fortune: Technology, Growth and Economic Development since the Industrial Revolution* (Cambridge, Mass., 1991), 241, 258; R. D. Gwynn, *Huguenot Heritage* (1985), 98–103, 164–6; though cf. Bernard Cottret, *The Huguenots in England: Immigration and Settlement c.1550–1700* (Cambridge, 1985), 238–9, 248, 263–4.

[49] E. Healey, *Coutts & Co. 1692–1992: The Portrait of a Private Bank* (1992), 7; A. L. Karras, *Sojourners in the Sun: Scottish Migrants in Jamaica and the Chesapeake, 1740–1800* (Ithaca, NY, 1992); G. Marshall, *Presbyterianism and Profits: Calvinism and the Development of Capitalism in Scotland 1560–1707* (Oxford, 1980).

between the Quakers and the European Jewish diaspora that linked London, continental Europe, and the Americas.[50]

Social scientists have recently been as prolific as historians in extolling the virtues of honesty, trust, and reciprocity. Econometricians routinely find that societies with higher levels of trust have lower transaction costs and thus operate more efficiently,[51] while the more flamboyant populists extol the almost unlimited advantages of trust.[52] Business schools now routinely offer electives in business ethics. Yet there is no one-to-one correlation between superior morality and business success, for the mosaic of any economy is made up of a wide variety of trades and industries, in none of which simple formulas—whether based on honesty or anything else—unequivocally produce success. It is far from obvious that an eighteenth-century England entirely populated by Quakers would have been more successful: what the market achieved was to ensure that their economic usefulness in specific trades was successfully leveraged by customers who did *not* need to share their moral character.

A Harvard Business School professor's ethics casebook[53] provides an illustration of how complex the moral economy of business remains, even in a period where business morality is more clearly defined in more elaborate commercial laws and regulations. Édouard Sakiz was chairman when Roussel-Uclaf developed a drug that safely induced abortion. Profits from the drug were likely to be small, and anti-abortion groups threatened international boycott of the company's other products if it went ahead. Mr Sakiz personally felt the drug was beneficial, but his employees were divided and the boycott threat was real. Moreover, 55 per cent of the company's shares were owned by a German company, Hoechst, run by a devout Catholic, though the second largest shareholder—with 36 per cent—was the French government (which believed the drug would be medically and socially beneficial). The choice was not between right and wrong but between two competing rights and there was no point in choosing one option if this merely ensured that Sakiz was fired. His way out of the dilemma owed more to Machiavelli than to conventional moralists. First he called a snap meeting of top management and persuaded them to drop the drug, announcing that they had done so, contrary to his personal preference, and because of pressure from

---

[50] N. Zahedieh, 'Credit, Risk and Reputation in Late Seventeenth-Century Colonial Trade', in O. U. Janzen (ed.), *Merchant Organization and Maritime Trade in the North Atlantic, 1660–1815* (Research in Maritime History, 15; St John's, Newfoundland, 1998), 53–74; M. Woolf, 'Foreign Trade and the London Jews in the Seventeenth Century', *Transactions of the Jewish Historical Society of England*, 24 (1974), 38–58.

[51] R. La Porta, F. Lopez-de-Silanes, A. Shleifer, and R. Vishny, *Trust in Large Organizations* (National Bureau of Economic Research Working Paper, No. 5864; 1998).

[52] F. Fukuyama, *Trust: The Social Virtues and the Creation of Prosperity* (1995); cf. D. Gambetta (ed.), *Trust-Making and Breaking Cooperative Relations* (Oxford, 1990).

[53] J. L. Badaracco Jnr., *Defining Moments: When Managers must Choose between Right and Right* (Boston, Mass., 1997).

anti-abortion groups. This provoked the French government into threatening to expropriate Roussel's proprietary rights and give them to another firm. Mr Sakiz then announced a change of policy: the company would directly distribute the drug. The anti-abortionists could not credibly attack the company (rather than the democratically legitimated French government), so Mr Sakiz had achieved the result he felt both desirable and ethically best: he (and his employees) kept their jobs, while doing the right thing. He had shielded his company from the tension between irreconcilable absolute moralities. Whether this promoted economic growth depends, of course, on other issues: on the complex direct and indirect effects of abortion on the economy and on the broader implications of delegating 'moral' decisions of this kind to democratically elected governments rather than leaving their resolution to competition between 'private-order' institutions such as anti-abortion pressure groups.

Quaker morality had the attraction—not shared by all other private-order institutions such as the Spanish Inquisition or the (armed) American anti-abortion lobby—of generally dealing with willing counter-parties in both personal and trading relationships. Its code of morality was imposed on self-selected volunteers who chose to join the Society of Friends and was commercially offered more widely—as in the bill-discounting relationship— only to willing customers who preferred its advantages in long-distance trade to any available alternative. Introducing state or theocratic compulsion of 'moral' or 'civil' behaviour may seem at first sight a superior solution, but the record of its extreme manifestations—from the Spanish Inquisition to the Soviet model—suggests that there is much to be said for limiting state power. This does not mean that central persuasion—whether of a Reithian BBC, a Blairite spin doctor, or a Japanese developmental state[54]—is always wrong or counter-productive, nor that punishing murderers or fining (or jailing the executives of) a corporation that monopolizes computer operating systems is necessarily foolish. The society where guardians do not have to enforce standards of some kind has yet to be invented: saints are always a minority and selfless Utopias are often planned but never achieved. The boundary between the state and the individual is never easy to define, but this age-old problem is more easily and often more creatively resolved where voluntary and competitive self-regulation successfully enables society to avoid the extremes of choices between the two.[55]

[54] C. Johnson, *MITI and the Japanese Miracle: The Growth of Industrial Policy, 1925–1975* (Stanford, Calif., 1982).
[55] J. Jacobs, *Systems of Survival: A Dialogue on the Moral Foundations of Commerce and Politics* (New York, 1994).

17

Civilizing Mammon: Laws, Morals, and the City in Nineteenth-Century England

PAUL JOHNSON

The massive economic and social changes ushered in by industrialization and urbanization created many practical fears and moral doubts about the competitive pressures of a market economy. Geoffrey Searle has recently produced a masterly survey of the way in which educated mid-Victorians 'sought enlightenment as they faced the conflicting claims of conscience and self-interest, religion and political economy', and concludes that the attempt to 'moralize' the market was largely a failure.[1] Yet, if this is true, it suggests that there was a developing social schizophrenia in Victorian society as the way in which people behaved increasingly ran counter to the moral beliefs that they held. This may indeed have been the case, but to establish or verify this requires the historian to look beyond the intellectual strategies developed by articulate mid-Victorians, and consider not just what they said and wrote about the market, but also what they did. The aim here is to explore developments in the moral and legal environment of the City of London in general, and the Stock Exchange in particular, during the nineteenth century.

The morality of market activity is not an easy thing to measure, or even identify. All too often the details of the deal are hidden, and, even when they are known, they may shed little light on the motives. Motives matter because identical outcomes may have entirely different origins and moral foundations. Take, for instance, the case of an insolvent debtor. Is he morally bound to repay old debts after discharging his legal obligations? This question was posed by Edwin Freedley, an American evangelical whose writings on commercial morality went through many editions in England. Freedley thought the answer depended on intent. If the debtor had acted with fraud, misrepresentation, carelessness, or extravagance, then, yes, he should repay. But if the insolvency arose from personal misfortune or commercial fluctuation, then there should be no repayment beyond legal requirements, otherwise 'the

This paper forms part of a larger research project on laws and markets in Victorian England supported by the British Academy.

[1] G. R. Searle, *Morality and the Market in Victorian Britain* (Oxford, 1998), p. x.

wheels of business would stop'.[2] It was not just evangelicals, but lawyers too, who paid attention to motives; successful prosecution of commercial fraud required that intent be proven.

A short essay cannot trace in detail the development of commercial morality across the nineteenth century. What follows is no more than an illustration of how conditions may have differed at the beginning and end of the century. The object is to consider whether the institutions and the actors in the City were, and remained, beyond the pale of a more general and polite bourgeois morality, or whether, by the century's end, the principles and practices of commerce and finance had become acceptable and accepted. Did the 'Mammon-Gospel of Supply-and-demand, Competition, Laissez-faire and Devil take the hindmost' remain, as viewed by Thomas Carlyle in 1843, 'one of the shabbiest Gospels ever preached', or was it civilized and reclothed in a secular garb of popular capitalism?[3] The empirical focus for this examination is two cases of Stock Exchange fraud that were separated by more than seventy years, each of which involved a current or prospective MP who had a public reputation for fighting fraud and corruption. The alleged offences, and the legal, parliamentary, and public responses, give an insight into the changing nature of commercial propriety and morality. These case studies are examined in Sections II and III below, but, before turning to the detail, the literature on commercial morality must first be surveyed, together with the way in which it has been studied by other historians.

I

In 1873 Walter Bagehot described the financial markets of the City of London as 'by far the greatest combination of economical power and economical delicacy that the world has ever seen'.[4] England was the 'greatest moneyed country in the world'; London, according to one of Bagehot's successors as editor of the *Economist*, was 'the capital city of banking and investment'.[5] The economical power of the City, and more generally the investment capital of London-based merchants, manufacturers, professionals, and managers, provided the financial core of Britain's formal and informal economic empire.[6] The City was also, by the century's end, fully incorporated within the status

---

[2] E. T. Freedley, *How to Make Money: A Practical Treatise on Business* (1859), 36. Evangelical views on bankruptcy were far from simple. Freedley's fellow Philadelphian Henry Boardman believed that all bankrupts were morally bound fully to repay all debts, even if creditors had compounded and the bankruptcy had been discharged. See H. A. Boardman, *The Bible in the Counting House* (1854), 136–7.

[3] Thomas Carlyle, *Past and Present*, bk. III, ch. 9, repr. in E. Jay and R. Jay, *Critics of Capitalism: Victorian Reaction to 'political economy'* (Cambridge, 1986), 67.

[4] Walter Bagehot, *Lombard Street* (14th edn., 1915), 3.

[5] Ibid. 4; F. W. Hirst, *The Stock Exchange* (1911), 243.

[6] L. E. Davis and R. A. Huttenback, *Mammon and the Pursuit of Empire* (Cambridge, 1988), 162–82.

and power hierarchies of the country. Successive generations of banking clans ascended social and political ladders. Between 1832 and 1918 the Rothschilds produced six MPs and gained a peerage; the Baring family accounted for twelve MPs and accumulated four peerages (Northbrook, Ashburton, Revelstoke, and Cromer).[7] Dynastic provenance helped in the social ascent, but it was not essential. Ernest Cassel was an entirely self-made financier who, by the early 1900s, was sufficiently esteemed to be accepted as a house guest by the Devonshires at Chatsworth, was a close friend and confidant of the Prince of Wales (the future Edward VII), and was consulted on financial and economic affairs by successive chancellors from Hicks Beach to Asquith.[8]

Yet, even as the denizens of the City reached these heights of prestige and influence, voices were raised as to the propriety of this magnificent financial edifice. 'We must', wrote Bagehot, 'examine the system on which these great masses of money are manipulated, and assure ourselves that it is safe and right.'[9] Bagehot's concern was more with technical matters relating to reserve regulations and the governance of the Bank of England, but others questioned the whole moral basis of the money and commodity markets. In the wave of anti-gambling literature that appeared in the late nineteenth century, links were repeatedly drawn between the speculative trading that formed the core of City market activity and the moral corruption of gambling. Speculation, said the Revd Joseph Parker in a sermon to his black-coated flock at the City Temple, London,

is falsely supposed to be the genius of commerce. An unbridled fancy would not hesitate to describe speculation as the very poetry of business. Many commercial Miltons fancy they are born to cultivate this Paradise Regained. Away with all such fantastic and mischievous nonsense! The Stock Exchange is the bottomless pit of London.[10]

Such opinion was not confined to anti-gambling circles. 'Public moralists' as politically diverse as Herbert Spencer and John Hobson could equally declaim against the evils of the City.[11] For Spencer, many directors of joint stock banks wilfully neglected their responsibilities and were 'near akin in morality to the speculators themselves'. He concluded that 'trade is essentially corrupt', and it was so because of 'the *indiscriminate respect paid to wealth*'.[12]

[7] Y. Cassis, *City Bankers, 1890–1914* (Cambridge, 1994), chs. 6, 7, esp. pp. 228–30, 269.

[8] P. Thane, 'Financiers and the British State: The Case of Sir Ernest Cassel', in R. P. T. Davenport-Hines (ed.), *Speculators and Patriots: Essays in Business Biography* (1986), 80–99. For a more general discussion of the social and political status of financiers, see J. Harris and P. Thane, 'British and European Bankers 1880–1914: An "Aristocratic Bourgeoisie"?', in P. Thane, G. Crossick, and R. Floud (eds.), *The Power of the Past: Essays for Eric Hobsbawm* (Cambridge, 1984), 215–34.   [9] Bagehot, *Lombard Street*, 18.

[10] Joseph Parker, *Gambling in Various Aspects* (5th edn., 1902), 12–13.

[11] The term 'public moralist' is taken from S. Collini, *Public Moralists: Political Thought and Intellectual Life in Britain, 1850–1930* (Oxford, 1991). Collini includes Spencer but not Hobson in the group of intellectuals he considers in this book, but Hobson equally fits the criterion of being one of the 'leading minds' of the period.

[12] Herbert Spencer, 'The Morals of Trade', in W. H. Lyttleton, *Sins of Trade and Business* (Oxford, 1891), 43–4, 50, 56.

Hobson took much the same line. 'The whole theory of modern commercial enterprise', he argued 'involves using other people's money, getting the advantage of this use for one's own self, and paying to the owner as little as one can'. Banks and finance companies used depositors' money in 'doubly speculative' ways 'which do not essentially differ from betting on the turf'.[13]

Spencer and Hobson were latecomers to a long nineteenth-century line of secular and religious critics of commercial morality, and these critics have themselves attracted a good deal of attention from historians. Victorian evangelicals, taking a lead from Thomas Chalmers, were forthright in condemning mammonism in general, and speculation in particular. Chalmers distinguished between 'legitimate' business that involved solid commerce, part of God's instrument for the development of His world, and the selfish and 'illegitimate' business of speculation and overtrading that would necessarily incur God's wrath and punishment as he visited the preventive check of bankruptcy on these earthly sinners.[14] Nowhere was the link between illegitimate trade, spiritual bankruptcy, and atonement drawn more clearly than in the work of the American Henry Boardman, who set himself the task of updating Chalmers for the new commercial conditions of mid-century:

The sorcery of wealth can be dissolved only by the BLOOD OF THE CROSS. And for yourselves—unless you are prepared to barter the 'TRUE RICHES' for the 'mammon of unrighteousness', that disastrous error which has consigned so many Merchants to irretrievable and eternal bankruptcy, you must admit the Gospel of Christ to its legitimate supremacy in the realm of Commerce, and ENTHRONE THE BIBLE IN ALL YOUR COUNTING-HOUSES.[15]

Boyd Hilton suggests that evangelical influence waned from mid-century, and he identifies the introduction of limited liability in 1856 as a key turning point. Up to this date, speculative behaviour carried with it the risk of retribution in the form of personal insolvency, since financial liability in partnerships and the majority of joint stock companies was unlimited. Thereafter, speculation became a one-way bet; profits potentially unlimited, but with the risk of loss restricted to the amount of capital invested in the venture. According to Hilton, limited liability legislation ensured 'that in future the blood of bankrupts should be sprinkled only, and not spilt'.[16] But Jane Garnett disagrees. She finds that limited liability legislation attracted relatively little comment in evangelical tracts, and instead argues that evangelical churchmen played an important role both before and after 1856 in constructing and

---

[13] John Hobson, 'The Ethics of Gambling', in B. Seebohm Rowntree (ed.), *Betting and Gambling: A National Evil* (1905), 17–18.

[14] B. Hilton, *The Age of Atonement: The Influence of Evangelicalism on Social and Economic Thought, 1785–1865* (Oxford, 1988), ch. 4. See also B. Hilton, 'Chalmers as Political Economist', in A. C. Cheyne (ed.), *The Practical and the Pious: Essays on Thomas Chalmers (1780–1847)* (Edinburgh, 1985), 141–56.

[15] Boardman, *Bible*, 284.   [16] Hilton, *Atonement*, 297.

reinforcing a broad set of ethical norms that were applicable not just to their own flock, but to the middle-class business community as a whole. Individual responsibility, honesty, and a renunciation of selfish accumulation at the expense of honourable conduct; these were the moral precepts that needed to be applied both for the spiritual good of the trader and the commercial gain of the nation.[17]

The behavioural implications of this evangelical morality were not dissimilar to those that were implicit within the 'culture of altruism', which, according to Stefan Collini, particularly flourished among the most articulate members of the educated class between 1850 and 1880, exactly the moment when Hilton finds the evangelical strictures on selfishness and commercial excess to be on the wane. Collini suggests, in a resolute challenge to prevailing historiographical norms about Victorian individualism, that 'the texture of moral response among the most prominent Victorian intellectuals was marked at least as much by an obsession with the role of altruism and a concern for the cultivation of feelings as it was by any commitment to the premises of self-interest and rational calculation'.[18] Searle has taken something from each of these approaches in order to trace the mental strategies and rhetorical devices adopted by many mid-Victorian thinkers and writers as they grappled with the practicalities of market transactions. He concludes that ultimately acquisitive individualism was held in check by the forces of Victorian 'authority': religion, political leadership, a disinterested civil service, and employer paternalism.[19]

There are, however, a number of methodological and interpretational problems evident in this historiography of Victorian morality, at least as applied to commercial matters. Garnett's evaluation of the reach of evangelical thought into the economic world is based on representative samples of writings on social ethics from each of the major Protestant evangelical denominations, with particular attention paid to fourteen individuals. She shows that some of the tracts enjoyed wide circulation; the Wesleyan Methodist William Arthur's *The Successful Merchant* sold an impressive 84,000 copies, although this occurred over a somewhat less impressive forty-eight-year period from publication to century's end. However, what this approach cannot reveal is whether evangelical ideas had an impact on commerce beyond a narrow group of evangelical businessmen. Garnett notes that nationally distributed denominational periodicals, sermons, lectures, and tracts circulated among merchants, small businessmen, shopkeepers, clerks, and commercial travellers; what she does not, and cannot, show is whether this literature was read by

---

[17] E. J. Garnett, 'Aspects of the Relationship between Protestant Ethics and Economic Activity in Mid-Victorian England', D.Phil. thesis (Oxford, 1986), ch. 1. See also J. Garnett and A. C. Howe, 'Churchmen and Cotton Masters in Victorian England', in D. J. Jeremy (ed.), *Business and Religion in Britain* (Aldershot, 1988), 72–94.
[18] Collini, *Public Moralists*, 62.   [19] Searle, *Morality*, ch. 11.

anything other than a small minority of such people, and, if read, whether it had any practical affect on their behaviour.[20]

Hilton casts his evidential net much wider, but he likewise assumes rather than demonstrates the practical influence of evangelical ideas on commerce. His method is to deduce the importance of the works of key thinkers such as Chalmers from the extent to which similar ideas and similar language pervaded the 'lower level' of socio-economic debate in Parliament and in tracts and magazines.[21] But how far these ideas, or even the language, had an entrée to Lombard Street is barely considered. Collini confines himself to the 'higher level' of debate generated by public moralists. Rather than assuming that prominent theories and ideologies of the day had a direct influence on society, he instead argues that 'those theories acquired their prominence partly because they gave a coherent form and foundation to attitudes and beliefs already widely, if unselfconsciously, entertained'.[22] Yet the extent of these belief systems remains unexplored. Collini's almost exclusive focus on the 'leading minds' of the day precludes any evaluation of more broadly based social norms and values.

There are several distinct reasons why a well-developed and fully articulated public morality may lie well removed from and have a diminished impact on behaviour. The actors may be an uneducated majority unfamiliar with the higher ideals. They may be aware of the ideals, but constrained by their economic and social circumstances to forgo morally superior but costly forms of behaviour. They may be aware of the ideals but consider them intellectually or philosophically invalid. Or they may consider the public morality as something that is appealing in a general sense, generically a good thing, but simply not appropriate to their particular time, place, and circumstance. While these possibilities are not denied in the historiography, neither are they explicitly accepted. There exists an underlying assumption that none of these four possible causes of a disjuncture between articulation and action really matters.

The two case studies that follow have been chosen because they involve individuals who were not constrained by ignorance, poverty, or philosophy from pursuing the goal of public probity and commercial morality. Indeed, both key actors had established personal reputations as fearless prosecutors of hypocrisy and financial irregularity. The cases, therefore, are not in any sense representative of the majority of trade on the Stock Exchange. It is their exceptionalism, in terms of the high public and parliamentary standing of the protagonists, that makes them such a rich historical source for the analysis of changing public and private attitudes to commercial morality across the course of the nineteenth century.

---

[20] Garnett, 'Aspects', pp. i, 272–86. [21] Hilton, 'Chalmers', 142.
[22] Collini, *Public Moralists*, 4.

II

In the early hours of Monday, 21 February 1814, a man wearing a staff officer's red military tunic adorned with gold star and medal hammered on the door of the Ship Inn at Dover. The stranger demanded pen, ink, paper, a post-chaise and four, together with an express horse and rider to take a message to Admiral Foley at the Deal garrison. The message was that Napoleon had been slain by Cossacks; the allied forces had saved Paris from destruction and entered the city; the white cockade (symbol of the Bourbons) was everywhere displayed; peace was imminent. The signature was that of Lieutenant-Colonel R. du Bourg, Aide-de-Camp to Lord Cathcart, ambassador to the Court of Russia and British military commissioner at the Czar's headquarters. Foley attempted to transmit this news to the Admiralty in London by means of semaphore telegraph, but a heavy mist made this impractical. Meanwhile Colonel du Bourg was proceeding to London in his chaise and four, dispensing the good news at each coaching inn, where payment for new horses was made from a large stock of gold napoleons (although the coachman at Dover, suspicious of dubious foreign coin, demanded and received payment in Bank of England £1 notes). By about 9 a.m. du Bourg had arrived at Marsh Gate, on the south side of Blackfriars Bridge, where he transferred into a hackney carriage and made off in the direction of Grosvenor Square. Around midday, striking confirmation of the news of peace was brought by another chaise and four, decorated with laurels and containing three French officers wearing white cockades, which drove over London Bridge, down Lombard Street, along Cheapside, and over Blackfriars Bridge. Throughout their passage, the occupants distributed small leaflets inscribed with 'Vive le Roi! Vivent les Bourbons!'

The rumour of victory and peace proved to be false, and at first sight the events of 21 February appear to be more farce than fraud. But for a short time, at least, the news of Napoleon's defeat was believed. Newspapers had been awash with speculation and rumour since late January, when Napoleon had ventured out of Paris. Reports of initial success for the allied forces filtered back to London; unsubstantiated news of Napoleon's death appeared in the *Courier* on 10 February. Four days later it was clear that this was nothing but false hope; by 18 February *The Times* acknowledged that Napoleon had secured an impressive victory over Blucher. The country was eager for good news; rumour piled on rumour.[23]

Nowhere did such rumours have a larger impact than on the Stock Exchange. Hopes and expectations had been driving up the value of government stock since the beginning of February. Consols were priced at 66½ on Monday 7th, and within a week reached 72, before falling back to 70 on

---

[23] Information about the personation of du Bourg, and other details of the fraud, are taken from J. B. Atlay, *The Trial of Lord Cochrane before Lord Ellenborough* (1897), 3–14.

Saturday 19th. Over the same period, Omnium (a mixture of government stock and public annuities) rose from $19\frac{1}{8}$ to $28\frac{3}{4}$ before falling to $26\frac{3}{4}$.[24] When the exchange opened at 10 a.m. on Monday 21st, prices rose rapidly on the strength of the news from Dover, with Omnium reaching $30\frac{1}{4}$. The absence of official verification created some disquiet, and prices were sliding around midday until confirmation appeared in the form of the three French officers and their handbills. Omnium touched 32, but after a messenger returned from government offices in the afternoon to report that the whole affair had been a fraud, prices sank back to their level of Saturday.

Trading on the exchange on Monday 21st had been heavy, though not much more so than over the previous two weeks of extremely volatile prices. Nevertheless the blatant and deliberate way in which the false rumour had been generated led the Committee of the Stock Exchange to instigate an enquiry. This investigation revealed that three people together accounted for sales on Monday 21st of over £1.1 million of Consols and Omnium, 'most of which had been purchased in the course of the week preceding'.[25] These three people were Thomas, Lord Cochrane, naval hero, Radical MP for Westminster and eldest son of the ninth Earl of Dundonald; his uncle the Hon. Andrew Cochrane-Johnstone, also an MP, and sometime army colonel and Governor of Domenica; and Richard Butt, former naval pay clerk, successful Stock Exchange speculator, and financial adviser to Lord Cochrane. The Stock Exchange investigation also found that du Bourg's hackney coach had taken him to 13 Green Street, Grosvenor Square, the recently established residence of Lord Cochrane. Furthermore, it was found that four of the £1 notes generously paid out by du Bourg on his journey from Dover had been paid to Butt by his stockbroker on the Saturday afternoon.

The Stock Exchange was variously praised and abused for publishing the result of its enquiry, which had no legal standing and which did not take evidence under oath. In the Commons the Whig Francis Horner congratulated the Stock Exchange on tracing the fraud to its source, and in *The Satirist* George Cruikshank viciously lampooned the conspirators. Meanwhile, William Cobbett, ever keen to support a fellow Radical, fulminated that:

under no wild democracy, under no military despotism, under no hypocritical and cunning oligarchy, under no hellish tyranny upheld by superstition, was there ever committed an act more unjust and more foul than what has, within these three weeks, been committed, in the city of London, through the means of the Press, against the three gentlemen.[26]

However, publication of this report pressurized Lord Cochrane into voluntarily swearing an affidavit about his movements on 21 February. He acknow-

[24] Atlay, *Trial*, 13.
[25] *Report of the Sub-Committee of the Stock Exchange Relative to the Late Fraud* (1814), 15.
[26] Parl. Deb. (1814), 27, c. 987 (20 May); *Cobbett's Weekly Political Register*, 26 Mar. 1814, 25/13, c. 385.

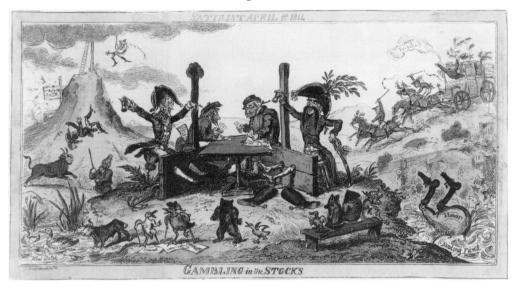

15. George Cruikshank, *Gambling in the Stocks* (1814). Cruikshank's satire on the Stock Exchange hoax. Cochrane (seated on a thistle) and de Berenger play dice, Cochrane-Johnstone and Butt play cards, even as they are entrapped in the stocks. In the foreground a bull, a bear, and two lame ducks trample Omnium and Consols underfoot; on the right, Honor dives head first into the Sinking Fund.

ledged that he knew well, and had breakfasted with, Cochrane-Johnstone and Butt, that he had traded down all his Omnium, and that a uniformed officer had visited his house. His defence, however, was that he had left general orders with his broker to sell whenever the price rose to one point over the purchase price, and had issued no direct, personal instructions to trade on the 21st. Furthermore the officer who had visited him was a Captain Random de Berenger, a distant acquaintance, who had earlier contacted Cochrane about joining him on a forthcoming naval mission.

De Berenger was a designer, inventor, rifleman, pyrotechnician, and insolvent debtor of Prussian birth, currently living under the rules of the King's Bench (as was, it subsequently emerged, one of the three men who purported to be a French officer). He was arrested in Leith in early April while trying to buy a passage out of the country, and in his possession were found a number of gold napoleons, together with bank notes that traced back to Cochrane-Johnstone and Butt: De Berenger and du Bourg were one and the same person.[27] With evidence in place, the Stock Exchange brought a prosecution against both major and minor players in the fraud. The case was heard before Lord Ellenborough in June 1814; the key charge was that Lord Cochrane,

---

[27] Atlay, *Trial*, 50.

Cochrane-Johnstone, and Butt had conspired, by disseminating false information, to raise the price of government funds 'with a wicked and fraudulent
intention' to 'cheat and defraud' the King's subjects.[28] The motive was made
plain by the chief prosecuting counsel, the Quaker Adolphus Gurney. For
several months prior to the fraud the three principal conspirators had been
speculating heavily on the Stock Exchange,[29] invariably as 'bulls'—that is, they
bought in the expectation of the price rising, so they could sell out at a profit.
They traded very large quantities, but needed very little cash so to do, because
transactions within each fortnightly Stock Exchange accounting period were
settled only at the end of the account. As long as equal amounts were bought
and sold, the only money that changed hands was the difference between the
buying and selling price, plus the broker's ⅛ per cent commission. The account
open at the time of the fraud (or 'hoax' as Lord Cochrane whimsically chose
to call it) had begun on 8 February and was due to close on the 23rd.[30]
Cochrane *et al.* were speculating heavily on an increase in price. According to
Adolphus Gurney, 'their purchases vastly exceeded their sales . . . they had
gone on plunging deeper and deeper until they were out of their depth'.[31] They
had contracted to buy more than £1 million of stock, in anticipation of selling
at a profit before 23 February. But news from France on the 14th kept prices
flat, while on the 18th confirmation of Napoleon's victory depressed prices. An
attempt to offload £1 million of stock onto a declining market would have sent
prices spiralling; the trio of conspirators faced 'an immense loss, perhaps
irrecoverable ruin', according to de Berenger.[32] The fraud was designed not to
make them vast sums (though their net profits, seized by the Stock Exchange
Committee and subsequently donated to various charities, totalled more than
£10,000), but to prevent even larger losses.[33]

Despite the efforts of a strong defence team, which included the future Lord
Chancellor Henry Brougham, the future Chief Justice of Common Pleas,
William Best (Lord Wynford), and 'by far the most successful advocate of his
day' and future Attorney-General, James Scarlett (Lord Abinger),[34] the special
jury of City men found for the prosecution. The chief conspirators were each
sentenced to twelve months' imprisonment in the Marshalsea, a fine of
£1,000, and an hour in the pillory outside the Royal Exchange.[35] The case is

[28] W. B. Gurney, *The Trial of Charles Random de Berenger, taken in shorthand* (1814), 7.
[29] Cochrane first traded on the Exchange in Nov. 1813. See *The Trial of Lord Cochrane* (1814),
32.
[30] *The calumnious aspersions contained in the report of the sub-committee of the Stock-Exchange
exposed and refuted* (1814), 32.
[31] Gurney, *Trial*, 40.
[32] Charles Random de Berenger, *The Noble Stock Jobber* (1816), 64.
[33] Atlay, *Trial*, 239. Cochrane-Johnstone in particular could not afford to lose, as he was already
in financial difficulty and evading arrest only by means of his privileges as an MP.
[34] *DNB* xvii. 891.
[35] *The Case of Thomas Lord Cochrane* (Edinburgh, 1814), 60. After parliamentary discussion it
was agreed to revoke the sentence of pillory.

remarkable for more than just its extraordinary genesis and the ensuing lordly dispute between three generations of Dundonalds and Ellenboroughs over the probity of court proceedings and the validity of the verdict.[36] The personal history of Lord Cochrane, the legal basis of the case, and the public and parliamentary reaction to the verdict all shed light on the nature of commercial morality in the early nineteenth century.

Cochrane had achieved both fame and fortune as a courageous and imaginative naval captain. He had been awarded the Order of the Bath for his heroic assault on the French fleet in the Aix roads in 1809, but had attracted the unbending hostility of the naval establishment by using his privilege as an MP to accuse his commander, Lord Gambier, of incompetence.[37] He was briefly MP for the rotten borough of Honiton in 1806, before winning one of the Westminster seats in 1807, where his fellow MP was the Radical Sir Francis Burdett. With support from Cobbett's *Political Register*, Cochrane launched a number of parliamentary attacks on the gross inefficiency of Admiralty administration and on the scale and extent of sinecures paid, under the guise of pensions, to many parliamentarians. He took an unambiguous personal stand against privilege and 'old corruption'; indeed, at an initially unsuccessful attempt to secure the seat of Honiton, he promised the electors: 'I shall never accept any sinecure or pension, or any grant of the public money; and that I will never ask or receive any such for any person whatever that may be in any way dependent on me.'[38] Cochrane's public profile, both as naval hero and as anti-corruption campaigner, made his fall from grace all the more poignant. He had claimed the moral high ground for himself, but, in the words of Mr Justice Leblanc in the preamble to the sentence, was found guilty of 'a crime, which, in its progress, was denoted by every unseemly characteristic; it was tainted with meanness, mendacity, and avarice'. Furthermore, Cochrane 'had not even the palliative of poverty as an apology for the sin'.[39]

Cochrane claimed that both the verdict and the sentence were politically motivated, and that Ellenborough had conducted the case with overt bias and political spite. This claim was accepted by Burdett and other Radicals, who commenced an active campaign to rescue Cochrane's reputation. The details

---

[36] Cochrane's grandson petitioned Parliament in 1877 to have the trial verdict set aside, and in 1890 republished, with amendment, Cochrane's autobiography, but did not alter a number of accusations levelled against the trial judge. Ellenborough's nephew and grandson replied personally in print and at length, as well as commissioning Atlay to write an account of the case. The last of these ripostes appeared a full century after the trial. See: Thomas, 10th earl of Dundonald, *Autobiography of a Seaman*, and Thomas, 11th earl of Dundonald and H. R. Fox Bourne, *Life of Thomas, 10th earl of Dundonald, completing the autobiography of a seaman* (2 vols., 1869; repr. in one volume in 1890); Henry Spencer Law, *Reviews of the 'Autobiography of a Seaman'* (1877); Lord Ellenborough (Edward Downes Law), *The Guilt of Lord Cochrane* (1914).

[37] C. Lloyd, *Lord Cochrane* (1947), 81–104.

[38] *The Case*, 2. On 'old corruption' in general, see P. Harling, *The Waning of 'Old Corruption'* (Oxford, 1996).

[39] *The Case*, 60.

of the case, however, hardly reveal a concerted Tory attack on radicalism. The prosecution was brought not by the government, but by the Stock Exchange, and the evidence of Cochrane's intimate knowledge of the 'hoax' was overwhelming. Cochrane does not appear to have viewed Stock Exchange speculation, or even the manipulation of stock prices through rumour-mongering, as morally wrong.[40] Although he was unrestrained in his critique of public corruption, and forthright in his renunciation of all public favours (something that his subsequent career proved to be a rhetorical flourish rather than a principled stand), he behaved in the market as he did in war, adopting morally dubious policies in the belief that the ends justified the means.[41]

The legal basis of the prosecution case also reveals a good deal about contemporary perceptions of commercial probity. Cochrane *et al.* were charged with conspiracy to defraud the King's subjects by deliberately manipulating stock prices. Yet, as Cobbett noted before the trial, 'Whether it be a *legal* offence to spread false reports for the purpose of gaining in the funds, remains to be shewn; but if it be a legal offence, it is one which the newspaper people have been accusing each other almost every week, for twenty years past.'[42] It was not just newspapers that generated false rumours; individuals did this too. Nathan Rothschild used the rumour mill to manipulate prices; when he possessed advance news (often from his private Paris–London pigeon post) calculated to make the funds rise, he would sell heavily, knowing that others would follow his lead, thereby allowing him to buy in at a much reduced price before the good news arrived and prices rose.[43] There were many ways of creating false rumours; Cochrane's scheme was more theatrical than most, but it seems certain that the Committee of the Stock Exchange tolerated many less blatant manipulations.

However, the prosecution managed to demonstrate that Cochrane's 'hoax' was not a victimless crime. On the day of the fraud the Accountant-General had purchased over £15,000 of Consols at inflated prices on behalf of the official trustee, who managed assets for public charitable trusts, orphans, and other dependants. Had this purchase been made at the price prevailing on the preceding Saturday, the same quantity of Consols could have been had for

---

[40] See the disquisition on Cochrane's motives in the anonymous *Letter to the Electors of Westminster on the Case of Lord Cochrane* (1814), 9–10.

[41] Part of Cochrane's dispute with Gambier over the naval action in the Aix roads arose because Cochrane wanted to use fire ships against the French fleet, which Gambier thought improper. Cochrane also developed in 1812 a 'top-secret' scheme for chemical warfare (using sulphur gas to poison garrison towns), and relentlessly pressed his ideas on the British government over the next four decades. In response to criticisms that such methods were immoral, he argued that such a plan might save lives by ending conflict more quickly than conventional warfare: Lloyd, *Lord Cochrane*, 105–13.

[42] *Cobbett's Weekly Political Register*, 18 June 1814, 25/25, col. 771.

[43] D. Morier Evans, *The City: Or, The Physiology of London Business* (1845), 51–3; John Francis, *Chronicles and Characters of the Stock Exchange* (1855), 300.

some £340 less. The case demonstrates that both within the Stock Exchange fraternity and among jurors in the King's Bench court there existed a clear conception of commercial probity. Concealing privileged information from the public, as Nathan Rothschild often did when he traded on the market, was legitimate, but knowingly creating and supplying false information was not.

The official response to Cochrane's crime was damning. He lost income, political position, and social status, as he was struck off the navy list, expelled from the Commons, and ejected from the Order of the Bath with ritualistic humiliation: his heraldic banner was torn down from the Chapel of Henry VII in Westminster Abbey and ignominiously kicked down the steps. The public response, however, was very different; within a few days of his expulsion from the House he was returned again by the electors of Westminster.[44] He was forthright in pursuing his personal grievances and claims for recompense, and in 1816 brought forward in the House a charge of 'partiality, misrepresentation, injustice and oppression' against Lord Chief Justice Ellenborough, the motion being lost by 89 votes to 0. From 1818 until the 1830s he served with the navies of Chile, Peru, Brazil, and Greece, but he maintained a long-running campaign to have his sentence quashed, making lengthy representations to the government in 1825 and 1830. His perseverance paid off. In May 1832 he was granted a free pardon and reinstated to his rank of rear-admiral and placed on half pay. In 1841 he was granted a naval pension for meritorious service, in 1847 was restored to the Order of the Bath, and in 1848–51 was appointed Commander-in-Chief of the North American and West Indian station. Not content with this, in 1856 he wrote to Palmerston requesting the restoration of his banner to Henry VII's chapel, repayment of his £1,000 fine, and restoration of half pay for the period 1814–32. This latter claim he bequeathed to his heirs, who in 1877 successfully petitioned for a Select Committee to investigate the claim. This Committee noted that his treatment since 1832 amounted to 'nothing less than a public recognition by those Governments of his innocence', and in the following year the grandson received an *ex gratia* payment of £5,000 in respect of the 'distinguished services' of his grandfather.[45]

From being the best-known fraudster of his day, Cochrane managed gradually to rewrite his personal history and reinvent himself. Although he regained his formal rank and honours, he never became fully accepted by the mid-Victorian élite. He was buried in 1860 in the nave of Westminster Abbey, but no cabinet minister or officer of the state attended the funeral, though his old friend Lord Brougham did.[46] Yet in popular standing Cochrane was a hero

---

[44] For details, see A. Aspinall, 'The Westminster Election of 1814', *EHR* 40 (1925), 562–9.
[45] Atlay, *Trial*, 241–54, 283–91, 369–77.
[46] J. W. Fortescue, *Dundonald* (1895), 201.

rather than a fraud, and his heroism grew over time, finally being lionized in one of G. A. Henty's historical tales.[47] In 1814 he had erred against the laws and morals of the day, but over time the public perception of his crime diminished. To some extent his naval exploits may have atoned for his sins, but attitudes towards commercial morality were changing. As the next section shows, Stock Exchange fraud in the late-Victorian period was no barrier to a public and parliamentary career.

III

On 14 January 1887 the Rae-Transvaal Gold Mining Company was registered at Companies' House with limited liability status. This was one of many prospecting companies floated during the 'Kaffir' speculation of 1886–7, and at first sight appeared to be no better or worse placed than any of its many competitors. However, in the judgement of the *Financial News*, one of the leading financial journals of the day,[48] this new company displayed 'every element of success' and was 'likely to prove a good speculation'. So confident was the *Financial News* of the prospects for the Rae-Transvaal that it offered no less than thirty-three recommendations for these shares between 18 January and 29 April 1887. Yet the performance of the company was lamentable; it spent only £138 on prospecting equipment and managed to sink a shaft to a depth of just 30 feet, it produced not an ounce of gold, never made a profit, and was liquidated on 22 May 1888. Shareholders lost everything; creditors received payments of less than 6d. in the £.[49]

The fortunes of this company, and the fate of the shareholders, were far from exceptional. The intriguing part is the way in which the company was formed, floated, and promoted by Harry H. Marks. In late 1886 Marks purchased a bankrupt 6,154-acre Transvaal farm for £10,300, and immediately sold it on for a notional £50,000 to a company he formed for the purpose, using a dummy (a stockbroker's clerk) to sign the appropriate deeds and checks in exchange for £200. Marks was paid with about 23,000 of the company's £1 shares. He then set about drawing up a prospectus for the company prior to registration and public flotation. The enthusiasm of the *Financial News* encouraged members of the public to apply for almost 8,000 shares, but this still left over 19,000 shares unallocated, so Marks generated a slew of bogus applications from, among others, his brother-in-law and his

---

[47] G. A. Henty, *With Cochrane the Dauntless* (1897). Henty makes no reference to the Stock Exchange fraud, but the incident is used as the centrepiece of a more recent novel of naval heroism. See P. O'Brian, *The Reverse of the Medal* (1986).

[48] Mr Pooter's son, Lupin, 'was riveted to the *Financial News* as if he had been born a capitalist' (George and Weedon Grossmith, *The Diary of a Nobody* (Bristol, 1892)).

[49] The details of the Rae-Transvaal company are taken from Henry Hess, '*The Critic*' *Black Book*, app. vol. (1901–2), 179–85.

brother-in-law's mistress. To encourage further public support for the issue he ensured that the shares were quoted at a false premium in the *Financial News*; this created an active market that allowed him and his dummy share-holders to offload their holdings at a profit. A total of 45,500 shares were foisted on the public, all at a price above their £1 par value.

The Rae-Transvaal was just one of many dubious deals carried out by Marks. He was deeply implicated in at least one other gold prospecting fraud, appears to have received bribes in excess of £17,000 from the corrupt financial empire of E. T. Hooley, and was described as 'a scoundrel on his own admission' and 'a dishonest rogue' by a judge in a libel case in 1903.[50] But Marks was no ordinary company fraudster. He was, in addition, managing editor of the *Financial News*, a member of the London County Council in 1889–91 and 1895–7, and Conservative MP for Tower Hamlets 1895–1900 and for Thanet 1904–10. Born in 1855 to the prominent Jewish theologian David Woolf Marks, Harry cut his journalistic teeth in the USA before bringing an aggressive American newspaper style to Britain. Under the editorship of Marks, the *Financial News* fearlessly exposed other people's fraud and corruption. Marks was responsible for revealing the financial misdeeds within the Metropolitan Board of Works, and it was largely for this reason that he secured election as one of the first cohort of LCC councillors.[51] But he was not content with the rewards of an editor's salary, and he used his position, as perhaps did other representatives of the financial press, to 'puff' companies in exchange for payment.[52] In the case of the Rae-Transvaal, however, he went much further, and conducted a massive fraud on the public.

From at least 1890 Marks's fraudulent activity was sufficiently well known to lead to public accusations and a number of (unsuccessful) suits by Marks for libel.[53] By 1903 Henry Hess was writing openly about the Rae-Transvaal scam that 'it has become a standing wonder to all who know the particulars, how Marks and those who subsequently joined him in the venture, escaped penal servitude'.[54] But this invective was not sufficient to prevent Marks from re-entering parliament in 1904, having retired in 1900 because of ill health. He retained his Thanet seat in 1906, much to the dismay of a dissident group of local Conservatives who in November wrote to the Speaker of the Commons itemizing Marks's past record and arguing that he was 'unfit to be a member of the House'. They followed this up with a pamphlet, circulated

[50] Ibid. 159–62; D. Porter, '"A trusted guide of the investing public": Harry Marks and the *Financial News*, 1884–1916', in Davenport-Hines (ed.), *Speculators and Patriots*, 8, 10; *The Times*, 26 Nov. 1906.

[51] *Men and Women of the Time* (15th edn., 1899), 722–3. Marks's articles exposing MBW corruption were reprinted in *The Metropolitan Board of Works: a brief account of the disclosures which have led to the appointment of a Royal Commission* (1888).

[52] The veteran financial journalist Charles Duguid believed that bribery was rife within the financial press. See Charles Duguid, *How to Read the Money Article* (1901), 103–6.

[53] Porter, 'Harry Marks', 8.   [54] Hess, *Black Book*, 179.

to every sitting MP, detailing a number of court cases from 1890 to 1904 in which the fraudulent actions of Marks had been exposed.[55] There was, however, never any attempt to prosecute him for market-rigging, or to unseat him from Parliament. At his death in 1916 he owned a country estate of 200 acres in Kent where he was a JP, had a London residence in Cavendish Square, and was a member of the Carlton, Royal Cinque Ports, and Royal Temple Yacht Clubs.

IV

The cases of Cochrane and Marks are as exceptional as the individuals themselves. Despite the almost baroque richness of the historical accounts that lend themselves to a form of 'thick description', it would be no more legitimate to take these two individual histories as emblematic of nineteenth-century commercial morality than it would be to take the careers of Nathan Rothschild and Alexander Baring as typical of the nineteenth-century bank manager. But the actions of Cochrane and Marks, and the manner in which they were treated by Parliament and the law, do indicate how stock-market dealings were viewed by a wider world, and they indicate this in a way that is different from, and more direct than, a study of the writings of selected evangelicals or intellectuals.

The parliamentary responses to Cochrane and Marks could not have been more different. Cochrane was unseated by a vote of 140 to 41, on the grounds that his conviction of conspiracy to defraud the King's subjects rendered him unfit for public office, regardless of his earlier service to King and country in the Royal Navy. The actions of the conspirators had been against the public interest, and had also undermined the reputation of the Stock Exchange. In the immediate aftermath of the hoax, *The Times* gave a clear indication of what was needed to restore public confidence in a damaged institution: 'let the Members of the Stock Exchange agree to exclude from their body every individual, who shall be known to enter into such speculations as now disgrace the market, and though their numbers may be somewhat diminished, their respectability and public benefit will be much more than proportionately increased.'[56] In the case of Marks, however, there was no attempt by either Parliament or the Conservative Party to distance themselves from his actions or to suggest how the public interest might be protected in the future from similar stock-market depredations. It might be easy to attribute the benign

---

[55] *The Times*, 26 Nov. 1906, 11 Nov. 1907. In addition to his commercial frauds, Marks was also publicly accused of extensive electoral bribery and malpractice. See J. C. Haig, 'The Case of Thanet, Illustrating the Methods of Mr H. H. Marks', in C. R. Buxton, *Electioneering Up-to-Date* (1906), 77–90.

[56] *The Times*, 14 Mar. 1814.

treatment of Marks to simple good fortune if his were a unique case, but in fact the mid- and late-Victorian Parliament consistently condoned dubious Stock Exchange dealing.[57] One of several other cases was that of Harry Seymour Foster, an exact contemporary of Marks. Foster, like Marks, was renowned for promoting worthless companies. Between 1878 and 1900 he formed sixty-six companies, of which only four were still in existence and paying dividends by 1902. He, like Marks, unsuccessfully pursued libel cases against newspapers that accused him of fraudulent commercial activity.[58] Yet this record was no barrier to political position; like Marks, he became an LCC councillor in 1889, sat as conservative MP for Lowestoft in 1892–1900, for North Suffolk in 1910, and for Portsmouth in 1924–9. For his good service to the Conservative Party Foster received a knighthood in 1918.[59]

These parliamentary responses can also be contrasted with public opinion. Although in 1814 *The Times* fulminated against Cochrane and his co-conspirators, the electors of Westminster did not. In July 1814 they nominated him as their sole candidate for the parliamentary seat made vacant by his expulsion from the House, and elected him by acclamation. At the hustings his proposer, Sir Francis Burdett, without any hint of irony assured the electors that Cochrane's presence in the House was essential 'for the purpose of laying the axe to the root of corruption', a sentiment that drew loud applause from the crowd.[60] Contrast this with the state of electoral politics in Thanet in 1906. A substantial group of Conservative constituents actively opposed the election campaign of Marks, on the grounds that he was 'of notorious character'. His electoral success owed rather more to the convivial banquets he provided for constituents, his extensive donations to local benefit clubs and friendly societies, his gifts to clergymen, and his use of *Financial News* staff as full-time election agents, than to popular approval for his personal conduct.[61] But once elected there was no move in the Commons to question either his alleged stock-market frauds or his alleged electoral malpractices, despite the publicity they received. In the early nineteenth century it seems that the majority of parliamentarians took a lead in identifying and censuring immorality on the Stock Exchange on the grounds that such behaviour was against the public interest; by the early twentieth century their complicity was eloquently articulated by their silence.

Identifying the reasons for a change in parliamentary attitudes to financial fraud is not a simple task, but one important factor must be the way in which many parliamentarians became direct beneficiaries of speculative company

[57] This readiness of politicians and aristocrats to endorse questionable commercial morality was brilliantly satirized by Anthony Trollope in *The Way We Live Now* (1875).

[58] Hess, *Black Book*, 218–19; *Secrets of Company Promoting* (1894), *passim*.

[59] M. Stenton and S. Lees, *Who's Who of British Members of Parliament, 1919–45* (Brighton, 1979).

[60] *The Times*, 12 July 1814.   [61] Haig, 'The Case of Thanet', 78–85.

promotions. In Georgian England, Stock Exchange activity was largely restricted to trade in government stock by a small number of wealthy investors. The Exchange had become formalized in its own building only in 1801; few people other than City professionals knew much about its workings. The railway mania of 1845 changed this; hundreds of new joint-stock companies were floated and tens of thousands of small investors were attracted into the market by the prospect of high dividends and capital gains. Lawyers were perhaps the biggest winners from this speculative boom,[62] but MPs also did very well. The new railway companies, most of which never built a yard of track or carried an ounce of freight, needed 'respectable' citizens on their boards to convey an appropriate picture of stability and probity to the investing public. By the end of 1845 over 150 MPs had 'made a traffic on their presumed responsibility' by becoming railway directors, thereby entitling themselves to advantageous share allocations and directorial remuneration.[63] The bond between the boardroom and Parliament grew in strength throughout Victoria's reign; in 1866, 216 MPs were company directors, a number that had risen by 1898 to 293, representing 44 per cent of the House of Commons.[64] Parliamentarians quite literally 'bought in' to the methods and morals of the stock exchange.

In terms of the law, Marks's Rae-Transvaal fraud was more calculated and more complex than Cochrane's 'hoax'. Cochrane supplied false information in the hope that the market would respond in a particular way. Marks, on the other hand, carried out a 'sting'—first he created what was, in effect, a false company, then he supplied false information about its prospects, using his privileged position as editor of the major financial newspaper of the day, and finally he created an artificial demand for the shares by making bogus applications. But perhaps the most important difference between the two incidents is that, whereas Cochrane's fraud was a unique event, Marks's scam was just one among hundreds of spurious company promotions of the mid- and late-Victorian period. Fraudulent company promotion had been clearly identified by the 1844 Select Committee on Joint Stock Companies as a problem requiring legislative action, but the minimal financial reporting requirements placed on joint-stock companies throughout the nineteenth century, and the consistent failure of the legislature to tighten the regulatory regime, allowed company promoters and directors to extract many millions of pounds from the incipient popular capitalism that was developing throughout Victoria's reign.[65]

---

[62] R. W. Kostal, *Law and English Railway Capitalism* (Oxford, 1994), pt. 1.

[63] D. Morier Evans, *The Commercial Crisis 1847–8* (1848), 5, 19 n.

[64] *The Joint-Stock Companies' Directory, 1866* (1866), 961–1266; *Directory of Directors for 1898* (1898), *passim.*

[65] H. C. Edey and P. Panitpakdi, 'British Company Accounting and the Law, 1844–1900', in A. C. Littleton and B. S. Yamey (eds.), *Studies in the History of Accounting* (Homewood, Ill., 1956),

In addition to the weakness of company and stock-market regulation, there was a relaxation from mid-century in the judicial treatment of commercial crimes. This had more to do with the emergence of the general joint-stock company after 1844 than with limited liability. In the joint-stock company there was a necessary divorce of ownership and control, and responsibility for incompetence or fraud was difficult to locate. When the private bank of Strachan, Paul, and Bates failed in 1855 and it was revealed that the partners (including the prominent evangelical Sir John Paul) had fraudulently used depositors' funds, they were held personally liable and were sentenced to four-teen years' transportation. But when, a year later, the joint-stock Royal British Bank folded, in part because the directors had granted themselves huge (and secret) unsecured loans, it was difficult to prove anything other than con-tributory negligence. Sentences ranged between three and twelve months, and most of the defendants managed to escape the full measure of even this modest punishment.[66]

Changes in social and economic circumstances always put pressure on inherited rules of morality. Keith Thomas has noted this tension during the seventeenth-century 'age of conscience'; it was no less severe during the nineteenth-century age of industry.[67] What is striking about this nineteenth-century experience is the ease with which the new commercial morality became accepted and adopted by middle-class society. Mammon became civilized well before the century's end, but this civilizing process was not one in which Mammon submitted to an inherited morality, whether evangelical or altruistic. Rather than the Bible being enthroned in the counting houses (the Stock Exchange Christian Association, founded in 1876, had only 250 members by 1901, or just over 3 per cent of those eligible to join),[68] it was the morality of Mammon that was exported to and enthroned in the wider world. It was incorporated into the civil law, acceded to in the criminal courts, and embraced by MPs, who boarded the speculative stock-market gravy train in their hundreds.

356–79; C. Gilmore and H. Willmott, 'Company Law and Financial Reporting: A Sociological History of the UK Experience', in M. Bromwich and A. Hopwood (eds.), *Accounting and the Law* (Hemel Hempstead, 1992), 159–90.

[66] D. Morier Evans, *Facts, Failures and Frauds* (1859), 103–53, 268–390.

[67] K. Thomas, 'Cases of Conscience in Seventeenth-Century England' in J. Morrill, P. Slack, and D. Woolf (eds.), *Public Duty and Private Conscience in Seventeenth-Century England: Essays Presented to G. E. Aylmer* (Oxford, 1993), 29–56.

[68] Charles Duguid, *The Story of the Stock Exchange* (1901), 255.

18

Civility and Empire

JOHN DARWIN

Civility is a subtle and ambiguous term with a long history, but its obvious current definition seems to be a code of behaviour designed to restrain the natural quarrelsomeness of individuals and promote social solidarity. Politeness and good manners lubricate social life and supply a diplomatic procedure for the negotiation of interpersonal conflicts. In reality, however, interpersonal courtesies depend upon a certain commonality of outlook: otherwise they can be maintained only by studied formality and the careful minimization of social contact. Hence the importance of other historic uses of civility to imply 'right conduct' in all those spheres of social action where individual preferences or idiosyncrasies were likely to jar against each other. Forms of greeting or social deference—the raising of hats, kissing, bowing, shaking hands, phrases of respect and recognition—were the most elementary expression of this. But civility could hardly thrive where personal habits were unregulated or uncodified—if attitudes to clothing, personal decoration, cleanliness, bodily functions, and the consumption of food, drink, and stimulants were left entirely to the anarchy of individual choice. Nor could civility easily be reconciled with widely divergent attitudes towards violence, the definition of crime, the status of women and children, or the formal requirements (rather than the actual practice) of sexual morality.

I

From this it is easy to see that civility, even in the narrow sense of politeness, is really a function of an entire complex of social relations. Codes of conduct and mutual obligation were as variable as the social structures and belief systems from which they sprang. When widely different societies made contact or were locked together by conquest or colonization, rival versions of civility competed for hegemony. For the participants in this struggle of civilities, the stakes were high. Civility's symbolic importance as the register of obligations and values conferred on apparently trivial adjustments of dress, gesture, or even hairstyle a much larger significance. In that sense, 'law' and 'culture' may both be seen as proxies for specific aspects of civility. Where communities were already under strain—as embattled minorities or defeated majorities—failure to uphold their established order of civility in its full rigour seemed to threaten the unravelling of the whole social fabric.

This syndrome is visible in the earliest phases of English imperial expansion into the Celtic societies of Wales and Ireland. English administrators were acutely aware that settler minorities faced a war of cultural attrition in which the first victim would be their English civility. The daily pressure of social and economic contact with the surrounding population, the attractions of conviviality, the lure of intermarriage, the temptation to profit by taking service under or holding land from the indigenous élite: all were likely to erode the distinctive ethos of the incomers and (as a consequence) to dissolve the bonds that held them together as a community. How seriously this danger was taken may be deduced from the recourse to legal rules. The Statute of Rhuddlan (1284)[1] and the Statute of Kilkenny (1366) were great regulatory dikes to guard a fragile English civility. 'Many English of the land,' declared the Statute of Kilkenny,

forsaking the English language, dress, style of riding, laws and usages, live and govern themselves according to the manners, dress and language of the Irish enemies, and had also contracted marriages and alliances with them whereby the land and liege people thereof, the English language, the allegiance due to the lord king and the English laws there are put into subjection and decayed . . .[2]

The statute was renewed in 1498 and supplemented in 1536 by a strict prohibition on the use of Irish customs and dress within the Pale.

The intolerance and even savagery that marked the enforcement of such regulations seem strangely at odds with the pretensions to cultural superiority that underlay English expansion then and later. Part of the explanation can be found in the peculiar nature of English civility. To grapple with that, we need to apply a simple twofold classification to the idea of civility. One view of civility would be to see it as a universal attribute of human communities, however small in scale or simple in structure. Every human group, it might be argued, requires rules of social engagement if it is not to disintegrate at its first dispute. Civility is merely a neutral label that describes the practices of social restraint detectable by any external observer willing or able to cast off his own cultural prejudices. The second view would narrow drastically the meaning of civility by refusing to see it as a universal social phenomenon. Civility was not instinctive but a conscious choice made under certain social conditions. It was incompatible with a society where individual status and behaviour were rigidly prescribed by religion or kinship obligations. Indeed,

[1] Sometimes the Statute of Wales. See R. R. Davies, *The Age of Conquest: Wales 1063–1415* (Oxford, 1991), 368 ff.
[2] Cited in J. A. Watt, 'The Anglo-Irish Colony under Strain 1327–1399', in A. Cosgrove (ed.), *The New History of Ireland*, ii. *Medieval Ireland* (Oxford, 1987), 387.

in societies where loyalty to kin took precedence over every other kind of social obligation, civility in its wider sense could hardly be practised at all. Civility was an acknowledgement that social membership of a polity (as opposed to a family, clan, tribe, caste, or ethnic group) depended upon the careful cultivation of habits, manners, and preferences designed to maximize harmonious social intercourse and its benefits. It was the ethos required by an open society, or, at the least, one whose scale, mobility, and forms of hierarchy permitted a degree of individual choice over what social obligations to assume.

If we adopt this second meaning of civility, we can see that its real function was to act as a social glue in communities where other forms of solidarity have been cast aside or drastically limited in scope. Such communities might be more efficient as producers and exchangers, but they were also likely to be more vulnerable to internal disruption than simpler societies if the bonds of social sympathy were snapped. Least of all could they tolerate community members who avowed (or were suspected of) prime loyalty, not to the welfare of the social collective as a whole, but to the codes of a particularistic sub-group or even of an outside authority. Hence the savage response of an increasingly open and mobile early modern English society to religious or ethnic groups who resisted absorption. Refusal, or inability, to conform was punished by exclusion or worse. From that point of view, even the institutional apparatus of slavery—the imposition of 'social death'—might be seen as the necessary counterpart to the practice of civility amongst an anomic planter class in the tropical dystopia of the English Caribbean.[3]

In early modern England there was no consensus on the reasons why other peoples rejected English notions of civility or clung to obsolete customs. Edmund Spenser, an apologist for English rule in Ireland, put into the mouth of 'Eudoxus' horrified bafflement at the social retrogression of English settlers there. 'Is it possible that an Englisheman brought up naturallye in suche swete civilytie as Englande affordes can finde suche likinge in that barbarous rudenes that he shoulde forgett his own nature and forgoe his own nacion?' gasps Eudoxus.[4] It was tempting to ascribe cultural backwardness to religious error—Edward I had denounced Irish laws as 'detestable to God'—a tendency that the Reformation may have encouraged. In the Elizabethan conquest of Ireland, the brutal expropriation of native Irish was sometimes justified on the grounds of their paganism. But English civility had also come to be equated with a whole pattern of governance with a law-making Parliament at its centre;[5] with the use of written legal instruments; with a view of crime as

---

[3] See R. S. Dunn, *Sugar and Slaves: The Rise of the Planter Class in the English West Indies, 1624–1713* (Chapel Hill, NC, 1972), 249–50.

[4] Quoted in H. Pawlisch, *Sir John Davies and the Conquest of Ireland* (Cambridge, 1985), 57.

[5] For the place of Parliament in Tudor political culture, see N. D. Jones, 'Parliament and the Political Society of Elizabethan England', in D. Hoak (ed.), *Tudor Political Culture* (Cambridge, 1995).

an offence against the ruler (rather than the victim); and increasingly with the prevalence of individuated property. It was instability in the succession of property under Gaelic custom, claimed Sir John Davies in 1603, that prevented a proper exploitation of the soil and a stable polity in Ireland: the survival of Gaelic tenures had been the root of English weakness and Irish disaffection.[6] In the later seventeenth century Locke formalized these insights into a powerful theoretical system, insisting that the great engine of social and political change lay in the emergence of individual property rights in response to economic necessity. But it was Hume who articulated most effectively what might be called the 'historicist revolution' in the idea of civility, supplying in the process one of the most important keys to British imperial thinking in the nineteenth and twentieth centuries.

Hume's achievement was to connect up the processes of economic transformation to which Locke had referred with an older idea of civility as the refinement of law, language, and manners. The full development of civility, he argued, depended upon reaching the highest stage of economic progress. That was possible only when men, who were naturally competitive in their economic relations, grasped that collective economic benefits required cooperation, the division of labour, and the recognition of interdependence. But these would emerge only when what Hume called the 'principles of justice' were adopted: the right to the undisturbed possession of property; the transfer of property only by consent; and the sacredness of promises.[7] Where these 'artificial virtues' were entrenched, the widest codified social intercourse became possible and civility, whose most obvious sign was a deference to the opinions of others, could flourish. The stages of economic development, from hunter-gathering through agriculture to the trade and manufactures of Hume's 'commercial economy', were thus also stages in the growth of civility—and civilization.

Hume's attractive formula, at once both reassuring and intelligible, was also readily compatible with one of the most powerful influences on Victorian imperial attitudes, the growth theory of classical political economy. Adam Smith and his followers were at pains to show how economic and social motives could interlock to produce different levels of civilization. It was the insecure condition of the post-Roman countryside, Smith speculated, that had encouraged a warrior outlook in the landed aristocracy and placed a premium on the control of men rather than the production of an agrarian surplus.[8] It was the social revolution by which great men came to prefer luxury consumption to the upkeep of unproductive warlike retinues, suggested

---

[6] Pawlisch, *Sir John Davies*, 61.

[7] J. B. Stewart, *The Moral and Political Philosophy of David Hume* (New York, 1963), 122. Hume's own opinions can be approached in his essay 'Of the Rise and Progress of the Arts and Sciences', in David Hume, *Selected Essays* (pbk. edn., Oxford, 1993), 56–77.

[8] Adam Smith, *The Wealth of Nations* (Everyman edn., 2 vols., 1933), 341–6.

Malthus,[9] which had triggered the eventual shift from an agrarian to a commercial society. Here was the grand theory, as opposed to the more mundane administrative necessity, that informed the passionate Victorian dislike of social systems, which seemed to depend on the idea of military service to a feudal lord or clan chief. Only towards the end of the nineteenth century, when a certain reaction set in among the British élite against industrialism and political economy, were 'tribalism' and 'feudalism' acknowledged as breakwaters against a dangerous tide of social change, and as reservoirs of a social virtue that could be adapted to imperial purposes. Even so, the most ardent proponents of 'princely rule' in India or of 'indirect rule' in colonial Africa found it difficult to deny that they were only a delaying tactic against economic change, which, for all its disadvantages, provided the wherewithal for colonial administration. Nor could they evade the paradox that to associate colonial rule with indigenous traditions was to deny its fundamental moral basis as an act of enlightened trusteeship.[10] So long as colonialism was identified with the task of 'civilization'—the diffusion of civility—commerce must be its *Doppelgänger*. In the last era of the Raj, the annual reports of the Government of India were still magnificently entitled *The Moral and Material Progress of British India*.

Not surprisingly, perhaps, there was usually a tension between notions of civility conventional in England (or Britain) and those that seemed to be favoured by the English (or British) living abroad in alien cultural settings. Expatriates were commonly suspected of being all too ready to discard the manners and morals laboriously cultivated at home. Long before either slavery or the slave trade was repudiated by British public opinion, the planter class in the British Caribbean were regularly impugned as greedy degenerates.[11] 'Nabobs' returning from India were excoriated for lawlessness and brutality in a popular play of 1772.[12] Burke's indictment of Warren Hastings portrayed him as a ruthless, amoral despot who had abandoned any vestige of English civility. An elaborate anti-imperialist critique, looking back, perhaps, to the earliest accounts of Europeans' maltreatment of Amerindians, contrasted the degraded incivility of the expatriate with the natural virtue of the subject peoples whom they ruled or exploited. This critique found full voice in the fierce debate over the future of South Africa and New Zealand in the 1830s

[9] 'If a taste for idle retainers and a profusion of menial servants had continued among the great landholders of Europe from the feudal times to the present,' remarked Malthus, 'the wealth of its different kingdoms would have been very different from what it now is' (T. R. Malthus, *The Principles of Political Economy*, ed. J. Pullen (Variorum edn., Cambridge, 1989), 35).

[10] 'Our duty to apply Western knowledge to the mitigation of African suffering and the betterment of African health is, perhaps, a crucial test for "trusteeship",' remarked W. M. Macmillan, the best-informed critic of British policy in colonial Africa. See his *Africa Emergent* (1938; Penguin edn., 1949), 228.

[11] S. Drescher, *Capitalism and Anti-Slavery* (1986), 18–19.

[12] See the extract from Isaac Foote's 'The Nabob' in P. J. Marshall, *Problems of Empire: Britain and India 1757–1813* (1968), 147–9.

and reached a devastating climax in the deadly phrases of the Devlin report into unrest in Nyasaland (now Malawi) in 1959.[13] The colonial government, said Devlin, was operating a 'police state'—an accusation that, only fourteen years after the defeat of Hitler, rang out like a pistol shot. The enormous emphasis that was laid in both India and the rest of the colonial empire, from the mid-nineteenth century onwards, upon the moral purity of British administrators, and the effort made to segregate them from what was seen as the corrupting influence of local society, may be seen in part as a response to the persistent allegation that mastery over alien peoples was incompatible with the practice of English civility. But to the anglophone liberals of the Indian National Congress, it was the 'unBritishness of British rule'—the Raj's betrayal of liberal values—that was its greatest crime.

II

Wherever British rule was extended overseas by British settlers, the fundamental question was whether the social and political institutions of the mother country could be successfully transplanted to an alien setting. In principle, at least, there was little choice in the matter. The migrants themselves (unless they were Irish Catholics) expected to carry with them the same civil rights as they enjoyed at home, since the alternative was likely to be an arbitrary executive on the one hand or frontier anarchy on the other. Not surprisingly, many clung tenaciously to familiar customs and habits (not least in diet and dress) in a strange and sometimes intimidating environment. 'Before the American war', complained an early historian of South Carolina, 'the citizens of the Carolinas were too much prejudiced in favour of British manners, customs and knowledge, to imagine that elsewhere than in England, anything of advantage could be obtained'.[14] For their part, the imperial authorities found it all but impossible to free themselves from a set of administrative precedents that stretched back to the earliest phases of medieval English expansion.[15] Everywhere, the assumption was that, where English settlers had colonized a no-man's-land or a region whose inhabitants lacked a sufficient conception of property, they carried with them the customs and precedents of English common law. (Thus the Assembly of South Carolina declared the Common Law of England in force throughout the colony in 1712.)[16]

[13] *Report of the Nyasaland Commission of Enquiry* (the Devlin Report), Cmnd. 814 (1959), para. 2.

[14] John Drayton, *A View of South Carolina as respects her Natural and Civil Concerns* (Charleston, S.C., 1802), 217.

[15] See A. F. Madden, '1066, 1776 and All That', in G. Williams and J. Flint (eds.), *Perspectives of Empire: Essays Presented to G. S. Graham* (1973).

[16] Drayton, *South Carolina*, 186.

But this did not mean that settler communities displayed a slavish attachment to the *version* of English civility currently in vogue in the metropolis. Migrants arrived at different times and brought with them a variety of traditions. In England itself, the political and intellectual upheavals of the seventeenth century and the growth of commercial society in the eighteenth produced widely different prescriptions for moral and social order. The result was the diversity strikingly evident in the social ethos of the Thirteen Colonies of mainland America. Secondly, settler societies soon became selective in the aspects of English civility that they wished to import. The Virginia assembly, remarked Jefferson, adopted the laws of England in 1661 'except so far as a "difference of condition" rendered them inapplicable'[17] — a rule that produced significant local variation. The idea of an established church and of the undivided inheritance of landed property through primogeniture, bastions of the civil social order in England, held little appeal on the other side of the Atlantic. One of the immediate consequences of the American revolution in Virginia was to change the laws of inheritance and sweep away the remains of the colonial religious establishment.

Indeed, the revolt of the American colonies raised the larger question of whether English notions of civility could be sustained if the political tie between mother country and colony were broken. If a common civility rested upon the seamless web of language, law, governance, and social custom, could it survive beyond the reach of English political authority? More important, could it be sustained without an institutional apparatus whose legitimacy had been derived from the Crown? One strand of English opinion was strongly attracted to the idea of a republican social virtue, democratic and egalitarian in spirit. Tom Paine derided the idea that formal government made any positive contribution to social order and civilization. Man's 'natural wants' and the system of 'social affections' implanted in him by nature, not the order imposed by governments, were the secret of social harmony — a truth revealed, argued Paine, in the American revolution.[18] A government should be merely the instrument a society used for its needs and 'the more perfect civilization is, the less occasion has it for government'.[19] While the monarchies of the Old World pursued the private interests of dynasty and courtiers at public expense, the representative governments established in America served the real needs of civil society. Far from jeopardizing the achievements of civility, Paine seemed to be saying, ending the political link with a corrupt and oppressive system at home was a giant step towards the progress of civilization and the diffusion of knowledge.

[17] See Thomas Jefferson, 'Notes on Virginia', in *The Life and Selected Writings of Thomas Jefferson*, ed. A. Koch and W. Peden (New York, 1944), 249.
[18] Thomas Paine, *The Rights of Man* (Thinkers Library edn., 1937), 135.
[19] Ibid. 136.

The first half of the nineteenth century saw a sea change in domestic British attitudes towards overseas settlement. Whereas earlier commentators had been inclined to regard colonization as either a means of refuge for a minority, a useful escape valve for the adventurous, or a dump for the anti-social, the cost and trouble of which were justified only by the commercial benefits it might yield, the 1830s and 1840s saw the growth of a much more positive estimate. Now, quite apart from its economic advantages in widening markets and supplies, colonization became a legitimate source of national pride, and the mark of a special British genius for building new societies. 'The great interest and purpose of England', declared Gladstone in 1852, 'was the multiplication of her race . . .'[20] Strikingly, this new view coincided not only with the final assault on slavery, abolished between 1833 and 1838, but with the attack on transportation, launched by Sir William Molesworth in 1838.[21] Significantly, Molesworth, while drawing upon the new theories of penal reform, directed his heaviest fire at the damage transportation was claimed to inflict upon the prospects of new colonial communities. What free immigrant, demanded Molesworth, would settle in a colony populated by criminals and ne'er-do-wells? Worse still, what respectable woman, the indispensable agent of demographic growth and social stability, would emigrate to places where both males and females were so disreputable.[22] It was left to a former Colonial Secretary, Earl Grey, who favoured keeping transportation, to restate the older, less flattering view of British migrants as adventurers and opportunists.[23]

Nevertheless, before long, sympathy for the idea of colonization had modulated into a warm endorsement of its social function. Critics of the *domestic* incivility wrought by industrialization and rapid urbanization were often attracted by the vision of a fresh start in a virgin landscape where lost social harmony and virtue—the basic ingredients of civility—could be rediscovered. By the 1880s, when renewed fear of social unrest sharpened the sense of a society undergoing fundamental change (the term 'industrial revolution' was coined by Arnold Toynbee in 1883), the value of settlement colonies as a safe haven for the ethos of an old rural order had caught the attention of conservatives as well. In 1886 James Anthony Froude prophesied that the ever-increasing drift to the towns would create a population of 'sickly, poor and stunted wretches whom no school teaching . . . could save from physical decrepitude'.[24] 'The experience of all mankind', he insisted, 'declares that a race of men sound in soul and limb can be bred and reared only in the exercise of

---

[20] Parl. Deb. (1852), 121, c. 956. For Cardwell's views, ibid. (1865), 169, cc. 911–14 (26 May).

[21] *Selected Speeches of Sir William Molesworth*, ed. H. E. Egerton (1903), 22–4, 90–143.

[22] Ibid. 73. For Molesworth's views on the effects of transportation on the balance of the sexes, see pp. 118–20.

[23] Earl Grey, *The Colonial Policy of Lord John Russell's Administration* (2 vols., 1853), ii. 79.

[24] J. A. Froude, *Oceana or England and her Colonies* (1886), 9.

plough and spade, in the free air and sunshine, with country enjoyments and amusements, never amidst foul drains and smoke blacks and the eternal clank of machinery.[25] Froude conjured up the nightmare of a degenerate urban mob unleashing a cycle of political corruption and imperial decline. The remedy he prescribed was colonial migration to those 'fairest spots upon the globe' picked out by the 'genius of England' where there was still 'soil and sunshine boundless and life-giving; where the race might for ages renew its mighty youth, bring forth as many millions as it would and . . . still have means to breed and rear them strong . . .'.[26] But such a future, Froude acknowledged, was incompatible with the old form of empire, since the 'English race do not like to be parts of an empire'. Instead there must be 'a "commonwealth" of Oceana held together by common blood, common interest, and a common pride in the great position that unity can secure'.[27] The price of safeguarding English civility against decay was to throw over entirely the old notion of empire as rule from the imperial centre.

The view that emigration made possible the survival of endangered moral and physical qualities in a freer, healthier, and more spacious environment remained a trope of imperial thinking and of emigration literature up until the 1960s and perhaps beyond. Its counterpart was a persistent colonial belief, already evident in colonial America, that, left to their own devices, settler societies embodied social virtues that the home environment had made it impossible to practise. Perhaps the most influential statement of this doctrine was Jefferson's great manifesto of agrarian populism. Trade and manufacture, said Jefferson, were necessary in Europe only because there the land was locked up against the people. But

those who labour on the earth are the chosen people of God. . . . Corruption of morals in the mass of cultivators is a phenomenon of which no age nor nation has furnished an example. It is the mark set on those, who, not looking up to heaven, to their own soil and industry as does the husbandman, for their subsistence, depend for it on casualties and caprice of customers. Dependence begets subservience and venality, suffocates the germ of virtue, and prepares fit tools for the designs of ambition.[28]

The same view of Old World civility that stressed its fragility, pretension, and artificiality can be found among colonial writers in nineteenth-century New Zealand. The absence of social rivalry, the modesty of consumption, and the ease with which even the poor could obtain a 'competence' in a setting where land was abundant were contrasted with the relentless competitive pressures in English society that made conspicuous consumption a tool of social ambition, and bred debt, snobbery, and social conflict.[29] The demotic civility of such a colonial Arcadia had no need of the elaborate social and political

---

[25] Ibid. 8.   [26] Ibid. 10.   [27] Ibid. 12.
[28] Jefferson, 'Notes on Virginia', 280.
[29] M. Fairburn, *The Ideal Society and its Enemies* (Auckland, 1986), chs. 2, 3.

superstructure of the Old World and was impatient of any formal code of manners prescribed by an élite—a trait Tocqueville had observed in American society.[30] Indeed antipathy towards the ostentation and rituals of social life 'at home' became almost a reflex in colonial attitudes and an enduring one. But the corollary was often a fierce intolerance of diversity, perhaps because a loose-knit and unhierarchical social order was ill-equipped to contain, absorb, or control social and cultural variation except by the crude device of exclusion. Hence the frequency with which what we might call (using Hume's classification) 'agrarian civility' in a colonial setting was accompanied by the apparatus of segregation or white supremacy, or by a battery of devices to repel racially undesirable migrants. The instinct of such communities might have been expressed in the speech William Faulkner puts into the mouth of the small-town Southern lawyer Gavin Stevens:

Only a few of us know that only from homogeneity comes anything of a people or for a people of durable and lasting value—the literature, the art, the science, that minimum of government and police which is the meaning of freedom and liberty, and perhaps most valuable of all a national character worth anything in a crisis . . .[31]

But the mainstream of British opinion was rarely sympathetic towards what it saw as the self-regarding parochialism of settler communities and their marked tendency towards a form of cultural autarky. Towards the largest settler state of all, the American republic, it displayed a persistent animus, jeering at the boorishness of American manners, or deploring the frontier incivility that, in Macaulay's phrase, administered 'a rude justice with the rifle and the dagger'.[32] Mid-Victorian British governments feared the political consequence of this incivility: the inability of the American executive to restrain its citizens from violations of international law and its susceptibility to gusts of crudely amplified popular prejudice.[33] Victorian mistrust of American society sprang from its apparent failure (except in the South) to produce a recognizable governing class whose more elevated notion of the public interest would serve as a barrier to the corrupt pursuit of private gain in the public sphere. To a society as preoccupied as Victorian Britain with the creation of a new gentlemanly class and the dissemination of a revised gentlemanly code, American indifference to these great projects proclaimed an inferior civility—and civilization.

Indeed, conservative opinion was inclined to see Britain's loss of the American colonies as rooted in a defective colonial social order. In the aftermath of the American revolution, when the authorities in London wrestled with the

[30] Alexis de Tocqueville, *Democracy in America*, ed. J. P. Mayer and Max Lerner (Fontana edn., 1968), ii. 784 ff.

[31] William Faulkner, *Intruder in the Dust* (1948; Penguin edn., 1960), 149.

[32] T. B. Macaulay, *The History of England from the Accession of James the First* (Everyman edn., 1906), i. 221.

[33] See L. M. Roeckell, 'British Interests in Texas 1825–1846', D.Phil. thesis (Oxford, 1993).

problem of governing the Loyalist settlements in the Canadian interior, they identified the central weakness of the old colonial system as the lack of an adequate reservoir of influence, patronage, and revenue at the disposal of the Crown.[34]

> The power of conferring honours and emoluments enables the Sovereign, in this country, to animate the exertions of individuals and to secure their attachment to the existing form of government, by all the fair objects of just and honourable ambition. The case was widely different in the colonies . . .[35]

The remedy lay in securing a Crown revenue (by the reservation of lands) and creating in the colonies a class that would enjoy 'some personal or hereditary distinctions of honour and nobility'. By these means, 'a juster and more effectual security against a republican or independent spirit' might be obtained.

The Constitution Act of 1791 was thus an attempt to craft an ersatz British society in the backwoods of Upper Canada. The Church of England was endowed with extensive 'clergy reserves' and successive governors tried to foster a pseudo-aristocratic order in which great proprietors would colonize large tracts with emigrant tenants and assume the role of a governing class. In Australia, schemes of this sort were irrelevant as long as New South Wales was merely a faraway gaol. But as soon as free settlement began to develop, governors in Sydney were instructed to fix it within limits as constricting as the English Pale in medieval Ireland. Within the 'Nineteen Counties' colonial civility was to be maintained by close settlement and a model of intensive agriculture designed to support the classic triptych of English rural life: landlord, tenant, and landless labourer.[36] If free settlers were allowed to spread into the vast interior, warned every imperial instinct, the outcome would be a cycle of civilizational degeneration. Labourers would flee their masters. Tenants would abandon their holdings. Agriculture would decline in competition with the loose, licentious life of pastoralism. Rentals, taxes, and social order would evaporate simultaneously. The general collapse of civility would signal the colony's slide into anarchy or demand an expensive and embarrassing reassertion of imperial authority.

In neither Canada nor Australia did the effort to impose an English-style social order work very well or last very long. Instead, under the influence of political economy, policy-makers and private projectors turned to an economic catalyst to promote the commercial society and progressive civility that Hume had seen as two sides of a single social process. The originator was

---

[34] 'Canada: Memorandum on Questions at Issue in Framing a New Constitution, 1789', in V. T. Harlow and A. F. Madden (eds.), *British Colonial Developments 1774–1834: Select Documents* (Oxford, 1953), 197–201.

[35] Ibid.

[36] For the best account, see M. Roe, *The Quest for Authority in Eastern Australia 1835–1851* (Parkville, 1965).

a disciple of Malthus, the radical scapegrace Edward Gibbon Wakefield. Wakefield's avowed object was to forestall the tendency of settlement colonies to drift into the agrarian self-sufficiency celebrated by Jefferson. In his famous manifesto *The Art of Colonization*, Wakefield proposed a simple formula by which the price of colonial land would be set at a level that only those with some capital could afford. Having invested his capital, the colonial farmer would have no option but to produce for the market—that is, for export— and to become both producer of foodstuffs and raw materials and a consumer of the manufactures and capital the mother country had to offer. The proceeds of the colonial land sale would meet the costs of importing the migrant labourers on whom Wakefield's commercial farmers would depend.[37] In this way the colony would be complementary to the economic needs of the mother country. Wakefield's scheme has usually been interpreted as a misconceived strategy of economic colonialism, but it can also be understood as a drastic remedy for the defects of colonial society excoriated in his fictional *Letter from Sydney* (1829).

Wakefield's argument in the *Letter* built on the contrast between the abundant natural resources of New South Wales and what he insisted was the narrowness, meanness, and vulgarity of colonial life. Cheap, plentiful, labour was the prerequisite for any advance of civilization, because cheap labour allowed the accumulation of wealth and

Wealth will bestow leisure; and leisure will bestow knowledge. Wealth, leisure and knowledge mean civilization. Schools and colleges will be established. The arts and sciences will flourish, because artists and discoverers will be paid and rewarded. Abstract truth will be sought because its pursuit will be rewarded, and this will make philosophers.[38]

But the reality in new countries, both America and Australasia, was that land was extremely cheap and labour consequently dear or unobtainable. The result was a pathological restlessness as labour migrated constantly in search of yet higher wages or even cheaper land. In America, claimed Wakefield,

I saw a people without monuments, without history, without local attachments . . . without any love of birthplace, without patriotism. . . . I learnt that with a new people, restlessness is a passion, insatiable whilst any means of indulging it remains; a disease incurable but by cutting away its source.[39]

Worse still, where a wealthy leisured class was lacking, 'tastes and habits, as well as modes and manners, must necessarily proceed from the lowest class'.[40] Wherever territory was disproportionate to population, concluded Wakefield,

[37] Wakefield's economic ideas were set out in *England and America* (2 vols., 1833), where the original essay on 'The Art of Colonization' appeared, and collected later in *The Art of Colonization* (1849).
[38] E. G. Wakefield, *A Letter from Sydney* (Everyman edn., 1929), 46.
[39] Ibid. 47.   [40] Ibid. 66.

a society was condemned to remain in the inferior condition of a 'new people' (a category that included the USA as well as the British colonies) who,

> though they continually increase in number, make no progress in the art of living; who, in respect to wealth, knowledge, skill, taste, and whatever belongs to civilization have degenerated from their ancestors . . . who, ever on the move, are unable to bring anything to perfection; whose opinions are only violent and false prejudices, the necessary fruit of ignorance . . . and who delight in a forced equality . . . which, to keep the balance always even rewards the mean rather than the great . . . we mean in two words a people who are rotten before they are ripe.[41]

Wakefield's ideas, as this suggests, were congenial to the prejudices of an aristocratic ruling class in Britain, and his economic prescription exerted considerable influence on imperial policy in the 1830s and 1840s, not least perhaps by reinforcing the attack on transportation. But it soon proved impossible to combine imperial control over colonial 'wastelands'—Wakefield's means of funding emigration—with the concession of local self-government in Australia and British North America. Agrarian populism of the kind Wakefield loathed remained a major political force in all the colonies of white settlement, even in late-Victorian New Zealand, proverbially the most loyal of colonies.[42] But it failed to engender the 'democratical spirit', the demotic incivility, that Wakefield believed would drive the Canadian and Australian colonists down the American road to separation and independence.

There were several reasons for this. The emerging colonial upper class, reared on imperial privilege in land and trade, may have been small and precarious, but it proved more resilient than Wakefield imagined. In Upper Canada it comfortably survived the populist revolt of 1837, partly because economic growth broadened the appeal of 'Toryism', and partly because it successfully exploited the visceral monarchism of Highlander and Irish Protestant settler communities (among whom the Orange Order had already been established).[43] The concession of 'responsible government' encouraged the conscious modelling of colonial parliamentarism on the British model. The social and economic dynamism of Victorian Britain, throwing up new urban, business, and religious élites, enhanced its cultural appeal and multiplied the sources of contact and influence between mother country and colony. Migrant communities, drawn from different parts of the United Kingdom, maintained closer links with those left behind than Wakefield's 'new-people' model imagined. But perhaps the most important reason why the problem of colonial civility seemed so much less important by the end of the nineteenth century—except where, as in South Africa, there was a

[41] Ibid. 68–9.
[42] See R. Arnold, *New Zealand's Burning: The Settler World of the mid 1880s* (Wellington, 1994); T. Brooking, *Lands for the People?* (Dunedin, 1996).
[43] See S. D. Clark, *Movements of Political Protest in Canada 1640–1840* (Toronto, 1959), chs. 16, 17, 18.

non-British settler majority—was that economic and social growth combined with the annihilation of distance by steamship and telegraph created ideal conditions for the more rapid and intensive exchange of images, ideas, information, and even values. Journalism, sport, and higher education were all channels through which these reciprocal influences could travel. And, as colonial societies expanded in scale, with larger and more sophisticated political, economic, and cultural institutions, the model of 'modernity' to which they most frequently turned was necessarily Britain, still, perhaps as late as the 1930s, the cynosure of economic and social progress. It might even be suggested that the consequence of this and of the huge volume of British migration that continued up to 1914 (and on a lesser scale in the interwar years) was the appearance of a broad-based 'Britannic' (rather than narrowly English or British) civility, a set of beliefs, values, and prejudices that served more effectively than the political apparatus of empire to promote the solidarity of what the most ardent Edwardian imperialists liked to call 'the younger nations in the Empire' or the 'oversea-Britons'.[44]

III

In a stimulating series of essays, Edward Shils defined civility as

a belief which affirms the possibility of the common good; it is a belief in the community of contending parties within a morally valid unity of society. . . . Civility is an attitude which recommends that consensus about the maintenance of the order of society should exist alongside the conflicts of interests and ideals . . .[45]

It was 'a restraint on the passion with which interests and ideals are pursued' and was incompatible with the dissolution of society 'into an aggregation of demanding individualities'.[46] In its most concentrated form, civility was 'the capacity for imagination and cognition of the properties of one's fellow-men and the capacity to entertain and give precedence to the inclusive collective self-consciousness within oneself over one's individual self-consciousness':[47] it was nourished by the idea of disinterested public service. It entailed 'a cognitive account of the structure or pattern of the whole society and a normative prescription to act for its benefit'.[48] Above all, it was indispensable to the proper functioning of a large, open, differentiated society.[49]

However inchoate its expression, a concept of civility recognizably similar to the definition advanced by Shils had become something of a political commonplace in England by Tudor times, perhaps earlier.[50] In a society so aware

---

[44] Lord Milner, *The Nation and the Empire* (1913), 437, 491.
[45] E. Shils, *The Virtue of Civility* (Indianapolis, 1997), 4.
[46] Ibid. 10.   [47] Ibid. 348.   [48] Ibid. 78.   [49] Ibid. 75.
[50] For a fascinating study of its diffusion in early modern England, see M. James, 'The Concept of Order and the Northern Rising', in his *Society, Politics and Culture: Studies in Early Modern England* (Cambridge, 1986), 270–307.

of its dependence on civility, and wracked in the seventeenth century by its apparent breakdown, there was good reason to worry about how it would fare under conditions of imperial expansion. Would English civility taken abroad wilt and wither in a harsher climate? If emigrant English communities lost their civility, what would prevent them from falling into anarchy or drifting into rebellion? Worse still, what assurance was there that repatriated English, returning from some imperial sojourn, would not contaminate the civility of the homeland with the degenerate customs and mentality picked up like an infection in foreign lands. This suspicion lay, as we have seen, at the heart of the violent criticism heaped on returning 'nabobs' from India in the eighteenth century, surfaced repeatedly in Victorian anxieties about the consequences of an Indian Empire,[51] and reached a crescendo of paranoia in J. A. Hobson's famous tract *Imperialism: A Study* published in 1902.

It was true, of course, that much of this later suspicion that civility at home and empire abroad were incompatible was focused on the imperialism of rule and not on the imperialism of settlement with which this essay has been mainly concerned. But it was foreshadowed in earlier fears about the behaviour of English communities and individuals released from the disciplines of home. It was sharpened by uncertainty about the active ingredients that a successful civility required. Civility seemed to depend upon a form of social alchemy wrought by an invisible hand. It was a volatile compound whose chemical structure defied close analysis and discouraged experimentation. As Burke famously claimed, it could not be designed to a blueprint. But the experience of empire forced thoughtful opinion in England to speculate about how civility could be preserved. Not surprisingly, the usual prescription was to model the institutions of the colony as closely as possible on those of England itself.

As we have seen, this was rarely a satisfactory solution. Sometimes it was simply impracticable. Sometimes the export of English institutions had unintended consequences in an alien setting. But by the nineteenth century it was also clear that the domestic version itself was too pluralistic to offer a simple guide to the colonial perplexed. The result was not (in general) to acknowledge that a distinctive civility existed in the colonies of settlement but to expand the notion of English (or British) civility to embrace the settler experience and on occasion to draw inspiration from it. To Hobson, the radical scourge of imperialism, the settlement colonies were a 'genuine expansion of nationality',[52] embodying social experiments and egalitarian values he was anxious to promote in Britain. The Edwardian imperialists searched for an idea of 'Britishness' that would appeal even to non-British settler communities. Glimpses of this ambitious project can be seen in the last age of imperial power between the wars and shreds survived into the 1960s in the

---

[51] For two classic examples, Richard Cobden, 'How Wars are Got up in India' (1853), repr. in *Political Writings of Richard Cobden* (2 vols.; 1867); Goldwin Smith, *The Empire* (Oxford, 1860).

[52] J. A. Hobson, *Imperialism: A Study* (3rd edn., 1938), 6.

pieties of 'Commonwealthmanship'. The peculiar ritualized informality of Commonwealth Conferences in the 1960s and 1970s may have represented a last brave attempt to preserve a form of imperial civility. But by that time the cultural self-confidence upon which a distinctive British vision of civil society had been built was ebbing rapidly away. Like two old warhorses from a bygone age, English civility and the British Empire stepped together into oblivion.

19

The Public and the Private in Modern Britain

BRIAN HARRISON

Private life 'is nothing if not a protean subject',[1] but it is integral to the history of civility, which maintains a delicate balance between the public and the private. The ramifications of privacy's complex history embarrass the lawyers. Law courts upholding privacy paradoxically expose it to publicity, and entangle lawyers in such diverse areas as trespass, nuisance, misrepresentation, and impersonation. Yet the lawyer's difficulty is the historian's opportunity, for to brave the apparent absurdity involved in chronicling the history of the hidden is to acquire an unfamiliar perspective on the British people, to whom Taine ascribed 'a corner of the mind and heart inviolably private, a kind of forbidden enclosure which is respected by everyone'.[2] It was 'the *privateness* of English life' that struck Orwell in 1940: 'all the culture that is most truly native centres round things which even when they are communal are not official.'[3]

Privacy rests upon a Judaeo-Christian respect for the individual's dignity and autonomy, but why should this be so prized in Britain? First, a pluralistic culture emerges from a Protestant (and still more from an evangelical) Christianity that cultivates a direct relationship between individual and creator. Secondly, free-market industrialization enhanced this pluralism, and was not supplanted by a Germanic collectivism. So prominent amateur wirelessmen could, for instance, inform the Post Office in 1922 that 'every Englishman is entitled to hear what is going on in the aether provided his listening apparatus does not annoy his neighbours'.[4] Thirdly, industrialization encouraged social ascent through the permeable class barriers of a hierarchical society. For Englishmen, first encounters inevitably entailed mutual appraisal; hence the need for 'reserve'. Tocqueville claimed in 1840 that, whereas in England 'everybody lives in constant dread lest advantage should be taken of his familiarity', democratic Americans have a 'natural, frank, and open' manner.[5] For

---

[1] K. Thomas, 'Behind Closed Doors', *New York Review of Books*, 9 Nov. 1989, 16.

[2] H. Taine, *Notes on England*, ed. and trans. E. Hyams (1957), 91.

[3] G. Orwell, 'The Lion and the Unicorn', in Orwell, *Collected Essays, Journalism and Letters*, ii (Harmondsworth, 1970), 77–8.

[4] Quoted in A. Briggs, *A History of Broadcasting in the United Kingdom*, i (1961), 129.

[5] A. de Tocqueville, *Democracy in America* (1840; trans. H. Reeve, ed. P. Bradley, New York, 1945), ii. 179.

Wallas, a fourth factor—climate—partly explained northern Europe's 'instinctive need of privacy', a subject that he thought 'would repay special and detailed study'.[6]

Privacy can be assigned six dimensions: from privacy of the person through privacy of 'personal space' to privacy in personal relations and residential patterns, and thence to privacy in social roles and public life. Respect for privacy of the person precludes degrading exhibitions of the body. Humanitarians from the late eighteenth century gradually curbed exhibitions of freaks and lunatics, and only the poorest Victorian beggar profited from displaying his deformities. Public hanging ended in 1868, capital punishment in 1965, and state schools banned the cane in 1987. Privacy usually attends bodily zones closest to sexual features,[7] but C. E. M. Joad noted in 1933 that different parts 'had been wicked in different ages'; a woman's ankle had once seemed intoxicating, yet now even the knee 'had ceased to be mildly exciting. As one extended the area which was exposed one also diminished the area which was wicked.'[8] Exposure of the same bodily part may be taboo in some contexts but not in others. The columnist Marje Proops in 1976, at just the time when Helene Hayman controversially suckled her baby at Westminster, pronounced it incongruous to discourage the practice in shops when bare breasts were so frequently exhibited in the press.[9]

On total nudity, social extremes diverged from centre. Poverty, overcrowding, and spontaneity made nude bathing common among working-class children before 1914—though working-class adults disliked being seen naked, even when undressing for intercourse.[10] At the opposite extreme, public-school changing rooms have never been known for reticence, nor did Churchill hesitate in 1942 to bathe naked at Palm Beach; Oxford dons and undergraduates disported themselves in Parson's Pleasure for another half-century.[11] Coyness prevailed most among intermediate groups socially insecure yet self-consciously 'respectable'. Chartist leaders in Warwick gaol were horrified at having to strip naked and bathe indiscriminately with other prisoners.[12] Respectable mid-Victorian artisans detested the Contagious Diseases Acts for subjecting alleged prostitutes to compulsory inspection. There seemed only three ways to curb venereal disease: restrain indiscriminate male sexuality by getting servicemen to marry or abstain, inspect a few suspected women, or inspect their more numerous male clients. The first option offered

---

[6] G. Wallas, *Human Nature in Politics* (1908), 50.

[7] On this my graduate student Richard Coombs refers me to D. Morris, *Manwatching: A Field Guide to Human Behaviour* (1977), 204.

[8] *Sun Bathing Review* (Summer 1933), 6.

[9] *Daily Mirror*, 15 Dec. 1976, 7.

[10] See e.g. Bertram Stevens's interesting discussion in *Sun Bathing Review* (July 1952), 24; but also R. Hoggart, *The Uses of Literacy* (1957; pbk. edn., Harmondsworth, 1958), 75.

[11] W. H. Thompson, *I was Churchill's Shadow* (1951), 83; *Daily Telegraph*, 31 Jan. 1992, 3.

[12] W. Lovett, *The Life and Struggles of William Lovett* (1876), 222.

no rapid cure; doctors, not yet themselves securely respectable, relished neither the second nor the third. 'I think that cleanliness is next to godliness', the Senior Surgeon of St Thomas's Hospital told a parliamentary committee in 1865, 'and I think that every man ought to wash underneath the foreskin', but only a minority did so.[13] Why not inspect the women instead? J. S. Mill thought women found inspection 'exceedingly degrading', whereas men 'are not lowered in their own eyes as much by exposure of their persons'.[14] An almost mystical reverence for the female body inspired Josephine Butler's attack on the Acts, claiming for every woman 'a Divine right, to protect the secrets of her own person'.[15] Such attitudes helped draw Victorian women towards becoming doctors.

By the 1930s a small, rationalistic, and self-consciously progressive Anglo-American middle-class group was turning respectability upside down by unveiling nudism or 'gymnosophy' as the route to moral progress. Its strange combination of puritanism and liberation owed much to German and Swiss health-cure movements, and combined medical self-help with an earnestly bucolic quest for the simple life. So colonial peoples who were now at last putting their clothes on witnessed the imperial race taking them off. In 1953 the forty-one British nudist clubs had 4,000 members, and their numbers tripled in the next twenty years.[16] But high interwar nudist ideals now shrivelled into suburban fenced-off clubs whose exclusiveness belied an earlier breadth of view. Puzzled when adolescent offspring seceded, nudists learned nothing from Kinsey, disliked the 'permissive society', and had no part in those three hedonistic clothes-shedding highlights of 1970 when 'Oh Calcutta!' opened at the Roundhouse, the Isle of Wight pop festival shocked respectable local opinion, and anarchist students demonstrated nude at Keele. Still more disconcerting, the nudists' hitherto austerely air-brushed organ *Health and Efficiency* suddenly in the late 1960s became explicitly pornographic. Health and high-mindedness were the nudist vision, not sex and fun. If nudist success is measured by area of flesh exposed, triumph occurred in the 1970s with its combination of sexual emancipation and overseas travel. Yet only in the few overseas beaches known to initiates were clothes totally shed. Besides, nudists were more than mere sunbathers: they did not seek less clothing, but no clothes at all.

Some societies defend privacy in its second dimension, personal space, by invoking veils and masks, but more effective are formal styles of address,

[13] Select Committee appointed to Inquire into the Pathology and Treatment of the Venereal Disease, *Parliamentary Papers*, 1867–8 (4031), xxxvii, Q. 3929 (Samuel Solly), cf. QQ. 5675–7 (J. W. Trotter).
[14] Royal Commission on the . . . Contagious Diseases Act, *Parliamentary Papers*, 1871 (408), xix, Q. 20,008.
[15] Select Committee of the House of Commons on the Contagious Diseases Acts, *Parliamentary Papers*, 1882 (340), ix, Q. 5379.
[16] *British Naturism*, 46 (Nov. 1975), 11.

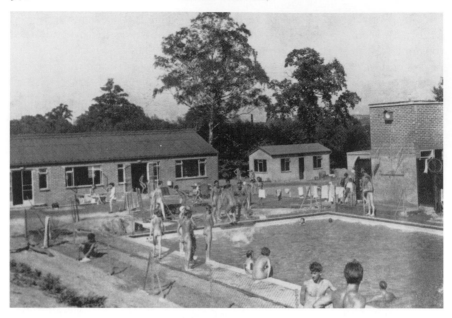

16. North Kent Sun Club, from *Health and Efficiency* (May 1960), 23. Behind the swimming pool is a brick-built pavilion; beside it are the sanitary block and showers.

guarded speech, curbed emotions, a remote manner, restrained and stylized correspondence, avoidance of 'difficult' conversational topics, firm but unspoken rules of conduct and dress. Unlike glad-handing Americans or 'Latin' and perhaps 'Celtic' temperaments, Englishmen when sober do not 'give themselves away'. Privacy of personal space was for W. H. Auden a frontier 'some thirty inches from my nose',[17] but acceptable distances fluctuate with fashion. The informality of the Romantic Age, of the Nineties, the Twenties, and the Sixties, seemed in the 1990s (with help from Diana, Princess of Wales) to be returning. After the 1960s men and women were more likely to kiss in public, though English men embraced the *abrazo* only when heterosexually secure on the sports field.

Cameras threaten personal space. The well-known late-Victorian Whitby photographer Frank Sutcliffe, pursuing subjects in remote local communities, found many who thought it unlucky to be drawn or photographed.[18] Such reticence now seems merely quaint. By the 1880s parliamentary candidates were giving electors their photographs, and those of prominent politicians were being sold in 1886, the year when Lord Randolph Churchill's

[17] W. H. Auden, *About the House* (1966), 14.
[18] M. Hiley, *Frank Sutcliffe: Photographer of Whitby* (1974), 63.

lost anonymity disturbed his prized annual continental holiday.[19] Writing in 1951, the Duke of Windsor thought privacy's disappearance 'one of the most inconvenient developments since . . . my boyhood'; the press had then rarely published likenesses, and 'we were not often recognized in the street; when we were, the salutation would be a friendly wave of the hand or, in the case of a courtier or family friend, a polite lifting of the hat'.[20] His grand-father's *incognito* low-life London forays of the 1860s were now impossible. In 1936 there was even a fuss when he was photographed walking in a London street beneath an umbrella instead of taking the Daimler.[21] Television made things worse, and the later diaries of the actor Kenneth Williams, too famous for anonymity but too poor to buy privacy, often grumble at 'the moron's nudge and the cretin's wink'.[22] Add to this the camera's mounting sophistication: 'where ever you are,' said Prince Charles in 1994,

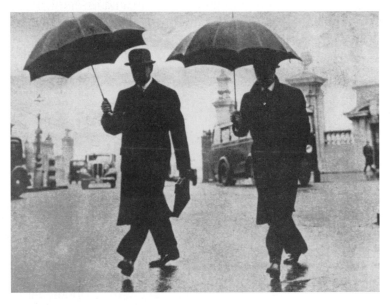

17. Some thought King Edward VIII (*right*, with Sir Lionel Halsey) should not have walked the London streets beneath an umbrella in 1936. In his memoirs, where the photograph was reproduced, the duke of Windsor recalled an MP telling Mrs Simpson at a dinner party, 'We can't have the King doing this kind of thing. He has the Daimler.'

[19] *Photographic News*, 25 Mar. 1880, 145–6; 10 Sept. 1886, 585; 22 Oct. 1886, 681.
[20] Duke of Windsor, *A King's Story* (1951; Reprint Society, 1953), 42.
[21] Ibid. 261.
[22] *The Kenneth Williams Diaries*, ed. R. Davies (1993; pbk. edn., 1994), 317, 579; see also 314, 444, 572.

'there's somebody hiding behind something, somewhere; and with these immense cameras now, with these huge lenses and magnification, you can sit a mile away and photograph through windows and everything else. And they do'.[23]

Privacy's second and third dimensions—in personal space and personal relations—are intertwined, as emerges from focusing on the sexual component of personal relations. Closer understanding of homosexuality paradoxically discourages males from close public bodily contact, just as alertness to paedophilia discourages adults from publicly embracing children. One consistency persists: it remains 'hard to find a society where people seek absolutely no form of concealment when engaging in sexual intercourse or relieving themselves'.[24] None the less, after the 1950s a cumulative national striptease extended what could be displayed and still more what could be publicly discussed. The twentieth century concomitantly eroded those intense same-sex friendships between the heterosexually inclined that under the old regime had provided inlets for enlightenment and outlets for emotion. Advanced late-Victorian feminists such as W. T. Stead and Josephine Butler wanted more honesty about sex, and the conversation in mixed company of interwar feminist or Bloomsbury intellectuals was still more explicit; in 1936 Molly Hamilton claimed that the post-war generation 'is, or tries to be, proud and not ashamed of its body'.[25] Nor did the *Lady Chatterley* trial in 1960 initiate sexuality's irruption into respectable fiction: already by 1949 Orwell was predicting that 'this modern habit of describing love-making in detail' would eventually be viewed rather 'as we do things like the death of Little Nell'.[26]

Privacy's further retreat on sexuality since the 1960s has been dramatic and cumulative. Each dimension has its own timetable. With Mrs Gaskell's *Ruth* in 1853 the Victorians opened up prostitution. The crusade against the CD Acts did the same for venereal disease. Christabel Pankhurst and her mother deplored doctors' collusion with husbands to conceal their infection from the wife, and Christabel published suffragette articles on venereal disease in 1913 that the *Standard* thought tackled 'questions which should never be discussed except between doctor and patient'.[27] Birth control was first publicly discussed in 1872,[28] but the public then associated condoms with prostitution. Not till the 1920s did some feminists publicly endorse this reform, hitherto having tactically concealed their support, and by the 1950s birth control had become sufficiently uncontroversial for doctors to lend their public support. The 1960s gradually extended it to unmarried couples, and the 1980s saw AIDS converting even Roman Catholics to the condom as the

[23] *Guardian*, 30 June 1994, 3.
[24] Thomas, 'Behind Closed Doors', 16.
[25] In R. Strachey (ed.), *Our Freedom and its Results* (1936), 267.
[26] Letter to Richard Rees, in Orwell, *Collected Essays*, iv (1970), 546.
[27] *Standard*, 4 Oct. 1913, 7.
[28] In the *Fortnightly Review*, according to G. M. Young, *Portrait of an Age*, ed. G. Kitson Clark (1977), 157, 378.

government's preventative.[29] Next out of the closet stepped abortion, never inaccessible to those who could afford expensive West End doctors or find a backstreet abortionist. Campaigning for the Abortion Act (1967) enhanced publicity, with Diane Munday even informing the public about her own abortion.[30] There followed menstruation and the menopause, covert basis for Victorian anti-suffragism and source of Victorian woman's unexplained 'delicacy'.[31] In 1924 Virginia Woolf privately confessed to a prudery that 'for 10 years led me to make sanitary towels out of Kapok down rather than buy them'.[32] Adverts for them soon proliferated in the press and by the late twentieth century were regaling prime-time television viewers. In 1943 an MP publicly deployed the menopause against registering the women's age group between 45 and 50 for war work,[33] and even thirty years later experts could note that the subject had 'received relatively little attention in the medical literature'.[34] Here Thatcher may ultimately win a reluctant feminist accolade: 'what she's done', said Shirley Williams in 1987, 'has been to lay to rest for ever the belief that women can't make decisions in the middle of the menopause'.[35]

Twentieth-century research into sexuality in itself threatened privacy, yet homosexuals owe much to it. 'To seek out the most vital facts of life is still in England a perilous task,' wrote Havelock Ellis in 1899,[36] but progressive figures from Carpenter to Russell to Jenkins saw that, while socialism might extend state control over the economy and welfare, its liberal affinities might curb restraints on personal conduct. But homosexuality must first emerge from the closet. The 'masonic secret' of public-school homosexuality was still being husbanded as late as the 1950s,[37] and adult homosexuals led a double life or fled abroad. Their ironic detachment from heterosexual society could prompt major artistic achievement. Jo Orton's oft-observed bizarre contrast between private and public generated high farce; his diary in 1967, for instance, describes a 'frenzied homosexual saturnalia' occurring in a Holloway Road public lavatory while 'no more than two feet away the citizens of Holloway moved about their ordinary business'.[38] The cautious and rationalistic Homosexual Law Reform Society focused on extending private freedom through political change, and its Sexual Offences Act (1967) distinguished

---

[29] *The Times*, 6 Dec. 1986, 1.

[30] K. Hindell and M. Simms, *Abortion Law Reformed* (1971), 113.

[31] See B. Harrison, *Separate Spheres: The Opposition to Women's Suffrage in Britain* (1978), 61–4.

[32] Letter to Mary Hutchinson, in V. Woolf, *Letters*, ed. N. Nicolson, vi (1980), 505.

[33] *House of Commons Debates*, 24 Sept, 1943, cc. 605–7 (Dr Russell Thomas).

[34] S. M. McKinlay and J. B. McKinlay, 'Selected Studies of the Menopause', *Journal of Biosocial Science*, 5 (1973), 534.

[35] Interview with Janet Watts, *Observer*, 24 May 1987, 20.

[36] H. Ellis, *Studies in the Psychology of Sex*, i (3rd edn., Philadelphia, 1910), p. xi (preface to first edition).

[37] See the letter from 'Dayschoolmaster', *Times Educational Supplement*, 20 Dec. 1957, 1607.

[38] *The Orton Diaries*, ed. J. Lahr (1986), 106 (4 Mar. 1967).

between sexual conduct in private, where surveillance should cease, and sexual conduct affecting the public interest (as in prostitution and child abuse), where surveillance should tighten. For flamboyant Gay Liberation after 1970, however, new lifestyles could become feasible only when publicized. Like the teetotal, socialist, suffragist, and pacifist movements before it, Gay Liberation encouraged supporters to 'come out', thereby in effect dissolving the 1967 Act's dichotomy between the public and the private. Only a few hundreds attended Gay Liberation's first annual London festival in 1970, but 160,000 were there by 1995. 'It may be a celebration,' said one participant, 'but the simple act of being here is a political statement.'[39] Politicians could now gradually come out too: Maureen Colquhoun in the mid-1970s as the first confessedly lesbian MP, Chris Smith (a self-professed homosexual since 1984) as the first confessedly homosexual cabinet minister in 1997.

The nuclear family was now under attack: its 'narrow and tawdry secrets' were, for the Reith Lecturer in 1967, 'the source of all our discontents'.[40] There followed a gradual and often reluctant acquiescence in sexual diversity. The simplistic dichotomy between male and female—with its psychological, sartorial, and career stereotypes—slowly blurred, and in the early 1950s Roberta Cowell's was the first of many much-publicized trans-sexual revelations. This national striptease was not unreservedly libertarian in tendency. Feminism and the 'Yorkshire ripper' in the 1980s escalated publicity about rape, which after 1991 a wife could impute to her husband.[41] In the 'homosexual terrorism'[42] of the 1990s OutRage 'outed' allegedly homosexual bishops. By then politicians' sexuality was so widely discussed as to destabilize the Major governments, and concurrent revelations about children's homes rendered the paedophile a hate figure. The 1967 Act did nothing for Joe Orton, for whom Morocco remained a place of resort. 'Well, you're legal now,' said his agent after the Bill's enactment; 'it's only legal over twenty-one,' he replied; 'I like boys of fifteen.'[43] By 1995 the Scout Association was issuing guidance on how to identify and report abuse.[44] Sexual technique, too, was unveiled. The American writer Philip Roth did wonders for masturbation in *Portnoy's Complaint* (1969), afforced in the following year by Brian Aldiss's *The Hand-Reared Boy* and revived in 1994 by the much-discussed suicide of the Conservative MP Stephen Milligan. As for 'oral sex', Maureen Kirby in Margaret Drabble's *The Ice Age* (1977), a novel set in the 1960s, 'thought it was a good new invention' and was rather surprised that Derek Ashby, her architect employer, was so good at it, 'because he must be at least forty-five';[45] it was a novelty that President Clinton amply readvertised in 1998.

[39] Jeremy Philpott, quoted in *Observer*, 25 June 1995, 6. For 1970 statistics, see *Independent*, 23 June 1995, 19.
[40] Edmund Leach, *Listener*, 30 Nov. 1967, 695.
[41] *Independent*, 24 Oct. 1991, 34.   [42] *Daily Telegraph*, 1 Dec. 1994, 16 (leader headline).
[43] *Orton Diaries*, 233 (4 July 1967).   [44] *Daily Telegraph*, 24 Oct. 1995, 5.
[45] M. Drabble, *The Ice Age* (1977; pbk. edn., 1978), 219.

Privacy in its fourth dimension, residential patterns, subdivides between home, neighbourhood, town, and overall environment. Early seventeenth-century law courts knew that 'the Englishman's home is his castle'.[46] Thereafter the state—collecting taxes, providing services, preventing cruelty—battled continuously with what Orwell in 1940 saw as England's non-political variant of libertarianism. 'The most hateful of all names in an English ear', he said, 'is Nosey Parker'.[47] Power supplies, television, piped water, and indoor plumbing made homes simultaneously more self-sufficient but less private, given that safety, health, and debt collection justified entry by outsiders. Telephone and Internet also bypass the front door. Stephen Spender was astonished in old age that complete strangers would telephone for an interview—an intrusion he would not have dreamt of inflicting when young.[48] Sex pests made 180,000 reported calls in 1980, unwanted commercial calls mounted thereafter, and political canvassers' calls escalated in election year 1992.[49] As for the Internet, its computer viruses must be among the least welcome of modern intruders into the home.

What of privacy inside the home? A tenth of English households from the sixteenth to the early nineteenth century contained kin outside the current nuclear family, and nearly a quarter of early Victorian Preston's households contained a lodger. Furthermore, in a society with wide wealth differentials, the poor lose privacy because overcrowded, the rich because underemployed. 'There were many things we might not do, not because they were wrong in themselves, but "because of the maids"', Gwen Raverat recalled.[50] Courtroom details of the scandal that ruined Dilke's political career reveal the domestic ubiquity of servants; this led Campbell-Bannerman in conversation to designate politicians only by place of residence.[51] The domestic servant's disappearance benefited the privacy of both master and servant; servants still exist, but they do not live in. Homes are now much less crowded: persons per room in England and Wales fell from 0.9 in 1921 to 0.5 in 1981.[52] Wartime housing scarcity and post-war marriage boom combined to ensure that probably more British households contained two lineally related married couples in 1947 than at any time since the seventeenth century.[53] But affluence has subsequently mechanized the home, expelled its servants and lodgers, and narrowed the

---

[46] L. C. Orlin, *Private Matters and Public Culture in Post-Reformation England* (Ithaca, NY, 1994), 2–3.

[47] Orwell, 'The Lion and the Unicorn', in Orwell, *Collected Essays*, ii. 78.

[48] F. du Sorbier (ed.), *Oxford, 1919–1939* (Paris, 1991), 50.

[49] For sex pests, see *The Times*, 21 Dec. 1983, 11. For canvassers, see D. E. Butler and D. Kavanagh, *The British General Election of 1992* (1992), 239.

[50] G. Raverat, *Period Piece* (1952; pbk. edn., 1960), 102.

[51] J. Wilson, *CB: A Life of Sir Henry Campbell-Bannerman* (1973), 131.

[52] M. Anderson, *Family Structure in Nineteenth Century Lancashire* (Cambridge, 1971), 2, 46. A. H. Halsey (ed.), *British Social Trends since 1900* (2nd edn., 1988), 365.

[53] M. Anderson, 'The Social Implications of Demographic Change', in F. M. L. Thompson (ed.), *The Cambridge Social History of Britain 1750–1950*, ii (1990), 59–60.

range of relatives jointly housed. Smaller families can spread themselves within houses designed for larger. In all twentieth-century industrial countries the number of households has grown faster than population, a trend boosted in Britain since the 1960s by the spread of one-parent families and by the tendency for Britain's growing proportion of pensioners to live alone. Households consisting of two people or less in England and Wales rose from just over a fifth in 1911 to more than a half in 1981, and after the 1960s the proportion of one-bedroom houses completed rose steadily.[54]

The domesticated ideal focused national stability, personal aspiration, and recreational taste on the home. Even the Victorian country house was becoming more private,[55] and a nation whose formal and informal clubs had long sheltered people from bad weather now turned the home itself into a club. This happened through interlinked social changes, many of which worked outwards from the middle classes. Industrialization from the late eighteenth century distanced work from home; affluence from the late nineteenth century enhanced home comforts; thereafter feminism and birth-control rendered home-based companionship between the sexes both desirable and feasible. Working-class communal values had always owed more to austerity than to conviction,[56] and Conservatives after 1945 fostered the individualism of semi-detached owner-occupation, whose privacy was increasingly extended by access to a mobile room (the family car) and a private cinema (the television). Feminist hopes went unrealized: despite Gilman, Besant, and Sylvia Pankhurst, the home retained its kitchen and did not shrivel into a private enclave within a commune run by professionalized and paid cooks and cleaners. The mechanized and individuated kitchen/scullery supplanted communal laundry, wash house, and bakery; the suburban back garden extended the backyard's prized seclusion. Institutionalization concomitantly retreated— fewer barracks, boarding schools, workhouses, orphanages, asylums, nunneries, monasteries, clubs, and residential hotels, and more privacy inside those that remained. With some justice, Galbraith warned the 1950s of Sallust's association between 'private affluence' and 'public squalor'.

The home's all-purpose rooms gradually subdivided, for open-plan interiors captured only the fashionable few. Indoor bathrooms and lavatories promoted hygiene; separate bedrooms liberated and diversified home-based self-improvement, sexuality, and recreation. House plans reflected changed relations between the sexes; husbands more rarely took their recreation in study, library, and billiard or smoking room, still less in pub and club. While separate taxation, progressively extended from the early 1970s, could in theory

---

[54] D. Coleman and J. Salt, *The British Population* (Oxford, 1992), 234. Halsey (ed.), *British Social Trends since 1900*, 118, 388.

[55] M. Girouard, *The Victorian Country House* (1971), 10.

[56] For more on this point, see B. Harrison, 'Class and Gender in Modern British Labour History', *P&P* 124 (Aug. 1989), 143–4.

have enhanced privacy between partners on money matters, shared budgeting now seemed preferable. By 1983 nine-tenths of working wives knew their husband's income,[57] a far cry from their Victorian predecessors' Friday-night fight to share a male-controlled pay packet of unknown size. If anything, husbands were keener than wives on the ideal of the home-as-retreat, for they rarely carried workplace friendships into family life, and disliked returning from work to find neighbours there whom the wife had befriended during the day.[58]

Children in Orwell's dystopia discipline their parents: 'the family had become in effect an extension of the Thought Police.'[59] There has been no British equivalent of Pavlik Morosov, the Soviet hero-child murdered by peasants in 1932 for exposing his parents as enemies of the state. Still, twentieth-century British children have in some ways accumulated privacy. Homes with more rooms per person gave them 'rooms of their own', especially after the 1960s when central heating and double glazing made more rooms continuously habitable. Thereafter privacy issues became central to disputes between parents and teenagers. Furthermore, home-generated privacy criteria were exported to boarding schools and universities, undermining teachers' semi-parental relationship with pupils. For the young, privacy's yearned-for advent marks childhood's departure; for the old, privacy's dreaded disappearance marks second childhood's advent. On the other hand, children's privacy suffered after 1945 in two ways: smaller families were recreationally less self-sufficient, and fears of traffic accidents and child molestation kept children indoors.

Privacy from neighbours amidst overcrowding requires tact. According to a census enumerator in 1871, 'families that had occupied different rooms in the same little house . . . referred me from one to another, or tapped at each other's doors to attract the attention of the inmates, without intruding on one another, and with an evident delicacy that would have well become a higher station'.[60] Yet the frosted glass and unobtrusive side entrances shielding the publican's and pawnbroker's customers represented a mere nod towards privacy in a working-class existence that was substantially public. The shared facilities (lavatories, bakehouses, markets, water pumps, wash houses, courtyards, and alleys), the ever-open door, the colourful and often dramatic social life of the street, the swarming children, the street-corner gossip networks for continuous mutual help and scrutiny—all these created a face-to-face society out of Victorian urban anonymity. But not for long: a century later, urban social fragmentation had gone so far, and had generated such problems, that

[57] Gallup poll, reported in *The Times*, 18 May 1983, 2.
[58] P. Willmott, *The Evolution of a Community* (1963), 62–3. M. Tebbutt, *Women's Talk? A Social History of 'Gossip' in Working-Class Neighbourhoods, 1880–1960* (Aldershot, 1995), 106, 116.
[59] G. Orwell, *Nineteen Eighty-Four* (1949; pbk. edn., 1955), 109–10.
[60] 'The Experiences of an Enumerator', *Morning Advertiser*, 11 Apr. 1871, 4.

Anglo-American commentators on the city yearned to rebuild a sense of community; planning for 'defensible space' could rescue a neighbourhood from its predators, said Oscar Newman in 1972.[61] By the 1990s those substitute neighbours, the security cameras, were working in the same direction.

Middle-class socialists romanticized and over-politicized Victorian slum life. To some it offered warm security; to others, narrow vendettas. Immediate escape was difficult, but psychological space could be generated between self and neighbour. 'With advance in the social scale,' wrote Seebohm Rowntree in 1901, 'family life becomes more private'.[62] From 1872 the ballot, un-English and unfashionable in its secrecy, freed voters from self-interested local pressures and buttressed respectability against intimidation and corruption. Through 'keeping himself to himself', pursuing self-sufficiency, and advertising status in front parlour and Sunday best—the respectable artisan might risk ridicule, loneliness, boredom, and failure, but he had a world of suburban semi-detachment to win. Transport changes and municipal slum-clearing planners ensured that twentieth-century cities carried further the suburban trail thus blazed. Turning themselves inside out, they supplanted the shared space of the inner-city cellular street plan by suburban privacy[63] with its associated investment in family relationships. Owner-occupation simultaneously pursued ribbon development's compromise between privacy and community, culminating in the owner-occupied 'semi' and 'starter home'. After 1945 urban neighbourliness was eroded further by high-rise housing, paid work for married women, standardized retailing, and traffic-ridden streets. The pace of its demise varied with house design, street layout, and region; friendships between neighbours sprouted more readily in north than in south. A late-1950s Dagenham householder with East End communities in mind spoke of 'suburbanitis, a withdrawing, a shutting of the door'.[64]

Yet inner-city life had never been inevitably public; crowded living can reduce visibility. Town-dwellers have less of a character to lose, and can shake off the organic rural intrusiveness of squire, parson, and paternalist employer. Nineteenth-century authority tried to replicate its rural control through urban slum clearance, policeman, clergyman, and social worker. It failed: in London, said Charles Booth in 1902, 'to ask no questions is commonly regarded as the highest form of neighbourliness'.[65] Uniformity in belief and conduct

---

[61] O. Newman, *Defensible Space* (1973), 2–4, 204.

[62] B. S. Rowntree, *Poverty* (1901), 77.

[63] I carry some of these themes further in B. Harrison, 'Traditions of Respectability in British Labour History', in Harrison, *Peaceable Kingdom* (1982), 157–216.

[64] Quoted in Willmott, *Evolution of a Community*, 67; cf. 74–6, 79–80, 122–3 for regional contrasts, street layout, and house design, together with B. Kuper, *Privacy and Private Housing* (n.p., c.1968), 7–9.

[65] C. Booth, *Life and Labour of the People in London. Third Series: Religious Influences*, vii (1902), 429.

inevitably weakened as the urban population of England and Wales grew by 50 per cent between 1901 and 1981, steadily absorbing a higher proportion of the total population.[66] Absconding apprentices, criminals in flight, recalcitrant employees, youths seeking adventure, terrorists seeking an impact, all—together with the new idea and the new social movement—relished the big city's relative freedom.

In overall environmental context, however, privacy was increasingly endangered. J. S. Mill, peering through the turmoil of mid-Victorian material progress to his ideal of 'a stationary condition of capital and population', recognized in 1848 that 'it is not good for man to be kept perforce at all times in the presence of his species': that solitude 'is essential to any depth of meditation or of character', especially 'solitude in the presence of natural beauty and grandeur'.[67] Yet late-Victorian tourists were soon littering Lakeland moors with empty soda-water bottles and newspapers, and by the Edwardian period had ravaged Devon rock pools 'undisturbed since the creation of the world'.[68] The successive cumulation of 'country cottage', 'week-end cottage', 'mobile home', and 'second home' undermined the privacy that had been their initial objective. Interwar charabancs, shanty towns, ribbon development, and petrol garages generated the case for rural planning that prevailed in 1947, together with the associated high-rise housing strategy. But the line could not be held: by the 1990s sprawling city life and inter-city travel ensured that only the Netherlands and Belgium within Europe surpassed Britain for night-time light pollution. In the thirty years up to 1995 city-generated noise destroyed an area of tranquillity the size of Wales.[69] Noise levels were increasing too, especially beneath Heathrow's flight paths in the 1950s or near Birmingham's 'Spaghetti Junction' after it opened in 1972. Furthermore, the more urbanized the population the more intrusive seemed any given level of noise, generating by the 1970s the concept of the 'noise abatement zone'.

In its fifth dimension, privacy's incidence reflects social role—whether by occupation, gender, or social class. Many occupations were once moulded by the ideal of discreet personal service—from shop assistants to professional people, and especially domestic service, the largest female occupation until 1961. Nineteenth-century country-house plans aimed to segregate servants, but in the employer's presence a silent efficiency was required. Through privacy, too, one moved up socially—by joining exclusive structures: trade unions, employers' organizations, professional bodies and clubs, each with its

[66] Halsey (ed.), *British Social Trends since 1900*, 326.

[67] J. S. Mill, *Principles of Political Economy*, in *Collected Works of J. S. Mill*, ed. J. M. Robson, iii (Toronto, 1965), 756. William Thomas of Christ Church, Oxford, kindly supplied this reference.

[68] For Devon, see E. Gosse, *Father and Son* (1907; pbk. edn., 1949), 110. For the Lake District, see M. Pattison, *Love in a Cool Climate* (Oxford, 1985), 92, writing in 1881.

[69] *Daily Telegraph*, 26 Nov. 1996, 10 (light pollution); *The Times*, 1 Dec. 1995, 8 (areas of tranquillity).

private rituals and language. It was through professional bodies and learned associations that middle-class influence extended. Each offered personal and confidential service, publicized not through advertising but through colleagues' formal endorsement and clients' recommendation. 'I cared in the highest degree for the approbation of such men as Lyell and Hooker, who were my friends,' wrote Darwin; 'I did not care much about the general public.'[70] Intermediate structures such as the University Grants Committee and research councils fended off direct parliamentary control; until recently, professional confidentiality, in medicine, for example, could deny crucial information even to the client.

Until the 1960s even many feminists saw gender roles as complementary. Politics, business, diplomacy, and war were for the men; family life and good works for the women. Their sexual innocence was assumed, so that interwar working-class wives entrusted even birth control to the husband.[71] Respectable Victorian women did not move about freely, least of all unaccompanied. Paid work was normally approved only for women (spinsters, widows) without male protection. Women often chose paid work that in some sense grew out from their domestic function, and employers took over the male relative's protective role by segregating female from male employees.[72] Women were silent in the churches: Annie Besant might secretly speak impromptu from her husband's pulpit in the 1870s, but she felt guilty and told nobody.[73] The very thought of public speaking terrified many women later proficient on the platform. If they did speak, they must avoid being 'shrill', and their cause (philanthropic, educational, humanitarian) must be suitable. Indirect female influence, however, as confidante and spouse was preferred. A genuinely private family seclusion could have generated major female achievement, but sociability pervaded private life just as confidentiality pervaded public life. Florence Nightingale's *Cassandra* memorably deplored the private sphere's unending, intellectually fragmenting round of trivial conversation and petty commitments—the requirement to 'say something' every two minutes, but nothing of consequence.[74]

There were escape routes. The Brontë sisters, George Eliot, and Harriet Martineau initially published under assumed male names or anonymously, with what Charlotte Brontë described as 'a kind of ostrich-longing for concealment'.[75] Virginia Woolf, analysing women's literary underachievement,

---

[70] F. Darwin (ed.), *The Life and Letters of Charles Darwin* (1887), i. 67; cf. ii. 219.
[71] On this, see K. Fisher's remarkable D.Phil. thesis, 'An Oral History of Birth Control Practice c.1925–50: A Study of Oxford and South Wales' (Oxford, 1997).
[72] C. Hakim, 'A Century of Change in Occupational Segregation 1891–1991', *Journal of Historical Sociology* (Dec. 1994), 448.
[73] A. H. Nethercot, *The First Five Lives of Annie Besant* (1961), 63.
[74] R. Strachey, '*The Cause*' (1928), 408, cf. 401.
[75] Discussing *Villette* with G. M. Smith on 3 Nov. 1852, quoted in E. C. Gaskell, *The Life of Charlotte Brontë* (1857), ii. 265.

thought 'anonymity runs in their blood. The desire to be veiled still possesses them.' Beatrice Webb before marrying Sidney bifurcated her day into 'the thoughtful part' (private study from 5.0 to 8.0 a.m.) and 'the active part' (normal social life for the rest of the day).[76] Martineau and Nightingale capitalized on women's alleged frailty by deploying the invalid's couch. This brought a genuine privacy free from domestic distraction, and hence a chance to mould national policy. 'It would seriously injure your influence if you were known to have influence,' Jowett told Nightingale in 1865,[77] whereas feminists argued that women's influence would become more responsible if exercised publicly. The bicycle, the teashop, and the motor car gradually ousted the chaperon and broadened woman's sphere; yet attitudes changed more slowly, for women's magazines, home mechanization, and Freudian psychology long confirmed twentieth-century women in an unpaid, houseproud, and maternal professionalism. Furthermore, in moving into paid work after the 1940s, many middle-class women saw their earnings as pin money; full-blown careers did not come till later.

Still stranger to us is the aristocratic amalgam of privacy and publicity. Daylight was shed only occasionally on a magic that was resolutely husbanded through reticence and discretion. Josephine Butler, Millicent Fawcett, and the Countess of Warwick might seek more openness, but they were outwitted by mutual self-interest within the élite, an acquiescent press and police force, and a ready resort to the law courts. So Edward VII's *amours*, the interwar mistresses of Mosley and the Prince of Wales, the homosexuality of Lady Astor's son Bobbie Shaw, Harold Macmillan's unorthodox married life, and the premarital pregnancy of his daughter all remained under wraps. As late as 1974 Earl Mountbatten could advise Prince Charles that 'a man should sow his wild oats and have as many affairs as he can before settling down. But for a wife he should choose a suitable and a sweet-charactered girl before she meets anyone else she might fall for.'[78]

Analysis of privacy's five social dimensions since the late eighteenth century has shown privacy retreating in all but the fourth, where the impact of changing residential patterns is equivocal. Privacy in the sixth dimension, public life, persisted well into the democratic age, but is also now retreating fast. This discussion has so far been primarily concerned with the experience of privacy, but to consider public life entails considering changing attitudes to privacy as well, together with shifts in the boundary between public and private. This is aristocratic decline viewed from an unfamiliar aspect. At least until the 1960s a rearguard defence of élite values against popular pressures was mobilized

---

[76] V. Woolf, *A Room of One's Own* (1929; pbk. edn., New York, 1957), 52; B. Webb, *My Apprenticeship* (2nd edn., n.d.), 105 (24 Apr. 1883).

[77] Quoted in Sir E. Cook, *The Life of Florence Nightingale* (1914), ii. 97.

[78] Letter of 14 Feb. 1974, quoted in J. Dimbleby, *The Prince of Wales: A Biography* (1994), 205.

within clublike male-dominated political institutions. In the most famous club of all, the House of Commons, etiquette reigned supreme: there 'nothing could be easier than to say the wrong thing, either with the wrong levity or the wrong seriousness'.[79] Women MPs from Astor to Thatcher refrained from invading its male inner sanctum, the smoking room. In the Oxford Union women could not become full members till 1963, and it was not till the 1970s that Oxford colleges went mixed. The two party conferences were not televised till 1955, the fourteen-day rule (precluding media discussion of matters coming up in Parliament) lasted till 1956, and the media were deterred from fully covering general elections till 1959. Not until 1978 was the House of Commons broadcast; not until 1989 was it televised, and not until 25 October 1996 was a mobile phone first inadvertently allowed to ring on the floor of the House.

Many critics of governmental privacy merely huddled into disapproving enclaves of group privacy. Nonconformist quietists were wary of a state that had persecuted their ancestors. Besides, for them the Almighty's all-seeing eye was a more powerful discipline than any state regulation. The Reformation had replaced the communal privacies of confessional and religious order by the more personal privacies of domesticity and individual self-scrutiny. The Englishman's anti-Catholic distaste for priestly intrusion into family relationships fed into his longer-lasting individualist distaste for tax collectors or welfare inspectors, however well intentioned: they might prise spouse from spouse and child from parent. And, however integral to effective planning a governmental 'population policy' might be, the idea has never caught on. Such quietism had its regional aspect, with nineteenth-century industrialists and provincials aiming to ward off an allegedly parasitic metropolis. Libertarian objection prevented any national census till 1801, then repeatedly curbed its questions; got the income tax abolished in 1816; then after its reintroduction in 1842 sought until the 1870s to phase it out; and continuously employed accountants and tax lawyers to skirmish against the Inland Revenue, with the 'black economy' as their ultimate weapon. 'According to the prevailing code,' wrote Barbara Wootton in 1955, 'a man's income is one of his private economic parts: reference to it is subject to a powerful social taboo'.[80] Arrogant and ignorant taxmen, bureaucrats, and politicians were as repugnant to John Citizen in Strube's cartoons of the 1930s as to Giles's inoffensive family man of the 1950s. Wartime identity cards were abolished in 1952, and in the 1960s concern about governmental threats to privacy was fuelled by the advent of the computer.

Victorian working people, too, were wary of a state that had often intervened clumsily in their affairs. Though remarkably tolerant of well-intentioned but often ill-informed or insensitive middle-class intruders within

---

[79] Virginia Woolf (1932), in her *The London Scene* (New York, 1975), 40.
[80] B. Wootton, *The Social Foundations of Wage Policy* (1955), 28.

their homes—Bible women, charity workers, health advisers, and canvassers—they gave short shrift to Home Secretaries opening their letters or inspecting their pubs; such espionage was un-English. 'It is almost impossible to persuade the poor that workshop and factory inspectors are acting in *their* interest,' wrote Miss Loane in 1907. 'Lads and lasses alike go home after a surprise visit and, shouting with laughter, relate how they have helped their employers "do" the N-Spectre, or how he "*nearly* cotched 'em".'[81] Many working people felt 'a quite insurmountable aversion towards embarking upon anything which would necessitate coming in contact with officials, filling up forms, etc.'.[82] The interwar means test was hated for similar reasons: it seemed callously to expose prized possessions to public view, encouraged mutual spying among neighbours, and structured benefits so as to subvert family solidarity. For Beveridge, a means-tested universal system of public assistance 'would not lead to abolition of want, because the citizens would in many cases suffer want rather than submit to investigation of their needs and means'; so the means test's demise was 'fundamental' to his welfare scheme of 1942.[83] Thereafter, trade-union wariness of law and government eventually destroyed corporatist planning, especially of incomes.

During the twentieth century these group privacies from government declined concomitantly with reticence in public figures. Whereas Rousseau in 1756 saw himself as 'pitilessly assailed' by 'idle people' keen to visit a celebrity,[84] nineteenth-century authors grew more calculating. Anonymity in print was already retreating in the 1820s, first in the quarterlies, then in the weeklies, and much later in the dailies, where the anonymous leading article persists.[85] By the 1860s open authorship had become a progressive cause; a secular and democratic society wanted everything made plain. Besides, journalists were becoming more respectable, so authors were less likely to lose status through being identified. Anonymity's last major bastion fell in June 1974, when the *Times Literary Supplement* succumbed. Biography, which for the Victorians was an improving medium, had by then become less reticent. A thin stream of indiscreet society memoirs—Greville's diaries, and the memoirs of Almeric Fitzroy and Margot Asquith—had earlier hinted at concealed realities, yet, despite Lytton Strachey's iconoclasm in *Eminent Victorians* (1918), Roy Harrod was still reluctant as Keynes's biographer in 1951 'to pry among the inner eddies of his subject's emotions'.[86] Appropriately, Michael Holroyd's

[81] M. Loane, *The Next Street but One* (1907), 88.

[82] Florence, Lady Bell, discussing Middlesbrough workers in her *At the Works* (1907; Nelson edn., 1911), 175.

[83] W. H. Beveridge, *The Pillars of Security* (1943), 121–2. My colleagues Drs R. McKibbin and John Stevenson helped me generously on this.

[84] J.-J. Rousseau, *The Confessions* (1781; trans. J. M. Cohen, Harmondsworth, 1953), 396.

[85] O. Maurer, 'Anonymity vs Signature in Victorian Reviewing', [University of Texas] *Studies in English*, 27/1 (June 1948), provides valuable background.

[86] R. F. Harrod, *The Life of John Maynard Keynes* (1951; pbk. edn., 1972), 430.

Lytton Strachey (1967–8) broke this barrier, and by 1980 the *Dictionary of National Biography* had freed E. M. Forster and Somerset Maugham to become homosexuals.[87]

Americans invented both the phrase and the reality of 'public relations'. His biographer was 'doubtful' whether Lord Lansdowne, the late-Victorian Unionist statesman, 'ever gave a press interview during his long life. He certainly never posed for a press photograph.'[88] In 1870 the word 'interview' still seemed too American to shed its inverted commas,[89] but by the 1880s statesmen were besieged by publicity and even by tourists. In the 1930s a press photographer like Edward J. Dean felt no apparent scruple about infringing the privacy of the famous,[90] and on 9 September 1951 the *Sunday Pictorial*'s front page featured the sick King George VI leaving his clinic: 'Why are we proud to print this picture? Because it is news, because it is human, because it is symbolic.' In the 1960s Labour politicians began exposing the inner sanctum: the cabinet. For Castle, publishing cabinet ministers' diaries could 'only strengthen the democratic process'.[91] A government that had once eavesdropped on its citizens now found the roles reversed, and in the 1990s overseas precedents and pressures brought even MI5 blinking into the limelight. The distinction between publicity and notoriety had long been dissolving. The Edwardian militant suffrage movement set precedents for the Campaign for Nuclear Disarmament's direct-action offshoot in the 1960s, and since the 1970s the IRA has plumbed further sensationalist depths. Publicity of any sort was now relished, if only for fifteen minutes. After firing blank shots at the Queen in 1981, the teenager Marcus Sarjeant allegedly told his captors 'I wanted to be somebody. I wanted to be famous.'[92]

For the élite the best form of defence was attack. Powerful people can stage the frequency, timing, and circumstances of their appearance, and can deploy their charm and glamour in interviews. Seeking these was, after all, only a more public form of the autograph craze, already well under way in the 1820s. So monarchs, while ruthless towards unauthorized disclosure—by Queen Elizabeth II's once-loved nanny Marion Crawford ('Crawfie'), for example— took the initiative. They broadened admission to the thanksgiving of 1872 and to twentieth-century Buckingham Palace garden parties, allowed the coronation to be televised in 1953, and authorized two television programmes: 'Royal Family' in 1969 and 'Elizabeth R.' in 1992. Politicians have been equally shrewd, from mid-Victorian private briefings of journalists to the Wilsons' televised guided tour of 10 Downing Street in 1969 and Thatcher's televised

---

[87] E. T. Williams, 'prefatory note', to E. T. Williams and C. S. Nicholls (eds.), *The Dictionary of National Biography 1961–1970* (1981), p. vi.
[88] Lord Newton, *Lord Lansdowne: A Biography* (1929), 493.
[89] *The Times*, 10 Mar. 1870, 11.
[90] See E. J. Dean, *Lucky Dean: Reminiscences of a Press Photographer* (1944).
[91] *The Castle Diaries 1964–70* (1984), p. vii (preface).
[92] S. Tendler, 'The Teenager who Wanted Fame', *The Times*, 15 Sept. 1981, 30.

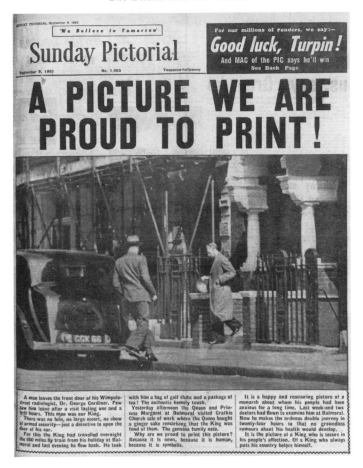

18. *Sunday Pictorial*, 9 September 1951, 1

glimpse into her wardrobe in 1986. Conservatives acquiesced more readily in publicity than mid-century Labour, with its residual rationalistic puritanism. Public-relations officers 'do not exist in order to build up the personalities of Ministers,' Attlee told journalists in 1949. 'They exist in order to explain Government policy,' disarmingly adding that 'I should be a sad subject for any publicity expert'.[93] Yet politics could no longer tolerate the Asquiths, McKennas, and Harold Nicolsons who were too fastidious to cultivate the press. Besides, pressmen now questioned whether public figures deserved the privacy the ordinary citizen enjoyed—given that publicity so frequently benefits them politically, financially, or in other ways, and is known in advance

[93] H. Nicolson, *Diaries and Letters 1945–1962*, ed. N. Nicolson (1968), 163 (14 Jan. 1949).

to be the price of influence. Privacy laws, said Rupert Murdoch in 1997, 'are for the protection of people who are already privileged'.[94]

'The further we go back into history,' wrote Marx, 'the more the individual . . . seems to depend on and belong to a larger whole.'[95] Privacy is indeed fragile within the tight social structures generated by primitive man's contest with a harsh environment, though in its environmental dimension privacy may benefit from dispersed pre-industrial patterns of settlement. Brandeis and Warren, pioneering the idea of protecting privacy by law in 1890, echoed Marx's chronology, but not his reasoning or terminology. For them, 'the intensity and complexity of life, attendant upon advancing civilization' made privacy more necessary. For them, 'political, social, and economic changes entail the recognition of new rights', and the common law 'in its eternal youth, grows to meet the demands of society'.[96] For us their equation between progress and privacy is questionable, and their high hopes of the law seem inflated; besides, they were apparently unaware that some pre-industrial societies value privacy,[97] whereas some modern societies do not. Privacy is vulnerable within utopias, and twentieth-century autocrats offer utopian justifications for regressing to oppressively organic structures. Post-war international declarations designed to prevent further Hitlers include privacy among the political rights they endorse. MPs debating how to uphold privacy in the 1960s often cited Orwell's *Nineteen Eighty-four*, where Winston Smith's sex act with Julia, unobserved and unsanctioned by Big Brother, constitutes 'a blow struck against the Party . . . a political act'.[98]

There are yet more tensions between privacy and democracy, which acquiesces in small-scale privacies higher up—governmental secrecy aimed at warding off war or terrorism, for example—in order to uphold large-scale privacies lower down, most notably the citizen's privacy from the state. Besides, democracy's components are disparate. Privacy is compatible with some (with democracy's valuation of human diversity and autonomy, for example, or its need to curb governmental power)—but is less so with others (its need for equitable legislation, for example, and for an informed and participatory electorate). At the end of the twentieth century, British democracy remained beset by the tension between the citizen's right to know and his need to attract reticent talent into public life. That Victorian arch-democrat Joseph Chamberlain was still able to safeguard his privacy at Highbury as zealously as any

[94] *Daily Telegraph*, 8 Oct. 1997, 5, addressing News Corporation's annual meeting in Adelaide on 7 Oct.
[95] K. Marx, *The Grundrisse*, ed. D. McLellan (1971), 17. Professor McLellan kindly provided me with this reference.
[96] S. D. Warren and L. D. Brandeis, 'The Right to Privacy', *Harvard Law Review*, 4/5 (15 Dec. 1890), 196, 193.
[97] In her refreshingly broad approach to privacy, K. J. Day gathers interesting evidence in her 'Perspectives on Privacy: A Sociological Analysis', Ph.D. thesis (Edinburgh, 1985), 39.
[98] Orwell, *Nineteen Eighty-Four*, 104.

Whig aristocrat; a century later the radical sociologist Howard Kirk in Bradbury's *The History Man*, enthusiastically writing a book on 'the defeat of privacy', was outraged to find his student Felicity Phee reading the typescript: 'you'd no business to do that,' he told her, 'it's not quite finished. It's private.'[99]

Domestic privacy may even become so attractive as to deny public life both volunteers and voters. For Lord John Russell in 1858 British domesticity ensured that 'we have not the public life which was common in some ancient republics' or in the USA.[100] He was unconcerned, because the home then seemed a stabilizing influence; besides, an aristocratic society could justifiably assume that a sense of public duty was widely diffused. Yet the warlike virtues integral to aristocracy are now unfashionable, and their decline has been accompanied, not by a new rank-ordering of public loyalties, but by the retreat into privacy. E. M. Forster knew that 'all society rests upon force', but thought that 'all the great creative actions, all the decent human relations' occur only 'during the intervals when force has not managed to come to the front'.[101] A temperament continuously preoccupied with politics may indeed lack cultivation and balance. Yet political indifference also has its drawbacks: Tocqueville rightly warned us that despotism 'immures' the citizen 'each in his private life' and thrives on a quietist social atomization.[102] The Labour Party could never have captured the British left without access to virtues less private than Bloomsbury's. By the end of the twentieth century, prominent British politicians from more than one party were coming full circle, and were seeking to transcend domesticity by restoring to civility some of its original humanist and public-spirited content.

[99] J. L. Garvin, *The Life of Joseph Chamberlain*, ii (1933), 493; M. Bradbury, *The History Man* (1975; pbk. edn., 1985), 91.

[100] Speech to friends of the Manchester Athenaeum, *The Times*, 23 Oct. 1858, 12.

[101] E. M. Forster, 'What I Believe' (1939), in his *Two Cheers for Democracy* (1951; pbk. edn., 1970), 78.

[102] A. de Tocqueville, *The Ancien Regime and the French Revolution* (1856; trans. S. Gilbert, pbk. edn., 1966), 29.

20

The Published Writings of Keith Thomas, 1957–1998

GILES MANDELBROTE

This list sets out to include all Keith Thomas's publications, as well as interviews containing substantial quotation. Unpublished lectures, papers, and reports, letters to the press, and Keith Thomas's unsigned 'Annual Report' as President of Corpus Christi College, Oxford (printed in *The Pelican Record* since 1987), have been omitted, as have publications about him. Books and articles are listed first, followed by reviews. Items marked * are unsigned.

1957

Reviews

*D. Grant, *Margaret the First: A Biography of Margaret, Duchess of Newcastle 1623–1673*, in *Schoolmaster*, 29 March, 604.

H. J. Randall, *Bridgend: The Story of a Market Town*, in *Transactions of the Honourable Society of Cymmrodorion*, session 1956, 136–7.

G. L. Mosse, *The Holy Pretence*, in *Oxford Magazine*, 5 December, [back cover].

1958

'Women and the Civil War Sects', *P&P* 13: 42–62. Reprinted, with corrections and additions, in Trevor Aston (ed.), *Crisis in Europe 1560–1660: Essays from Past and Present* (London: Routledge & Kegan Paul, 1965), 317–40.

Review

D. M. Stenton, *The English Woman in History*, in *Oxford Magazine*, 13 March, 379.

I am very grateful to Arnold Hunt, J. R. Maddicott, Scott Mandelbrote, and the editors, for suggesting a number of additions to this list. I would also particularly like to thank Keith Thomas himself for his cooperation and for allowing me access to his own notes and files.

1959

'The Double Standard', *Journal of the History of Ideas*, 20: 195–216. Reprinted, with revisions, in Philip P. Wiener and Aaron Noland (eds.), *Ideas in Cultural Perspective* (New Brunswick: Rutgers University Press, 1962), 446–67, and in Maryanne Cline Horowitz (ed.), *Race, Gender, and Rank: Early Modern Ideas of Humanity* (Rochester, NY: University of Rochester Press, 1992), 137–58.

Reviews

R. H. Tawney, *Business and Politics under James I*, in *Oxford Magazine*, 26 February, 281–2.

*P. M. Handover, *The Second Cecil*, in *The Economist*, 18 July, 151.

P. Williams, *The Council in the Marches of Wales under Elizabeth I*, and W. Rees, *An Historical Atlas of Wales*, in *Transactions of the Honourable Society of Cymmrodorion*, session 1959, 115–18.

*M. Lee, *John Maitland of Thirlestane and the Foundation of the Stewart Despotism in Scotland*, in *The Economist*, 5 December, 964.

1960

Reviews

J. H. M. Salmon, *The French Religious Wars in English Political Thought*, in *Journal of Ecclesiastical History*, 11: 136–7.

*P. R. Kemp and C. Lloyd, *The Brethren of the Coast*, in *The Economist*, 11 June, 1089–90.

*S. G. E. Lythe, *The Economy of Scotland in its European Setting 1550–1625*, in *The Economist*, 2 July, 31.

*W. A. Aiken and B. D. Henning, *Conflict in Stuart England: Essays in Honour of Wallace Notestein*, in *The Economist*, 30 July, 470–1.

*F. G. Bengtsson, *The Life of Charles XII, King of Sweden, 1697–1718*, in *The Economist*, 27 August, 796–7.

R. A. Marchant, *The Puritans and the Church Courts in the Diocese of York 1560–1642*, in *Oxford Magazine*, 10 November, 87–8.

1961

*'In My Father's House', *Oxford Magazine*, 19 January, 143.

*'Admissions', *Oxford Magazine*, 26 January, 163.

*'The Association of University Teachers', *Oxford Magazine*, 2 February, 183.

*'Isis and the Proctors', *Oxford Magazine*, 9 February, 203–4.

*'Graduate Accommodation', *Oxford Magazine*, 16 February, 223.

*'Open Scholarships', *Oxford Magazine*, 23 February, 239.

*'The New Proctors', *Oxford Magazine*, 2 March, 259–60.
*'The Delegacy of Lodgings', *Oxford Magazine*, 9 March, 283.
*'The Colleges and the Schools', *Oxford Magazine*, 27 April, 299–300.
*'The Classics as Literature', *Oxford Magazine*, 11 May, 331–2.
*'A Business School for Oxford?', *Oxford Magazine*, 18 May, 347–8.
*'Dons and the W. E. A.', *Oxford Magazine*, 25 May, 363.
*'The Future of the College System', *Oxford Magazine*, 1 June, 379–80.
*'Rhodes House', *Oxford Magazine*, 19 October, 1–2.
*'Open Secrets', *Oxford Magazine*, 26 October, 25.
*'Teaching and Research', *Oxford Magazine*, 2 November, 41.
*'Open Scholarships', *Oxford Magazine*, 9 November, 57.
*'A Long Vacation Term', *Oxford Magazine*, 23 November, 89.
*'Committees', *Oxford Magazine*, 30 November, 105–6.
*'College Entrance', *Oxford Magazine*, 7 December, 121–2.

Reviews

G. Donaldson, *The Scottish Reformation*, in *Oxford Magazine*, 19 January, 151, 153.
G. E. Aylmer, *The King's Servants*, and S. T. Bindoff, J. Hurstfield, and C. H. Williams (eds.), *Elizabethan Government and Society: Essays Presented to Sir John Neale*, in *Guardian*, 17 February, 6.
J. S. Bromley and E. H. Kossmann, *Britain and the Netherlands*, in *Oxford Magazine*, 11 May, 343.
E. E. Evans-Pritchard, *Anthropology and History*, in *Oxford Magazine*, 1 June, 387–8.
R. Ashton, *The Crown and the Money Market 1603–1640*, in *Oxford Magazine*, 15 June, 420–2.
C. Blitzer, *An Immortal Commonwealth: The Political Thought of James Harrington*, in *Oxford Magazine*, 15 June, 428.
Christopher Hill, *The Century of Revolution 1603–1714*, in *Guardian*, 16 June, 6.
F. J. Fisher (ed.), *Essays in the Economic and Social History of Tudor and Stuart England in Honour of R. H. Tawney*, in *Oxford Magazine*, 16 November, 83.
C. V. Wedgwood, *Thomas Wentworth, Earl of Strafford: A Revaluation*, in *Guardian*, 17 November, 8.

1962

Reviews

K. Samuelsson, *Religion and Economic Action*, in *Oxford Magazine*, 1 February, 166.
C. H. and K. George, *The Protestant Mind of the English Reformation*, in *Oxford Magazine*, 8 February, 180–1.

A. Simpson, *The Wealth of the Gentry 1540–1660: East Anglian Studies*, in *Oxford Magazine*, 1 March, 230.

J. H. Hexter, *Reappraisals in History*, in *Oxford Magazine*, 15 March, 264–5.

I. Coltman, *Private Men and Public Causes: Philosophy and Politics in the English Civil War*, in *Oxford Magazine*, 17 May, 313.

L. H. Carlson (ed.), *The Writings of Henry Barrow, 1587–1590*, and *The Writings of John Greenwood, 1587–1590*, in *Oxford Magazine*, 1 November, 42–3.

1963

'History and Anthropology', *P&P* 24: 3–24.

Reviews

E. M. Carus-Wilson (ed.), *Essays in Economic History*, ii, iii, in *Oxford Magazine*, 28 February, 221.

G. D. Ramsay (ed.), *John Isham, Mercer and Merchant Adventurer*, in *Oxford Magazine*, 28 February, 222.

1964

'Work and Leisure in Pre-Industrial Society', *P&P* 29: 50–62.

1965

'The Social Origins of Hobbes's Political Thought', in K. C. Brown (ed.), *Hobbes Studies* (Oxford: Basil Blackwell), 185–236.

Reviews

J. A. and Olive Banks, *Feminism and Family Planning in Victorian England*, in *Economic History Review*, 2nd ser., 17: 600–1.

'Some Contributions to Medical History', *Archives*, 7: 98–100.

1966

'The Tools and the Job', *Times Literary Supplement*, 7 April, 275–6.

Reviews

*Michael Walzer, *The Revolution of the Saints*, in *Times Literary Supplement*, 14 April, 331.

M. F. Bond (ed.), *The Manuscripts of the House of Lords*, NS xi. *Addenda, 1514–1714*, in *Archives*, 7: 178–9.

Hannah Gavron, *The Captive Wife*, in *New Statesman*, 13 May, 691, 694. Reprinted as 'Captive Wife' in Karl Miller (ed.), *Writing in England Today: The Last Fifteen Years* (Harmondsworth: Penguin Books, 1968), 288–92.

A. B. Ferguson, *The Articulate Citizen and the English Renaissance*, in *Review of English Studies*, NS 17: 306–8.

1967

Reviews

C. H. Josten (ed.), *Elias Ashmole (1617–1692)*, i–v, in *Oxford Magazine*, 10 March, 271–2.

S. E. Prall, *The Agitation for Law Reform during the Puritan Revolution*, in *History*, 52: 206–7.

H. R. Trevor-Roper, *Religion, the Reformation, and Social Change*, in *Guardian*, 1 September, 5.

1968

Reviews

Ronald Fraser (ed.), *Work*, and Peter Hollowell, *The Lorry-Driver*, in *Listener*, 29 February, 276–7.

E. R. Foster (ed.), *Proceedings in Parliament, 1610*, i, ii, in *EHR* 83: 351–5.

1969

'Another Digger Broadside', *P&P* 42: 57–68. Reprinted in Charles Webster (ed.), *The Intellectual Revolution of the Seventeenth Century* (London and Boston: Routledge & Kegan Paul, 1974), 124–37.

'The Date of Gerrard Winstanley's *Fire in the Bush*', *P&P* 42: 160–2. Reprinted in Charles Webster (ed.), *The Intellectual Revolution of the Seventeenth Century* (London and Boston: Routledge & Kegan Paul, 1974), 138–42.

Review

F. J. Levy, *Tudor Historical Thought*, in *Review of English Studies*, NS 20: 80–1.

1970

'Wizards', *Listener*, 5 March, 306–8.

'Witches', *Listener*, 12 March, 339–42.

'The Relevance of Social Anthropology to the Historical Study of English

Witchcraft', in Mary Douglas (ed.), *Witchcraft Confessions and Accusations* (A.S.A. monographs, 9; London: Tavistock Publications), 47–79. Translated into Polish (1977), *Odrodzenie i Reformacja w Polsce*, 22: 27–56.

Reviews

Histoire Mondiale de la Femme, iv, in *EHR* 85: 220.
J. L. Axtell (ed.), *The Educational Writings of John Locke*, in *EHR* 85: 363–6.

1971

Religion and the Decline of Magic: Studies in Popular Beliefs in Sixteenth and Seventeenth Century England (London: Weidenfeld & Nicolson). Reprinted as a paperback by Penguin Books 1973; reprinted as a Peregrine Book 1978. Extracts published in translation in Marina Romanello (ed.), *La Stregoneria in Europa (1450–1650)* (Bologna: Il Mulino, 1975), 177–95, 203–34; as 'Die Hexen und ihre soziale Umwelt', in Claudia Honegger (ed.), *Die Hexen der Neuzeit: Studien zur Sozialgeschichte eines kulturellen Deutungsmusters* (Frankfurt am Main: Suhrkamp Verlag, 1978), 256–308; and as 'L'eclisse della magia', *Prometeo*, 3 (September 1985), 42–53. Translated into Italian (Milan: Mondadori, 1985), Dutch (Amsterdam: Agon, 1989), Portuguese (São Paulo: Companhia das Letras, 1991), and Japanese (Tokyo: Hosei University Press, 1993).

Reviews

R. Ashton (ed.), *James I by his Contemporaries*, in *EHR* 86: 411.
B. Rosen (ed.), *Witchcraft*, in *EHR* 86: 411–12.

1972

'The Levellers and the Franchise', in G. E. Aylmer (ed.), *The Interregnum: The Quest for Settlement 1646–1660* (London and Basingstoke: Macmillan), 57–78. Revised and corrected reprint in paperback, 1974.
'Notes and Comments' (contribution drawing attention to publications by Margaret Spufford and Tapan Raychaudhuri), *P&P* 54: 141–2.

Reviews

Winfried Förster, *Thomas Hobbes und der Puritanismus. Grundlagen und Grundfragen seiner Staatslehre*, in *EHR* 87: 189.
Reinhart Koselleck and Roman Schnur (eds.), *Hobbes-Forschungen*, in *EHR* 87: 417–19.
Christopher Hill, *The World Turned Upside Down*, in *New York Review of Books*, 30 November, 26–9.

Wayne Shumaker, *The Occult Sciences in the Renaissance*, in *Times Higher Education Supplement*, 29 December, 12.

1973

Reviews

Peter Burke (ed.), *A New Kind of History from the Writings of Lucien Febvre*, and Marc Bloch, *The Royal Touch*, in *New Statesman*, 20 April 1973, 585–6.

L. C. Knights, *Public Voices: Literature and Politics with Special Reference to the Seventeenth Century*, in *Review of English Studies*, NS 24: 208–10.

Antonia Fraser, *Cromwell: Our Chief of Men*, in *Listener*, 7 June, 760–1.

French Fogle (ed.), *Complete Prose Works of John Milton*, v. *1648?–1671*, in *EHR* 88: 635–6.

Lawrence Stone, *Family and Fortune*, in *Listener*, 16 August, 222.

Fernand Braudel, *Capitalism and Material Life, 1400–1800*, in *New York Review of Books*, 13 December, 3–4.

1974

Reviews

G. E. Aylmer, *The State's Servants: The Civil Service of the English Republic 1649–1660*, in *Guardian*, 3 January, 12.

Paul Boyer and Stephen Nissenbaum, *Salem Possessed: The Social Origins of Witchcraft*, in *New York Review of Books*, 8 August, 22–3.

Herbert M. Atherton, *Political Prints in the Age of Hogarth*, in *Times Higher Education Supplement*, 20 September, p. v.

Neil McKendrick (ed.), *Historical Perspectives: Studies in English Thought and Society in Honour of J. H. Plumb*, in *Times Higher Education Supplement*, 8 November, 15.

1975

'An Anthropology of Religion and Magic, II', *Journal of Interdisciplinary History*, 6: 91–109. Reprinted in Brian P. Levack (ed.), *Anthropological Studies of Witchcraft, Magic and Religion* (Articles on Witchcraft, Magic and Demonology, 1; New York and London: Garland Publishing, 1992), 133–51.

Reviews

Perry Anderson, *Passages from Antiquity to Feudalism* and *Lineages of the Absolutist State*, and Immanuel Wallerstein, *The Modern World-System*, in *New York Review of Books*, 17 April, 26–8.

E. P. Thompson, *Whigs and Hunters*, and Douglas Hay *et al.*, *Albion's Fatal Tree*, in *New Statesman*, 10 October, 443–4.

Kenneth A. Lockridge, *Literacy in Colonial New England*, in *History*, 60: 399–400.

Charles Webster, *The Great Instauration*, and Michael Hunter, *John Aubrey and the Realm of Learning*, in *Guardian*, 27 November, 18.

1976

Rule and Misrule in the Schools of Early Modern England (Stenton Lecture, University of Reading, 1975; Reading: University of Reading).

Age and Authority in Early Modern England (Raleigh Lecture on History, British Academy, 1976; London: British Academy). Reprinted in *Proceedings of the British Academy*, 62 (1977), 205–48.

Reviews

Eileen Power, *Medieval Women*, in *New Statesman*, 16 January, 73–4.

Lloyd de Mause (ed.), *The History of Childhood*, in *New Statesman*, 16 April, 511–12.

Edward Shorter, *The Making of the Modern Family*, in *New Statesman*, 28 May, 716–17.

Margaret Spufford, *Contrasting Communities: English Villagers in the Sixteenth and Seventeenth Centuries*, in *History*, 61: 271–2.

William H. McNeill, *Plagues and Peoples*, in *New York Review of Books*, 30 September, 3–4.

Marina Warner, *Alone of All Her Sex: The Myth and the Cult of the Virgin Mary*, and Geoffrey Ashe, *The Virgin*, in *New York Review of Books*, 11 November, 10–13.

1977

'The Place of Laughter in Tudor and Stuart England' (Neale Lecture, University College, London, 1976), *Times Literary Supplement*, 21 January, 77–81.

'Stregoneria, Magia e Superstizione in Inghilterra', *Ricerche di Storia Sociale e Religiosa*, NS 11: 141–9.

Reviews

Peter Laslett, *Family Life and Illicit Love in Earlier Generations*, and Lawrence Stone, *The Family, Sex and Marriage in England 1500–1800*, in *Times Literary Supplement*, 21 October, 1226–7 (and Letter, 30 December, 1528).

1978

Edited (with Donald Pennington), *Puritans and Revolutionaries: Essays in Seventeenth-Century History Presented to Christopher Hill* (Oxford: Clarendon Press). Contributed 'The Puritans and Adultery: The Act of 1650 Reconsidered', pp. 257–82.

'The United Kingdom', in Raymond Grew (ed.), *Crises of Political Development in Europe and the United States* (Princeton, NJ: Princeton University Press), 41–97.

Obituary

**'Mr J. P. Cooper', *The Times*, 22 April, 16.

Reviews

A. G. Dickens (ed.), *The Courts of Europe: Politics, Patronage and Royalty 1400–1800*, in *New York Review of Books*, 26 January, 18–20.

Alan Macfarlane (ed.), *The Diary of Ralph Josselin, 1616–1683*, in *History*, 63: 125–6.

Norbert Elias, *The Civilizing Process: The History of Manners*, and P. R. Gleichmann, J. Goudsblom, and H. Korte (eds.), *Human Figurations: Essays for Norbert Elias*, in *New York Review of Books*, 9 March, 28–31.

Emmanuel Le Roy Ladurie, *Montaillou*, Lucien Febvre, *Life in Renaissance France*, and Edward Britton, *The Community of the Village: A Study in the History of the Family and Village Life in Fourteenth-Century England*, in *New York Review of Books*, 12 October, 52–4.

1979

Reviews

Quentin Skinner, *The Foundations of Modern Political Thought*, in *New York Review of Books*, 17 May, 26–9.

Isaiah Berlin, *Against the Current: Essays in the History of Ideas*, in *Observer*, 22 July, 36.

1980

Reviews

Frank E. and Fritzie P. Manuel, *Utopian Thought in the Western World*, in *Sunday Times*, 6 January, 43.

E. S. de Beer (ed.), *The Correspondence of John Locke*, i–iv, in *EHR* 95: 845–51.

John Boswell, *Christianity, Social Tolerance, and Homosexuality*, in *New York Review of Books*, 4 December, 26–9.

1981

Reviews

Henry S. Salt, *Animals' Rights Considered in Relation to Social Progress*, and James Turner, *Reckoning with the Beast: Animals, Pain, and Humanity in the Victorian Mind*, in *New York Review of Books*, 30 April, 47–8.

Marina Warner, *Joan of Arc: The Image of Female Heroism*, and Frances Gies, *Joan of Arc: The Legend and the Reality*, in *New York Review of Books*, 25 June, 7–12.

Muriel St Clare Byrne (ed.), *The Lisle Letters*, 6 vols., in *Sunday Times*, 19 July, 43. Reprinted ('The True Voice of Tudor England') in *The Reception of the Lisle Letters 1981–1982: A Selection of Reviews from England and the United States in Chronological Order from Publication Date to Presentation of the Carey-Thomas Award* (London: Secker & Warburg; Chicago, Ill.: University of Chicago Press, [1983]), 29–30.

1982

Review

Lawrence Stone, *The Past and the Present*, in *Times Literary Supplement*, 30 April, 479.

1983

Man and the Natural World: Changing Attitudes in England 1500–1800 (London: Allen Lane). (A revised version of the George Macaulay Trevelyan Lectures, University of Cambridge, 1979.) Excerpt published as 'No Compassion for "the Brute Creation"', *History Today*, 33 (April), 5–10. Reprinted as a paperback by Penguin Books 1984. Translated into French (Paris: Gallimard, 1985), Portuguese (São Paulo: Companhia das Letras, 1988), Swedish (Stockholm: Ordfront Förlag, 1988), Japanese (Tokyo: Hosei University Press, 1989), Dutch (Amsterdam: Agon, 1990), and Italian (Turin: Einaudi, 1994).

The Perception of the Past in Early Modern England (Creighton Trust Lecture, University of London, 1983; London: University of London [issued 1984]).

'Meeting the Challenge', a contribution to a symposium on 'the new history', *Times Higher Education Supplement*, 4 November, 13.

'Interview with Keith Thomas' (interviewed by Francis Brooks), *Australian Historical Association Bulletin*, 36: 24–6.

Reviews

Ivan Illich, *Gender*, in *New York Review of Books*, 12 May, 6–10 (and Letter in reply to Fritz Staal, 29 September, 65–6).

Contribution to 'History Books of the Year', *History Today*, 33 (December), 50.

1984

Reviews

Antonia Fraser, *The Weaker Vessel: Woman's Lot in Seventeenth-Century England*, in *Sunday Times*, 6 May, 40.

Daniel Boorstin, *The Discoverers*, in *New York Review of Books*, 10 May, 20–2 (and Letter, 19 July, 45).

Barbara Stafford, *Voyage into Substance: Art, Science, Nature and the Illustrated Travel Account, 1760–1840*, in *New York Times Book Review*, 14 October, 22–3.

Barbara J. Shapiro, *Probability and Certainty in Seventeenth-Century England*, in *Journal of Ecclesiastical History*, 35: 636–7.

Fernand Braudel, *Civilization and Capitalism, 15th–18th Century*, iii. *The Perspective of the World*, in *New York Review of Books*, 22 November, 41–4.

Contribution to 'History Books of the Year', *History Today*, 34 (December), 54.

1985

'The Utopian Impulse in Seventeenth-Century England', *Dutch Quarterly Review of Anglo-American Letters*, 15: 162–88. Reprinted in Dominic Baker-Smith and C. C. Barfoot (eds.), *Between Dream and Nature: Essays on Utopia and Dystopia* (DQR Studies in Literature, 2; Amsterdam: Rodopi, 1987), 20–46.

1986

'The Meaning of Literacy in Early Modern England', in Gerd Baumann (ed.), *The Written Word: Literacy in Transition* (Wolfson College Lectures, Wolfson College, Oxford, 1985; Oxford: Clarendon Press), 97–131.

Compiled (with H. M. Colvin), *The Canterbury Quadrangle 1636–1986: An Anthology* (Oxford: Bocardo Press, privately printed for St John's College, Oxford).

'Foreword' to Michael Carrithers *et al.*, *Founders of Faith* (Oxford: Oxford University Press), p. [v].

Review

J. G. A. Pocock, *Virtue, Commerce, and History*, in *New York Review of Books*, 27 February, 36–9.

1987

'Numeracy in Early Modern England' (Prothero Lecture, Royal Historical Society, London, 1986), *Transactions of the Royal Historical Society*, 5th ser., 37: 103–32.

Reviews

Gertrude Himmelfarb, *Marriage and Morals among the Victorians*, in *New York Review of Books*, 28 May, 26–8.
Roy Porter, *Mind-Forg'd Manacles* and *A Social History of Madness*, in *Times Literary Supplement*, 4 December, 1339–40.

1988

History and Literature (Ernest Hughes Memorial Lecture, University College of Swansea, 1988; Swansea: University College of Swansea [issued 1989]).
'Foreword' to *Corpus Christi College, Oxford: Biographical Register 1880–1974*, compiled by P. A. Hunt, ed. N. A. Flanagan (Oxford: Corpus Christi College), pp. vii–x.
'The Past in Clearer Light, a Beacon on our Future' (on the humanities), *Times Higher Education Supplement*, 2 December, 13, 16.
Vergangenheit, Zukunft, Lebensalter: Zeitvorstellungen im England der frühen Neuzeit (Kleine Kulturwissenschaftliche Bibliothek, 10; Berlin: Verlag Klaus Wagenbach). A translation, by Robin Cackett, of 'The Perception of the Past in Early Modern England', 'Age and Authority in Early Modern England', and 'The Utopian Impulse in Seventeenth-Century England'.

Review

Edmund S. Morgan, *Inventing the People: The Rise of Popular Sovereignty in England and America*, in *New York Review of Books*, 24 November, 43–5.

1989

'Children in Early Modern England', in Gillian Avery and Julia Briggs (eds.), *Children and their Books: A Celebration of the Work of Iona and Peter Opie* (Oxford: Clarendon Press), 45–77.

Reviews

John Boswell, *The Kindness of Strangers: The Abandonment of Children in Western Europe from Late Antiquity to the Renaissance*, in *Times Literary Supplement*, 25 August, 913–14.
Roger Chartier (ed.), *A History of Private Life*, iii. *Passions of the Renaissance*, in *New York Review of Books*, 9 November, 15–19.

1990

'Yours', in Christopher Ricks and Leonard Michaels (eds.), *The State of the Language* (new edn., London and Boston, Mass.: Faber & Faber), 451–6.

'The Future of the Past' (on history in the National Curriculum), *Times Literary Supplement*, 8 June, 610, 621.

'Historians don't have any Ideas of their Own' (interviewed by Peer Vries), *Leidschrift*, 6: 99–113.

'The Human Carnivore: Changing Attitudes to Meat-Eating in England 1500–1990', *The Society of Food Writers News*, 4: 8–11.

Reviews

Carole Fink, *Marc Bloch: A Life*, in *Observer*, 14 January, 45.

Linda Colley, *Lewis Namier*, in *New York Review of Books*, 14 June, 46–8.

Michelle Perrot (ed.), *A History of Private Life*, iv. *From the Fires of Revolution to the Great War*, in *Observer*, 1 July, 57.

Fernand Braudel, *The Identity of France*, ii. *People and Production*, in *Observer*, 16 December, 4.

1991

'Ways of Doing Cultural History', in Rik Sanders, Bas Mesters, *et al.* (eds.), *Balans en Perspectief van de Nederlandse Cultuurgeschiedenis: De Verleiding van de Overvloed* (Amsterdam and Atlanta, Ga.: Rodopi), 65–81.

'Introduction' to Jan Bremmer and Herman Roodenburg (eds.), *A Cultural History of Gesture from Antiquity to the Present Day* (Cambridge: Polity Press), 1–14.

'Foreword to paperback edition' of Elizabeth Rawson, *The Spartan Tradition in European Thought* (Oxford: Clarendon Press), pp. v–vi.

'Foreword' to R. M. Hare *et al.*, *Founders of Thought: Plato, Aristotle, Augustine* (Oxford: Oxford University Press), pp. v–vi.

'Foreword' to François Laroque, *Shakespeare's Festive World: Elizabethan Seasonal Entertainment and the Professional Stage* (Cambridge: Cambridge University Press), pp. xiii–xiv.

Reviews

Carlo Ginzburg, *Ecstasies: Deciphering the Witches' Sabbath*, in *Observer*, 20 January, 59.

Lawrence Stone, *Road to Divorce: England 1530–1987*, in *New York Review of Books*, 7 March, 30–3.

Max Oelschlaeger, *The Idea of Wilderness*, in *Observer*, 26 May, 61.

Tessa Watt, *Cheap Print and Popular Piety, 1550–1640*, and Natascha Würzbach,

The Rise of the English Street Ballad, 1550–1650, in *Times Literary Supplement*, 23 August, 5–6.

E. P. Thompson, *Customs in Common*, in *Observer*, 27 October, 61.

Contribution to 'Books of the Year', *Observer*, 24 November, 4.

Antoine Prost and Gérard Vincent, *A History of Private Life*, v. *Riddles of Identity in Modern Times*, in *Observer*, 15 December, 48.

Vincent Scully, *Architecture: The Natural and the Manmade*, in *New York Times Book Review*, 29 December, 1, 26.

1992

'Introduction' to C. C. W. Taylor (ed.), *Ethics and the Environment* (Oxford: Corpus Christi College), 1–11.

'Foreword' to Quentin Skinner *et al.*, *Great Political Thinkers* (Oxford: Oxford University Press), pp. v–vii.

'Foreword' to John Dunn *et al.*, *The British Empiricists* (Oxford: Oxford University Press), pp. v–vii.

'Ik ben niet zo geïnteresseerd in mijn mening, maar in wat men vroeger dacht' (interviewed by Peter de Brock), *Folia*, 3 April, 9, 12.

Reviews

Francis Fukuyama, *The End of History and the Last Man*, in *Observer*, 1 March, 63.

Carlo Cipolla, *Miasmas and Disease: Public Health and the Environment in the Pre-Industrial Age*, in *Guardian*, 19 March, 29.

A. H. Halsey, *The Decline of Donnish Dominion: The British Academic Professions in the Twentieth Century*, in *Guardian*, 26 March, 26.

David Underdown, *Fire from Heaven: The Life of an English Town in the Seventeenth Century*, in *Guardian*, 7 May, 24.

Peter Burke, *The Fabrication of Louis XIV*, in *Guardian*, 21 May, 26.

Bram Kempers, *Painting, Power and Patronage: The Rise of the Professional Artist in the Italian Renaissance*, and Clare Robertson, *'Il Gran Cardinale': Alessandro Farnese, Patron of the Arts*, in *Guardian*, 11 June, 26.

Jeremy Black, *The British Abroad: The Grand Tour in the Eighteenth Century*, in *Guardian*, 20 August, 22.

Linda Colley, *Britons: Forging the Nation 1707–1837*, and Peter Linebaugh, *The London Hanged: Crime and Civil Society in the Eighteenth Century*, in *New York Review of Books*, 19 November, 35–8 (and Letter in reply to Peter Linebaugh, 13 May 1993, 57).

David Cannadine, *G. M. Trevelyan: A Life in History*, in *Guardian*, 24 September, 24.

Roy Porter (ed.), *Myths of the English*, in *Observer*, 18 October, 61.

Contribution to 'Christmas Books', *Observer*, 29 November, Christmas books supplement, 2.

Eamon Duffy, *The Stripping of the Altars: Traditional Religion in England, c.1400–c.1580*, in *Observer*, 13 December, 51.

1993

'Cases of Conscience in Seventeenth-Century England', in John Morrill, Paul Slack, and Daniel Woolf (eds.), *Public Duty and Private Conscience in Seventeenth-Century England: Essays Presented to G. E. Aylmer* (Oxford: Clarendon Press), 29–56.

'Foreword' to A. L. Le Quesne *et al.*, *Victorian Thinkers* (Oxford: Oxford University Press), pp. v–vii.

'Foreword' to James McConica *et al.*, *Renaissance Thinkers* (Oxford: Oxford University Press), pp. v–vii.

'No Place at the Table' (on funding the humanities), *Times Higher Education Supplement*, 2 July, 8–9.

'The Humanities', in David Allen and Lynn Williams (eds.), *Higher Education Wales Research Conference: Proceedings* (Cardiff: University of Wales), 84–91.

'Greetings from Sir Keith Thomas', *Reed: The Quarterly Magazine of Reed College*, 72: 22.

Reviews

John Brewer and Roy Porter (eds.), *Consumption and the World of Goods*, in *Observer*, 7 March, 58.

Christopher Hill, *The English Bible and the Seventeenth-Century Revolution*, in *Guardian*, 9 March, G2, 8.

David McKitterick, *A History of the Cambridge University Press*, i. *Printing and the Book Trade in Cambridge, 1534–1698*, in *Observer*, 14 March, 60.

Robert Bartlett, *The Making of Europe: Conquest, Colonisation and Cultural Change, 950–1350*, in *Guardian*, 18 May, G2, 8.

Francis Haskell, *History and its Images*, in *Guardian*, 15 June, G2, 14–15.

B. H. G. Wormald, *Francis Bacon: History, Politics and Science*, in *Observer*, 11 July, 63.

Natalie Zemon Davis and Arlette Farge (eds.), *A History of Women in the West*, iii. *Renaissance and Enlightenment Paradoxes*, in *Observer*, 8 August, 54.

Lawrence Stone, *Uncertain Unions: Marriage in England 1660–1753* and *Broken Lives: Separation and Divorce in England 1660–1857*, in *New York Review of Books*, 4 November, 22–4.

Contribution to 'Christmas Books', *Observer*, 28 November, Christmas books supplement, 4.

1994

'College Life, 1945–1970', in Brian Harrison (ed.), _The History of the University of Oxford_, viii. _The Twentieth Century_ (Oxford: Clarendon Press), 189–215.

'Cleanliness and Godliness in Early Modern England', in Anthony Fletcher and Peter Roberts (eds.), _Religion, Culture and Society in Early Modern Britain: Essays in Honour of Patrick Collinson_ (Cambridge: Cambridge University Press), 56–83. Excerpt published as 'Coming Clean to the House of the Lord', _Church Times_, 29 July, 8.

'Trustee's Choice' (William Hogarth, 'The Graham Children', 1742), _National Gallery News_, March, 1.

Reviews

Georges Duby, _Love and Marriage in the Middle Ages_, in _Guardian_, 11 January, G2, 9.

Geneviève Fraisse and Michelle Perrot (eds.), _A History of Women in the West_, iv. _Emerging Feminism from Revolution to World War_, in _Observer_, 30 January, review section, 22.

John Dixon Hunt (ed.), _Garden History: Issues, Approaches, Methods_, in _Journal of Garden History_, 14: 63–4.

Margaret Aston, _The King's Bedpost: Reformation and Iconography in a Tudor Group Portrait_, in _Guardian_, 1 March, G2, 12–13.

Ilana Krausman Ben-Amos, _Adolescence and Youth in Early Modern England_, in _Guardian_, 10 May, G2, 14–15.

Lyndal Roper, _Oedipus and the Devil: Witchcraft, Sexuality and Religion in Early Modern Europe_, in _Guardian_, 31 May, G2, 8–9.

William Eamon, _Science and the Secrets of Nature: Books of Secrets in Mediaeval and Early Modern Culture_, in _Guardian_, 14 June, G2, 12–13.

Stephen Daniels, _Fields of Vision: Landscape Imagery and National Identity in England and the United States_, in _Ecumene_, 1: 311–13.

N. J. G. Pounds, _The Culture of the English People: Iron Age to Industrial Revolution_, in _Observer_, 17 July, review section, 20.

Joyce Appleby, Lynn Hunt, and Margaret Jacob, _Telling the Truth about History_, in _Guardian_, 6 September, G2, 12.

Steven Shapin, _A Social History of Truth: Civility and Science in Seventeenth-Century England_, in _London Review of Books_, 22 September, 14–15. (Reprinted in Science and Religion Forum, _Reviews_, 26 (February 1995), 14–19.)

Jonathan Goldberg, _Queering the Renaissance_ and _Sodometries: Renaissance Texts, Modern Sexualities_, in _New York Review of Books_, 22 September, 9–12.

Adrian Wilson (ed.), _Rethinking Social History: English Society 1570–1970 and its Interpretation_, in _Times Literary Supplement_, 14 October, 7–8.

Roy Porter, *London: A Social History*, in *Observer*, 30 October, review section, 21.

Contribution to 'Books of the Year', *Observer*, review section, 20 November, 5.

Richard Sennett, *Flesh and Stone: The Body and the City in Western Civilisation*, in *Guardian*, 2 December, G2, 26.

Richard Critchfield, *The Villagers: Changed Values, Altered Lives*, in *New York Times Book Review*, 25 December, 10–11.

1995

'English Protestantism and Classical Art', in Lucy Gent (ed.), *Albion's Classicism: The Visual Arts in Britain, 1550–1660* (Studies in British Art, 2; New Haven and London: Yale University Press for the Paul Mellon Centre for Studies in British Art and the Yale Center for British Art), 221–38.

'Presidential Addresses' (7 July 1994 and 6 July 1995), in The British Academy, *Annual Report 1993–95*, 7–15.

'Foreword' to R. T. W. Denning (ed.), *The Diary of William Thomas of Michaelston-super-Ely, near St Fagans, Glamorgan, 1762–1795* (South Wales Record Society Publications, 11; Cardiff: South Wales Record Society and South Glamorgan County Council Libraries and Arts Department), 7–8.

'Westminster's Past Glories', *The House Magazine*, 4 December, 22–3.

Reviews

John Boswell, *The Marriage of Likeness: Same-Sex Unions in Pre-Modern Europe*, in *Guardian*, 14 February, G2, 18.

Raphael Samuel, *Theatres of Memory*, i. *Past and Present in Contemporary Culture*, in *London Review of Books*, 20 April, 7–8.

Richard Grove, *Green Imperialism: Colonial Expansion, Tropical Island Edens and the Origins of Environmentalism, 1600–1860*, in *Observer*, 18 June, review section, 16.

Simon Schama, *Landscape and Memory*, in *New York Review of Books*, 21 September, 8–12.

1996

'James Edward Oglethorpe (1696–1785)', *Pelican Record*, 39/3: 12–27.

'Presidential Address' (4 July 1996), in The British Academy, *Annual Report 1995–96*, 7–11.

Reviews

Christopher Hill, *Liberty against the Law*, in *Guardian*, 24 May, *G2*, 12.

Nicholas Jardine, J. A. Secord, and E. C. Spary (eds.), *Cultures of Natural History*, in *Times Literary Supplement*, 6 September, 28–9.

Felipe Fernández-Armesto and Derek Wilson, *Reformation, Christianity and the World, 1500–2000*, in *The Times*, 19 September, 34.

Thomas Pakenham, *Meetings with Remarkable Trees*, in *Spectator*, 30 November, 54.

1997

'Health and Morality in Early Modern England', in Allan M. Brandt and Paul Rozin (eds.), *Morality and Health* (New York and London: Routledge), 15–34.

'Foreword' to D. D. Raphael *et al.*, *Three Great Economists: Smith, Malthus, Keynes* (Oxford: Oxford University Press), pp. v–viii.

'Foreword' to Roger Scruton *et al.*, *German Philosophers: Kant, Hegel, Schopenhauer, Nietzsche* (Oxford: Oxford University Press), pp. v–vii.

'James Edward Oglethorpe, Sometime Gentleman Commoner of Corpus', in John C. Inscoe (ed.), *James Edward Oglethorpe: New Perspectives on his Life and Legacy* (Savannah, Ga.: Georgia Historical Society), 16–34.

'Foreword' to R. B. Outhwaite, *Scandal in the Church: Dr Edward Drax Free, 1764–1843* (London and Rio Grande, Oh.: Hambledon Press), pp. xi–xii.

Reviews

Mark Kishlansky, *A Monarchy Transformed: Britain 1603–1714*, in *Guardian*, 30 January, *G2*, 10–11.

John Brewer, *The Pleasures of the Imagination: English Culture in the Eighteenth Century*, in *Guardian*, 22 May, *G2*, 12–13.

Eric Hobsbawm, *On History*, in *Guardian*, 10 July, *G2*, 16.

Richard Fletcher, *The Conversion of Europe*, in *The Times*, 4 September, 35.

Richard Evans, *In Defence of History*, in *New Statesman*, 17 October, 46–7.

Peter Mandler, *The Fall and Rise of the Stately Home*, James Lees-Milne, *Ancient as the Hills*, and David Littlejohn, *The Fate of the English Country House*, in *London Review of Books*, 13 November, 7–8.

1998

'Presidential Address' (4 July 1997), in The British Academy, *Annual Report 1996–97*, 7–11.

'Nothing can Replace Books' (interviewed by Suchitra Behal), *Hindu*, 4 January, magazine section, p. xiv.

Reviews

Peter Ackroyd, *The Life of Thomas More*, in *Guardian*, 12 March, G2, 14.

David F. Noble, *The Religion of Technology: The Divinity of Man and the Spirit of Invention*, in *New York Review of Books*, 17 December, 78–80.

INDEX

Index by Jackie Brind